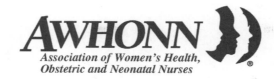

Association of Women's Health,
Obstetric and Neonatal Nurses

D1121045

HIGH-RISK & CRITICAL CARE
OBSTETRICS

Third Edition

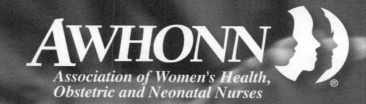

AWHONN
Association of Women's Health,
Obstetric and Neonatal Nurses

HIGH-RISK & CRITICAL CARE
OBSTETRICS

Third Edition

Editors

Nan H. Troiano, RN, MSN
Director, Women's and Infants' Services
Sibley Memorial Hospital
Johns Hopkins Medicine
Washington, D.C.

Carol J. Harvey, RNC, C-EFM, MS
Clinical Specialist
High Risk Perinatal
Labor & Delivery
Northside Hospital
Atlanta, Georgia

Bonnie Flood Chez, RNC, MSN
President, Nursing Education Resources
Perinatal Clinical Nurse Specialist &
Consultant
Tampa, Florida

Wolters Kluwer | Lippincott Williams & Wilkins
Health
Philadelphia · Baltimore · New York · London
Buenos Aires · Hong Kong · Sydney · Tokyo

Acquisitions Editor: Bill Lamsback
Product Director: David Moreau
Product Manager: Rosanne Hallowell
Development and Copy Editors: Catherine E. Harold and Erika Kors
Proofreader: Linda R. Garber
Editorial Assistants: Karen J. Kirk, Jeri O'Shea, and Linda K. Ruhf
Creative Director: Doug Smock
Cover Designer: Robert Dieters
Vendor Manager: Cynthia Rudy
Manufacturing Manager: Beth J. Welsh
Production and Indexing Services: Aptara, Inc.

10 9 8 7 6 5 4 3 2 1

Library of Congress Cataloging-in-Publication Data
High-risk & critical care obstetrics / editors, Nan H. Troiano, Carol J. Harvey, Bonnie Flood Chez. – 3rd ed.
    p. ; cm.
  High-risk and critical care obstetrics
  Rev. ed. of: AWHONN's high-risk and critical care intrapartum nursing / [edited by] Lisa K. Mandeville, Nan H. Troiano. 2nd ed. c1999.
  Includes bibliographical references and index.
   ISBN 978-0-7817-8334-7 (pbk. : alk. paper)
   I. Troiano, Nan H. II. Harvey, Carol J. III. Chez, Bonnie Flood. IV. AWHONN's high-risk and critical care intrapartum nursing. V. Title: High-risk and critical care obstetrics.
   [DNLM: 1. Obstetrical Nursing—methods. 2. Critical Care. 3. Delivery, Obstetric—nursing. 4. Obstetric Labor Complications—nursing. 5. Pregnancy Complications—nursing. 6. Pregnancy, High-Risk. 7. Pregnancy. WY 157]

  618.20231–dc23
                                        2011040224

*To my mother, Bonnie Lee Chappell Hamner; to my
brother, Philip David Hamner; and in loving memory
of my father, Harold Max Hamner. Finally, to Bogart,
my companion throughout, and Bacall.*
                    —Nan H. Troiano

*In loving memory of my parents, Mildred and
Richard Harvey; to my husband, Scott Sneed;
and to my sisters by birth and by choice.*
                    —Carol J. Harvey

*To my dad, Dr. William A. Flood;
and to my George and Semi.*
                    —Bonnie Flood Chez

Since publication of the second edition of this text in 1999, we continue to appreciate the challenges and rewards associated with providing care to this unique patient population. Time has granted us the benefit of a rapidly expanding knowledge base derived from ongoing research and clinical experience related to the care of pregnant women who experience significant complications or become critically ill during pregnancy. Time has also gifted us with an appreciation for the value of advanced practice collaboration among clinicians who care for these women and their families. Therefore, this edition includes extensive revisions that reflect evidence-based changes in clinical practice for specific complications, and new chapters have been added that address foundations for practice, adjuncts for clinical practice, and selected clinical guidelines.

One of the most challenging aspects of perinatal care continues to be meeting the clinical and psychosocial health care needs of an increasingly diverse obstetric patient population. A general overview of today's obstetric population depicts women who, in general, are older, larger in body habitus, more likely to have existing comorbid disease, more prone to high-order multiple gestations, known to have an increased incidence of operative intervention, less likely to attempt vaginal birth after a previous Cesarean birth, apt to have high expectations for care in terms of outcomes, and predisposed to complex clinical situations that may generate ethical issues related to their care.

It remains true that most pregnant women are without identified complications and proceed through pregnancy, labor, delivery, and the postpartum period without problems. Accordingly, obstetric care remains based on a wellness-oriented foundation. However, maternal mortality remains unacceptably high and there has been a renewed commitment to addressing this problem. Significant complications may develop at any time during pregnancy without regard for a woman's *identified* risk status. Unfortunately, this very phrase has evolved into being synonymous with labels such as *high risk* or *at risk*. However, we believe that use of such terms to designate levels of risk should be appreciated as being reasonably imprecise and nonspecific. We should avoid any suggestion that categorical boundaries exist for patients or for the clinicians who care for them. For example, there are women who manifest medical conditions during pregnancy who, absent appropriate recognition and management, may be more prone to adverse obstetric outcomes. However, it is also recognized that this same population of pregnant women may, with appropriate management, experience no adverse perinatal outcomes above those of the general population.

Further, providing care to this unique population and their families within our evolving health care delivery system presents additional challenges to us as a society. Efforts to reform health care continue to attempt to address the concepts of accessibility, affordability, quality, responsibility, safety, and cost-effectiveness. Debate will no doubt continue regarding what is the best way to achieve reform measures.

This edition is reflective of these and other associated challenges. However, the most significant intent of the format of this text is to promote appreciation for the importance of a collaborative approach to the care of this specific obstetric population. Therefore, for the first time, most chapters are co-authored by nurse and physician experts in their respective areas of practice.

The first section is devoted to discussion of foundations for practice. It includes an overview of the state of our specialty, the importance of collaboration in clinical practice, and the complexities of practice that often include ethical dilemmas that must be considered in the overall care of the patient and her family.

The second section presents information on adjuncts often used in the clinical care of this patient population. We hope that this information proves useful for clinicians caring for obstetric patients with significant complications or who are critically ill during the intrapartum setting, as well as for those who provide consultation for such patients on other services. The third section presents comprehensive critical concepts and current evidence-based information regarding specific clinical entities in obstetric practice. The fourth section includes practice resources in the form of clinical guidelines, in an attempt to provide clinicians with references and tools to optimize clinical care of this special obstetric population.

On a personal note, we the editors feel that it is important to acknowledge that the evolution of this text over the past several years reflects the reality of accommodating to changes and challenges in our paths, much like the population of women for whom we provide care and our colleagues who care for them. We all have our personal stories. The interval between publication of the second and third editions bears witness to personal and professional stories for us all. During this period of time, we have: celebrated years of remission from breast cancer; finished 60-mile Komen Foundation walks in Washington, DC, and

Boston; lost beloved members of our family; grieved the loss of 10 precious pets; supported co-authors with professional and family tragedies and triumphs; changed jobs; endured the economy; found new love; gained energy and renewal because of the support of family and friends, and navigated significant challenges in order to bring this project to completion.

We are grateful for the overwhelmingly positive feedback from those who have read previous editions and provided us with direction to take this third edition to the next level. We are in debt to the wonderful group of contributing authors for sharing their special expertise and time. It has been an honor to work with these colleagues, AWHONN, and Lippincott Williams & Wilkins on this project.

Nan H. Troiano
Carol J. Harvey
Bonnie Flood Chez

CONTRIBUTORS

Julie M.R. Arafeh, RN, MSN
Obstetric Simulation Specialist
Center for Advanced Pediatric and Perinatal Education
Lucile Packard Children's Hospital
Stanford, California

Suzanne McMurtry Baird, RN, MSN
Assistant Director, Clinical Practice
Women's Services
Texas Children's Hospital
Houston, Texas

Michael A. Belfort, MD, PhD
Professor and Chair, Obstetrics and Gynecology
Baylor College of Medicine
Houston, Texas
Obstetrician/Gynecologist-in-Chief
Texas Children's Hospital
Houston, Texas

Frank A. Chervenak, MD
Given Foundation Professor and Chairman
Department of Obstetrics and Gynecology
New York Weill Cornell Medical Center
New York, New York

Bonnie Flood Chez, RNC, MSN
President, Nursing Education Resources
Perinatal Clinical Nurse Specialist and Consultant
Tampa, Florida

Steven L. Clark, MD
Medical Director, Women's and Children's Clinical
    Services
Clinical Services Group
Hospital Corporation of America
Nashville, Tennessee

Patricia Marie Constanty, RN, MSN, CRNP
Clinical Nurse Specialist and Perinatal Nurse Practitioner
Labor and Delivery and High Risk Obstetrics
Thomas Jefferson University Hospital
Philadelphia, Pennsylvania

Deborah Anne Cruz, RN, MSN, CRNP
Clinical Nurse Specialist and Perinatal Nurse Practitioner
Labor and Delivery and High Risk Obstetrics
Thomas Jefferson University Hospital
Philadelphia, Pennsylvania

Gary A. Dildy III, MD
Director of Maternal-Fetal Medicine
MountainStar Division
Hospital Corporation of America
Nashville, Tennessee;
Clinical Professor
Department of Obstetrics and Gynecology
Louisiana State University School of Medicine
New Orleans, Louisiana;
Attending Perinatologist
Maternal Fetal Medicine Center at St. Mark's Hospital
Salt Lake City, Utah

Karen Dorman, RN, MS
Research Instructor
Maternal–Fetal Medicine
University of North Carolina School of Medicine
Chapel Hill, North Carolina

Patrick Duff, MD
Professor and Residency Program Director
Department of Obstetrics and Gynecology
University of Florida
Gainesville, Florida

Bonnie K. Dwyer, MD
Assistant Clinical Professor, Affiliated, Stanford
    University
Division of Maternal–Fetal Medicine
Department of Obstetrics and Gynecology
California Pacific Medical Center
San Francisco, California

Sreedhar Gaddipati, MD
Assistant Clinical Professor of Obstetrics and
    Gynecology
Columbia University
College of Physicians and Surgeons
Medical Director, Critical Care Obstetrics
Division of Maternal–Fetal Medicine
New York, New York

Lewis Hamner, III, MD
Division of Maternal Fetal Medicine
Kaiser Permanente
Georgia Region
Atlanta, Georgia

Carol J. Harvey, RNC-OB, C-EFM, MS
Clinical Specialist
High Risk Perinatal
Labor and Delivery
Northside Hospital
Atlanta, Georgia

Nan Hess-Eggleston, RN, BSN
Clinical Nurse Specialist—Women's and Infants'
    Services
Sibley Memorial Hospital
Johns Hopkins Medicine
Washington, DC

Washington C. Hill, MD, FACOG
First Physician Group of Sarasota
Medical Director, Labor and Delivery
Director, Maternal–Fetal Medicine
Sarasota Memorial Hospital;
Department of Clinical Sciences
OB-GYN Clerkship Director—Sarasota Campus
Florida State University, College of Medicine;
Clinical Professor
Department of Obstetrics and Gynecology
University of South Florida, College of Medicine
Tampa, Florida

Maribeth Inturrisi, RN, MS, CNS, CDE
Coordinator and Nurse Consultant, Regions 1 and 3
California Diabetes and Pregnancy Program
Assistant Clinical Professor, Family Health Care
    Nursing
University of California
San Francisco, California;
Sweet Success Nurse Educator
Physician Foundation Sweet Success Program
California Pacific Medical Center
San Francisco, California

Thomas M. Jenkins, MD
Director of Prenatal Diagnosis
Legacy Center for Maternal–Fetal Medicine
Portland, Oregon

Renee' Jones, RNC-OB, MSN, WHCNP-BC
Nurse Practitioner
The Medical Center of Plano
Women's Link–Specialty Obstetrical Referral Clinic
Plano, Texas

Betsy B. Kennedy, RN, MSN
Assistant Professor of Nursing
Vanderbilt University School of Nursing
Nashville, Tennessee

Ellen Kopel, RNC-OB, MS, C-EFM
Perinatal Nurse Consultant
Tampa, Florida

Stephen D. Krau, RN, PhD, CNE, CT
Associate Professor of Nursing
Vanderbilt University School of Nursing
Nashville, Tennessee

Nancy C. Lintner, RNC, MS, CPT
Clinical Nurse Specialist and Nurse Consultant/
    Educator
Diabetes and Pregnancy Program
University of Cincinnati Physicians/Greater Cincinnati
    Obstetrics & Gynecologists
University of Cincinnati Medical School/Division of
    Maternal–Fetal Medicine
Cincinnati, Ohio

Marcy M. Mann, MD
Maternal Fetal Medicine Specialist
Atlanta Perinatal Consultants
Center for Perinatal Medicine
Northside Hospital
Atlanta, Georgia

Brian A. Mason, MD, MS
Associate Professor
Wayne State University
St. John's Hospital / Medical Center
Detroit, Michigan

Laurence B. McCullough, PhD
Center for Medical Ethics and Health Policy
Baylor College of Medicine
Houston, Texas

Keith McLendon, MD
Staff Anesthesiologist
Northside Anesthesiology Consultants
Northside Hospital
Atlanta, Georgia

Richard S. Miller, MD, FACS
Professor of Surgery
Medical Director, Trauma Intensive Care Unit
Vanderbilt University School of Medicine
Nashville, Tennessee

Jeffrey P. Phelan, MD, JD
Director of Quality Assurance
Department of Obstetrics and Gynecology
Citrus Valley Medical Center
West Covina, California;
President and Director of Clinical Research
Childbirth Injury Prevention Foundation
City of Industry, California

Amy H. Picklesimer, MD, MSPH
Division of Maternal–Fetal Medicine
Greenville Hospital System University Medical Center
Greenville, South Carolina

Donna Ruth RN, MSN
Nursing Professional Development Specialist
Nursing Education and Professional Development
Vanderbilt University Medical Center
Nashville, Tennessee

George R. Saade, MD
Professor, Department of Obstetrics and Gynecology
Divisions of Maternal–Fetal Medicine and Reproductive
    Sciences
Director, Maternal–Fetal Medicine Fellowship Program
The University of Texas Medical Branch
Galveston, Texas

Shailen S. Shah, MD
Director of Operations, Antenatal Testing Unit
Virtua Health System
Assistant Professor, Department of Obstetrics and
    Gynecology
Thomas Jefferson University
Philadelphia, Pennsylvania

Baha M. Sibai, MD
Professor of Clinical Obstetrics and Gynecology
Maternal–Fetal Medicine
Department of Obstetrics and Gynecology
University of Cincinnati
Cincinnati, Ohio

Melissa C. Sisson, RN, MN
Director of Women's Services
Northside Hospital
Atlanta, Georgia

Kimberlee Sorem, MD
Maternal–Fetal Medicine Specialist
Medical Director
Physician Foundation Sweet Success Program
California Pacific Medical Center
San Francisco, California

Mary Ellen Burke Sosa, RNC, MS
President, Perinatal Resources, Rumford, Rhode Island
Per Diem Staff Nurse, LDR, Kent Hospital, Warwick,
    Rhode Island
Diabetes Nurse Educator, Division of Maternal–Fetal
    Medicine
Women & Infants' Hospital
Providence, Rhode Island

Nan H. Troiano, RN, MSN
Director, Women's and Infants' Services
Sibley Memorial Hospital
Johns Hopkins Medicine
Washington, DC

Patricia M. Witcher, RNC-OB, MSN
Clinical Nurse Specialist
Labor and Delivery, High Risk Obstetrics
Northside Hospital
Atlanta, Georgia

ACKNOWLEDGMENTS

The editors gratefully acknowledge the unparalleled support of colleagues who have played an instrumental role in making this third edition possible. In the years between the second and third editions, we have had the privilege of working collaboratively with valued colleagues, mentors, fellows, residents, and students in our respective practice environments. We thank them all for their untiring dedication to the health and safety of all pregnant women and their unborn children, and specifically to this unique subset of pregnant women.

We have also been privileged to participate in perinatal education programs and consulting opportunities throughout the United States and other countries. We appreciate that this demonstration of commitment to education, clinical practice, and research represents our best hope for collectively advocating for safe and effective perinatal care. Ultimately, it represents the foundation for true "collaboration" in practice. It also reminds us that we have made friends with, listened to, and benefitted from the wisdom of those who are on the "front lines" every day. These networking opportunities have resulted in deep and lasting relationships that are part of the very fabric of this book.

Further, there have also been individuals who have contributed their special expertise to this third edition. Among these:

- Susan Drummond, RN, MSN, for helping us to identify and appreciate content related to patient safety that continued as a theme throughout this text and to Frank H. Boehm, MD for lending his expertise and wisdom to her efforts.
- A. Scott Johnson, Esq., for providing guidance related to understanding legal implications for practice.
- Patricia Witcher, RNC-OB, MSN, for authoring some of the most challenging chapters and for ghost-writing additional ones with her amazing talent.
- Fay Rycyna, our AWHONN rock of support throughout this entire project, who never lost faith that the finish line was in sight.

On a personal note, the editors and a core group of contributing authors thank the wonderful people of Arley, Alabama, particularly those who comprise the communities of Rock Creek and Smith Lake, for providing the perfect place from which this project was launched. Memories remain rich and vivid of time spent enjoying the tranquil beauty and warm hospitality that surrounded us there as we continued to nurture this endeavor over time.

Finally, we acknowledge the patients and families for whom we have provided care and from whom we learned valuable lessons. Your "stories" are reflected in the content and spirit of this book and will continue to affect the care provided to others.

Nan H. Troiano
Carol J. Harvey
Bonnie Flood Chez

CONTENTS

PART IV: CLINICAL CARE GUIDELINES
NAN HESS-EGGLESTON, NAN H. TROIANO, CAROL J. HARVEY, AND BONNIE FLOOD CHEZ

PART I

Foundations for Practice

CHAPTER 1

Obstetric Practice: State of the Specialty

Jeffrey P. Phelan, Bonnie Flood Chez, and Ellen Kopel

Women with obstetric complications or critical illness in pregnancy represent an estimated 1 to 3 percent of the overall obstetric population requiring intensive care services in the United States each year.[1] The health status of these patients reflects that of the general population, which has been changing rapidly due, in part, to an increased incidence of obesity in all age groups. Obesity-related complications such as hypertensive disorders, diabetes, and other medical conditions directly and indirectly present significant health risks for pregnant women. In addition, the likelihood of developing co-morbid disease increases proportionately with maternal age. While there has always been, and will continue to be, a modest percentage of women who are or will become critically ill during pregnancy, current demographic trends support a greater propensity for this to occur. A snapshot of today's pregnant woman in the U.S. depicts an expectant mother who is older (the average age of first-time mothers was 3.6 years older in 2007 than in 1970), heavier (in 2009, 24.4 percent of women of childbearing age in the U.S. met the criteria for obesity, which is a body mass index above 30), and more likely to have a Cesarean birth (31.8 percent of all births in 2007 were Cesarean) than at any previous time.[2,3]

This chapter is intended to provoke thought and generate discussion about the challenges facing perinatal clinicians in identifying and providing care to this subset of women whose pregnancy complications may evolve from and are intertwined with contemporary societal and/or obstetric trends.

MATERNAL AGE

Older gravidas are more likely to have preexisting medical conditions and are more prone to both chronic and pregnancy-related diabetic and hypertensive disorders.[2] As well, older gravidas are more likely to experience high-order multiple gestations. Approximately 5 percent of pregnancies among women ages 35 to 44, and more than 20 percent in women age 45 and older, result in multiple gestations, thereby increasing the risk of complications.[1] Furthermore, women in their thirties are also more likely than younger women to conceive multiples. Overall, an increasing number of pregnancies (approximately 1 in 100) occur later in the childbearing years and are achieved using assisted reproductive technology (ART), which increases the likelihood of multi-fetal gestations.[4] Perinatal morbidity and mortality are significant threats arising from multiple gestation and evidence suggests that the impact on maternal health, in particular, is significant and may result in the need for maternal critical care exceeding three times that for women with a singleton pregnancy.[5] As familiarity with ART increases and media attention continues to focus on high-order multiple gestations, it is reasonable to anticipate that these numbers will continue to rise, along with the numbers of expectant mothers requiring more intensive care.

OBESITY

Not only is the childbearing population affected by obesity in disproportionate numbers, but recent data show that weight gain during pregnancy is well beyond recommended amounts. In 2009, the Institute of Medicine issued updated guidelines for weight gain during pregnancy.[6] The maximum recommended weight gain of 40 pounds was intended for the minority of pregnant women who begin their pregnancies underweight; however, this recommendation is currently exceeded by 21 percent of the total gravid population.[1] There are significant clinical and logistical implications in caring for overweight or obese pregnant women in a manner equivalent to the care of gravid women of normal weight. Under ordinary circumstances, an obese patient's size may present challenges as basic as finding a bed suitable to accommodate increased maternal body habitus and having other properly sized equipment readily available to monitor maternal and fetal status. Additional personnel may be needed to carry out procedures or assist in safe transfers. A complete discussion of obesity in pregnancy is presented in Chapter 22.

CESAREAN BIRTH

Since 1996—when trial of labor (TOL) and vaginal birth after Cesarean (VBAC) were most widely utilized, induction rates had not yet reached current levels, and with a near-complete cessation of attempts at vaginal breech delivery—Cesarean birth rates have increased 54 percent.[1] Factors that have contributed to this increase include the rising rate of repeat Cesarean delivery, Cesarean birth by patient request, and population demographics. Maternal age is a compounding factor due to issues discussed previously and also because breech/malpresentation increases proportionately with maternal age (occurring almost twice as often in those age 40 and older as compared with pregnant women younger than age 20).[1] Despite the fact that Cesarean delivery has become commonplace, there continue to be risks with this procedure. Two of the four most common preventable errors related to maternal deaths include failure to pay sufficient attention to alterations in maternal vital signs following Cesarean delivery and hemorrhage following the procedure.[7]

PROFESSIONAL ISSUES

Patient safety and the importance of collaboration, communication, and teamwork among professional staff are "high-visibility" topics in perinatal care. Although it specifically addressed factors influencing infant death and injury during delivery, the Joint Commission Sentinel Event Alert, Issue 30, in 2004 brought increased attention to issues related to patient safety in a manner that no longer allowed them to be overlooked by institutions. These patient safety–related topics are particularly applicable to high-risk and critical care obstetrics, where there is even greater need for collaboration and effective communication and less of a margin for error. Collaboration in clinical practice is discussed further in Chapter 2.

In January 2010, the Joint Commission issued Sentinel Event Alert 44: Preventing Maternal Death.[7] Based on the 2008 Hospital Corporation of America (HCA) study, which evaluated causes of maternal death among 1.5 million births within 124 hospitals over 6 years, the Alert noted that most maternal deaths were not preventable. Further, it suggested that, although some deaths might have been prevented by improved individual care, precise figures indicating the frequency of preventable deaths should be examined carefully and with caution. According to this study, the most common preventable causes of maternal death include:

- failure to adequately control blood pressure in hypertensive women
- failure to adequately diagnose and treat pulmonary edema in women with preeclampsia
- failure to pay sufficient attention to maternal vital signs following Cesarean delivery
- hemorrhage following Cesarean birth.[7]

Sentinel Event Alert 44 highlights the clinician's responsibility to be alert to changes in patient status and respond accordingly in a timely manner. In particular, the report emphasizes that from 1991 through 2003, severe morbidity in pregnancy was 50 times more common than maternal death in the U.S. Consequently, it is essential that institutions have plans in place to identify and manage high-risk and critically ill obstetric patients. Joint Commission National Patient Safety Goal 16 (recognize and respond to changes in a patient's condition) is clearly applicable to the care of women during labor and birth. As such, the Provision of Care, Treatment and Services standard PC.02.01.19 requires the hospital to:

- have a process for recognizing and responding as soon as a patient's condition appears to be worsening
- develop written criteria describing early warning signs of a change or deterioration in patient condition and to seek further assistance
- inform the patient and family how to seek assistance when they have concerns about the patient's condition.

Whenever possible, it is optimal to conduct multidisciplinary care planning when there is relevant history or current evidence of potential complications. Management for the particular patient can be outlined more specifically at this time, including details of where she will be cared for and by whom, what equipment and supplies should be on hand, and any other contingencies relevant to her anticipated course. Ideally, this should be accomplished well in advance of the need for specialty services and should serve as a helpful guide to ongoing care throughout the patient's hospitalization.

The physical location of the patient in the hospital should not dictate the care the patient receives. The Joint Commission (2010) recommendation for "comparable standards of care" sets the expectation that "patients with comparable needs receive the same standard of care, treatment, and services throughout the hospital."[8] The methods for accomplishing this will necessarily differ from one institution to another, based on the frequency and level of experience with patients of varying acuities, access to specialty and subspecialty providers, equipment, and staffing. Competence in core procedural skills for critical care clinicians varies as well. Techniques to develop or maintain skills may derive from multiple sources, including didactic instruction with or without follow-up supervised application, computerized on-line independent study, and/or task training through the use of medical simulation.

Although the focus is often on the gravid patient, it is important to note that the overwhelming majority of obstetric ICU admissions (approximately 75 percent) occur in the postpartum period, a time when the patient may have been discharged from the acute care setting and is under less intense observation.[1] Again, it is essential that clinicians remain alert to changes in patient status throughout the course of a patient's hospitalization. Mother-baby units typically are not considered care environments of high acuity, yet the patient care and teaching provided in these areas are integral to maternal health and safe outcomes. It is imperative that postpartum units are provided the education, staffing, equipment, and tools necessary to ensure patient safety during hospitalization and throughout the postpartum period and transition to home. Maternal death is defined as that which occurs within 42 days following delivery or pregnancy termination, and this is a period of particular vulnerability.[7] Thorough patient assessment and teaching before discharge are vital to early recognition of symptoms such as infection and hemorrhage. Care providers in triage and emergency departments should be attentive to the possibility that a woman of childbearing age who presents for urgent care may be experiencing complications from a recent pregnancy. Extending relevant education to personnel in these areas is crucial to accurate patient assessment, diagnoses, and treatment.

LOGISTICAL ISSUES

Although between 0.1 and 0.8 percent of obstetric patients are admitted to an intensive care unit (ICU), it is important to recognize that the total number of pregnant women requiring intensive or critical care services is greater. Patients often receive critical care outside of the ICU in highly specialized labor and delivery units (L&D) that are prepared to handle such cases with skilled maternal-fetal medicine subspecialists and registered nurses specially trained in critical care obstetrics. Further, it should be noted that a large percentage of maternal mortality occurs without the patient ever reaching an ICU.[9] Early admission of critically ill obstetric patients to the appropriate intensive care environment may decrease perinatal mortality and morbidity.

Although many pregnant women receive some form of critical care in the hospital, provision of consistent care to critically ill pregnant women is challenging. The model for delivery of care to critically ill obstetric patients varies from institution to institution and depends on various factors, including the availability of highly skilled physicians and nurses. From the physician's perspective, care of the critically ill obstetric patient depends, to a large extent, on the availability of maternal-fetal medicine subspecialists and critical care intensivists, or pulmonary subspecialists in a particular hospital. The relative scarcity of these specialized physicians is a limiting factor. Many maternal-fetal medicine subspecialists choose to limit their practices to outpatient services or to a select number of deliveries. To be available 24 hours a day, 7 days a week for the sickest of patients does not lend itself to satisfying the ever-expanding overhead of the subspecialist or to lifestyle enhancement. Critical care intensivists are often even less accessible than maternal-fetal medicine subspecialists, many having limited their practices to university-based programs where there is immediate availability of residents and subspecialty fellows in training. In many community hospitals, the intensivists' shoes have been primarily filled by pulmonary subspecialists. By working in a practice comprised of at least four physicians, this group of subspecialists is often best able to provide clinically effective care while maintaining a reasonable work-life balance.

Staffing

Ideally, the hospital ICU has a multidisciplinary team with a thorough understanding of the complexities of care associated with a critically ill pregnant woman.[10] This multidisciplinary team should include nurses, physicians, respiratory therapists, pharmacists, anesthesiologists, and other non-medical support personnel. The cornerstone of caring for the critically ill obstetric patient is a dedicated physician or group of physicians and well-trained registered nurses. The critically ill obstetric patient admitted to the ICU is more likely to receive uniform care through a dedicated critical care intensivist or group of intensivists. Under these circumstances, coordination of care may be transferred to their purview for the window of time the peripartum patient is in the ICU. Throughout her ICU stay, the patient's primary obstetric physician may continue to provide specialty consultation and help maintain continuity of care for the patient and her family. As ICU patients require multidisciplinary care, there should be clear delineation of the roles of subspecialists with a primary medical physician and team leader identified. This model for provision of care in an ICU is effective in enhancing patient outcomes and is associated with less ICU and hospital mortality and shorter hospital stays.[11]

Environment of Care

The complexities of the critically ill gravida mandate highly skilled nursing care. It is prudent for institutions to develop plans for how care will be provided to this unique patient population. Crucial to the success of such plans is the inclusion of educational preparation for core staff expected to deliver clinical care.

Logistics also require that essential resources are available to address both maternal and neonatal needs. If a facility is not equipped or prepared to provide care to this patient population, a plan for appropriate consultation, referral, and transport to another facility should be in place. It is also important to note that if maternal transport is unsafe or not possible due to clinical circumstances, arrangements for neonatal transport may be necessary. In situations where delivery may be imminent, transfer should be delayed. It is mandatory to adhere to federal guidelines and the Emergency Medical Treatment and Labor Act (EMTALA) related to the transfer of patients from one facility to another.

Determining the optimal care setting is a challenging decision based on factors previously addressed as well as specific clinical circumstances and maternal and/or fetal status. Additional considerations in determining the optimal clinical setting may include the gestational age of the fetus and the anticipated duration of ICU services. Factors affecting the decision about delivery method may include, but are not limited to, the degree of patient instability, interventions required, staffing and expertise available, anticipated duration of ICU stay, and probability of success.

A critically ill gravida in the ICU has an increased likelihood of operative vaginal delivery. Additionally, in ICU patients with underlying cardiac or neurologic complications, operative vaginal delivery is often recommended to shorten the second stage of labor. Adequate analgesia is required, and it is important to note that assessment of pain may be complicated by the patient's altered mental status and/or intubation. Regional analgesia is preferred but may not be possible because of coagulopathy, hemodynamic instability, or difficulties with patient positioning. Parenteral opioids can be used instead of regional analgesia but provide less effective relief. Suboptimal treatment of pain may result in maternal or fetal hemodynamic changes that must be anticipated and managed.

Cesarean delivery in the ICU is also challenging and carries significant disadvantages compared with performance of this procedure in an operating room. As with vaginal delivery, there may be inadequate physical space for the necessary equipment and personnel. In addition, ICUs have the highest rate of hospital-acquired infections, increasing the risk of nosocomial infection with drug-resistant organisms.[12,13] Cesarean delivery in the ICU should, therefore, be limited to those cases in which transport to the operating room or delivery room cannot be achieved safely or expeditiously, or when a perimortem Cesarean must be performed.

ETHICS

The complexities of providing perinatal care to a critically ill gravida from both nursing and medical perspectives are captured throughout this book. There are no simple solutions, and the breadth of such patients' illnesses is beyond the capabilities of many institutions. As a rule, these patients have, in addition to their primary clinical problem, multiorgan dysfunction. As such, any care and treatment are inherently complicated, and the impact on the fetus must be considered at each step in the clinical process and with every intervention and medication administered. Striking a balance between what is best for the mother and what is best for the fetus is a common clinical challenge in these circumstances. Further discussion on ethical decision making in critical care obstetrics can be found in Chapter 3.

COSTS OF CARE

Perinatal clinicians appreciate the need for clinical competence as a requirement to enhancing the care of the critically ill pregnant woman. On a personal level, however, issues confronting clinicians include not only the requirements of additional training, skill, and experience but also increased expectations of responsibility and accountability for the individual nurse or physician. Providing care to these patients can become quite complex and is mentally, physically, and emotionally demanding. Recovery time for clinicians dealing with intense clinical circumstances should be considered. In the event of maternal or fetal death, the opportunity to process what occurred and to grieve, if necessary, should be provided for all members of the team.

Ongoing issues with reimbursement make it impossible to ignore the overall financial impact of these issues on health care providers and institutions. One paramount issue is the ever-present concern over litigation. Some specialists may decline to consult on a critically ill pregnant patient due to fear of potential medical–legal consequences. Certainly, legal claims and increased insurance premium costs have affected the number of providers who choose to be involved in obstetric care in general and critical care obstetrics in particular. Whether through health care reform, professional society initiatives, or legislative action, it is clear that steps must be taken to reduce costs and mitigate risk in order to optimize maternal-fetal care.

SUMMARY

In addition to focusing on the care of high-risk and critically ill obstetric patients, it is equally important to consider ways to reduce the number of patients who fall into these categories. Comprehensive pre- and inter-conception health care is essential; however, public perception of and access to well-woman care currently fall short of what is needed to generate meaningful improvement. Increasing regular access to preventive health care for women in their childbearing years (including health education and counseling intended to improve a woman's health before and between pregnancies) has been part of the Centers for Disease Control and Prevention's (CDC's) Preconception Health and Health Care Initiative since 2004.[14] Counseling should be tailored to the individual's needs and risk factors and also should give consideration to age-related and racial disparities. The age-related propensity for complications has been discussed; however, it is important to note that black women are four times more likely to experience pregnancy-related death than are women of other races.[15] This population requires greater study, with focus on intervention to bridge the gap to safer pregnancy and birth.

In addition to managing medical issues that may exist before pregnancy, it is also important to identify and address behavioral, lifestyle, and social risk factors during pre- and inter-conception counseling. For example, although the short- and long-term health risks of smoking are well known, approximately 22 percent of women in their reproductive years smoke, and approximately 10 percent of women giving birth report smoking during pregnancy.[16] Smoking, alcohol and drug use, and nutrition are some examples of factors that directly affect the health of women of childbearing age and may contribute to the development and progression of diseases that influence maternal morbidity and mortality. A greater focus on counseling and treatment to modify behaviors, and provision of information on family planning, pregnancy spacing, and the importance of prenatal care may be useful methods for preventing some high-risk and critical-care perinatal cases.

REFERENCES

1. American College of Obstetricians and Gynecologists. (ACOG, 2009). *Critical care in pregnancy: ACOG Practice Bulletin, 100,* 1–8. Retrieved from http://mail.ny.acog.org/website/SMIPodcast/CriticalCare.pdf
2. Martin, J. A., Hamilton, B. E., Sutton, P. D., Ventura, S. J., Mathews, T. J., Kirmeyer, S., et al. (2010). Births: Final data for 2007. *National Vital Statistics Reports, 58*(24), 1–86. Hyattsville, MD: National Center for Health Statistics.
3. Centers for Disease Control and Prevention (CDC, 2011). *Behavioral risk factor surveillance system.* Retrieved from http://www.marchofdimes.com/peristats
4. American Society for Reproductive Medicine. (ASRM, 2010). *Oversight of assisted reproductive technology* (p. 4). Birmingham, AL: Author. Retrieved 2011, from http://www.asrm.org/uploadedFiles/Content/About_Us/Media_and_Public_Affairs/OversiteOfART%20%282%29.pdf
5. Baskett, T. F., Colleen, M. B., & O'Connell, M. (2009). Maternal critical care in obstetrics. *Journal of Obstetrics and Gynaecology Canada, 31*(3), 218–221.
6. Institute of Medicine (IOM, 2009). *Weight gain during pregnancy: Reexamining the guidelines.* Washington, DC: National Academies Press.
7. Joint Commission. (2010). *Sentinel event alert, Issue 44: Preventing maternal death.* Washington, DC: Author. Retrieved from http://www.jointcommission.org/sentinel_event_alert_issue_44_preventing_maternal_death/
8. Joint Commission. (2010). *Leadership standards for hospitals: Standards and rationales* (LD.04.03.07). Washington, DC: Author. Retrieved from http://www.jcrinc.com/common/Documents/OnlineExtras/JCLS09/JCLS09_H.pdf
9. Hazelgrove, J. F., Price, C., Pappachan, V. J., & Smith, G. B. (2001). Multicenter study of obstetric admissions to 14 intensive care units in Southern England. *Critical Care Medicine, 29,* 770–775.
10. Graves, C. R. (2004). Organizing a critical care obstetric unit. In G. A. Dildy, M. A. Belfort, G. R. Saade, Phelan, J. P., Hankins, G. D. V., and Clark, S. L. (Eds.), *Critical care obstetrics* (4th ed., pp. 13–16). Malden, MA: Blackwell Science.
11. Pronovost, P. J., Angus, D. C., Dorman, T., Robinson, K. A., Dremsizov, T. T., & Young, T. L. (2002). Physician staffing patterns and clinical outcomes in critically ill patients: A systematic review. *JAMA, 288*(17), 2151–2162.
12. Weber, D. J., Sickbert-Bennett, E. E., Brown, V., & Rutala, W. A. (2007). Comparison of hospital-wide surveillance and targeted intensive care unit surveillance of healthcare-associated infections. *Infection Control and Hospital Epidemiology, 28*(12), 1361–1366.
13. Edwards, J. R., Peterson, K. D., Andrus, M. L., Dudeck, M. A., Pollock, D. A., Horan, T. C. National Healthcare Safety Network Facilities (2008). National healthcare safety network (NHSN) report, data summary for 2006 through 2007, issued November 2008. *American Journal of Infection Control, 36,* 609–626.
14. Centers for Disease Control and Prevention (CDC, 2006, April 21). Recommendations to improve preconception health and health care—United States. *MMWR, 55*(RR06), 1–23. Retrieved from http://www.cdc.gov/mmwr/preview/mmwrhtml/rr5506a1.htm
15. Berg, C. J., Chang, J., Callaghan, W. M., & Whitehead, S. J. (2003). Pregnancy-related mortality in the United States, 1991–1997. *Obstetrics & Gynecology, 101*(2), 289–296.
16. Centers for Disease Control and Prevention (CDC, 2008). Smoking prevalence among women of reproductive age—United States, 2006. *MMWR, 57,* 849–852.

CHAPTER 2

Collaboration in Clinical Practice

Nan H. Troiano, Shailen S. Shah, and Mary Ellen Burke Sosa

The current health care delivery system challenges all of us to provide care that is patient-centered, efficient, effective, safe, and easily accessible. To meet these challenges, quality and safety become priorities for everyone. Optimal collaboration between nurses and physicians holds promise as a strategy to improve patient care and create healthy work environments. In fact, there is arguably a need to optimize all interactions in a multidisciplinary health care team.

Collaboration between nurses and physicians is a complex process. Traditionally, the term *collaboration* has been used to reflect interpersonal interaction, and it implies collective action toward a common goal in a spirit of trust and harmony.[1–6] In the context of health care, collaboration often refers to the way in which physicians and nurses interact with one another in relation to clinical decision making.[7,8] Each of these health care professions has information the other needs in order to practice at an optimal level. In the interest of quality clinical care and patient safety, neither profession can stand alone; thus, good collaboration skills are not only desirable but essential. This chapter provides an overview of the history of collaboration and describes benefits of collaboration, obstacles to collaboration, and strategies to improve nurse–physician collaboration in clinical practice.

HISTORY OF COLLABORATION

One inherent characteristic of the relationship between nurses and physicians is that they care for patients both independently and together. With respect to gender and the historic origins and roots of each profession, most physicians were male and most nurses female. Thus, traditional gender expectations of the time became deeply associated with the physician and nurse roles and were strictly followed, both formally and informally, in the hospital setting.

Various wars, epidemics, and societal evolution expanded roles for women. The role of the nurse expanded as well, and the education of nurses moved out of the hospitals and into colleges. Nurses subsequently assumed administrative and teaching roles. Columbia University awarded the first master's degree in the clinical specialty of nursing in 1956.[9] The role of the "bedside nurse" became increasingly filled by personnel other than registered nurses (usually licensed practical nurses), and prompted the Surgeon General in the early 1960s to appoint a group of nurses to review nursing needs.[10] The report, *Toward Quality in Nursing*, noted increased responsibilities of professional nurses, changing medical practices, and specified levels of preparation for professional nurses. The report contained a number of recommendations, one of which was to study the nursing education system with respect to nursing skills and responsibilities to provide for patient care of the highest quality. Another was to provide federal funding for student loans and scholarships toward advanced education for professional nurses. In addition, recommendations were also made to increase and improve the quality of education programs and to support an increase in nursing research.

The role of the advanced practice nurse evolved over time and increased the dialogue and legislative activity regarding collaboration between nurses and physicians.[11] The American Nurses Association (ANA) and the National League for Nursing (NLN) obtained funding for an independent study on nursing. The National Commission for the Study of Nursing and Nursing Education in the United States was formed in 1967 to assess the status of recommendations from the Surgeon General's report. The commission's work lasted several years and the final report, *An Abstract for Action,* was published in 1971.[12] One of the major recommendations of the report was to establish the National Joint Practice Commission between medicine and nursing "to discuss and make recommendations concerning the congruent roles of the physician and the nurse in providing quality health care, with particular attention to the rise of the nurse master clinician; the introduction of the physician's assistant; and the increased activity of other professions in areas long assumed to be the concern solely of the physician and/or the nurse."[13] The Commission's director proposed that nursing and medicine work out their respective roles through joint discussions, and the term *joint practice* was born. Not initially well received, the term has evolved over time to *collaborative practice.*

The American Medical Association (AMA) recognized the need for discussion about collaborative practice and issued a position statement in 1970 regarding the role of the nurse in expanded practice.[14] The ANA in 1980 defined collaboration as "a true partnership, in which the power on both sides is valued by both, with recognition and acceptance of separate and combined practice spheres of activity and responsibility, mutual safeguarding of the legitimate interests of each party, and a commonality of goals that is recognized by both parties."[15]

Rising costs of medical care and insurance, the nursing shortage of the 1980s, and the availability of advanced practice nursing degrees brought about further discussions regarding collaborative practice.[16] Nursing practice continued to expand with advanced degrees such as certified nurse-midwifery, nurse-anesthetist, clinical nurse specialist, and nurse practitioner. In addition, doctoral degrees became available for an increased number of nurses in the United States. This posed an even larger debate between nurses and physicians, as the business of taking care of patients moved forward from physicians only to nurses and physicians both looking for how to deal with these changes. The AMA and the ANA conducted a series of hearings between 1993 and 1994 in an attempt to reach agreement on nurse–physician professional relationships and establish an acceptable definition of the term "collaboration." They agreed on the following definition: "Collaboration is the process whereby physicians and nurses plan and practice together as colleagues, working interdependently within the boundaries of their scopes of practice with shared values and mutual acknowledgment and respect for each other's contribution to care for individuals, their families, and their communities." A study was published in 1996, where both physicians and nurses had the opportunity to evaluate services "delivered in collaborative obstetrics and gynecology practices to determine whether patients perceived a difference in the delivery of services in a variety of practice settings."[17] This study demonstrated that patients accepted a collaborative practice model and determined that it offered a number of positive outcomes. The authors also noted that the model of care based on

partnership between physician and non-physician professionals was not new and that, "The creation of collaborative models of care in which professionals work within their scopes of practice to meet patients needs *without duplication* may improve efficiency and patient outcomes."

BENEFITS OF COLLABORATION

Nurse–physician collaboration is a key factor in nurses' job satisfaction, retention, and job valuation.[18-22] Decreased risk-adjusted mortality and length of stay, fewer negative patient outcomes, and enhanced patient satisfaction have also been associated with better nurse–physician collaboration.[7,23,24]

A number of instruments with published psychometrics have been used in research to measure nurse–physician collaboration.[25] These instruments include:

- Collaborative Practice Scale (CPS)
- Collaboration and Satisfaction about Care Decisions (CSACD)
- ICU Nurse–Physician Questionnaire
- Nurses Opinion Questionnaire (NOQ)
- Jefferson Scale of Attitudes toward Physician Nurse Collaboration.

These instruments have been recommended for use because they have undergone initial reliability and validity testing. The ICU Nurse–Physician Questionnaire and the CSACD measure collaboration of the same construct dimensions for both nurses and physicians. The CPS measures different aspects of collaboration between nurses and physicians. The CMSS component of the NOQ measures nurse perception of collaboration, but physicians were not included in the initial survey development. The Jefferson Scale has been used primarily to compare attitudes toward collaboration between countries and cultures.

Two themes have been identified with respect to this subject. First, registered nurses have initiated much of the research on collaboration and, second, ICUs have been the site of much of the research.

A number of factors may help explain these phenomena. A study by Kurtz suggested that physicians may prefer not to be interactive and would subsequently avoid group involvement.[26] Sexton and colleagues described a significant disparity in nurse and physician perceptions of teamwork and communication.[27] Larson identified a disparity in nurse and physician perceptions of current and ideal authority of nurses.[28] Others have described the inequity of power and authority between nurses and physicians.[29,30]

The professional education of nurses and physicians does not generally include interdisciplinary experiences in communication, planning, and decision-making.[31] Nurses and physicians may practice professionally as they have been frequently taught, using primarily independent decision-making on the part of physicians and more interdependent decision-making with coordination and communication functions on the part of nurses.[32,33] Thus, nurses and physicians perceive the value and need for collaboration differently, and this may affect their interest in research on the subject.

Factors have also been identified that may explain why most research with respect to collaboration has been conducted in an ICU setting. Knauss and colleagues demonstrated the importance of communication and coordination in the achievement of positive patient and fiscal outcomes in the ICU.[23] This led to additional studies conducted in ICUs, possibly because of the higher rates of patient acuity, mortality, and the potential for clinical practice errors to occur in that setting. The critical care setting requires immediate medical and nursing intervention, active dialogue, and communication to respond to patients' rapidly changing physiologic parameters. Low staffing ratios, smaller units, the presence of experienced and specialized nurses, and close proximity among staff members are factors that potentially influence collaboration in an ICU. Arguably, these same factors exist in the obstetric care setting, especially when the patients have significant complications or are critically ill. The study of collaboration within the construct of patient safety and in a variety of clinical care settings may provide an added impetus for change in nurse–physician collaboration that transcends historical and sociological constraints. This change in patterns of collaboration between nurses and physicians may ultimately lead to better clinical communication and patient outcomes.

BARRIERS TO EFFECTIVE COLLABORATION

Two fundamental obstacles to improved nurse–physician collaboration have been identified: disruptive physician behavior and unacceptable nurse conduct.[34] Disruptive behavior has captured the attention of health care providers and leaders as well as the general public. This is due in part to the increased focus on the role of culture as a contributing factor in medical errors.[35] To a great extent, health care organizations devoted their initial patient safety efforts to training and to redesigning clinical processes, such as medication administration. However, there is little evidence to suggest that error rates have decreased significantly as a result of these efforts.

The health care industry has begun to acknowledge that human interaction is an important but largely ignored source of error. Conflict appears to be ubiquitous in human relationships; yet, few people would argue that conflict in the workplace is desirable. The complexities of modern medicine and of the technologies involved clearly require the combined knowledge, skills, and collaboration of many different health professionals.

Disruptive Behaviors in the Workplace

Since the 1990s, recognition of negative workplace behaviors has increased.[36,37] These disruptive behaviors include use of verbally abusive language, intimidation tactics, sexual comments, racial slurs, and ethnic jokes. Additional disruptive behaviors include shaming or criticizing colleagues in front of others; threatening colleagues with retribution, litigation, violence, or job loss; and throwing instruments, charts, or other objects.[38] These behaviors, in part, reflect a broader problem. In a poll conducted by *U.S. News and World Report,* 89% of Americans identified incivility as a serious social problem and 78% agreed that it had worsened in the past 10 years.[39]

Personal interactions are a critical component of a culture of safety and quality. For this reason, the Joint Commission has developed standards that address disruptive behavior. The Joint Commission generally defines disruptive behavior as those that have the capacity to intimidate staff, affect staff morale, or lead to staff turnover.[40] Behavior deemed disruptive may be verbal or nonverbal, and could involve the use of rude language or facial expressions, threatening manners, or even physical abuse. Leaders are expected to create and maintain a culture of safety and quality throughout the health care organization. Safety and quality thrive in an environment that supports teamwork and respect for other people. Disruptive behavior that intimidates others and affects morale or staff turnover can be harmful to patient care. Specific elements of performance related to The Joint Commission Standards on this subject are listed in Box 2-1. In addition, the Joint Commission issued a Sentinel Event Alert related to prevention of behaviors that undermine a culture of safety.[40] Specifically, the agency warned that rude language and hostile behavior are not only unpleasant but pose a serious threat to patient safety and the overall quality of care.

Data continue to be published regarding the prevalence and impact of disruptive behavior. Veltman specifically addressed disruptive behavior in obstetric practice in a study in which hospital labor and delivery units were surveyed to determine rates of disruptive and intimidating behavior by health care providers and how this behavior threatens patient safety.[41] In this study, disruptive behavior was reported in 60.7 percent of responding labor and delivery units. Physicians

Box 2-1. ELEMENTS OF PERFORMANCE: THE JOINT COMMISSION STANDARD LD.03.01

- Leaders regularly evaluate the culture of safety and quality using valid and reliable tools.
- Leaders prioritize and implement changes identified by the evaluation.
- Leaders provide opportunities for all individuals who work in the hospital to participate in safety and quality initiatives.
- The hospital has a code of conduct that defines acceptable, disruptive, and inappropriate behavior.
- Leaders create and implement a process for managing disruptive and inappropriate behavior.
- Leaders establish a team approach among all staff at all levels.
- All individuals who work in the hospital, including staff and licensed independent practitioners, openly discuss issues of safety and quality.
- Literature and advisories relevant to patient safety are available to all who work in the hospital.
- Leaders define how members of the population(s) served can help identify and manage issues related to safety and quality in the hospital

TABLE 2-1

Number of Deliveries Per Month and Occurrence of Disruptive Behavior

Number of Deliveries per Month (Respondents)		Incidents of Disruptive Behavior on Unit	
1–99	(30 hospitals)	13/30	(43.3%)
100–199	(8 hospitals)	6/8	(75%)
200–299	(3 hospitals)	2/3	(66%)
300–399	(6 hospitals)	5/6	(83%)
>400	(9 hospitals)	8/9	(88%)
Total: 56 hospitals responding		34/56	(60.7%)

administrators' perceptions of its effects on providers and its impact on clinical outcomes.[42] Surveys were distributed to 50 hospitals across the country, and results from more than 1,500 survey participants were evaluated. Nurses were reported to have behaved disruptively almost as frequently as physicians. Most respondents perceived disruptive behavior as having negative or worsening effects, for both nurses and physicians, on stress, frustration, concentration, communication, collaboration, information transfer, and workplace relationships. Even more disturbing were the respondents' perceptions of negative or worsening effects of disruptive behavior on adverse events, medical errors, patient safety, patient mortality, quality of care, and patient satisfaction.

STRATEGIES TO IMPROVE COLLABORATION

Despite the challenges of battling non-collaborative habits, true collaboration between nurses and physicians is possible and vital, not only for the benefit of patients, but also for the satisfaction of health care providers.[18] Collaboration between physicians and nurses is rewarding when responsibility for patient well-being is shared. Professionalism is strengthened when all members take credit for group successes.

Various strategies have been described to improve collaboration. Lindeke and Sieckert identify three categories of collaborative strategies, namely self development, team development, and communication development.[18] These strategies can enhance nurse–physician collaboration and promote positive patient and nurse outcomes.[18] An overview of elements related to these three strategies is presented in Table 2-2. The authors note that collaboration may occur within long-term relationships between health professionals. In such cases, collaboration has a development trajectory that evolves over time as team members leave or join the group and/or organization structures change. On

(obstetricians, anesthesiologists, family practitioners, pediatricians, and neonatologists) accounted for most of the disruptive behavior. However, registered nurses (midwives and certified registered nurse anesthetists) and nurse administrators also were reported as demonstrating disruptive behaviors. The survey results indicated that some hospital medical staffs are more effective in ameliorating disruptive behavior. When asked whether nurses on the unit had quit or had transferred out of the unit because of others' disruptive behavior, 39.3 percent responded affirmatively. Adverse outcomes were felt to be directly linked to disruptive or intimidating behavior in 41.9 percent of respondents. The number of deliveries per month and occurrence of disruptive behavior in hospitals participating in the survey are presented in Table 2-1.

Unacceptable Nurse Conduct

Disruptive behavior is not limited to physicians. It is important to acknowledge that nurses also bear responsibility in determining the tenor of nurse–physician relationships, with poorly structured clinical communication and unprofessional behavior particular sources of frustration for physician colleagues.

A study conducted by Rosenstein and O'Daniel utilized surveys to examine the disruptive behavior of both physicians and nurses, as well as both groups' and

TABLE 2-2

Categories of Collaborative Strategies

Self development strategies	Develop emotional maturity.
	Understand the perspectives of others.
	Avoid compassion fatigue.
Team development strategies	Build the team.
	Negotiate respectfully.
	Manage conflict wisely.
	Avoid negative behaviors.
	Design facilities for collaboration.
Communication development strategies	Communicate effectively in emergencies.
	Use electronic communication thoughtfully.
	• Project openness with a friendly, courteous tone.
	• Evaluate the content of received messages before reacting.
	• Clarify your understanding of messages, critique the message and not the sender.
	• Send messages with only pertinent details, pay attention to what the receiver will find useful and avoid jargon.
	• Summarize issues without being repetitive; be as brief as possible.

Adapted from Lindeke, L.L., & Sieckert, A.M. (2005). Nurse-physician workplace collaboration. *OJIN, 10,* 1, Manuscript 4.

other occasions, collaboration between nurses and physicians may involve fleeting encounters in patient arenas. In these settings, there is no chance to collaborate effectively, and a given interaction may leave lasting positive or negative impressions on those involved or on those who witness a particular nurse–physician interaction.[18] The Nursing Executive Center identifies specific tactics and strategies to revitalize the nurse–physician relationship and strengthen collaboration.[34] An overview of suggested tactics is presented in Table 2-3.

Professional organizations have also embraced a commitment to address issues related to collaboration in clinical practice. In 2001, the American Association of Critical-Care Nurses (AACN) made a commitment to actively promote the creation of healthy work environments that support and foster excellence in patient care wherever acute and critical care nurses practice.[43]

TABLE 2-3

Tactics and Strategies to Revitalize the Nurse–Physician Relationship

Tactic #1	*Create Leadership Alliances*	Nursing-Medical Leadership Linkage
Tactic #2	*Address Unacceptable Behavior*	All-Staff Conduct
Tactic #3	*Build Trust in Organization*	Complaint Feedback Loops
Tactic #4	*Provide Tools for New Graduates and New Hires*	Communication Coaching
Tactic #5	*Commit to Clear Standards of Responsiveness & Preparedness*	Nurse–Physician Service Contracts
Tactic #6	*Nurse Leaders Educate Physicians about Nursing Department Operations*	Nursing-Driven Physician Education
Tactic #7	*Nursing and Physician Leaders Collaborate*	Hospital-Wide Nurse–Physician Committee
Tactic #8	*Establish Opportunities for Multidisciplinary Learning*	Interprofessional Health Care Education
Tactic #9	*Nursing and Medical Leadership Collaborate to Improve Communication*	Communication Improvement Campaign
Tactic #10	*Physicians and Nurses Conduct Joint Rounds*	Clinical Expertise Sharing
Tactic #11	*Hospital Sponsors Unit-Based Clinical Practice Committees*	Unit-Based Interdisciplinary Committees

Adapted from The Advisory Board Company. Nursing Executive Center. *The case for strengthening nurse–physician relations.* Washington, DC: Author.

TABLE 2-4

AACN Standards for Establishing and Sustaining Healthy Work Environments

Skilled Communication	Nurses must be as proficient in communication skills as they are in clinical skills.
True Collaboration	Nurses must be relentless in pursuing and fostering true collaboration
Effective Decision-Making	Nurses must be valued and committed partners in making policy, directing and evaluating clinical care and leading organizational operations.
Appropriate Staffing	Staffing must ensure the effective match between patient needs and nurse competencies.
Meaningful Recognition	Nurses must be recognized and must recognize others for the value each brings to the work of the organization.
Authentic Leadership	Nurse leaders must fully embrace the imperative of a healthy work environment, authentically live it and engage others in its achievement.

Adapted from the American Association of Critical-Care Nurses. (2005). *AACN standards for establishing and sustaining healthy work environments.* Aliso Viejo, California: Author. Retrieved January 15, 2011, from http://www.aacn.org/WD/HWE/Docs/HWEStandards.pdf

Box 2-2. CRITICAL ELEMENTS IN TRUE COLLABORATION

- The health care organization provides team members with support for and access to education programs that develop critical communication skills, including self-awareness, inquiry/dialogue, conflict management, negotiation, advocacy, and listening.
- Skilled communicators focus on finding solutions and achieving desirable outcomes.
- Skilled communicators seek to protect and advance collaborative relationships among colleagues.
- Skilled communicators invite and hear all relevant perspectives.
- Skilled communicators call upon goodwill and mutual respect to build consensus and arrive at common understanding.
- Skilled communicators demonstrate congruence between words and actions, holding others accountable for doing the same.
- The health care organization establishes zero-tolerance policies that ensure effective information sharing among patients, families, and the health care team.
- Skilled communicators have access to appropriate communication technologies and are proficient in their use.
- The health care organization establishes systems that require individuals and teams to formally evaluate the impact of communication on clinical, financial, and work environment outcomes.
- The health care organization includes communication as a criterion in its formal performance appraisal system, and team members demonstrate skilled communication to qualify for professional advancement.

Mounting evidence suggests that unhealthy work environments contribute to medical errors, ineffective delivery of care, and conflict and stress among health professionals. Negative, demoralizing, and unsafe conditions in workplaces cannot be allowed to continue. The creation of healthy work environments is imperative to ensure patient safety, enhance staff recruitment and retention, and maintain an organization's financial viability. Six standards were identified for establishing and sustaining healthy work environments and are listed in Table 2-4. The standards are neither detailed nor exhaustive. They are designed to be used as a foundation for thoughtful reflection and engaged dialogue about the current realities of each work environment. The standards represent evidence-based and relationship-centered principles of professional performance. Each standard is considered essential because studies show that effective and sustainable outcomes do not emerge when any standard is considered optional.

Critical elements required for successful implementation accompany each standard. Elements related to the standard on pursuing and fostering true collaboration are presented in Box 2-2.

SUMMARY

Despite the need for further study, many organizations are energetically pursuing initiatives to improve collaboration between nurses and physicians. The organization provides the context in which nurse–physician communication occurs. The organization determines the structure in which these professionals interact, the professional development opportunities of the employed nurses, the group and individual power dynamics, and the cultural norms of behavior. The organization decides the number and required qualifications of direct-care staff, the availability of role modeling to refine communication skills, the authority of the nurse when involved in a conflict with a physician, and the valuing of nurses' clinical practice. Organizational theory is useful in guiding an analysis of the relationship between nurse–physician communication in context using the structural, human resource, political, and cultural perspectives of organizational behavior. It has become increasingly apparent that organizational investment in strategies to strengthen collaboration in clinical practice is essential to meet quality clinical care and patient safety expectations.

REFERENCES

1. Stein-Parbury, J. S., & Liaschenko, J. (2007). Understanding collaboration between nurses and physicians as knowledge at work. *American Journal of Critical Care, 16*(5), 470–478.
2. Mitchell, P. H., Shannon, S. E., Cain, K. C., & Hegyvary, S. T. (1996). Critical care outcomes: Linking structures, processes, and organizational and clinical outcomes. *American Journal of Critical Care, 5,* 353–363.
3. Van Ess Coeling, H., & Cukr, P. L. (2000). Communication styles that promote perceptions of collaboration, quality, and nurse satisfaction. *Journal of Nursing Care Quality, 14*(2), 63–74.
4. Corser, W. D. (1998). A conceptual model of collaborative nurse-physician interactions: The management of traditional influences and person tendencies. *Scholarly Inquiry for Nursing Practice, 12*(4), 325–346.
5. McMahan, E. M., Hoffman, K., & McGee G. W. (1994). Physician-nurse relationships in clinical settings: A review and critique of the literature, 1966–1992. *Medical Care Review, 51,* 83–112.
6. D'Amour, D., Ferrada-Videla, M., San Martin-Rodriquez, L., & Beaulieu, M. D. (2005). The conceptual basis for interprofessional collaboration: Core concepts and theoretical frameworks. *Journal of Interprofessional Care, 19*(Suppl. 1), 116–131.
7. Shortell, S. M., Zimmerman, J. E., Rousseau, D. M., Gillies, R. R., Wagner, D. P., Draper, E. A., et al. (1994). The performance of intensive care units: Does good management make a difference? *Medical Care, 32,* 508–525.
8. Baggs, J. G., Ryan, S. A., Phelps, C. E., Richeson, J. F., & Johnson, J. E. (1993). The association between interdisciplinary collaboration and patient outcomes in a medical intensive care unit. *Heart Lung, 21,* 18–24.
9. Columbia University School of Nursing. (2010). *Columbia University School of Nursing: A brief history.* Retrieved from http://www.nursing.hs.columbia.edu/about-school/history.html
10. Report of the Surgeon General's Consultant Group on Nursing. (1963). *Toward quality in nursing: Needs and goals.* Washington, DC: Department of Health, Education, and Welfare, Public Health Service Publication No. 922. Retrieved from http://eric.ed.gov/PDFS/ED021994.pdf
11. Wolf, K. A. (2009). The slow march to professional practice. In A. M. Baker (Ed.), *Advanced practice nursing.* Sudbury, MA: Jones & Bartlett Learning.
12. Christy, T. E., Poulin, M. A., & Hover, J. (1971). An appraisal of an abstract for action. *The American Journal of Nursing, 71,* 1574–1581.
13. Ritter, H. A. (1983). Collaborative practice: What's in it for medicine? *Nursing Administration Quarterly, 7,* 31–36.
14. American Medical Association Committee on Nursing. (1970). Medicine and nursing in the 1970s. *JAMA, 213*(11), 1881–1883.
15. American Nurses Association. (1993). *Testimony to the physician practice review commission.* Silver Spring, MD: Author.
16. Burchell, R. C., Smith, H. L., Tuttle, W. C., & Thomas, D. A. (1982). Collaborative practice in obstetrics/gynecology: Implications for cost, quality, and productivity. *American Journal of Obstetrics and Gynecology, 144,* 621–625.
17. Hankins, G. D. V., Shaw, S. B., Cruess, D. F., Lawrence, H. C. 3rd, & Harris, C. D. (1996). Patient satisfaction with collaborative practice. *Obstetrics & Gynecology, 88,* 1011–1015.
18. Lindeke, L. L., & Sieckert, A. M. (2005). Nurse-physician workplace collaboration. *OJIN, 10,* 1, Manuscript 4.
19. LeTourneau, B. (2004). Physicians and nurses: Friends or foes? *Journal of Healthcare Management, 49*(1), 12–14.
20. Baggs, J. G., & Ryan, S. (1990). ICU nurse physician collaboration and nursing satisfaction. *Nursing Economics, 8*(6), 386–392.
21. Baggs, J. G., Schmitt, M., Mushlin, A., Mitchell, P. H., Eldredge, D. H., Oakes, D., et al. (1992). Association between nurse physician collaboration and patient outcomes in three intensive care units. *Critical Care Medicine, 27*(9), 1991–1998.
22. Chaboyer, W., Majman, J., & Dunn, S. (2001). Factors influencing job valuation: A comparative study of critical care and non-critical care nurses. *International Journal of Nursing Studies, 38,* 153–161.
23. Knaus, W., Draper, E., Wagner, D., & Zimmermann, S. (1986). An evaluation of outcome from intensive care in major medical centers. *Annals of Internal Medicine, 104,* 410–418.
24. Larrabee, J., Ostrow, C. L., Withrow, M. l., Janney, M. A., Hobbs, G. R. Jr., & Burant, C. (2004). Predictors of patient satisfaction with inpatient hospital nursing care. *Research in Nursing & Health, 27,* 254–268.
25. Dougherty, M. B., & Larson, E. (2005). A review of instruments measuring nurse-physician collaboration. *JONA, 35*(5), 244–253.
26. Kurtz, M. W. (1980). A behavioral profile of physician's managerial roles. In R. Schenke (Ed.), *The physician in management.* Washington, DC: Artisian.
27. Sexton, J., Thomas, E., & Helmreich, R. I. (2000). Error, stress and teamwork in medicine and aviation: Cross sectional surveys. *BMJ, 320,* 745–749.
28. Larson, E. (1993). The impact of physician-nurse interaction on patient care. *Holistic Nursing Practice, 13*(2), 38–46.
29. Haddad, A. (1991). The nurse-physician relationship and ethical decision-making. *AORN, 53*(1), 151–156.
30. Keenan, G., Cooke, R., & Hillis, S. (1998). Norms and nurse management of conflict: Keys to understanding nurse-physician collaboration. *Research in Nursing & Health, 21*(1), 59–72.
31. Fagin, C. M. (1992). Collaboration between nurses and physicians: No longer a choice. *Academic Medicine, 67*(5), 295–303.
32. Zungolo, E. (1994). Interdisciplinary education in primary care: The challenge. *Nursing and Health Care, 15,* 288–292.
33. Barrere, C., & Ellis, P. (2002). Changing attitudes among nurses and physicians: A step toward collaboration. *Journal for Healthcare Quality, 24*(3), 9–15.
34. The Advisory Board Company. Nursing Executive Center. *The case for strengthening nurse–physician relations.* Washington, DC: Author.
35. Porto, G., & Lauve, R. (2006). Disruptive clinician behavior: A persistent threat to patient safety. *Patient Safety and Quality Health.* Retrieved from http://www.psqh.com/julaug06/disruptive.html
36. Felbinger, D. M. (2008). Incivility and bullying in the workplace and nurses' shame responses. *Journal of Obstetric, Gynecologic, Neonatal Nursing, 37*(2), 234–242.
37. Lutgen-Sandvik, P., Tracy, S. J., & Alberts, J. K. (2007). Burned by bullying in the American workplace: Prevalence,

perception, degree, and impact. *Journal of Management Studies, 44,* 837–862.

38. Pfifferling, J. H. (2003). Developing and implementing a policy to deal with disruptive staff members. *Oncology Issues, 18,* 1–5.

39. Marks, J. (1996). The American uncivil wars: How crude, rude, and obnoxious behavior has replaced good manners and why that hurts our politics and culture. *U.S. News & World Report, 22*(April 14), 66–72.

40. Joint Commission. (2008). *Sentinel Event Alert, issue 40: Behaviors that undermine a culture of safety.* Retrieved from http://www.jointcommission.org/sentinel_event_alert_issue_40_behaviors_that_undermine_a_culture_of_safety/

41. Veltman, L. (2007). Disruptive behavior in obstetrics: A hidden threat to patient safety. *American Journal of Obstetrics & Gynecology, 196*(6), 587.e1–587.e5.

42. Rosenstein, A. H., & O'Daniel, M. (2005). Disruptive behavior & clinical outcomes: Perceptions of nurses & physicians. *Nursing Management, 36*(1), 18–28.

43. American Association of Critical-Care Nurses. (2005). *AACN standards for establishing and sustaining healthy work environments.* Aliso Viejo, CA: Author. Retrieved from http://www.aacn.org/WD/HWE/Docs/HWEStandards.pdf

CHAPTER 3

Ethical Challenges

Frank A. Chervenak, Laurence B. McCullough, and Bonnie Flood Chez

In both medicine and nursing, there is a clinically based framework for bioethics applicable to the practice of high-risk and critical care obstetrics.[1,3] Some ethical crises that arise in acute clinical situations may be addressed only *after* they have occurred. In contrast, the concept of *preventive ethics* has evolved as a valuable clinical resource for anticipatory thought. Preventive ethics appreciates that the potential for ethical conflict exists in certain clinical situations and encourages the adoption of ethically justified strategies to reduce the frequency with which such conflicts occur. Preventive ethics assists clinicians to collaboratively establish a framework for clinical judgment and decision-making that is integral to the specialty and the patients and families it serves. This decision-making framework evolves from defining:

- the fundamental ethical principles of medicine and nursing, such as beneficence and respect for autonomy;
- how these two principles should interact in obstetric judgment and practice, with emphasis on the core concept of the fetus as a patient;
- different concepts of the ethical principles of justice; and
- ethical issues in responsible resource management that emphasize the virtues of health care professionals.

MEDICAL ETHICS AND NURSING ETHICS

Medical and nursing ethics involves the disciplined study of morality in the respective professions. Professional morality concerns the obligations of physicians, nurses, and health care organizations, within any given area of specialty care, and the patients and families served. It also includes the reciprocal obligations placed on patients and families.[4] Like any other social skill or knowledge, morality evolves by learning from the examples of those around us, so it is important not to confuse medical and nursing ethics with the many sources of morality in a pluralistic society. These include, but are not limited to: law, our political heritage as a free people in the United States, the world's religions (all of which can be found in the U.S.), ethnic and cultural traditions, families, the traditions and practices of medicine and nursing (including education and training), and personal experience. Medical ethics, since the eighteenth century European and American Enlightenments, has been secular.[5] It makes no reference to God or revealed tradition, but to what rational discourse requires and produces. At the same time, secular medical ethics is not intrinsically hostile to religious beliefs. Therefore, ethical principles and virtues should be understood to apply to all clinicians, regardless of their personal religious and spiritual beliefs.[6] Since the emergence of nursing as a profession in the nineteenth century, nursing ethics, too, has been understood to be secular in nature.

The traditions and practices of medicine and nursing constitute an obvious source of morality for physicians and nurses because they are based on the obligation to protect and promote the health-related interests of the patient. This obligation defines for physicians and nurses what morality in medicine ought to be, but in very general, abstract terms. Providing a more concrete, clinically applicable account of that obligation is the central task of medical and nursing ethics, using ethical principles that guide decision-making and behavior in the clinical setting.[4]

Beneficence

The principle of beneficence requires that clinicians "do good." Its application requires one to act in a way that

---

Adapted from Chervenak, F. A., & McCullough, L. B. (2008). Ethics in obstetrics and gynecology. The Global Library of Women's Medicine. Retrieved from http://www.glowm.com/index.html?p=glowm.cml/section_view&articleid=491

is expected reliably to produce the greater balance of benefit over harm in the lives of others.[6] To put this principle into clinical practice requires a reliable account of the benefit and harm relevant to the patient's care. In obstetrics, the definition of "patient" may include the pregnant woman and also the fetus. Further, what is good for the pregnant woman may not always be good for the fetus. For example, treatment of a pregnant woman's illness may require medications that are potentially harmful to the fetus, yet delaying treatment may seriously harm the pregnant woman. Overall, benefits and harms should be reasonably balanced against each other when not all of them can be achieved in a particular clinical situation, such as a maternal request for an elective Cesarean delivery.[7]

Beneficence-based clinical judgment has an ancient pedigree, with its first expression found in the Hippocratic Oath and accompanying texts.[8] It makes an important claim: to interpret reliably the health-related interests of the patient from the perspective of the health care professions. This perspective is provided by accumulated scientific research, clinical experience, and reasoned responses to uncertainty.[9] Rigorous evidence-based, beneficence-based judgment does not emanate from the individual clinical perspective of any particular physician or nurse. It should not be based merely on the clinical impression or intuition of an individual clinician. Rather, the clinical benefits that can be achieved for the patient in practice are grounded in the competencies of medicine and nursing. Benefits include the fact that physicians and nurses are competent to seek for patients the prevention/management of: disease, injury, or handicap; unnecessary pain and suffering; and premature or unnecessary death. Pain and suffering become unnecessary when they do not result in the achievement of other benefits of medical care (e.g., allowing a woman to labor without effective analgesia).[4]

A related term, nonmaleficence, means that health care practitioners should also prevent causing harm and is best understood as expressing the limits of beneficence. This is also known as *"Primum non nocere"* or "first, do no harm." This commonly invoked dogma is really a Latinized misinterpretation of the Hippocratic texts, which emphasized beneficence while avoiding harm when approaching the limits of medicine.[4] Nonmaleficence should be incorporated into beneficence-based clinical judgment when the physician or nurse approaches the limits of beneficence-based clinical judgment. In other words, when the evidence for expected benefit decreases and the risks of clinical harm increase, then the clinician should proceed with great caution. This becomes an especially important clinical ethical consideration in critical-care obstetrics when the patient is gravely ill. For example, the use of advanced technology for the intended purpose of extending and saving life is considered to be good; however, when this technology merely prolongs dying or when quality of life is poor, a controversy between beneficence and nonmalfience occurs. In these situations, the physician and nurse should be especially concerned to prevent serious, far-reaching, and irreversible clinical harm to the patient.

It is important to note that there is an inherent risk of paternalism in beneficence-based clinical judgment. Paternalism overlooks any individual's potential for self-determination. In other words, beneficence-based clinical judgment, if it is *mistakenly* considered to be the sole source of moral responsibility and therefore moral authority in medical care, invites the unwary physician or nurse to conclude that beneficence-based judgments can be imposed on the patient in violation of her autonomy. Paternalism is a dehumanizing response to the patient and, therefore, should be avoided in the practice of high-risk and critical care obstetrics.

The preventive ethics response to this inherent paternalism is for the physician to explain the diagnostic, therapeutic, and prognostic reasoning that leads to his or her clinical judgment about what is in the interest of the patient so that the patient can assess that judgment for herself. This general rule can be put into clinical practice in the following way: The physician should disclose and explain to the patient the major factors of this reasoning process, including matters of uncertainty. In neither medical law nor medical ethics does this require that the patient be provided with a complete medical education.[10] The physician should then explain how and why other clinicians might reasonably differ from his or her clinical judgment. The outcome of this process is that beneficence-based clinical judgments take on a rigor that they sometimes lack, and the process of their formulation includes explaining them to the patient. Awareness of this feature of beneficence-based clinical judgment provides an important preventive ethics antidote to paternalism by increasing the likelihood that one or more of these medically reasonable, evidence-based alternatives will be acceptable to the patient. This feature of beneficence-based clinical judgment also provides a preventive ethics antidote to "gag" rules that restrict physicians' communications with the managed care patient.[11] All beneficence-based alternatives must be identified and explained to all patients, regardless of how the physician is paid, especially those who are well established in evidence-based obstetrics and gynecology.

Nurses have an especially important role to play in collaboration with their physician colleagues before, during, and after information is presented. Knowing what has been discussed with the patient and family provides a unique follow-up opportunity for communication among clinicians, should the patient or family express a lack of understanding and the need for further explanation.

One advantage in carrying out this approach to communication is the increased likelihood of compliance.[12] Another advantage is that the patient is provided a better-informed opportunity from which to make a decision about whether to seek a second opinion. This approach should make such a decision less threatening to the clinician who has already shared with the patient the limitations on clinical judgment.

Respect for Autonomy

In contrast to the principle of beneficence, there has been increasing emphasis in the medical and nursing ethics literature on the principle of respect for autonomy.[6] This principle requires one always to acknowledge and carry out the value-based preferences of an adult, competent patient, unless there is compelling ethical justification for not doing so (e.g., prescribing antibiotics for viral respiratory infections). The pregnant patient increasingly brings to her medical care her own perspective on what is in her best interest. Because each patient's perspective on her best interests is a function of her values and beliefs, it is impossible to specify the benefits and harms of autonomy-based clinical judgment in advance. Indeed, it would be inappropriate for the clinician to do so, because the definition of her benefits and harms and their balancing are the prerogative of the patient. Not surprisingly, autonomy-based clinical judgment is strongly antipaternalistic in nature.[4]

To understand the moral demands of this principle, three sequential autonomy-based patient behaviors are most relevant to clinical practice, including:

- absorbing and retaining information about her condition and the alternative diagnostic and therapeutic responses to it;
- understanding the information (i.e., evaluating and rank-ordering those responses and appreciating that she could experience the risks of treatment); and
- expressing a value-based preference.

The physician and nurse have important roles to play in each of these. They are, respectively:

- to recognize the capacity of each patient to deal with medical information (and not to underestimate or overestimate that capacity);
- to provide information (i.e., disclose and explain all medically reasonable alternatives), recognizing the validity of the patient's values and beliefs;
- to assist the patient in her evaluation and ranking of diagnostic and therapeutic alternatives for managing her condition; and

- to elicit and implement the patient's value-based preference without interference.[4]

Respect for autonomy is inherent in the doctrine of informed consent. The legal obligations of the physician regarding informed consent were established in a series of cases during the twentieth century. In 1914, *Schloendorff v The Society of The New York Hospital* established the concept of simple consent (i.e., whether the patient says "yes" or "no" to medical intervention).[10,13] To this day, in the medical and bioethics literature, this decision is quoted: "Every human being of adult years and sound mind has the right to determine what shall be done with his body, and a surgeon who performs an operation without his patient's consent commits an assault for which he is liable in damages."[13] The legal requirement of consent further evolved to include disclosure of information sufficient to enable patients to make informed decisions about whether to say "yes" or "no" to medical intervention.[10]

There are two accepted legal standards for such disclosure. The *professional community* standard defines adequate disclosure in the context of what the relevantly trained and experienced clinician tells patients. The *reasonable person* standard, which has been adopted by most states, goes further and requires the physician to disclose "material" information defined as: what any individual in the patient's condition needs to know and what the layperson of average sophistication should not be expected to know. Patients need to know what the physician thinks is clinically salient (i.e., the physician's beneficence-based clinical judgment). This reasonable person principle has emerged as the ethical standard. As such, the physician should disclose to the patient her or the fetus's diagnosis (including differential diagnosis when that is all that is known), the medically reasonable alternatives to diagnose and manage the patient's condition, and the short-term and long-term benefits and risks of each alternative. In contrast, the nurse's responsibility is to verify that the signature of each individual granting consent belongs to the person who signs the consent documents. In addition, if the patient expresses additional questions related to the physician-provided informed consent, the nurse is responsible for notifying the physician of the patient's questions and concerns.

Advance Directives
A particularly important dimension of informed consent in clinical practice involves what has come to be known as an advance directive.[14] Spurred by the famous case of Karen Quinlan in New Jersey in 1976, all states have enacted advance directive legislation.[15,16] Advance directives play a major role in respect for the autonomy of critically ill pregnant women in end-stage disease.

Box 3-1. ETHICAL DIMENSIONS OF AUTONOMY

- A patient may exercise her autonomy now in the form of a request for or refusal of life-prolonging interventions.
- An autonomy-based request or refusal, expressed in the past and left unchanged, remains in effect for any future time during which the patient is determined to be without autonomy.
- A past autonomy-based request for or refusal of life-prolonging interventions should therefore translate into physician and nurse obligations at the time the patient becomes unable to participate in the informed consent process. In particular, refusal of life-prolonging therapeutic intervention should translate into the withholding or withdrawal of such interventions, including artificial nutrition and hydration.

The basic idea of an advance directive is that an autonomous patient can make decisions regarding her medical management in advance of a time when she might become incapable of making health care decisions. The relevant ethical dimensions of autonomy are presented in Box 3-1.

Living Will. The living will or directive to clinicians is an instrument that permits the patient to make a direct decision, usually to refuse life-prolonging medical intervention in the future. The living will becomes effective when the patient is considered to be "qualified," usually terminally or irreversibly ill, and is not able to participate in the informed consent process as judged by her attending physician. Court review is not required. Obviously, terminally or irreversibly ill patients who are able to participate in the informed consent process retain their autonomy to make their own decisions. Some states prescribe the wording of the living will, and others do not. The reader should become familiar with the legal requirements in the applicable jurisdiction. A living will, to be useful and effective, should be as explicit as possible. The reader should become familiar with hospital policies on advance directives, which should reflect and implement applicable law. Such policies also play the crucial role of assuring physicians and nurses that the organization will support them when they implement such policies.

Power of Attorney for Health Care. The concept of a durable power of attorney or medical power of attorney is that any autonomous adult, in the event that the person later becomes unable to participate in the informed consent process, can assign decision-making authority to another person. The advantage of the durable power of attorney for health care is that it applies only when the patient has lost decision-making capacity, as judged by her physician. Court review is not required. It does not, as does the living will, also require that the patient be terminally or irreversibly ill. However, unlike the living will, the durable power of attorney does not necessarily provide explicit direction, only the explicit assignment of decision-making authority to an identified individual or "agent." Obviously, any patient who assigns durable power of attorney for health care to someone else has an interest in communicating her values, beliefs, and preferences to that person. In order to protect the patient's autonomy, the physician and nurse can and should play an active role in encouraging this communication process so that there will be minimal doubt about whether the person holding durable power of attorney is faithfully representing the wishes of the patient.

The main clinical advantages of these two forms of advance directives are that they encourage patients to think carefully in advance about their request for or refusal of medical intervention and help to prevent ethical conflicts and crises in the management of terminally or irreversibly ill patients who have decision-making capacity. Unfortunately, the use of advance directives is not as widespread as it should be.[17] The reader is encouraged to think of advance directives as powerful, practical strategies for preventive ethics for end-of-life care, and to encourage patients to consider them seriously, especially obstetric patients who may require admission to a critical care unit during or after pregnancy. The use of advance directives prevents the experience of increased burden of decision making in the absence of reliable information about the patient's values and beliefs.[18]

Futility

An especially important and related ethical issue concerns clinical judgments of futility. Patients or their family members sometimes request or even demand inappropriate management.[19,20] This does not necessarily relieve physicians and nurses from an ethical duty to advocate for treatment that has been recommended clinically. A preventive ethics strategy may guide clinicians in formulating a response by ascertaining a patient's answers to selected questions.[21] A list of potentially helpful questions is presented in Table 3-1.

BENEFICENCE AND RESPECT FOR AUTONOMY: INTERACTION IN CLINICAL PRACTICE

The ethical principles of beneficence and respect for autonomy play a more complex role in obstetric clinical judgment and practice. There are obviously beneficence-based and autonomy-based obligations to the pregnant patient. One is the physician's and nurse's clinical

TABLE 3-1

Preventive Ethics Strategy: Example Questions and Ethical Implications

Sample Question	Ethical Implications
Is the intervention reliably expected to achieve the intended, usual anatomic or physiologic effect?	If in reliable (especially evidence-based) beneficence-based clinical judgment, it is not expected to do so, then the physician should not offer it. There is no obligation to offer or to perform medical interventions that are futile in this strict sense, such as providing a feeding tube for a patient with cancer cachexia. This is known as anatomic or physiologic futility.
Is the intervention reliably expected to have its usually intended anatomic or physiologic effect, but the patient is reliably not expected to survive the current admission and not to recover the ability to interact with the environment before death occurs?	If this is the patient's prognosis even with intervention, then the physician should not offer it and should recommend against it, explaining that intervention in such circumstances will only prolong the patient's dying process and not benefit the patient by restoring interactive capacity before death occurs. This is known as imminent-demise futility.
Is the intervention reliably expected to have some minimal clinical benefit, defined as maintaining some minimal level of ability to interact with the environment and thus grow and develop as a human being? Is the patient in a persistent or permanent vegetative state?	If, in reliable beneficence-based clinical judgment, it is not expected to do so, then the physician should not offer the intervention and should recommend against it. This approach respects patients or surrogate decision makers who are vitalists (those who value the preservation of life at any cost). The physician should explain that preserving life at all costs is not a value in medical ethics and never has been. Moreover, the intervention in question, whether it is initiated or continued, will just sustain a false hope of recovery. This is known as clinical or overall futility.
What if agreement cannot be reached?	If the patient or the patient's surrogate persists in the demand, then the clinician should consult with colleagues and then the Ethics Committee, which should have a clear policy on responding to demands by patients or their surrogates for futile intervention.

perspective on the pregnant woman's health-related interests, which provides the basis for the physician's and nurse's shared beneficence-based obligations to her. The other is the patient's own perspective on those interests, which provides the basis for the autonomy-based obligations of the physician and nurse to her. In contrast, because of an insufficiently developed central nervous system, the fetus cannot meaningfully be said to possess values and beliefs. Thus, there is no basis for saying that a fetus has a perspective on its interests. There can therefore be no autonomy-based obligations to any fetus. Hence, the language of fetal rights has no meaning and therefore no application to the fetus in obstetric clinical judgment and practice, despite its popularity in public and political discourse in the United States and other countries. Obviously, the physician and nurse have a perspective on the fetus's health-related interests, and the physician can have beneficence-based obligations to the fetus, *but only when the fetus is a patient*. Because of its importance for obstetric clinical judgment and practice, the ethical concept of the fetus as a patient requires detailed consideration.[4]

The Ethical Concept of the Fetus as a Patient

The ethical concept of the fetus as a patient is essential to obstetric clinical judgment and practice. Developments in fetal diagnosis and management strategies to optimize fetal outcome have become widely accepted. This has considerable clinical significance because, when the fetus is a patient, directive counseling (recommending a form of management for fetal benefit) is appropriate. Conversely, when the fetus is not a patient, nondirective counseling (offering but not recommending a form of management for fetal benefit) is appropriate. However, there can be uncertainty about when the fetus is a patient. One approach to resolving this uncertainty is to argue that the fetus is or is not a patient in virtue of personhood, or some other form of independent moral status. Unfortunately, this approach often fails to resolve the uncertainty, and alternative thinking may be necessary.

The Independent Moral Status of the Fetus
One prominent approach for establishing whether or not the fetus is a patient has involved attempts to show

whether or not the fetus has independent moral status. This means that one or more characteristics that the fetus possesses, in and of itself, exist independent of the pregnant woman or any other factor. This would generate obligations to the fetus on the part of the pregnant woman and her clinicians. Many fetal characteristics have been nominated for this role, including moment of conception, implantation, central nervous system development, quickening, and the moment of birth. It should come as no surprise that there is considerable variation among ethical arguments about when the fetus acquires independent moral status. Some take the view that the fetus has independent moral status from the moment of conception or implantation. Others believe that independent moral status is acquired in degrees, thus resulting in "graded" moral status. Still others hold, at least by implication, that the fetus never has independent moral status as long as it is *in utero*.[22,23]

Despite an ever-expanding theological and philosophical literature on this subject, there has been no closure on a single authoritative account of the independent moral status of the fetus. For closure ever to be possible, debates about issues such as final authority within and between theological and philosophical traditions would have to be resolved in a way satisfactory to all, an inconceivable intellectual and cultural event. If it cannot be considered feasible to understand the ethical concept of the fetus as a patient in terms of independent moral status, an alternative approach may be adopted that does make it possible to identify ethically distinct senses of the fetus as a patient and their clinical implications for directive and nondirective counseling.

The Dependent Moral Status of the Fetus

A second sense of the concept of the fetus as a patient begins with the recognition that being a patient does not require that one possess independent moral status. Rather, being a patient means that one can benefit from the applications of the clinical skills of the physician or nurse. Put more precisely, a human being without independent moral status is properly regarded as a patient when two conditions are met: that 1) a human being is presented to a health care professional, and 2) there exist clinical interventions that are reliably expected to be efficacious. That is, they are reliably expected to result in a greater balance of clinical benefits over harms for the human being in question.[24] This is the sense in which the ethical concept of the fetus as a patient should be understood, the dependent moral status of the fetus.

Beneficence-based obligations to the fetus exist when the fetus is reliably expected *later* to achieve independent moral status as a child and person.[4] That is, the fetus is a patient when the fetus is presented for medical interventions, whether diagnostic or therapeutic,

that reasonably can be expected to result in a greater balance of benefits over harms for the child and person the fetus can *later* become during early childhood. The ethical significance of the concept of the fetus as a patient, therefore, depends on links that can be established between the fetus and its later achieving independent moral status.

The Viable Fetal Patient.

One such link is viability. Viability, however, must be understood in terms of both biological and technological factors. It is only by virtue of both factors that a viable fetus can exist *ex utero* and thus achieve independent moral status. A viable fetus is of sufficient maturity to survive into the neonatal period, given the availability of the requisite technological support.

Viability exists as a function of biomedical and technological capacities, which vary in different parts of the world. As a consequence, there is, at the present time, no worldwide, uniform gestational age to define viability. In the United States, we believe viability presently occurs at approximately 24 weeks of gestational age.[25,26] For infants born between 23(0/7) and 24(6/7) weeks' gestation and with a birth weight of 500 to 599 g, survival and outcome are extremely uncertain. For these infants born in the so-called "gray zone" of infant viability, the line between patient autonomy and medical futility is blurred, and medical decision-making becomes even more complex and needs to embrace careful consideration of several factors. These factors include appraisal of prenatal data and the information obtained during consultations with the parents before delivery; evaluation of the patient's gestational age, birth weight, and clinical condition upon delivery; ongoing reassessment of the patient's response to resuscitation and intensive care; and continued involvement of the parents in the decision-making process after delivery.

When the fetus is a patient, directive counseling for fetal benefit is ethically justified and must take account of the presence and severity of fetal anomalies, extreme prematurity, and obligations to the pregnant woman. In clinical practice, directive counseling for fetal benefit involves one or more of the following:

- recommending against termination of pregnancy
- recommending against nonaggressive management
- recommending aggressive management.

Aggressive obstetric management includes interventions such as fetal surveillance, tocolysis, operative delivery, or delivery in a tertiary care center when indicated. Nonaggressive obstetric management excludes such interventions. It is very important to appreciate in obstetric clinical judgment and practice that the strength of directive counseling for fetal benefit varies according to the presence and severity of anomalies. As a rule, the more severe the fetal anomaly, the less directive counseling should be for fetal benefit. In particular, when lethal anomalies such as anencephaly can be diagnosed with certainty, there are no beneficence-based obligations to provide aggressive management. Such fetuses are dying patients, and the counseling, therefore, should be nondirective in recommending between nonaggressive management and termination of pregnancy, but directive in recommending against aggressive management for the sake of maternal benefit.[27] By contrast, third trimester abortion for Down syndrome, or achondroplasia, is not ethically justifiable, because the future child with high probability will have the capacity to grow and develop as a human being.[28,29]

Directive counseling for fetal benefit in cases of extreme prematurity of viable fetuses is appropriate. In particular, "just-viable" fetuses can be defined as those with a gestational age of 24 to 26 weeks, for whom there are significant rates of survival but high rates of mortality and morbidity. These rates of morbidity and mortality can be increased by nonaggressive obstetric management, whereas aggressive obstetric management may favorably influence outcomes. Thus, it appears that there are substantial beneficence-based obligations to just-viable fetuses to provide aggressive obstetric management. This is all the more the case in pregnancies beyond 26 weeks of gestational age. Therefore, directive counseling for fetal benefit is justified in all cases of extreme prematurity of viable fetuses, considered by itself. Of course, such directive counseling is appropriate only when it is based on documented efficacy of aggressive obstetric management for each fetal indication. For example, such efficacy has not been demonstrated for routine Cesarean delivery to manage extreme prematurity.

Any directive counseling for fetal benefit must occur in the context of balancing beneficence-based obligations to the fetus against beneficence-based and autonomy-based obligations to the pregnant woman. Any such balancing must recognize that a pregnant woman is obligated only to take reasonable risks of medical interventions that are reliably expected to benefit the viable fetus or child later. A unique feature of obstetric ethics is that the pregnant woman's autonomy influences how a viable fetus ought to be regarded in the context of the individual clinical presentation.

Obviously, any strategy for directive counseling for fetal benefit that takes account of obligations to the pregnant woman must be open to the possibility of conflict between recommendations by the physician or nurse and a pregnant woman's autonomous decision to the contrary. Such conflict is best managed preventively through the informed consent process as an ongoing dialogue throughout a woman's pregnancy, augmented as necessary by negotiation and respectful persuasion.[30]

The Previable Fetal Patient. The only possible link between the previable fetus and the child it can become is the pregnant woman's autonomy. This is because technological factors cannot result in the previable fetus becoming a child. The link, therefore, between a previable fetus and the child it can become can be established only by the pregnant woman's decision to confer the status of it being a patient. The previable fetus, therefore, has no claim to the status of being a patient independent of the pregnant woman's autonomy. The pregnant woman is free to withhold, confer, or, having once conferred, withdraw the status of being a patient on or from her previable fetus according to her own values and beliefs. The previable fetus is presented to the physician as a function of the pregnant woman's autonomy.[4]

Counseling the pregnant woman regarding the management of her pregnancy when the fetus is previable should be nondirective in terms of continuing the pregnancy or having an abortion if she refuses to confer the status of being a patient on her fetus. In contrast, if she does confer such status, at that point beneficence-based obligations to her previable fetus come into existence, and directive counseling for fetal benefit becomes appropriate. Just as for viable fetuses, such counseling must take account of the presence and severity of fetal anomalies, extreme prematurity, and obligations owed to the pregnant woman.

For pregnancies in which the woman is uncertain about whether to confer such status, it is proposed that the fetus be provisionally regarded as a patient. This justifies directive counseling against behavior that can harm a fetus in significant and irreversible ways (e.g., substance abuse, such as alcohol) until the woman settles on whether to confer the status of patient on the fetus.

In particular, nondirective counseling is appropriate in cases of what can be termed "near-viable" fetuses, that is, those that are 23 weeks of gestational age.[25,26,31] In these instances, aggressive obstetric and neonatal management should be regarded as clinical investigation (i.e., a form of medical experimentation), not a standard of care. There is no obligation on the part of a pregnant woman to confer the status of patient on a near-viable fetus, because the efficacy of aggressive obstetric and neonatal management has yet to be proven.[26]

THREE CONCEPTS OF JUSTICE

Ethical concerns about justice arise when resources are scarce. Justice directs a sense of fairness to all and requires that, in the distribution of resources, each should receive what is due to him or her. Different concepts of justice define "due" in different ways. Each strives to result in a fair distribution of benefits for all.

Utilitarianism

Utilitarianism is a theory of justice that makes central the obligation to produce the greatest good for the greatest number in the management of scarce resources. To be successful in guiding practical, day-to-day decisions about the allocation of resources, utilitarianism requires an account of the greatest good. For society overall, it has been difficult, if not impossible, to define what the greatest good is. For medicine in particular, the issue of how scarce and expensive medical resources are distributed has challenged the profession for decades. For example, some critics argue that too much money is being spent in trying to save infants who are not likely to gain sufficient benefits and may have extremely bad outcomes.[32] The value of utilitarianism is the balance it seeks to achieve among benefits and burdens of scarce resources, so that inequalities do not become inequities (i.e., unfair). Critics of utilitarianism have pointed out that sometimes utilitarianism results in inequities (i.e., shared distributions of benefits and burdens).[14]

Libertarianism

Another concept of justice, libertarianism, has been developed to address this problem. Libertarians argue that in a market that places different values on different services and products, and in which there is an equal opportunity to develop one's talents, those who provide more highly valued services rightly earn more than those who provide less valued (although not necessarily less intrinsically valuable) services. Thus, libertarian theories emphasize fairness of process, rather than equality of outcomes.

Egalitarianism

The third concept of justice is egalitarian. This concept was developed to protect vulnerable and disadvantaged members of society, who may lose out in a utilitarian distribution of scarce resources. This concept of justice corrects for unfair outcomes in the form of undue burdens on those least able to protect themselves.

These three and other concepts of justice remain in unresolved competition.[33] It is fair to say that the medical ethics literature is strongly influenced by a concept of justice that calls for fair equality of opportunity (an element of libertarian justice) and protection of the least well off (an element of egalitarian justice). However, it is also fair to say that no single concept of justice shapes health care policy in the United States. This lack of a conceptually coherent health care policy is a long-standing feature of American health care policy. In particular, the United States has yet to create a universal right to health care, although there are selective entitlements (e.g., for the elderly [Medicare], the medically indigent [Medicaid], and qualified veterans).

RESPONSIBLE RESOURCE MANAGEMENT AND PROFESSIONAL VIRTUES

The practice of obstetrics is coming under increasingly powerful economic constraints, particularly by managed care and resource-management strategies imposed by hospital managers and used by private and public payers and by health care organizations to control the cost of medical care. Two main business tools are used to achieve this goal: 1) creating conflicts of interest in how physicians are compensated, diplomatically called "sharing economic risk," and 2) increasingly strict control of clinical judgment and practice through such means as practice guidelines, critical pathways, physician report cards, and retrospective chart review. These business tools generate ethical challenges to obstetrician-gynecologists and obstetric nursing professionals that seriously threaten the virtues that define the fiduciary character of medicine and nursing as professions.[34]

In medicine and nursing, the physician-fiduciary or nurse-fiduciary is expected, as a matter of routine and habit, to fulfill obligations to protect and promote patients' interests rather than pursue their own personal interests. Professional virtues are those traits and habits of character that routinely focus the concern and behavior of an individual on the interests of others, and thereby habitually blunt the motivation to act on self-interest. There are four virtues that constitute the clinician-patient relationship based on the concept of clinician as fiduciary.[4]

Self-Effacement

The first virtue, self-effacement, requires the physician and nurse to blunt self-interest and focus concerns on the interests of the patient. It negates the adverse impact of discrepancies in clinicians' and patients' behaviors, demography, or morals. Self-effacement prevents biases and prejudices arising from these differences that could have an adverse impact on the plan of care for the patient.

Self-Sacrifice

The second virtue, self-sacrifice, speaks to the demanding part of the work of physicians and nurses to sacrifice time, energy, and personal obligations and accept reasonable risks to themselves. As one example, clinicians manifest this virtue in their willingness to care for patients with infectious diseases such as hepatitis, HIV infection, and tuberculosis, all of which pose a potential threat to the clinician's personal health. Irrespective of the financial model for professional compensation, this virtue of self-sacrifice obligates physicians and nurses to turn away from economic self-interest and focus on the patient's need for relief when the two are in conflict.

Compassion

Another virtue, compassion, motivates the physician and nurse to recognize and seek to alleviate the stress, discomfort, pain, and suffering associated with a patient's disease or illness or its outcome. Compassion sustains the moral relationship with the patient that is initiated with self-effacement and self-sacrifice. Its components are silent empathy (e.g., purposeful silence when a patient shares her pain with the clinician), expressive compassion (e.g., "I am so sorry that your baby died."), and helping the patient find a new identity in the suffering by making sense of it in her own right (e.g., "Why do *you* think your baby died?").

Integrity

The aforementioned response is strengthened by the fourth virtue, integrity. This virtue imposes an intellectual discipline on clinical judgments made by the physician and nurse about the patient's problems and how to address them. Integrity includes a life-long commitment to excellence in the care of patients via well-formed clinical judgment. Clinical judgment is rigorous when it is based on the best available scientific information or, when such information is lacking, on consensus clinical judgment. Thus, integrity is an antidote to the pitfalls of bias, subjective clinical impressions, and unexamined clinical "common sense" that can undermine evidence-based practice. Integrity provides the basis for the clinician's ethical response to the business tool of control of clinical judgment and practice.

The task of medical ethics is to identify both the application and the limits of these four virtues. The concept of legitimate self-interest provides the basis for these limits. Legitimate self-interest includes protecting the conditions for practicing medicine well, fulfilling obligations to persons in the clinician's life other than the patient, and protecting activities outside clinical practice that the clinician finds deeply fulfilling.

RESOURCE MANAGEMENT: THE CLINICIAN AS FIDUCIARY

Fee-for-service unconstrained by fiduciary obligations could and has led to harm to patients from nonindicated over-utilization of resources. It is a violation of the standard of care to subject patients to unnecessary active intervention in order to achieve personal economic gain.

On the other hand, resource management unconstrained by fiduciary obligations puts patients at risk of harm by denying access to the standard of care. This will occur if patients are subjected to unnecessary risk from withholding appropriate care and intervention in order to reduce cost.[34,35]

Financial incentives to the clinician and supervision of clinician decision-making that strictly controls utilization of services are the business tools used by managed care. Forms of payment by managed care organizations, such as capitation and withhold, deliberately impose an economic conflict of interest on the physician.[36] Every time the physician uses a resource (consultation, diagnostic testing, surgical procedures, and so on), the physician pays an economic penalty. The ethical challenge occurs when the patient's interests are subordinated to the pursuit of financial rewards and thereby harmed by this underutilization.

The virtue of self-sacrifice prohibits the physician from making the avoidance of such financial risk the *primary* consideration. Avoiding financial risk as one's primary consideration involves an ethically pathological process that leads naturally and quickly to the abandonment of self-effacement (economically driven managed care for some patients but not for others), compassion (patients' health-related concerns do not matter but are only a means to maximize revenues), and integrity (the standard of care is sacrificed to maximize revenues). Importantly, clinicians are not sanctioned by society to engage in the destruction of medicine as a fiduciary profession.

Physicians should not assume that managed care organizations and other payers are unwilling to negotiate contracts to reduce the severity of economic conflicts of interest. Physicians should therefore make a good faith effort to negotiate these matters. If the organization refuses to negotiate, and the economic risk of not signing the contract is very significant, then the physician should voluntarily accept the ethical responsibility to be alert to and manage these conflicts of interest well. First, integrity requires that the physician avoid the self-deception of underestimating potential influence on clinical judgment and practice by the conflict of interest. Second, once these contracts are signed, the virtues add an important dimension to total quality management: diligent monitoring of conflicts of interest to prevent them from resulting in substandard care should be among the physician's "accountabilities." Third, the realities of managed care mean that, for the near term at least, increasing financial sacrifice may be required to protect the integrity of medicine as a fiduciary profession. Fourth, in group practice, there should be a fair sharing of economic self-sacrifice. In particular, individual efforts to tune the system to one's economic advantage in a group (for example, avoiding the care of high-risk pregnancies), and to the disadvantage of colleagues should be avoided.

The second business tool of managed care, increasingly strict control of clinical judgment and practice, is a heterogeneous phenomenon. Some managed care organizations are poorly capitalized and poorly managed. They compete by price, with little or no attention given to the quality of their services. A "bottom line" mentality dominates, with economic savings and net revenue maximization the overriding values. These poorly managed companies have little or no understanding of or interest in the fiduciary nature of medicine, and so their controls of clinical judgment and practice are driven almost entirely by economic considerations.

Physicians and other health care practitioners subject to management controls by such companies face the very difficult challenge of trying to get such managed care organizations to constrain their economic interests by their fiduciary obligations, a daunting but not impossible task. The concerns of ethics, especially to protect the integrity of the fiduciary enterprise, may frequently be swept aside when they are not ignored altogether. Nonetheless, physicians and nurses in such organizations are the ultimate bulwark on which patients and society must be able to rely.

A physician-controlled managed care organization provides no immunization against the ethical challenges of the business tools of managed care. Physician-owned provider entities do not provide a solution in and of themselves to the ethical threats of conflict of interest and control of clinical judgment and practice. The virtue-based arguments previously cited will apply to these new entities without exception.

There is no conclusive evidence that preserving medicine and nursing as fiduciary professions is impossible, even given the economic power of managed care organizations, other payers, and hospital managers.[37] Ethics teaches us that business and economic power are not absolute and should always be called to account for their consequences. Society has not given managed care organizations the moral authority or permission to destroy the fiduciary character of medicine and nursing as a consequence of the pursuit of economic interest and power. Nor has society given physicians and nurses moral authority or permission to cooperate willfully with this destruction. Quite the opposite, society counts on physicians and nurses, because ultimately society can count on no one else to preserve and advocate for the fiduciary character of the medical profession.

CRITICALLY APPRAISING THE NORMATIVE ETHICS LITERATURE

Normative ethics uses analyses and argument to discuss the behavior and character required of clinicians in an ethically appropriate practice of obstetrics and gynecology. Normative ethics differs from descriptive ethics, which uses qualitative and quantitative research to describe clinicians' behavior and attitudes, an important point of departure for normative ethics.[9] There is a four-step approach to evidence-based medicine that is applicable to that of argument-based medical ethics. These are: (a) asking a focused question, (b) making a valid argument, (c) identifying the results of arguments, and (d) bringing the results of argument to clinical practice.[9]

Does the Argument Address a Focused Ethics Question?

A focused question may address a number of possible domains, including:

- theoretical issues, such as whether the fetus is a patient or a person;
- clinical issues for a specific patient population, such as the management of cancer during pregnancy;
- research issues for a specific population, such as surgical management of fetal spina bifida;
- organizational culture issues, such as quality improvement and cost control; and
- public policy issues, such as partial-birth abortion.

The ethical significance of the focused question should be explained. Its significance can be theoretical as well as clinical. The target perspective of the issue can be clinicians, scientific investigators, patients, patient's families and other support networks, payers, health care organization leadership, and scholars and public officials concerned with health policy. The relevance of this consideration is that the target audience for the use of the results of the argument should be clear.

Are the Results of the Argument Valid?

The validity of the result in an ethics argument has two parts: assembling a reliable and comprehensive account of the facts of the matter, and identifying and clarifying concepts relevant to evaluating the ethical implications of this information.

Arguments organize these concepts into a coherent set of reasons that together support a conclusion for how one should or should not act. Reasons in arguments are expressed in terms of appeals to one or more general ethical frameworks.[38]

DeGrazia and Beauchamp have identified and critically assessed five basic appeals.[39] The first appeal is to tradition and practice standards, the quality of which is a function of the ethical analysis and argument that support traditional beliefs and current practice standards. The second appeal is to ethical principles, such as respect for autonomy, beneficence, nonmalficence, and justice.[6] When these principles are "specified" (i.e., clarified in their relationship to clinical reality), they provide compelling action guides. The third appeal is general ethical theory, of which there are two types predominant in the argument-based medical ethics literature: consequentialism (the justification of a course of action depends on whether consequences of the right sort result from it) and deontological approaches (the justification of a course of action is grounded in considerations other than consequences). The fourth appeal is casuistry, which involves appeal to relevantly similar cases and applying the reasoning about these paradigm cases to the case at hand. The fifth appeal is to what is called "reflective equilibrium," which starts with considered judgments (those most likely to be free of bias) and explores their joint implications for the principles that should together guide decision making and behavior. A sixth appeal can be virtue based. This involves traits of character that clinicians should cultivate as fiduciary professionals responsible for the care of patients and the management of health care organizations.[1]

Some appeals are not acceptable in argument-based ethics. Sulmasy and Sugarman provide a useful account of these mistaken forms of reasoning in argument-based ethics.[40]

First, historical practices do not by themselves justify conclusions. That something has been done or not done in the past (e.g., abortion) even if commonly done or prohibited, does not by itself justify continuing to do it or prohibiting it. Second, majority opinions do not entail argument-based opinions, including majority opinions reported in well-designed surveys. The results of such studies provide important starting points for ethical analysis and argument but are no substitute for them. Third, the fact that something is permitted by law does not make it ethically permissible. The law is an important starting point for ethical analysis and argument, but should not be taken uncritically as the final word. The abortion controversy amply illustrates this point.

Fourth, the opinions of experts do not in and of themselves count as the conclusions of well-reasoned arguments. Argument-based ethics arguments and books should not be judged solely on the basis of their source (an individual physician, a clinical colleague, a research group, or a professional association) no matter how prominent and accomplished.[41] Instead, these works should be held to standards of intellectual rigor that are in their own way as demanding as those of evidence-based medicine and other standards for evaluating the medical and scientific literature. Fifth, the fact that something is biologically true does not by itself establish well-reasoned conclusions. It is an error to think that ethics can simply be derived from human biology.

Finally, it is often said that there is no right or wrong answer in ethics. This is a disservice to clinicians turning to the argument-based medical ethics literature. There are well argued and poorly argued positions, and they can be reliably distinguished. The latter appeal to gut feelings, unexamined common sense, free-floating intuition, and unsystematic clinical ethical judgment and decision-making. This is in contrast to judgment and decision-making that meet standards of careful reflection and argument (the hallmarks of argument-based medical ethics). Much of the current "pro-life" versus "pro-choice" public discourse about the ethics and public policy of abortion suffers from this shortcoming.

The literature of argument-based ethics in obstetrics and gynecology, as in many other specialties, is now very large, making it highly unlikely that there is no relevant literature to consider. Relevant literature should be cited and analyses and arguments from this literature should be presented clearly and accurately. In the basic and clinical science literature, investigators are increasingly expected to elucidate the search strategies, including key words, databases, bibliographies, and other sources used. This same standard should begin to be met by the argument-based ethics literature.

In preventing readers' bias, it is helpful to identify the disciplines represented among the authors.[41] The argument-based medical ethics literature is distinctive in that work of high quality by non-clinicians should influence the clinical judgment and decision making of clinicians, just as work on infectious diseases of the reproductive tract by microbiologists or on the pharmacokinetics of gynecologic cancer chemotherapy by pharmacologists rightly influences clinical judgment and practice. Argument-based ethics scholarship therefore should not be dismissed when only some or even none of the authors are clinicians.

At the same time, the reader should beware of positive or negative bias toward an argument, based on the reputation of the author(s) or of the journal. Just as in the basic and clinical sciences, the standing of authors and journals in obstetrics and gynecology or in the field of bioethics is no guarantee of quality in argument-based medical ethics.

What are the Results of the Argument?

The results of argument-based ethics are the conclusions of ethical analysis and argument. As emphasized, they should be clearly stated and easy to find in the argument.

How Should the Clinician Apply the Results In Clinical Practice?

The results of argument-based medical ethics can be helpful in at least three ways. First, they may have important practical implications, especially if the results incorporate evidence to support the clinical utility of acting on the conclusions of the paper. Second, they may have important theoretical implications which do not depend on whether an intervention was performed and evaluated. Identifying such theoretical implications results in critical assessment and revision of ethical frameworks and appeals based on them. Finally, readers of the normative ethics literature of obstetrics and gynecology should ask themselves how they should change their thinking (clinical judgment and reasoning), attitudes (toward patients, their families, and legal institutions), clinical practice, or organizational culture. This is a crucial step in the method of evidence-based reasoning and therefore in the methods of argument-based ethics, because the fourth step relates directly to improving the quality of patient care, teaching, research, and organizational culture.

SUMMARY

This chapter provides a comprehensive discussion and ethical framework for high-risk and critical care obstetric clinical judgment and practice. Professionalism can be defined in part by practicing with ethical competence and also being accountable for the ethical conduct of one's work. Both are critical factors in creating and sustaining the clinician–patient relationship. This framework emphasizes preventive ethics (i.e., an appreciation that the potential for ethical conflict is inherent in clinical practice), and the use of such clinical tools as informed consent and negotiation to minimize such conflict from occurring. This framework comprehensively appeals to the ethical principles of beneficence, respect for autonomy and justice, and the professional virtues of self-effacement, self-sacrifice, compassion, and integrity. Finally, this framework can be used to critically evaluate the literature of ethics in obstetrics.

REFERENCES

1. American College of Obstetricians and Gynecologists. (2004). *Ethics in obstetrics and gynecology* (2nd ed.). Washington, DC: Author.
2. Association of Professors of Gynecology and Obstetrics. (1994). *Exploring medical-legal issues in obstetrics and gynecology.* Washington, DC: APGO Medical Education Foundation.
3. FIGO Committee for the Study of Ethical Aspects of Human Reproduction. (1997). *Recommendations of ethical issues in obstetrics and gynecology.* London: International Federation of Gynecology and Obstetrics.
4. McCullough, L. B., & Chervenak, F. A. (Eds.). (1994). *Ethics in obstetrics and gynecology.* New York: Oxford University Press.
5. Engelhardt, H. T., Jr. (1995). *The foundations of bioethics* (2nd ed.). New York: Oxford University Press.
6. Beauchamp, T. L., & Childress, J. F. (2008). *Principles of biomedical ethics* (6th ed.). New York: Oxford University Press.

7. Chervenak, F. A., & McCullough, L. B. (1996). An ethically justified algorithm for offering, recommending, and performing cesarean delivery and its application in managed care practice. *Obstetrics & Gynecology, 87,* 302–305.
8. Hippocrates. (1976). Oath of hippocrates. In O. Temkin & C. L. Temkin (Eds.), *Ancient medicine: Selected papers of Ludwig Edelstein.* Baltimore: Johns Hopkins University Press.
9. McCullough, L. B., Coverdale, J. H., & Chervenak, F. A. (2004). Argument-based medical ethics: A formal tool for critically appraising the normative medical ethics literature. *American Journal Obstetrics Gynecology, 191,* 1097–1102.
10. Faden, R. R., & Beauchamp, T. L. (1986). *A history and theory of informed consent.* New York: Oxford University Press.
11. Brody, H., & Bonham, V. L., Jr. (1997). Gag rules and trade secrets in managed care contracts: Ethical and legal concerns. *Archives of Internal Medicine, 157,* 2037–2043.
12. Wear, S. (1998). *Informed consent: Patient autonomy and clinician beneficence within health care* (2nd ed.). Washington, DC: Georgetown University Press.
13. *Schloendorff v. The Society of the New York Hospital,* (1914) 211 N.Y. 125, 126, 105 N.E. 92, 93.
14. Post, S. G. (2003). *Encyclopedia of bioethics* (3rd ed.). New York: Macmillan Reference.
15. *In re Quinlan,* 355 A.2d 647 (N.J. 1976), *cert. denied sub nom.*
16. Meisel, A., & Cerminara, K. L. (2004). *The right to die: The law of end-of-life decision making* (3rd ed.). New York: Aspen Publishers.
17. SUPPORT Investigators. (1995). A controlled trial to improve care for seriously ill hospitalized patients. *JAMA, 274,* 1591–1598.
18. Braun, U. K., Beyth, R. J., Ford, M. E., & McCullough, L. B. (2008). Voices of African American, Caucasian, and Hispanic surrogates on the burdens of end-of-life decision making. *Journal of General Internal Medicine, 23*(3), 267–274.
19. *Truman v. Thomas,* 611 P.2d 902 (Cal. 1980).
20. Brett, A., & McCullough, L. B. (1986). When patients request specific interventions: Defining the limits of the physician's obligations. *The New England Journal of Medicine, 315,* 1347–1351.
21. Rabeneck, L., McCullough, L. B., & Wray, N. P. (1997). Ethically justified, clinical comprehensive guidelines for percutaneous endoscopic gastrostomy tube placement. *Lancet, 349,* 496–498.
22. Callahan, S., & Callahan, D. (Eds.). (1984). *Abortion: Understanding differences.* New York: Plenum Press.
23. Annas, G. J. (1987). Protecting the liberty of pregnant patients. *The New England Journal of Medicine, 316,* 1213–1214.
24. Chervenak, F. A., & McCullough, L. B. (1997). Ethics in obstetrics and gynecology: An overview. *European Journal of Obstetrics & Gynecology and Reproductive Medicine, 75,* 91–94.
25. Chervenak, F. A., & McCullough, L. B. (1997). The limits of viability. *Journal of Perinatal Medicine, 25,* 418–420.
26. Chervenak, F. A., McCullough, L. B., & Levene, M. I. (2007). An ethically justified clinically comprehensive approach to peri-viability: Gynaecological, obstetric, perinatal, and neonatal dimensions. *The Journal of Obstetrics & Gynaecology, 27,* 3–7.
27. Chervenak, F. A., & McCullough, L. B. (1990). An ethically justified, clinically comprehensive management strategy for third-trimester pregnancies complicated by fetal anomalies. *Obstetrics & Gynecology, 75,* 311–316.

28. Chervenak, F. A., McCullough, L. B., & Campbell, S. (1995). Is third trimester abortion justified? *British Journal of Obstetrics and Gynaecology, 102,* 434–435.

29. Chervenak, F. A., McCullough, L. B., & Campbell, S. (1999). Third trimester abortion: Is compassion enough? *British Journal of Obstetrics and Gynaecology, 106,* 293–296.

30. Chervenak, F. A., & McCullough, L. B. (1990). Clinical guides to preventing ethical conflicts between pregnant women and their physicians. *American Journal of Obstetrics & Gynecology, 162,* 303–307.

31. Lucey, J. F., Rowan, C. A., Shiono, P., Wilkinson, A. R., Kilpatrick, S., Payne N. R., et al. (2004). Fetal infants: The fate of 4172 infants with birth weights of 401 to 500 grams—the Vermont Oxford Network experience (1996–2000). *Pediatrics, 113*(6), 1559–1566.

32. Wilder, M. A. (2000). Ethical issues in the delivery room: Resuscitation of extremely low birth weight infants. *The Journal of Perinatal & Neonatal Nursing, 14,* 44–56.

33. Chervenak, F. A., & McCullough, L. B. (2002). Professionalism and justice in the leadership of academic medical centers. *Academic Medicine, 77,* 45–47.

34. Chervenak, F. A., McCullough, L. B., & Chez, R. (1996). Responding to the ethical challenges posed by the business tools of managed care in the practice of obstetrics and gynecology. *American Journal of Obstetrics and Gynecology, 175,* 524–527.

35. Council on Ethical and Judicial Affairs of the American Medical Association. (1995). Ethical issues in managed care. *JAMA, 273*(4), 330–335.

36. Spece, R. G., Shimm, D. S., & Buchanan, A. E. (Eds.). (1996). *Conflicts of interest in clinical practice and research.* New York: Oxford University Press.

37. Chervenak, F. A., & McCullough, L. B. (2003). Physicians and hospital managers as cofiduciaries of patients: Rhetoric or reality. *Journal of Healthcare Management, 48,* 173–179.

38. Brody, B. A. (1988). *Life and death decision making.* New York: Oxford University Press.

39. DeGrazia, D., & Beauchamp, T. L. (2010). Philosophy. In J. Sugarman & D. P. Sulmasy (Eds.), *Methods in medical ethics.* Washington, DC: Georgetown University Press.

40. Sulmasy, D. P., & Sugarman, J. (2010). The many methods of medical ethics (or thirteen ways of looking at a blackbird). In J. Sugarman & D. P. Sulmasy (Eds.), *Methods in medical ethics.* Washington, DC: Georgetown University Press.

41. Owen, R. (1982). Reader bias. *JAMA, 247,* 2533–2534.

PART II

Clinical Practice Adjuncts

CHAPTER 4

Invasive Hemodynamic and Oxygen Transport Monitoring During Pregnancy

Nan H. Troiano and Sreedhar Gaddipati

Invasive hemodynamic monitoring is a significant adjunct often used in the care of critically ill patients. Data obtained from this process may enhance the ability of critical care clinicians to assess a patient's hemodynamic and oxygen transport status, formulate diagnoses, develop and implement appropriate plans of care, and evaluate patient responses over time.

Since its introduction into clinical practice over three decades ago, the flow-directed balloon-tipped pulmonary artery (PA) catheter has played an integral role in the management of critically ill patients in a number of specialties, including obstetrics.[1–5] Intra-arterial catheters and PA catheters represent the two fundamental modalities for invasive hemodynamic assessment. This chapter reviews the fundamental principles related to invasive central hemodynamic and oxygen transport monitoring during pregnancy. Clinical case excerpts are presented to reinforce select principles regarding interpretation of data. More thorough discussion of clinical applications of these principles as they relate to the care of patients with specific obstetric complications is presented elsewhere in this text.

CARDIAC ANATOMY AND PHYSIOLOGY

Delivery of adequate oxygen, nutrients, and other vital substances in the blood to tissues is necessary for cellular function that sustains life. The role of the cardiovascular system is to pump these substances through the vascular bed by contraction of the heart. Normal cardiac anatomy is depicted in Figure 4-1.

Atria are low-pressure chambers that serve as reservoirs of blood for the ventricles. The right atrium receives venous blood via the superior and inferior vena cavae and coronary sinus from the systemic bed.

The left atrium receives oxygenated blood returning to the heart from the pulmonary bed via the four pulmonary veins. Approximately 70 to 80 percent of blood flows passively from the atria to the ventricles during early ventricular diastole, known as protodiastole. During the later phase, the atria contract and pump an additional 20 to 30 percent of blood into the ventricles. Loss of atrial systole, also referred to as *atrial kick*, in an otherwise normal heart usually has only minimal effect. However, in a patient with impaired left ventricular filling, left atrial systole is very important and may account for more than 50 percent of left ventricular filling.

The ventricles provide the force necessary to circulate blood through the lungs and the rest of the body. The right ventricle pumps deoxygenated blood into the pulmonary circulation via the pulmonary artery. The left ventricle, much thicker than the right, pumps oxygenated blood into the systemic circulation via the aorta. The left side of the heart functions as a higher pressure system than the right side. Under normal circumstances, the right ventricle ejects approximately 50 to 60 percent of its end-diastolic volume with each cardiac contraction, whereas the left ventricle ejects 60 to 70 percent.

Atrioventricular valves consist of the tricuspid valve on the right and mitral valve on the left. During diastole, valve leaflets open, which allows unidirectional blood flow into the respective ventricle. As ventricular pressure increases during systole, valve leaflets close, which prevents retrograde flow. Semilunar valves consist of the pulmonic valve on the right and aortic valve on the left. Open during ventricular systole, each of these valves allows unidirectional blood flow to the respective arterial outflow tract. Following systole, as arterial pressures increase, each valve closes to prevent retrograde flow during diastole.

FIGURE 4-1 Normal cardiac anatomy.

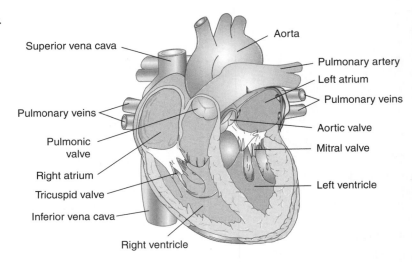

DETERMINANTS OF CARDIAC OUTPUT

Cardiac output is the amount of blood ejected from the heart per unit of time. It is determined by four variables: preload, afterload, contractility, and heart rate.

Preload

Preload refers to the tension or load on a muscle as it begins to contract. In the context of the cardiovascular system, preload is the length of the ventricular muscle fiber at end-diastole. The principal factor that determines muscle fiber length is the volume of blood in the ventricles at the point of maximal filling. Therefore, ventricular end-diastolic volume (EDV) is used as a reflection of preload for the intact heart. The pressure-volume curves in Figure 4-2 depict the influence of preload on the mechanical performance of the left ventricle during diastole (*lower curves*) and systole (*upper curves*). The solid lines on the curves represent the normal pressure-volume relationships during diastole and systole. Note that the uppermost curve in the figure has a rapid ascent, which indicates that small changes in EDV are associated with large changes in systolic pressure. For this reason, the most effective measure for preserving adequate cardiac output is to maintain an adequate EDV.

The intrinsic ability of the heart to adapt to alterations in the volume of blood returning to the heart is commonly known as the Frank-Starling phenomenon. The graph that is most often used to depict this relationship is known as a *ventricular function curve* (Fig. 4-3). Within certain physiologic limits, the more the ventricles are filled with blood during diastole, the greater the quantity of blood that will be ejected during systole.

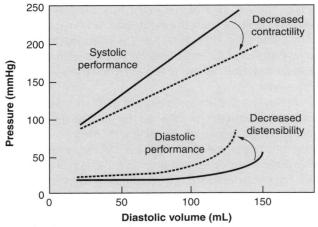

FIGURE 4-2 Pressure–volume curves for the intact ventricle. Solid lines represent normal pressure-volume relationships. Dotted lines represent abnormal pressure-volume relationships.

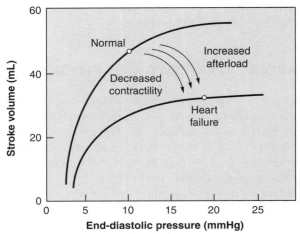

FIGURE 4-3 Ventricular function curve.

Conversely, when the amount of blood returning to the ventricles is diminished, cardiac output may be impaired. For example, this may be evident in the patient with significant blood loss or hypotension who has decreased circulating blood volume or venous return to the heart.

The stretch imposed on cardiac muscle is determined not only by the volume of blood in the ventricular chambers but also by the tendency of the ventricular wall to distend or stretch at a given volume within the chamber. This property is described as the *compliance* of the ventricle. Compliance is determined by the relationship between changes in end-diastolic pressure (EDP) and end-diastolic volume. The lower curve in Figure 4-3 illustrates this concept. As the ventricle becomes less compliant (e.g., in ventricular hypertrophy), there is less change in diastolic volume relative to the change in diastolic pressure. Early in the process, the EDV remains normal, but the EDP increases above normal. As the compliance decreases further, the increase in EDP eventually reduces venous return to the heart, thereby causing a reduction in EDV.[6]

Afterload

Afterload is the resistance or load that opposes ventricular ejection of blood during systole. The right ventricle pumps against pressure or resistance in the pulmonary vasculature, whereas the left ventricle pumps against the higher pressure or resistance in the systemic circulation. In contrast to preload, afterload and cardiac output have an inverse relationship. Within certain physiologic limits, the lower the afterload or resistance applied against the ventricles during systole, the greater the cardiac output. Conversely, patients with clinical conditions such as pulmonary or systemic hypertension, in which pressure in the pulmonary or systemic vessels respectively is increased, are at risk for decreased cardiac output. Forces that contribute to ventricular wall tension or afterload are listed in Box 4-1.

Because afterload is a transmural force, it is influenced by the pleural pressures at the outer surface of

Box 4-1. FORCES THAT CONTRIBUTE TO VENTRICULAR TENSION OR AFTERLOAD

- Transmural wall tension
- Systolic pressure
  - Pleural pressure
  - Outflow impedance
- Chamber radius
  - End-diastolic volume
- Vascular compliance
- Vascular resistance

the heart. Negative pleural pressures increase transmural pressure and increase ventricular afterload, whereas positive pleural pressures have the opposite effect. Negative pressures surrounding the heart may impede ventricular emptying by opposing the inward displacement of the ventricular wall during systole.[7] This action is responsible for the decrease in systolic blood pressure that occurs during the inspiratory phase of spontaneous breathing. Positive pleural pressures can promote ventricular emptying by facilitating the inward displacement of the ventricular wall during systole.

Contractility

Contractility, also known as the inotropic state of the heart, is the intrinsic ability of the heart muscle to shorten or develop tension independent of variations in preload and afterload. Not easily measured in clinical situations, contractility may nonetheless be inferred by a change in cardiac output when afterload and preload remain constant. Under conditions of altered catecholamine production or following administration of medications that alter inotropic response, the Frank–Starling curve shifts upward with a higher cardiac output for a given filling pressure. Conversely, with decreased contractility, the heart pumps less well at a given filling pressure. Thus, patients with compromised heart function at higher pressures under normal conditions have less reserve and are more prone to heart failure when stressed.

Heart Rate

Heart rate affects the strength of myocardial contraction and thus cardiac output. For example, at faster rates, the force of contraction is strong. At slower rates, the force is weaker. This intrinsic property of the heart muscle may be attributable to rate-driven variations in sarcoplasmic calcium concentration. It should be noted that an increased heart rate also results in decreased diastolic filling time and may thereby decrease preload. If continued over a period of time, this may lead to decreased cardiac output. In addition, a pause between heart contractions results in increased force of the next contraction, also known as rest potentiation, which may increase cardiac output. For these reasons, rate-related changes in the force of contraction, preload, and cardiac output interact in a complex manner.

OXYGEN TRANSPORT PHYSIOLOGY

The ability of cells to function normally depends on a continuous supply of adequate oxygen and nutrients. When oxygen transport is impaired, the patient is at increased risk for end-organ dysfunction or failure. Thus, evaluation of oxygen transport is essential in the care of obstetric patients with significant complications or who are critically ill. Key concepts related to oxygen transport include oxygen content, affinity, delivery, and consumption.

Oxygen Content

Oxygen is transported to the tissues in two ways: dissolved under pressure in plasma and bound to hemoglobin in red blood cells. The oxygen dissolved in plasma makes up approximately 1 to 2 percent of the total oxygen content, whereas oxygen bound to hemoglobin makes up the remaining 98 to 99 percent.

The role of hemoglobin in the transport of oxygen is significant. Hemoglobin is composed of four subunits, each consisting of a protein chain with a heme group attached to a histidine residue. One molecule of oxygen is loosely bound with one of the six coordinate valencies of each of the heme iron atoms. Thus, each molecule of hemoglobin is associated with four molecules of oxygen. The kinetics of the association are such that all of the molecules of oxygen bind at the same rate. When a hemoglobin molecule is combined with oxygen, it is called *oxyhemoglobin*. The saturation of hemoglobin with oxygen is the ratio of oxyhemoglobin to the total amount of hemoglobin capable of transporting oxygen (Fig. 4-4).

Although it represents only a small fraction of total oxygen content, oxygen dissolved in plasma plays a crucial role. The ability of oxygen to combine with hemoglobin in the lungs, later to be released at the tissue level, is affected by oxygen in the plasma. This reversible binding of oxygen to hemoglobin is an important concept in oxygen transport and allows for the loading of oxygen in the lungs and unloading at the tissue level.

Oxygen Affinity

Affinity refers to the ability of oxygen to bind to hemoglobin. Both the uptake and the release of oxygen from hemoglobin molecules are represented visually by the oxyhemoglobin dissociation curve, depicted in Figure 4-5.

The curve portrays the relationship between the partial pressure of oxygen (PaO_2) in arterial blood and the saturation of hemoglobin (SaO_2). The sigmoid shape of the normal curve is the result of:

- the increased affinity of hemoglobin for oxygen as more oxygen molecules combine with it, despite large alveolar PO_2 changes (the flat, upper portion of the curve) and
- the rapid unloading of oxygen from hemoglobin, with small changes in PaO_2 (the steep, lower portion of the curve).

The position of the curve is defined more precisely by a reference point known as the P_{50}. This point represents the PaO_2 at which hemoglobin is 50 percent saturated. Under normal conditions in nonpregnant people, the P_{50} is 26.3 mmHg (see Fig. 4-5).

The P_{50} is not fixed in those who are critically ill. If the affinity and P_{50} change, the oxyhemoglobin dissociation curve shifts to the right or left. Conditions known to change oxygen affinity are described in Table 4-1. Decreased oxygen affinity, resulting in a right shift of the oxyhemoglobin dissociation curve, means that at any given PaO_2, there is decreased saturation. Thus, oxygen is released more readily to tissues. Conversely, increased oxygen affinity, resulting in a left shift of the

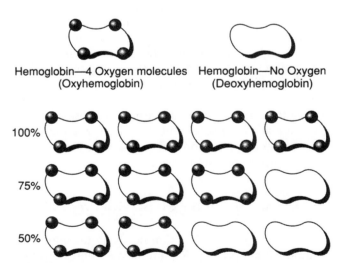

FIGURE 4-4 Percent saturation of hemoglobin.

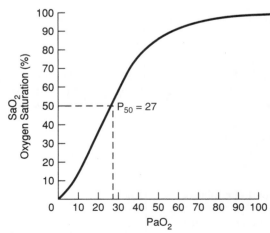

FIGURE 4-5 Oxyhemoglobin dissociation curve.

TABLE 4-1

Conditions Known to Change Oxygen Affinity to Hemoglobin

Conditions that Increase Affinity (Left Shift)	Conditions that Decrease Affinity (Right Shift)
High pH (alkalemia)	Low pH (acidemia)
Hypothermia	Fever
Decreased $PaCO_2$	Increased $PaCO_2$
Decreased 2,3 DPG	Increased 2,3 DPG
• Stored bank blood	• Anemia
• Hypothyroidism	• Chronic hypoxemia
• Hypophosphatemia	• Hyperthyroidism
• Chronic acidemia	• Chronic alkalemia
	• Some hormones

curve, means that at any given PaO_2, there is increased saturation. This results in oxygen binding more tightly to hemoglobin.

It should be noted that pregnancy also affects the position of the oxyhemoglobin curve. The maternal curve normally shifts to the right, whereby oxygen is released more quickly from hemoglobin. The fetal curve normally shifts to the left, resulting in increased affinity of oxygen for hemoglobin. This concept is depicted in Figure 4-6.

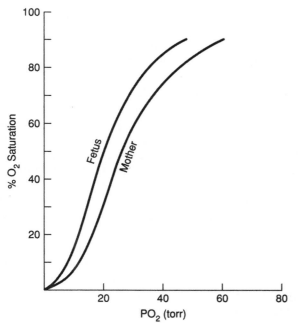

FIGURE 4-6 Maternal and fetal shifts in the oxyhemoglobin dissociation curve. From Clark, S. L., Cotton, D. B., Hankins, G. D. V., & Phelan, J. B. (Eds.). (1991). *Critical care obstetrics.* New York: Blackwell Scientific Publications, p. 106. Used with permission.

Oxygen Delivery

Oxygen delivery (DO_2) is the amount of oxygen delivered to the tissues per unit of time. The delivery of oxygen from the lungs to the tissues depends on cardiac output as well as on the content of oxygen in arterial blood (CaO_2). It should be recalled that cardiac output is dependent on preload, afterload, contractility, and heart rate. Arterial oxygen content is determined by the arterial concentration of hemoglobin, the arterial saturation of hemoglobin (SaO_2), and the amount of oxygen dissolved under pressure in plasma within the arteries (PaO_2).

Factors that increase cardiac output (e.g., uterine contractions, increased metabolism, and certain medications) also increase DO_2. In addition, factors that increase total oxygen content (e.g., transfusion of packed red blood cells) increase DO_2. Such conditions may include hypovolemia, hypoxemia, anemia, and administration of certain medications. When oxygen supply is threatened, the body attempts to compensate in order to maintain delivery to the tissues by first increasing cardiac output. It should be noted that cardiac output may increase severalfold above normal in healthy people under stressful circumstances.

Oxygen Consumption

Oxygen consumption (VO_2) refers to the amount of oxygen consumed by the tissues each minute. At rest, VO_2 is approximately 25 percent of the total oxygen available. Oxygen consumption is increased by numerous conditions as well as by interventions, therapeutic procedures, and various other stressors. It should be noted that VO_2 also increases significantly during normal pregnancy.

The normal relationship between DO_2 and VO_2 is such that sufficient reserve exists to maintain VO_2 *independent* of DO_2 over a wide range of delivery values. However, situations may develop whereby prolonged decreased DO_2, below a critical threshold, eventually results in a linear fall in VO_2. This is known as *delivery dependent* VO_2 because the amount of oxygen consumed is limited by the amount of oxygen delivered. In such circumstances, VO_2 does not become independent of DO_2 except at very high levels of oxygen delivery, if at all. This pathologic response is related to the fixed oxygen-extraction ratio present in some critically ill patients.

CENTRAL HEMODYNAMIC ASSESSMENT

Invasive hemodynamic monitoring may be accomplished via use of a central venous or pulmonary artery catheter. The description, assessment capabilities, indications, and associated complications for each follow.

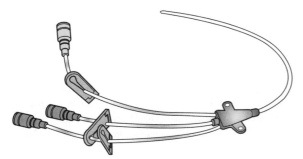

FIGURE 4-7   Central venous pressure (CVP) catheter.

Central Venous Pressure Catheter

The central venous pressure (CVP) catheter is a single- or multiple-lumen catheter advanced through a peripheral or central vein until the tip is in the proximal superior vena cava (Fig. 4-7). Central venous access is most commonly obtained via either the internal jugular or subclavian vein. The internal jugular vein is preferred during pregnancy because of the increased risk of pneumothorax with subclavian placement attempts during pregnancy.

Use of this catheter permits evaluation of right preload (expressed in mmHg as CVP), as well as access for administration of fluid or medications. The primary limitation with respect to central hemodynamic assessment is that right ventricular function may not accurately reflect left ventricular function. Thus, clinical use of the CVP may be misleading and possibly deleterious in certain clinical situations. In addition, a CVP catheter does not permit evaluation of data regarding other determinants of cardiac output or oxygen transport parameters. For these reasons, use of a CVP catheter for assessment of hemodynamic function in a critically ill obstetric patient is seldom, if ever, indicated. However, CVP catheters may be utilized for reasons other than assessment of hemodynamic function. Box 4-2 lists potential indications for use of a CVP catheter.[8]

Complications of central venous access that can occur during insertion and monitoring include pneumothorax,

Box 4-2. POTENTIAL INDICATIONS FOR USE OF A CENTRAL VENOUS PRESSURE CATHETER

- Rapid administration of large volumes of fluids
- Administration of medications that would irritate or damage a peripheral vein
- Total parenteral nutrition
- Hemodialysis
- Gaining venous access when peripheral vein cannulation is not possible

venous air embolism, inadvertent arterial puncture, and infection. Although pneumothorax has been reported in 1 to 5 percent of a general patient population undergoing central venous catheterization, Clark and associates observed no pneumothorax when the internal jugular approach was used in a compilation of obstetric and gynecologic patients.[2] Strategies to reduce the risk of central line–associated bloodstream infection (CLABSI) are presented later in this chapter.

Pulmonary Artery Catheter

The pulmonary artery (PA) catheter, also known as a Swan-Ganz catheter, is a balloon-tipped, flow-directed, multiple-lumen catheter (Fig. 4-8). The basic, standard PA catheter is a flexible, flow-directed, polyvinylchloride, Teflon, silicone elastomer, polyurethane, or proprietary polymer blend catheter that contains at least three lumens and a thermistor bead. Catheters are also available with additional lumens that permit extra central venous infusion ports, evaluation of right ventricular function, continuous mixed venous oxygen saturation assessment, and continuous measurement of cardiac output. The size of these catheters varies (7 to 8 French), depending on the number and type of additional options. It should be noted that French units are used in the measurement of the internal diameter of tubing or a catheter. Each French unit equals one-third of a millimeter.

The PA catheter is inserted into the pulmonary artery through a percutaneous introducer placed in a central vein. Characteristic waveforms may be visualized as the catheter tip passes through various cardiac structures (Fig. 4-9). Following insertion, the catheter rests in the pulmonary artery with the balloon tip deflated.

Use of this catheter permits continuous evaluation of pressures within the central vein (CVP) and pulmonary artery (PAP). Intermittent inflation of the balloon permits evaluation of pulmonary capillary wedge pressure (PCWP). This provides information regarding left preload by simulating closure of the pulmonic valve. This concept is illustrated in Figure 4-10. Intermittent evaluation of cardiac output may also be conducted utilizing thermodilution technology. Other hemodynamic data may be derived through calculations based on the preceding basic parameters.

Normal hemodynamic values during pregnancy are presented in Table 4-2.[9] These values are considered normal for peripartum women who are not in labor and not experiencing other acute or critical illness. Significant changes in these values occur with the onset of labor as well as other stressful conditions. Of most interest is a significant increase in cardiac output, usually at least 50 percent above the pregnancy baseline. This increase in cardiac output factors into mathematical formulas used to calculate other derived hemodynamic parameters,

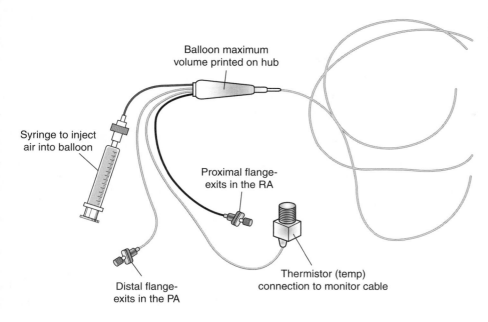

FIGURE 4-8 Pulmonary artery (PA) catheter.

Balloon maximum volume printed on hub

Syringe to inject air into balloon

Proximal flange-exits in the RA

Thermistor (temp) connection to monitor cable

Distal flange-exits in the PA

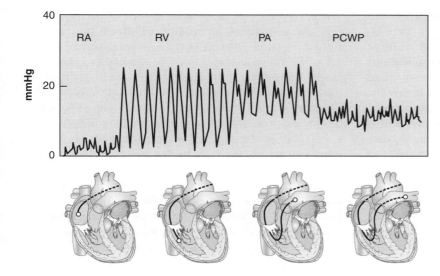

FIGURE 4-9 Characteristic waveforms during pulmonary artery (PA) catheter insertion.

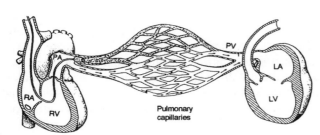

FIGURE 4-10 Pulmonary artery (PA) catheter location during assessment of pulmonary capillary wedge pressure (PCWP). From Darovic, G. O. (1987). *Hemodynamic monitoring: Invasive and noninvasive clinical application.* Philadelphia: W.B. Saunders Company. Used with permission.

TABLE 4-2

Normal Hemodynamic Values in Pregnancy at Rest

Parameter	Value and Standard Deviation
Cardiac output (L/min)	6.2 ± 1.0
Systemic vascular resistance (dyne/sec/cm^{-5})	1210 ± 266
Pulmonary vascular resistance (dyne/sec/cm^{-5})	78 ± 22
Mean pulmonary artery pressure (mmHg)	13 ± 2
Central venous pressure (mmHg)	3.6 ± 2.5
Left ventricular stroke work index (g/m/m^{-2})	48 ± 6

TABLE 4-3

Hemodynamic Parameters and Calculation Formulas

Parameter	Formula
Systemic vascular resistance (SVR)	$[(MAP - CVP) \div CO] \times 80$
Pulmonary vascular resistance (PVR)	$[(MPAP - PCWP) \div CO] \times 80$
Left ventricular stroke work index (LVSWI)	$LVSW \div BSA$
• Mean arterial pressure (MAP)	$(Systolic\ BP + [2 \times Diastolic\ BP]) \div 3$
• Stroke volume (SV)	$(CO \div HR) \times 1000$
• Left ventricular stroke work (LVSW)	$MAP \times SV \times 0.0136$

BP = blood pressure; BSA = body surface area; CO = cardiac output, HR = heart rate; MPAP = mean pulmonary artery pressure; PCWP = pulmonary capillary wedge pressure.

including systemic vascular resistance (SVR), pulmonary vascular resistance (PVR), and left ventricular stroke work index. (The formulas used to calculate derived hemodynamic assessment parameters are presented in Table 4-3.) Adjustment of these normal values is extremely important in the clinical setting when caring for the critically ill obstetric patient.

Pulmonary artery catheterization is not without risks, but few are life-threatening. Most complications are nonspecific and seen with all types of intravascular catheters. However, some are specific to PA catheters. Onset of ventricular dysrhythmias is the most common complication specific to PA catheters. It has been reported to occur in a nonobstetric patient population in approximately 50 percent of insertions when the catheter is passed through the right side of the heart.[10,11] These dysrhythmias are almost always benign and resolve when the catheter is either advanced into the pulmonary artery or is withdrawn. Right bundle branch block may also occur but usually disappears within 24 hours of insertion. Pulmonary artery rupture is a rare complication, with 10 cases reported in the first 10 years of PA catheter use.[12]

Technical Issues

Certain technical issues related to invasive hemodynamic assessment require attention when caring for the obstetric patient. These issues include prevention of catheter-associated clot formation, the method used for assessment of cardiac output, and timing of data collection. (For more information, see *Guidelines for the Care of Critically Ill Obstetric Patients* elsewhere in this text.)

Any catheter placed in the intravascular system, where it is exposed to components of blood that include clotting factors, is continuously or intermittently flushed to prevent clot formation on its tip or side. Continuous infusion usually is preferred for the purpose of flushing central hemodynamic catheters. The most common type of flush system is the continuous, in-line flush valve. Such valves are standardized to deliver 3 milliliters per hour (3 mL/hr) of solution when the intravenous solution is placed under 300 mmHg pressure via a pressure bag. Because pregnant women are in a hypercoagulable state and are at increased risk for clot formation, an additional precaution is warranted. Heparinized solutions, concentrated at a rate of 1:1 to 2:1 heparin/solution ratio, are used to provide a safety net during pregnancy.[13–15] Use of heparin in the flush solution for central hemodynamic catheters in pregnant patients may differ from the policy for care of nonpregnant patients in an intensive care unit (ICU).

A small percentage of patients who receive intravenous unfractionated heparin for the treatment of deep vein thrombosis or pulmonary embolism develop heparin-induced thrombocytopenia (HIT). For this reason, many ICUs have decreased or stopped adding heparin to flush solutions. Decreased heparin exposure from the flush solution in a pressure line is associated with an HIT rate of 0.5 percent. During pregnancy, the risk of HIT (less than 0.1 percent) from heparinized flush solutions is lower than in the nonpregnant population.[16] Thus, heparin typically is used in pressure lines for obstetric patients to prevent clot formation and catheter occlusion.

Cardiac output is most often assessed at the bedside using the thermodilution method. The temperature of the injectate solution is an issue when caring for a critically ill pregnant woman. Numerous studies report favorable correlation between room temperature and iced injectate solutions for thermodilution cardiac output assessment in the absence of either low or high cardiac output states. This normal range has most often been defined as an expected cardiac output of greater than 4.0 liters per minute (L/min) but less than 8.0 L/min. However, correlation is poor in patients with low or high cardiac output states.[17] Based on these findings, iced injectate is recommended if cardiac output is 3.5 L/min or less, or greater than 8 L/min. Women in the perinatal period most often are expected to have a cardiac output greater than 8.0 L/min during an acute or critical illness. For these reasons, it is recommended that iced injectate be used when assessing cardiac output by thermodilution.

Another critical issue when assessing central hemodynamic function in the pregnant patient relates to when data are obtained. Maternal cardiac output increases as early as 10 weeks of gestation and peaks at 50 percent over prepregnant levels by the end of the second trimester. Several factors are associated with additional changes in cardiac output. For example, Clark and colleagues described the effect of maternal position on cardiac output in late pregnancy.[9] Labor also alters cardiac output. Depending on the stage and phase of labor, cardiac output increases up to 40 percent. In addition, approximately 300 to 500 mL of blood is expelled into the maternal central circulation with each uterine contraction, increasing preload and thus further increasing cardiac output. During the first hour after delivery, cardiac output again increases approximately 22 percent. The effects of pain and administration of various medications during the intrapartum period may also significantly influence cardiac output. Generally, cardiac output returns to prepregnant levels in healthy women by 2 to 4 weeks after delivery. For these reasons, it is important to avoid assessing cardiac output and other hemodynamic parameters during a uterine contraction. The position of the patient during assessment should be noted and supine positioning avoided. In addition, these issues must be considered when considering use of a PA catheter with the capability for continuous cardiac output (CCO) assessment. Such catheters do not permit exclusion of

data acquired during uterine contractions; therefore, the quality of data may be affected and the usefulness of the information in provision of care compromised. Data are needed to determine the reliability during pregnancy of measurements obtained from PA catheters with CCO capabilities. Published data related to this subject are not currently available.

OXYGEN TRANSPORT ASSESSMENT

Technical adjuncts that enhance the ability to assess the oxygen transport status of critically ill patients include the pulse oximeter and continuous mixed venous oxygen saturation (SvO_2) PA catheter.

Pulse Oximetry

Oximetry is an optical method for measuring oxygenated hemoglobin in blood. It is based on the ability of different forms of hemoglobin to absorb light of different wavelengths. Oxyhemoglobin (HbO_2) absorbs light in the red spectrum, and deoxygenated or reduced hemoglobin (RHb) absorbs light in the near-infrared spectrum. If a light beam composed of red and infrared wavelengths is passed through a blood vessel, the transmission of each wavelength will be inversely proportional to the concentration of HbO_2 and RHb in the blood. This concept, referred to as reflective spectrophotometry, is depicted in Figure 4-11. The oxygen saturation is then calculated as the ratio of HbO_2 to total hemoglobin in the sample.

This calculation of oxygen saturation uses only two forms of hemoglobin and therefore neglects

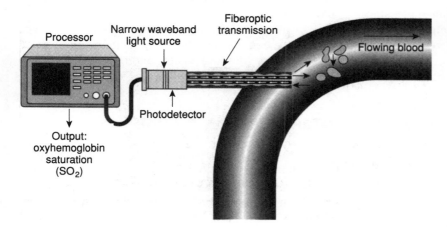

Principles of Reflection Spectrophotometry
Fiberoptic catheter oximetry (in vivo)

Processor

Narrow waveband light source

Fiberoptic transmission

Flowing blood

Photodetector

Output: oxyhemoglobin saturation (SO_2)

FIGURE 4-11 Reflective spectrophotometry. Continuous measurement of blood oxygen saturation in the high-risk patient. From Schweiss, J. F. (1986). *Introduction and historical perspective*. Mountain View, CA: Abbott Critical Care. Reproduced with permission.

methemoglobin and carboxyhemoglobin. The cooximeters for in vitro use have multiple wavelengths of light and can detect all forms of hemoglobin. Thus, use of the cooximeters permits evaluation of *fractional* saturation, whereas the type of pulse oximeter used clinically in most patients measures *functional* saturation.

Original oximeters suffered from two limitations. The first related to interference from light absorption by pigments and other tissue elements. The second was the inability to differentiate hemoglobin in the arteries from that in the veins. These limitations were reduced by oximeters that measure light transmission through pulsatile vessels only. These pulse oximeters are the type widely utilized in clinical practice today. The photodetectors in pulse oximeters can sense an alternating light input from arterial pulsations and a steady light input from veins and other nonpulsatile elements. Only the alternating light input is selected for analysis, thus eliminating contribution from other sources. This explains why pulse oximeters are not influenced by tissue thickness or pigments.

Mixed Venous Oxygen Saturation PA Catheter

The venous oxygen saturation (SvO_2), or the percentage of saturation of venous hemoglobin, reflects the overall balance between oxygen delivery and oxygen consumption of perfused tissues. This variable is dependent on the interactions of oxygen transport and consumption. Measurement of SvO_2 is determined by the saturation of hemoglobin in the pulmonary artery, the least oxygenated point in the cardiovascular system. This blood originates from the superior vena cava, the inferior vena cava, and the coronary sinus, and reflects a mixture of venous saturation from various organ systems. It is thus called mixed venous blood because it represents oxygen saturation of the body, rather than one organ or area.

SvO_2 values may be obtained intermittently or continuously. Intermittent analysis of SvO_2 is made from blood samples obtained from the distal lumen of a standard pulmonary artery catheter. The sample is drawn slowly to prevent blood that has been reoxygenated from being aspirated into the sample.

Continuous measurement of SvO_2 is obtained with a special PA catheter, first introduced in 1981 by Abbott Critical Care Systems. The catheter was equipped with a fiberoptic light source and receiver to measure pulmonary artery hemoglobin saturation. There are now several systems available for the continuous measurement of SvO_2. Each system consists of a microprocessor capable of in vitro calibration and memory storage for retroactive correction vis-à-vis a reference calibration. Analysis of the reflected light intensity and calculation

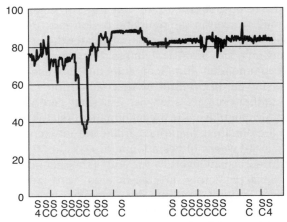

FIGURE 4-12 Continuous SvO_2 tracing. The acute drop in baseline maternal SvO_2 at the start of the tracing was associated with maternal repositioning and uterine contraction.

of oxyhemoglobin saturation is achieved by the microprocessor. The ratio of saturated and desaturated hemoglobin is measured, and a numeric value is displayed by the monitor. In addition, a continuous recording of SvO_2 may be visualized on the digital display of the monitor. An example of a continuous SvO_2 tracing is presented in Figure 4-12. The normal value for SvO_2 is between 60 and 80 percent, although higher values are common during pregnancy secondary to the higher cardiac output associated with pregnancy.

SvO_2 monitoring permits more thorough assessment of oxygen transport status in critically ill patients. Specific data that may be obtained with this technology and the formula for calculating each parameter are presented in Table 4-4.

SvO_2 provides invaluable information to the clinician regarding a patient's oxygen supply and ability to meet oxygen demands that accompany significant complications and stressors. If the patient has physiologic conditions that increase oxygen demand and the oxygen delivery system is marginal in meeting those needs, increasing the oxygen demand with clinical care activities may exceed the patient's ability to effectively cope. When SvO_2 is decreased, care should be taken to consider activities or conditions that may further compromise oxygen delivery. Table 4-5 lists conditions and activities that increase oxygen consumption.

INTERPRETATION OF DATA

Interpretation of hemodynamic and oxygen transport data requires knowledge of the normal values and trends during pregnancy and is facilitated by the use of a systematic approach to synthesize complex information. Information obtained by invasive monitoring should

TABLE 4-4

Oxygen Transport Parameters and Calculation Formulas

Parameter		Formula
Arterial oxygen content (CaO$_2$)	mL/dL	$(1.34 \times Hgb \times SaO_2) + (PaO_2 \times 0.0031)$
Oxygen delivery (DO$_2$)	mL/min	$(CaO_2 \times \text{cardiac output}) \times 10$
Venous oxygen content (CvO$_2$)	mL/dL	$(1.34 \times Hgb \times SvO_2) + (PvO_2 \times 0.0031)$
Arteriovenous oxygen difference (avDO$_2$)	mL/dL	$CaO_2 - CvO_2$
Oxygen consumption (VO$_2$)	mL/min	$(avDO_2 \times \text{cardiac output}) \times 10$
Oxygen extraction ratio (O$_2$ER)	%	$VO_2 \div DO_2$

Hgb = hemoglobin; PaO$_2$ = arterial oxygen tension in plasma; PvO$_2$ = venous oxygen tension in plasma; SaO$_2$ = arterial oxygen saturation; SvO$_2$ = venous oxygen saturation.

always be integrated with information obtained from review of the patient's history, underlying disease processes, clinical physical assessment findings, and laboratory data. It should be noted that abnormalities in centrally obtained hemodynamic and oxygen transport data may precede clinical manifestations. Thus, data may be used in such circumstances to prevent complications.

Hemodynamic Profile

Interpretation of a patient's hemodynamic profile begins with assessment of cardiac output. This is done to ascertain whether the overall amount of blood ejected from the heart per minute is sufficient to meet the patient's current demands. It should be recalled that cardiac output is a significant component to the formula for determining oxygen delivery. If cardiac output is not sufficient, the patient may exhibit clinical evidence of end-organ dysfunction or failure. During the intrapartum period, evidence of compromised maternal oxygen transport may be reflected by adverse changes in the fetal heart rate.

Following assessment of cardiac output, each of the four determinants of cardiac output should be evaluated. Preload, reflective of EDV, is the first determinant that should be assessed. If discrepancy exists between the right and left preload values (CVP and PCWP respectively), it should be recalled that the left ventricle should be the focus of any evaluation of hemodynamic function in the critically ill pregnant woman. Thus, PCWP is more helpful in providing information in an acute setting regarding central volume status. At this point, the clinician should be able to determine if the patient is centrally "wet," "dry," or normovolemic. When integrated with knowledge of the patient's underlying disease process, this information is often valuable.

The next determinant that should be assessed is afterload. It should be recalled that afterload is resistance that the ventricles must overcome to eject blood during systole. Alterations in right or left afterload values (PVR and SVR respectively), may represent the cause of a hemodynamic problem or may indicate a compensatory response to another problem. For example, a hypertensive patient may have elevated left afterload (SVR)

TABLE 4-5

Percentage Increase in Resting Oxygen Consumption (VO$_2$) Associated with Conditions and Activities

Conditions	%
Fever (each 1°C)	10
Fractures (each)	10
Agitation	18
Chest trauma	25
Work of breathing	40
Critically ill in emergency department	60
Severe infection	60
Shivering	50–100
Sepsis	50–100
Head injury, sedated	89
Head injury, not sedated	138
Burns	100

Activities	%
Dressing change	10
Electrocardiogram	16
Physical exam	20
Visitors	22
Bath	23
Chest x-ray	25
Endotracheal suctioning	27
Nasal intubation	25–40
Turn to side	31
Chest physiotherapy	35
Weigh on sling scale	36

From White, K. M. (1993). Using continuous SvO$_2$ to assess oxygen supply/demand balance in the critically ill patient. *Clinical Issues in Critical Care Nursing, 4*(1), 134–147.

that is causing increased left preload (PCWP) and is thus placing the patient at risk for pulmonary edema. The cornerstone for therapy would be administration of an agent to decrease left afterload. In contrast, a patient who is centrally "dry," as may be present with severe preeclampsia, may be vasoconstricting to compensate for the hypovolemia and decreased cardiac output. The cornerstone for therapy for this patient would be administration of intravascular fluid to expand vascular volume. Administration of an agent to decrease afterload in this patient would be deleterious to her overall condition.

Contractility and heart rate are evaluated next. Left ventricular function, indicated by the LVSWI, is often elevated in critically ill patients. This represents a valuable compensatory response in the healthy heart to alterations in preload and afterload. Contractility is increased in order to maintain adequate cardiac output and oxygen delivery. The same is true for elevations in the heart rate. When contractility is decreased, the patient is said to be in left ventricular failure. Most often this indicates loss of a valuable compensatory function, placing the patient at significant risk for hemodynamic failure and cardiopulmonary arrest. Interventions are targeted toward inotropic support. This may be accomplished by administration of medications, such as dobutamine hydrochloride, or by administration of intravascular fluids to optimize preload and, thus, ventricular stretch and cardiac output.

Oxygen Transport Data

Following assessment of the hemodynamic profile, the patient's oxygen delivery (DO_2) is evaluated. A determination should be made whether the overall DO_2 is sufficient to meet the patient's needs. It should be recalled that oxygen demand increases during pregnancy, labor, and other stressful circumstances. With certain disease processes, correction of oxygen deficit to specific end-organs may require supranormal levels of DO_2. It is important to remember that calculation of arterial oxygen content (CaO_2) requires a current hemoglobin in order for values to most accurately reflect the patient's oxygenation status. Because the amount of oxygen dissolved under pressure in plasma accounts for such a small percentage of the total, in the absence of a current arterial blood gas value, the PaO_2 is often deleted from the calculation formula. If the DO_2 is low, the cause should be ascertained and intervention directed toward correction of the underlying problem. For example, if cardiac output is normal but hemoglobin is low, the CaO_2 will also be low, thus producing a low DO_2. Intervention would include transfusion of packed red blood cells (PRBCs) to correct anemia or optimize oxygen carrying capacity.

Oxygen consumption (VO_2) is evaluated next. It should be recalled that VO_2 is increased in normal pregnancy.

Labor and other stressful conditions increase VO_2 further. When VO_2 is increased, it is important to identify possible reasons. Interventions may include administration of medication to relieve pain or reduce fever. When VO_2 is decreased, it is important to assess the patient for evidence of end-organ dysfunction or failure. In the presence of organ failure, oxygen extraction by tissues in the affected organ is severely impaired or eliminated.

In addition to assessment of oxygen delivery and consumption, it is important to note the patient's ongoing amount of oxygen reserve. Routine interventions as well as special procedures should be planned according to the patient's ability to meet the concomitant increase in oxygen demand.

FETAL ISSUES

Oxygen Transport

Because of the high oxygen diffusion gradient during pregnancy, oxygen diffuses from the maternal alveoli into the red blood cells at a more rapid rate. Oxygenated red blood cells pass through maternal arteries into the intervillous spaces of the placenta. Oxygen then diffuses from the placenta to fetal tissues. Each of these steps results in a progressive decrease in the partial pressure of oxygen.[18]

Based on the theory of venous equilibration, it is apparent that the uterine venous PO_2 is the major determinant of umbilical venous PO_2. The oxygen saturation of uterine venous blood is affected by three variables: oxygen saturation of maternal arterial blood (SaO_2), oxygen carrying capacity of maternal blood (CaO_2), and uterine blood flow. Any decrease in maternal oxygen delivery (DO_2) thus decreases uterine venous PO_2 and umbilical venous PO_2.

Uterine contractions reduce uterine blood flow because of a significant increase in uterine vascular resistance. In addition to the effect of uterine activity, a number of maternal conditions can impair oxygen delivery to the fetus. In essence, any condition that decreases maternal uterine venous PO_2 will also decrease oxygen transport to the fetus.

Adaptive Responses to Hypoxemia

In an otherwise healthy fetus, an initial response to decreased oxygen supply is elevation of the baseline fetal heart rate (FHR). Fetal tachycardia may develop as the fetus increases cardiac output in an attempt to compensate. However, fetal cardiac output is near maximum normally; therefore, this response may have only temporary value.

Should fetal hypoxemia continue, late decelerations of the FHR may develop. In the early stages, in an otherwise healthy fetus, late decelerations may have a reflexive component. However, if compromise in oxygen transport continues, a multifactorial basis for the decelerations develops, including direct fetal myocardial depression, which interferes with conduction of impulses. This may be related to a chain of events that began with chemoreceptor stimulation at the level of the aortic arch, the medulla, or both.

As hypoxemia continues, fetal compensatory mechanisms may become depleted, resulting in the development of acidemia. As acidemia develops, the centers controlling FHR variability (FHRV) become depressed and FHRV decreases. Therefore, the combination of an abnormal baseline FHR, recurrent late decelerations, and absent FHRV is considered a Category III electronic FHR monitor tracing. (For more information, see *Guidelines for Fetal Monitoring* elsewhere in this text.) The risks of continued labor must be seriously balanced against the risks of delivery.

CLINICAL CASE EXCERPT

The following brief case excerpt illustrates a systematic approach to interpretation of hemodynamic and oxygen transport data.

Brief History

This patient, a primigravida at 35 and 3/7 weeks gestation, was admitted with a diagnosis of severe preeclampsia. Induction of labor was initiated secondary to worsening preeclampsia and HELLP syndrome (**H**emolysis, **E**levated **L**iver enzymes, **L**ow **P**latelet count). Magnesium sulfate was administered for seizure prophylaxis, and oxytocin was infusing intravenously for induction of labor. Significant maternal hypertension (systolic pressure above 160 mmHg and diastolic pressure above 110 mmHg) did not resolve following administration of hydralazine. The patient subsequently developed persistent oliguria refractory to administration of an intravenous crystalloid fluid bolus (1,000 mL total volume). (A more thorough discussion of hypertensive disorders in pregnancy including severe preeclampsia, eclampsia, and HELLP syndrome is presented in Chapter 7.)

A decision was made to proceed with central hemodynamic and oxygen transport monitoring in order to more clearly discern the etiology for these clinical manifestations. A fiberoptic pulmonary artery catheter was inserted via a central venous introducer placed in the right internal jugular vein. Initial maternal assessment findings are presented in Table 4-6. Fetal heart rate and

TABLE 4-6

Case Excerpt: Maternal Hemodynamic and Oxygen Transport Assessment Findings

Assessment		*Initial Findings*	*Findings After Intervention*
Vital signs	Blood pressure	200/118 mmHg	158/94 mmHg
	Heart rate	120	92
	Respiratory rate	28	20
	Temperature	98.8° F	98.8° F
	SaO_2	92% (on supplemental oxygen by mask)	99% (on room air)
Hemodynamic values*	CVP	4 mmHg	4 mmHg
	PAP	36/18 mmHg	36/18 mmHg
	PCWP	18 mmHg	12 mmHg
	CO	4.1 L/min	8.6 L/min
	SVR	2751	1032
	PVR	117	111
	LVSWI	32	145
Oxygen transport values[†]	CaO_2	11 mL/dL	12 mL/dL
	DO_2	451 mL/min	1032 mL/min
	CvO_2	8 mL/dL	10 mL/dL
	$avDO_2$	3 mL/dL	2 mL/dL
	VO_2	123 mL/min	172 mL/min
	O_2ER	27%	16%

BSA = body surface area; CaO_2 = arterial oxygen content; CO = cardiac output; CvO_2 = venous oxygen content; CVP = central venous pressure; DO_2 = oxygen delivery; LVSWI = left ventricular stroke work index; O_2ER = oxygen extraction ratio; PAP = pulmonary artery pressure; PCWP = pulmonary capillary wedge pressure; PVR = pulmonary vascular resistance; SVR = systemic vascular resistance; VO_2 = oxygen consumption.

*Hemoglobin = 9.3; BSA = 2.1 m².

[†]SvO_2 = 61% before intervention; 84% after intervention.

FIGURE 4-13 Fetal heart rate (FHR) and uterine activity at the time initial central hemodynamic and oxygen transport data were obtained.

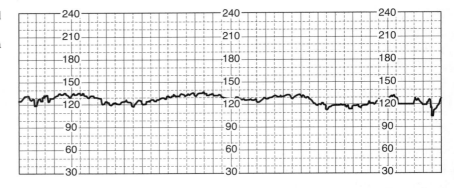

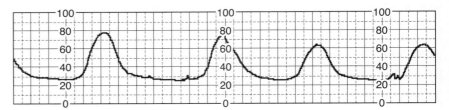

uterine activity at the time these data were obtained are presented in Figure 4-13.

Interpretation of Data

As noted previously in this chapter, it is important to utilize a systematic approach when interpreting hemodynamic and oxygen transport data. In addition, information should be placed in context with the patient's specific clinical situation and disease process. Collaboration between the patient's nurse and physician is imperative in order to synthesize data, formulate diagnoses, create an appropriate plan of care, initiate interventions, and evaluate patient responses.[19] Interpretation of initial hemodynamic data indicated the patient had a significantly low cardiac output (CO 4.1 L/min). Analysis of the determinants of CO revealed a high left preload (PCWP 18 mmHg), high right and left afterload (PVR 117 and SVR 2751, respectively), and significantly impaired left ventricular contractility (LVSWI 32). Interpretation of oxygen transport data indicated that the patient also had a significantly low oxygen delivery (DO$_2$ 451 mL/min). Analysis of determinants of oxygen delivery indicated that the primary cause of the patient's critically low DO$_2$ was low cardiac output. The mixed venous oxygen saturation (SvO$_2$), indicative of oxygen saturation of hemoglobin returned to the heart via the venous system, was significantly low for an obstetric patient. Most likely this was related to the critically low cardiac output state. Interpretation of FHR data included a normal baseline rate, minimal FHR variability, absence of FHR accelerations, and presence of recurrent late decelerations of FHR.

Nursing diagnoses, based on interpretation of these assessment findings, included decreased cardiac output, impaired maternal and fetal oxygen transport, impaired gas exchange, and activity intolerance related to inadequate oxygen reserve. Desired outcomes included optimization of cardiac output, maternal and fetal oxygen transport and gas exchange, and optimization of oxygen reserve.

To develop a plan of care, the patient's physician was contacted and the assessment findings and nursing diagnoses were discussed. Collaboration resulted in a plan of care intended to achieve the desired outcomes. Interventions to optimize cardiac output focused on reduction of left preload and left afterload as well as improvement of left ventricular contractility. Dobutamine was administered by intravenous infusion for inotropic support. (A more thorough discussion of pharmacologic agents utilized for inotropic support is presented in Chapter 6.) The method of action is stimulation of beta receptors in the heart muscle, which increases contractility, thereby increasing stroke volume and cardiac output. The initial dosage was 2.5 mcg/kg/min. In the absence of an appreciable increase in SvO$_2$, the dosage was increased to 5 mcg/kcg/min. Assessment of the ECG tracing revealed no tachydysrhythmias or ventricular ectopy. Hydralazine was administered intravenously to reduce left afterload. Oxytocin was discontinued, pending additional evidence of improved maternal hemodynamic and oxygen transport status. Within 15 minutes following the change in dobutamine dosage, the continuous SvO$_2$ monitor indicated a significant improvement, and hemodynamic and oxygen transport data were obtained (see Table 4-6).

Evaluation of the patient's response to interventions ensued. Interpretation of these data indicates significant improvement in left preload and left ventricular contractility, resulting in improved cardiac output. In addition, oxygen delivery increased significantly, which in turn increased the patient's oxygen reserve. Arterial oxygen saturation improved to 99 percent and remained at that level following discontinuation of supplemental oxygen by mask. Severe hypertension and oliguria also resolved. Subsequent fetal assessment findings included a normal FHR baseline, moderate FHR variability, and absence of FHR decelerations. Following a short period of rest, oxytocin was reinitiated and induction of labor continued. The patient's labor progressed well, and she subsequently had a spontaneous vaginal delivery without complications.

PREVENTION OF CENTRAL LINE–ASSOCIATED INFECTION

The potential for central line–associated bloodstream infection (CLABSI) is of considerable concern in any clinical setting. Research over the last decade has focused on a number of factors that reduce the incidence of infections related to central line placement. Four major risk factors are associated with increased rates of CLABSI:

- cutaneous colonization at the insertion site
- moisture under the dressing
- length of time the catheter remains in place
- the technique of care and placement of the central line.[20]

The Joint Commission's most current National Patient Safety Goals include implementation of best practices or evidence-based guidelines to prevent central line–associated bloodstream infections.[21,22] Resources related to best practices and current recommendations on this subject appear in Table 4-7.

TABLE 4-7

Sources of Guidelines and Scientific Resources Useful in Preventing Central Line–Associated Bloodstream Infections

Association for Professionals in Infection Control and Epidemiology, Inc.	http://www.apic.org
Infectious Diseases Society of America	http://www.idsociety.org
Society for Healthcare Epidemiology of America	http://www.shea-online.org

CONCLUSION

Invasive central hemodynamic and oxygen transport monitoring enhance the ability of clinicians to assess the pregnant woman who has significant complications or who is critically ill. Data may be used to plan and implement care as well as to evaluate patient responses to various interventions. However, monitoring equipment alone is not sufficient to improve patient outcomes. It is imperative that clinicians caring for critically ill pregnant women have a thorough understanding of how to correctly interpret data within the context of pregnancy and to integrate information with the complete clinical picture.

REFERENCES

1. Swan, J. H. C., Ganz, W., Forrester, J., Marcus, H., Diamond, G., & Chonette, D. (1970). Catheterization of the heart with use of a flow-directed balloon-tipped catheter. *The New England Journal of Medicine, 283,* 447–451.
2. Clark, S. L., Horenstein, J. M., Phelan, J. P., Montag, T. W., & Paul, R. H. (1985). Experience with the pulmonary artery catheter in obstetrics and gynecology. *American Journal of Obstetrics & Gynecology, 152,* 374–378.
3. Clark, S. L., & Cotton, D. B. (1988). Clinical opinion: Clinical indications for pulmonary artery catheterization in the patient with severe preeclampsia. *American Journal of Obstetrics & Gynecology, 158,* 453–458.
4. European Society of Intensive Care Medicine. (1991). Expert panel: The use of the pulmonary artery catheter. *Intensive Care Medicine, 17,* I–VIII.
5. Dildy, G. A., III, & Clark, S. L. (2004). Pulmonary artery catheterization. In G. A. Dildy III, M. A. Belfort, G. R. Saade, J. P. Phelan, G. D. V. Hankins, & S. L. Clark (Eds.), *Critical care obstetrics* (4th ed.). Malden, MA: Blackwell Science.
6. Marino, P. L., & Sutin, K. M. (2006). *The ICU book* (3rd ed.). Baltimore: Lippincott Williams & Wilkins.
7. Dantzger, D. R., & Scharf, S. M. (1998). *Cardiopulmonary critical care* (3rd ed.). Philadelphia: W.B. Saunders Company.
8. Kaur, S., & Heard, S. (2000). Central venous catheter. In R. S. Irwin & J. M. Rippe (Eds.), *Manual of intensive care medicine* (3rd ed.). Philadelphia: Lippincott Williams & Wilkins.
9. Clark, S. L., Cotton, D. B., Lee, W., Bishop, C., Hill, T., Southwick, J. (1989). Central hemodynamic assessment of normal term pregnancy. *American Journal of Obstetrics & Gynecology, 161,* 1439–1442.
10. Ermakov, S., & Hoyt, J. W. (1992). Pulmonary artery catheterization. *Critical Care Clinics, 8,* 773–806.
11. Marino, P. L. (1998). The pulmonary artery catheter. In P. L. Marino (Ed.), *The ICU book* (2nd ed.). Baltimore: Williams & Wilkins.
12. Paulson, D. M., Scott, S. M., & Sethi, G. K. (1988). Pulmonary hemorrhage associated with balloon flotation catheter. *The Journal of Thoracic and Cardiovascular Surgery, 80,* 453–458.
13. Meyer, B. A., Little, C. J., Thorp, J. A., Cohen, G. R., & Yeast, J. D. (1995). Heparin versus normal saline as a peripheral line flush in maintenance of intermittent intravenous lines

in obstetric patients. *Obstetrics & Gynecology, 85*(3), 433–436.

14. Harvey, C. J., & Harvey, M. G. (2007). Hemodynamic monitoring of the critically-ill obstetric patient. In R. R. Wieczorek & M. C. Freda (Eds.), *March of Dimes nursing module* (2nd ed.). White Plains, NY: March of Dimes.

15. American Association of Critical Care Nurses. (1993). Evaluation of the effects of heparinized and nonheparinized flush solutions on the patency of arterial pressure monitoring lines: The AACN Thunder Project. *American Journal of Critical Care, 2*, 3–15.

16. Warkentin, T. E., & Greinacher, A. (2004). Heparin-induced thrombocytopenia: Recognition, treatment, and prevention: The seventh ACCP Conference on antithrombotic and thrombolytic therapy. *Chest, 126*(Supplement), 311S–375S.

17. Wallace, D. C., & Winslow, E. H. (1993). Effects of iced and room temperature injectate on cardiac output measurements in critically ill patients with decreased and increased cardiac outputs. *Heart & Lung, 22*, 55–63.

18. Belfort, M. A., Saade, G. R., Foley, M. R., Phelan, J. P., & Dildy, G. A., III. (2010). *Critical care obstetrics* (5th ed.). Boston: Wiley-Blackwell.

19. Baird, S. M., & Troiano, N. H. (2010). Critical care obstetric nursing. In M. A. Belfort, G. R. Saade, M. R. Foley, J. P. Phelan, & G. A. Dildy, III. (Eds.), *Critical care obstetrics* (5th ed.). Boston: Wiley-Blackwell.

20. Baird, S. M., & Troiano, N. H. (2010). Critical care obstetric nursing. In M. A. Belfort, G. R. Saade, M. R. Foley, J. P. Phelan, & G. A. Dildy, III. (Eds.), *Critical care obstetrics* (5th ed.). Boston: Wiley-Blackwell.

21. The Joint Commission. (2011). *National patient safety goals 2011.* Washington, DC: Author. Retrieved from http://www.jointcommission.org/standards_information/npsgs.aspx

22. Society for Healthcare Epidemiology of America. (2008). *Compendium of strategies to prevent healthcare-associated infections in acute care hospitals.* Arlington, VA: Author. Retrieved from http://www.shea-online.org/about/compendium.cfm

CHAPTER 5

Mechanical Ventilation During Pregnancy

Nan H. Troiano and Thomas M. Jenkins

Mechanical ventilatory support is one of the major supportive modalities used in critical care. An essential element of cardiopulmonary resuscitation, it can be lifesaving during a variety of acute and chronic disorders, when respiratory drive is depressed, or when the patient lacks the neuromuscular ability to breathe. Further, the lung is usually one of the essential organs involved in multiple organ-system dysfunction or failure. Thus, delivery of appropriate ventilatory support can be challenging. For a number of reasons, challenges are compounded when the need for ventilatory support occurs in a patient who is pregnant.

This chapter reviews indications for intubation and mechanical ventilatory support during pregnancy. Types and modes of both conventional and newer ventilatory adjuncts are presented. Issues related to use during pregnancy as well as specific care measures are also described. More thorough description of disease processes that may lead to respiratory or ventilatory failure during pregnancy may be found elsewhere in this text.

INDICATIONS

Patients with refractory hypoxemia or tissue hypoxia who are unable to ventilate sufficiently despite supplemental therapy will require intubation and mechanical ventilation. Mechanical assistance may be necessary because ventilation is inadequate to regulate pH, because adequate oxygenation cannot be achieved at the fraction of inspired oxygen (FiO_2) available without manipulating the mode of ventilation, or because activity of the ventilatory muscles places excessive demands for blood flow on an already compromised cardiovascular system. General guidelines for the diagnosis of respiratory failure are presented in Table 5-1.[1] It should be noted that determination of some of these criteria is based on results of pulmonary function tests, which quantify respiratory function by measuring lung volume during normal and maximal ventilation.

CONVENTIONAL TYPES OF MECHANICAL VENTILATORS

Generally, conventional ventilators can be divided into two types: volume-cycled and pressure-cycled. They are classified according to the mechanism that terminates the inspiratory phase. Both types are positive pressure systems. The specific ventilator selected for a given clinical situation may depend on a number of variables, including the models available in a specific institution and the familiarity or experience level of the patient's care providers with one type over another. Irrespective of which type or model is used, a mechanical device used to sustain life is only as good as its design and the health care team using it.

Negative Pressure

Early ventilators were negative pressure systems known as *iron lungs*. The patient's body was encased in an iron cylinder and negative pressure was generated, which enlarged the thoracic cavity. A modification of this system involves a suit or shell that is fitted over the patient's chest with a hose connecting the device to a negative pressure generator. In either model, lung inflation is accomplished by reducing the pressure in the container to below atmospheric pressure. This causes the pressure surrounding the chest to drop below the pressure in the lungs, and the chest expands. The lungs then expand and the pressure inside them becomes less than atmospheric. Atmospheric gases are drawn into the lungs until lung pressure and atmospheric pressure reach equilibrium. Inspiration then ends. Once subatmospheric pressure surrounding the chest is released, the natural elastic recoil of the thoracic cage and lungs causes lung pressure

TABLE 5-1

Acute Respiratory Failure: Indications for Endotracheal Intubation and Mechanical Ventilatory Assistance

Parameter	Indication for Ventilatory Assistance	
Mechanics	Respiratory rate (breaths/min)	>35
	Vital capacity (mL/kg body weight*)	<15
	Inspiratory force (cm/H_2O)	<−25
	Compliance (mL/cmH_2O)	<25
	FEV_1 (mL/kg body weight*)	<10
Oxygenation	PaO_2	<70
	$P_{(A-a)}O_2$ (torr)	>450
	Qs/Qt (%)	>20
Ventilation	$PaCO_2$	55
	Vd/Vt	0.60

FEV_1 = forced expiratory volume in 1 minute; $P_{(A-a)}O_2$ = alveolar-arterial oxygen tension gradient; Qs/Qt = shunt fraction; Vd/Vt = dead space to tidal volume ratio.
* = Use ideal body weight.
Reference:
Whitty, J. E. (2004). Airway management in critical illness. In G. A. Dildy, III, M. A. Belfort, G. R. Saade, J. P. Phelan, G. D. V. Hankins, & S. L. Clark, (Eds.). *Critical care obstetrics* (4th ed., pp. 43–59). Malden, MA: Blackwell Science.

to exceed atmospheric pressure. Thus, gas leaves the lungs until pressures are again equal.

Negative pressure ventilator systems are advantageous in that they mimic normal respiration. However, such systems are rarely used except in select out-of-hospital settings.

Positive Pressure

Volume-Cycled

Volume-cycled ventilators are the most frequently used type in most adult critical care settings. The basic principle behind this type of ventilator is that once a designated volume of air is delivered to the patient, inspiration is terminated.

At the moment of cycling, the time taken to deliver the volume, the pressure in the patient circuit (due to the resistance to air flow), and the flow rate may all vary from one respiratory cycle to the next. The only parameter that remains constant is the volume.

Traditionally, volume-cycling is accomplished with the use of a double-circuit ventilator.[2] In these systems, the primary circuit is usually a blower and the secondary circuit comprises a bellows assembly. The volume-cycling mechanism itself can be either pneumatically or electronically operated. Advances in ventilator technology have produced reliable timing and flow-sensing devices that are electronically integrated to measure air

volumes. These devices are now found in single-circuit, volume-cycled systems.

Use of a volume-cycled ventilator requires the clinician to set the volume, flow, and frequency of air delivered. The primary advantage to this type of system is that, despite changes in patient lung compliance, a consistent tidal volume (Vt) is delivered.

Pressure-Cycled

The pressure-cycled ventilator works on the basic principle that once a preset pressure is reached, inspiration is terminated. At this pressure point, the inspiratory valve closes and exhalation occurs passively. At the moment of cycling, the volume of air delivered, the time taken to deliver the volume, and the flow rate may all vary from one respiratory cycle to the next. The only parameter that remains constant is the preset cycling pressure. Pressure-cycling mechanisms in the ventilator may be pneumatic, electronic, or a combination of both.

Clinical judgment dictates the cycling pressure selected. Because the patient's lung condition is not known when ventilatory assistance begins, there is no simple way of predicting the initial pressure requirements. Once the preliminary settings are made, the ventilator is connected to the patient. The volume delivered at that pressure and flow rate is determined with a volume-measuring device. Final adjustments to the cycling pressure and flow rate are then performed based on patient assessment data. If the Vt is too low, the cycling pressure is increased. If the Vt is too high, the cycling pressure is reduced. Clinically, as a patient's lungs become less compliant, the volume of air delivered to the patient may decrease. Thus, to ensure adequate minute ventilation and to detect changes in lung compliance and resistance, inspiratory pressure, rate, and exhaled tidal volume must be monitored frequently.

Although volume-cycled ventilators remain the most frequently used type in most adult situations, pressure-controlled and time-cycled systems are increasingly chosen in select cases. Because high volumes and pressures can lead to lung damage, pressure-controlled ventilation allows the clinician to select and control mean airway pressure as well as peak airway pressure. This may be especially beneficial in patients refractory to conventional ventilation or those with acute respiratory distress syndrome.

Time-Cycled

The time-cycled ventilator works under the basic principle that once a preset time is completed, inspiration is terminated. Expiratory time is determined by inspiratory time and the rate of breaths per minute. This is expressed as inspiratory to expiratory ratio (I:E ratio). The typical I:E ratio is 1:2. This means that for every second of inspiration the ventilator delivers, it allows twice that time for expiration.

Time-cycled machines limit the pressure achieved in the system and cause the ventilator to cycle at a preset interval, thereby setting frequency. Tidal volume (Vt) is varied by adjusting the flow rate and inspiratory time, or by setting minute ventilation and frequency. Many ventilators, especially those used in neonatology, are pressure-limited but time-cycled, allowing the delivered Vt to be highly variable.

MODES OF MECHANICAL VENTILATION

The mode of ventilation generally refers to the interaction between the patient's ventilatory effort and mechanical assistance. There are a variety of modes from which to choose, once the type of ventilator has been selected. Conventional modes include control, assist-control (AC), intermittent mandatory ventilation (IMV), synchronized intermittent mandatory ventilation (SIMV), and continuous positive airway pressure (CPAP). A schematic representing the ventilatory pattern for each is presented in Figure 5-1.[2]

Control

With controlled mandatory ventilation (CMV), the ventilator delivers a preset Vt at a preset number of times per minute. The patient cannot spontaneously ventilate or "trigger" breaths; thus, the machine controls ventilation. This mode is restricted to patients who are apneic as a result of brain injury, sedation, or muscle paralysis. If the patient is conscious or is not paralyzed, this mode can provoke high anxiety and discomfort. Properly functioning ventilator alarms are crucial to the safe use of CMV.

Assist-Control

In the assist-control (AC) mode, the ventilator delivers a breath either when triggered by the patient's inspiratory effort or independently, if such an effort does not occur within a preset period of time. All breaths are delivered under positive pressure by the machine, but unlike CMV, the preset rate can be exceeded by the patient's triggering of additional breaths. This triggering is accomplished by setting a sensitivity detector that identifies a patient breath by the negative pressure the patient uses to initiate inspiration. Particular attention must be paid to proper adjustment of the level of sensitivity of the triggering mechanism. If the ventilator is too sensitive, it may autocycle, whereby it delivers a breath when the patient did not try to initiate inspiration. If it is not sensitive enough, it may require the patient to generate large negative pressure in order to receive additional breaths.

The primary complication associated with this mode of ventilation is respiratory alkalemia. Because every breath, whether triggered by the patient or independently delivered by the ventilator, is at the preset Vt, hyperventilation is possible. This effect may be exacerbated in the obstetric patient because of the compensated respiratory alkalemia that normally accompanies pregnancy. It should be recalled that alkalemia results in a left shift of the oxyhemoglobin dissociation curve, thus making it more difficult for oxygen to be released from hemoglobin to tissues. Concepts related to oxygen transport physiology are presented in Chapter 4.

Intermittent Mandatory Ventilation

Intermittent mandatory ventilation (IMV) allows interspersion of spontaneous breaths by the patient with machine breaths. Spontaneous breaths are at the patient's own Vt, and machine breaths are delivered at the preset Vt. IMV was first introduced in 1971 for use with neonates with respiratory distress syndrome (RDS), because conventional ventilators were unable to deliver the rapid breath rates associated with this condition. Shortly thereafter, it was proposed by Downs and colleagues as an alternative method for weaning adults from mechanical ventilation.[3]

A schematic representation of an IMV circuit is depicted in Figure 5-2.[4] The patient is connected to a common source of oxygen through two parallel circuits. The first contains a volume-cycled ventilator. The other contains a reservoir bag filled with the inhaled gas mixture. A unidirectional valve in the circuit allows the patient to breathe spontaneously from the reservoir bag when a ventilator breath is not being delivered. The pattern of ventilation is such that a machine breath may be delivered at the same time the patient is spontaneously breathing. This concept, referred to as "stacking of breaths," is uncomfortable for the patient and increases volume and pressure in the airway. Current IMV systems eliminate this problem by synchronizing patient and machine breaths.

Synchronized Intermittent Mandatory Ventilation

Synchronized intermittent mandatory ventilation (SIMV) allows spontaneous breathing between mechanically delivered ventilator breaths. In addition, when the ventilator delivers a breath, it will wait until the patient starts inhalation and synchronize the delivered breath. This technique was introduced because of concern that a mechanical breath might be superimposed on a spontaneous breath. It prevents stacking of breaths and concomitant increases in peak inspiratory pressure (PIP), mean airway pressure, and mean intrapleural pressure.

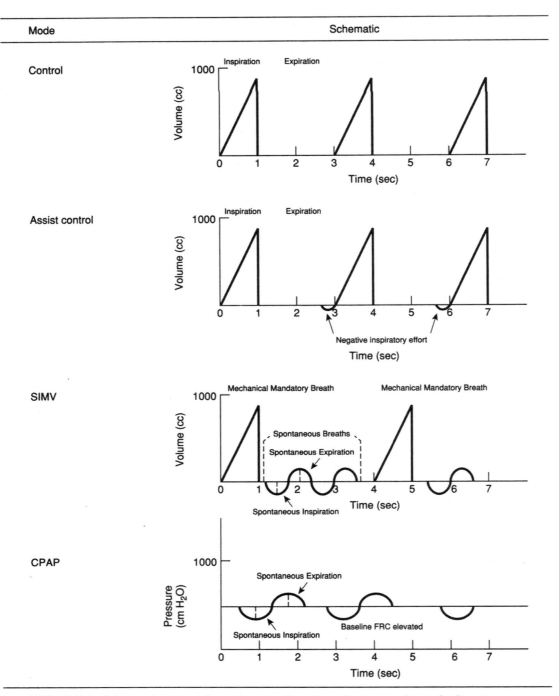

FIGURE 5-1 Schematic comparison of conventional ventilation modes and adjuncts.

It remains one of the most common modes used in obstetric critical care situations.

Continuous Positive Airway Pressure

In continuous positive airway pressure (CPAP), pressure at the airway opening is maintained above atmospheric level throughout the respiratory cycle during spontaneous breathing. CPAP may be delivered through a special mask to patients who do not have an endotracheal or tracheostomy tube. However, the mask must fit exactly so as to prevent air leaks. This mode of ventilation was first used as positive-pressure oxygen breathing to help keep the lungs expanded in patients with crushing chest injuries and to treat infants with RDS.

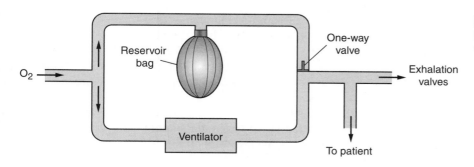

FIGURE 5-2 Schematic representation of an intermittent mandatory ventilation (IMV) circuit.

Gas exchange across the alveolar capillary membrane is promoted as functional residual capacity (FRC) is increased. However, the patient maintains a high level of work in breathing with this mode because she is responsible for all ventilatory effort. The CPAP mode is used more often during weaning from mechanical ventilatory assistance.

ADJUNCTS TO MECHANICAL VENTILATION

Pressure Support Ventilation

Pressure support ventilation (PSV) augments a patient's spontaneous breaths during mechanical ventilation. At the onset of every spontaneous breath, the negative pressure generated by the patient opens a valve that delivers the inspired gas at the desired pressure, usually 5 to 10 cm H_2O. This is designed to increase the Vt and reduce the work of breathing. In essence, the pressure boost is delivered to overcome resistance in the endotracheal tube and ventilator circuit tubing.

Newer microprocessor-driven mechanical ventilators include pressure-support modes that operate in conjunction with their demand-flow valve systems. The principal advantages of PSV are decreased work of breathing for the patient and improved subjective reports of comfort.

Positive End-Expiratory Pressure

Mechanical ventilation with positive end-expiratory pressure (PEEP) is designed for any pulmonary condition with widespread alveolar collapse. A pressure-limiting valve in the expiratory tubing prevents pressure in the airways from returning to atmospheric pressure at the end of expiration. This positive pressure in the alveoli at end-expiration helps prevent alveolar collapse and promotes gas exchange across the alveolar–capillary interface. This ventilatory adjunct increases the FRC, the lung volume at end-expiration. In select patients, this increases alveolar participation in gas exchange and allows the fractional concentration of inspired oxygen (FiO_2) to be lowered.

NEWER METHODS OF MECHANICAL VENTILATION AND OXYGENATION

The primary purposes of mechanical ventilation are to achieve adequate alveolar ventilation and to improve oxygen exchange. Traditionally, volume-limited ventilation used alone or with spontaneous breathing has been the only form of mechanical assistance commonly used in adults. In addition, enrichment of FiO_2 and the addition of positive end-expiratory pressure have been the principal means of improving oxygenation. Over time, newer techniques have been introduced to clinical practice. Because the majority of these newer modes are pressure-cycled, independent volume monitoring is highly desirable.

Pressure Control and Inverse I:E Ratio

It has been common practice in mechanically ventilated patients to allow at least as much time for exhalation as for inhalation. The rationale for this concept is to prevent the trapping of gas in the airways. However, gas exchange may be markedly improved when the I:E ratio is forced to values greater than 1:1. This principle is known as inverse ratio ventilation (IRV) or inverse I:E ratio ventilation. It has been applied clinically to neonates with hyaline membrane disease as well as adults with refractory acute respiratory distress syndrome and other forms of hypoxemia.

This method of ventilation may be accomplished in at least two ways. First, the rate of flow delivery during conventional volume ventilation may be decreased. More commonly, pressure-controlled ventilation is utilized. This involves maintenance of pressure at a controlled level for a fixed period of time.

The mechanism for the improvement of oxygenation with this method remains uncertain, although increased mean intrathoracic pressure and increased lung volume are most likely involved. Sustained tethering forces may recruit lung units that would otherwise remain collapsed, and units with very slow time constraints may be given sufficient time to ventilate.[5]

Advantages of IRV include improved oxygenation and reduced peak cycling pressures. A disadvantage of

IRV is a higher mean intrathoracic pressure, which may impede venous return and contribute to barotrauma. It should also be noted that patient cooperation is essential; thus, adequate sedation is crucial.

High-Frequency Ventilation

High-frequency ventilation (HFV) is a collective term that refers to modes of ventilation in which tidal volumes smaller than anatomic deadspace are moved at frequencies that range from 60 to 3,000 cycles per minute. High-frequency positive pressure ventilation (HFPPV) is identical in concept to conventional ventilation, with the exception that tidal volumes are very small and cycling frequencies are very fast. High-frequency jet ventilation (HFJV) works in a somewhat different way. With this method, a small-diameter injecting catheter is positioned in the central airway. This catheter then pulses gas along the axis of the lumen under high pressure at a rapid cycling rate, usually between 60 and 240 cycles per minute. HFJV is the most common type of HFV used in adult settings.

Yet another type of HFV is high frequency oscillation (HFO). This method works on the principle that very small volumes of gas (1 to 3 mL/kg) are moved back and forth by a piston at extremely high frequencies (500 to 3,000 cycles per minute).

All forms of HFV are characterized by lower peak airway pressures than conventional ventilation. Peripheral airway pressure is generally higher than measured central airway pressure, and mean alveolar pressure may not differ greatly from those observed during conventional ventilation. With rare exception, HFV does not produce cardiovascular side effects associated with conventional ventilation. HFV is generally utilized in carefully selected clinical situations, and data regarding use during pregnancy have not been reported.

Liquid Ventilation

Liquid ventilation involves instillation of a sterile perfluorocarbon into the lungs. The substance has a low surface tension and a very high solubility for oxygen and carbon dioxide. Oxygen is about 20 times more soluble in perfluorocarbons than in water, whereas carbon dioxide is about three times as soluble.[6] The first human trials of liquid ventilation were reported in 1989 and demonstrated the ability of perfluorocarbon to adequately support gas exchange in moribund infants.[7] Since that time, investigation has continued with respect to application in adult, pediatric, and neonatal populations.

The physiologic basis for use of liquid ventilation focuses on alteration of alveolar surface tension. The surface tension in the alveolus is a function of the air-fluid interfaces that line the alveoli. This tension can be reduced by filling the alveoli with fluid rather than gas because this eliminates the air-fluid interfaces.[8] Instillation of perfluorocarbon liquid may offer advantages to an injured lung for a number of reasons. Because perfluorocarbon is heavier than water, it tends to trickle down to the dependent regions of the lungs, which are usually more atelectatic.[9] In addition, instillation of liquid into the lungs physically opens and maintains the patency of dependent alveoli and provides a medium for gas exchange in areas of the lungs not previously ventilated.

Generally, there are two types of liquid ventilation. Total liquid ventilation (TLV) refers to replacement of the FRC of the lung by instillation of a perfluorocarbon liquid. Gas exchange is accomplished by inspiration and expiration of Vt of liquid.[10] This requires a special device to deliver and remove Vt of liquid and to extracorporeally oxygenate and remove carbon dioxide from the liquid. Partial liquid ventilation (PLV) involves intratracheal instillation of perfluorocarbon liquid equal to the FRC of the lungs during conventional mechanical ventilation.

ADVANCED MODES OF MECHANICAL VENTILATION

The primary goal of all ventilator modes is to maintain adequate oxygenation and ventilation, reduce the work of breathing, and improve patient comfort for the duration of respiratory compromise. This has led to the development of a variety of ventilation modes and applications that may reduce complications and shorten the duration of mechanical ventilation, resulting in improved patient outcomes.

Recent advances in ventilator modes have focused on three key areas.[11] First, modes have been developed that incorporate guaranteed control of both pressure and volume settings so as to obtain the benefits of both styles of ventilation. An example of this type of dual-control mode is pressure-regulated volume control (PRVC). Second, pressure style modes have been developed that allow spontaneous breathing to occur during both high-and low-pressure settings. This facilitates spontaneous breathing in the early phase of acute lung injury as well as during the weaning period. Examples of these modes include biphasic positive airway pressure (BiPAP) and airway pressure release ventilation (APRV). Third, advances in microcomputer technology have enabled the development of advanced closed-loop systems that allow the ventilator, as opposed to clinicians, the ability to manipulate ventilator variables based on feedback from patient data. Detailed descriptions of each of these modes are beyond the scope of this text.

Increasingly, critical care providers need to develop a sophisticated level of understanding of mechanical ventilation and accompanying respiratory physiology to ensure safe and effective management of patients ventilated by these advanced modes. Although physiological benefits have been identified, there are few reported large clinical studies that evaluate the efficacy of these modes; hence, further research is required.

COMPLICATIONS

Initiation of mechanical ventilatory assistance is accompanied by the potential for numerous complications (Box 5-1).

Cardiovascular

Mechanical ventilation results in major alterations in a patient's cardiopulmonary physiology. The normal transpulmonary pressure gradient, usually generated by a decrease in intrathoracic pressure, is functionally reversed, because an elevation in airway pressure is used to inflate the lungs during inspiration. As a result, mechanical ventilatory support results not only in efficient pulmonary excretion of carbon dioxide and adequate oxygenation of the pulmonary capillary blood, but also in perturbations in central hemodynamic and peripheral blood flow.[12]

One of the most significant risks of mechanical ventilation is decreased cardiac output. This may occur for several reasons. First, positive pressure ventilation can cause a reduction in venous return, resulting in reduced preload. Use of PEEP, especially at high levels, may exacerbate this effect. A second factor that may contribute to decreased cardiac output is related to right ventricular afterload. Pulmonary vascular resistance (PVR), the afterload that must be overcome by the right ventricle during systole, is increased as large tidal volumes and pressures are pushed into the lungs. This increase in volume and pressure stretches the intra-alveolar vessels and decreases their lumen size, thus increasing resistance to blood flow. Finally, two important factors impact left ventricular compliance and may decrease cardiac output. An increase in right ventricular afterload may over time lead to increased right ventricular preload. This increased volume of blood in the right ventricle may result in a shift of the interventricular septum to the left, thus reducing left ventricular compliance. The workload required of the left ventricle is thereby increased significantly. In general, from a cardiovascular standpoint, patients with normal to increased intravascular volume tolerate mechanical ventilation best.

Barotrauma

Barotrauma is a general term that refers to consequences of alveolar over-distention. Varied forms of barotrauma include interstitial emphysema, pneumomediastinum, pneumoperitoneum, subcutaneous emphysema, cyst formation, and pneumothorax. Generally, air can gain access to the pleural space in two ways. First, a disruption may occur in the visceral pleura, facilitated by obstructed airways, parenchymal inflammation, and necrosis. In addition, over-distention and rupture of individual alveoli may allow interstitial air to escape along bronchi and vessels to the mediastinum. From there, it enters soft tissues and may perforate the thin mediastinal pleura and cause a pneumothorax. If intrapleural air continues to gather in the closed intrathoracic cavity, a tension pneumothorax may result.

The patients most at risk for barotrauma usually have underlying lung disease, such as acute respiratory distress syndrome (ARDS), also known as acute lung injury (ALI), or chronic obstructive pulmonary disease (COPD). In addition, the risk of barotrauma is increased in patients with high mean inspiratory pressures (PIP) and who are receiving high levels of PEEP.

Clinical signs and symptoms of pneumothorax are presented in Table 5-2. Nursing management includes notification of the patient's physician and preparation for immediate insertion of a chest tube. Urgent decompression may be accomplished with a large-bore catheter-over-needle attached to a large syringe. A chest x-ray should also be obtained if a pneumothorax is suspected.

Box 5-1. COMPLICATIONS OF MECHANICAL VENTILATION

Cardiac
- Decreased cardiac output
- Dysrhythmias
- Decreased blood pressure

Pulmonary
- Tracheal injury
- Vocal cord injury
- Barotrauma
- Oxygen toxicity
- Hypoventilation
- Hyperventilation
- Atelectasis

Fluid imbalance

Infection

Gastrointestinal
- Stress ulcer
- Ileus

TABLE 5-2

Clinical Signs and Symptoms of Pneumothorax

Subtle	Pleuritic pain
	Shortness of breath
	Venous distention
	Accelerated rate of breathing
	Gradual increase in mean inspiratory pressure
	Unilateral decrease in breath sounds or chest movement
Acute or Severe	Bradycardia
	Shock-like appearance
	Cyanosis
	Loss of consciousness
	Tracheal and/or mediastinal shift
	Sudden rise in mean inspiratory pressure

Fluid Imbalance

Fluid retention, or development of a positive water balance, is fairly common in patients receiving mechanical ventilation. This condition occurs for a number of reasons. As increased intrathoracic pressure limits venous return, stretch receptors in the atria signal for additional antidiuretic hormone (ADH). This facilitates replenishment of intravascular volume. Compression of the atria from hyperinflated lungs may decrease atrial natriuretic factor (ANF), which in turn further increases ADH. In addition, hypotension caused by positive-pressure ventilation may decrease renal perfusion, redistribute renal blood flow, decrease glomerular filtration, and promote sodium retention.

The intrinsic advantage of this accumulation of fluid may be to promote cardiac output in the face of high intrathoracic pressures. However, the negative effects of central hypervolemia, including pulmonary vascular congestion and impaired gas exchange, should not be overlooked. As positive-pressure ventilation is discontinued, these fluid shifts usually reverse and may actually cause cardiac decompensation in the patient with poor hemodynamic reserve.

Infection

The major sites for health care–associated infections (HAIs) in the intensive care setting are the respiratory system, the urinary tract, and the bloodstream. Infections of the lungs and upper respiratory tract are increasingly common during mechanical ventilation. Based on current data from the Centers for Disease Control and Prevention (CDC), pneumonia accounts for approximately 15 percent of all HAIs and 26 percent of HAIs in adult and pediatric intensive care units.[13] Current estimates include a 6- to 20-fold increase in the incidence of pneumonia in patients receiving mechanical ventilation. In addition, patients with bacterial pneumonia are also at risk for bacteremia and thus are at significant increased risk for mortality.

A number of factors associated with the use of mechanical ventilation are responsible for the increased risk of infection. Endotracheal intubation prevents glottis closure, disrupts the laryngeal barrier, slows the mucociliary escalator, impedes secretion clearance, and provides an open pathway for large quantities of aspirated pharyngeal bacteria and fungi to inoculate the lung. In addition, patients exposed to respiratory therapy equipment have a higher risk for HAIs because of equipment contamination. Most cases of ventilator-associated pneumonia (VAP) are caused by repeated aspiration of pathogens that have colonized the mucosal surfaces of the oropharynx. These organisms usually reach the lungs in a liquid bolus, such as the condensate that accumulates in ventilator tubing. Intubated patients also often receive antacids through a nasogastric tube to decrease gastric acidity and prevent stress ulcers. However, as the pH of the gastric acid increases, the acid loses its bactericidal effect on gram-negative organisms. Thus, aspiration of gastrointestinal contents may initiate the colonization of bacteria, which results in pneumonia.

The CDC, in collaboration with other organizations, has developed guidelines for the prevention of VAP and other types of health care–associated pneumonia.[14] VAP data are reported to the CDC's National Healthcare Safety Network (NHSN) from health care facilities across the United States. In addition, the Joint Commission has included reduction of VAP as a National Patient Safety Goal and has endorsed strategies to achieve this goal.[15]

CLINICAL CARE ISSUES

Caring for an obstetric patient who requires mechanical ventilation presents unique challenges. Data related to patient characteristics and delivery rates associated with mechanical ventilation in an obstetric population have been reported.[16] Collected data included maternal demographics, medical condition that necessitated mechanical ventilatory support, delivery status, duration of ventilation, onset of parturition while receiving ventilation, mode of delivery, and maternal and early neonatal morbidity or death.[17] A summary of results from the study is presented in Table 5-3. The three most common diagnoses that led to complications and the need for mechanical ventilation were preeclampsia or eclampsia (43 percent), labor or preterm labor (14 percent), and pneumonia

TABLE 5-3

Characteristics of Obstetric Patients Requiring Mechanical Ventilation

Demographic and delivery characteristics in a group of 51 obstetric patients who needed mechanical ventilation

Characteristic	Value
Age* (years)	28 ± 7.4
Gravidity* (number)	3.0 ± 2.1
Parity* (number)	1.3 ± 1.9
Race (%)	
White	56
African American	38
Asian, other	6
Estimated gestational age on admission* (weeks)	31.6 ± 5.1
Length of stay* (days)	10.9 ± 3.6
Days on ventilator*	3.4 ± 3.6
Pulmonary artery catheter used (number)	33 (65%)
Undelivered on admission (number)	43
Delivered during admission (number)	37 (86%)
Vaginal delivery (number)	13 (35%)
Cesarean delivery (number)	24 (65%)
Labor during ventilation (number)	11 (30%)
EGA at delivery* (weeks)	32.6 ± 4.9
Birth weight* (grams)	2131 ± 1906
Neonatal intensive care nursery admission (number)	28 (76%)
Fetal/neonatal death (number)	4 (11%)
Maternal deaths (number)	7 (14%)

*Data expressed as mean ± standard deviation.

(12 percent). Overall, 43 (84 percent) of the 51 patients included in the study were cared for in a labor and delivery unit with critical care obstetric capabilities. Care was directed by a critical care perinatologist, a critical care obstetric nurse, with consultation and collaboration provided by other intensivists, depending on the patient's clinical situation.

Guidelines for care of the obstetric patient requiring mechanical ventilation are presented elsewhere in this text. A description of select clinical care issues follows.

Initial Settings and Goals

Following successful endotracheal intubation, the ventilator is connected to the patient. Initial ventilator settings are dependent on the patient's disease process and the overall plan of care. However, most often, a positive-pressure volume-cycled ventilator is used for the obstetric patient. The SIMV mode is often utilized during pregnancy. It should be recalled that, because of the normal compensatory respiratory alkalemia associated with pregnancy, use of assist-control may precipitate respiratory alkalemia more quickly than when used in non-pregnant women. General guidelines for initial settings and goals are presented in Table 5-4.[18]

Arterial blood gases are usually obtained within 15 to 30 minutes following initiation of ventilatory support. Initial settings are adjusted based on assessment data related to oxygenation and ventilation. Changes in ventilator settings are ordered by the patient's physician and made by respiratory therapy personnel. However, policies in individual institutions may address the issue of which professional personnel may make changes in settings in urgent situations.

Monitoring Ventilation and Oxygenation

In a critically ill obstetric patient, adequate oxygenation is essential for recovery. The quality of ventilation directly impacts the patient's oxygenation status. For these reasons, it is important to monitor both the ventilation and oxygenation status of all patients receiving ventilatory support. Common parameters used to assess

TABLE 5-4

General Guidelines for Initial Ventilator Settings and Goals

Initial Settings	Mode	SIMV
	Rate	12–14 breaths per minute (set)
	Tidal volume (Vt)	12–15 mL/kg
	PEEP	5 cm H_2O
	FiO_2	1.0 (depends on reason for intubation)
Goals	PaO_2	>60
	SaO_2	>95%
	$PaCO_2$	27–32
	FiO_2	<0.50

FiO_2 = fraction of inspired oxygen; $PaCO_2$ = arterial carbon dioxide pressure; PaO_2 = arterial oxygen pressure; PEEP = post end-expiratory pressure; SaO_2 = arterial oxygen saturation; SIMV = synchronized intermittent mandatory ventilation.

TABLE 5-5

Common Parameters Used to Assess Ventilation and Oxygenation Status

Parameter		Formula
Arterial oxygen content (CaO_2)	mL/dL	$(1.34 \times Hgb \times SaO_2) + (PaO_2 \times 0.0031)$
Venous oxygen content (CvO_2)	mL/dL	$(1.34 \times Hgb \times SvO_2) + (PvO_2 \times 0.0031)$
Arteriovenous oxygen difference ($avDO_2$)	mL/dL	$CaO_2 - CvO_2$
Oxygen delivery (DO_2)	mL/min	$CaO_2 \times CO \times 10$
Oxygen consumption (VO_2)	mL/min	$avDO_2 \times CO \times 10$
Oxygen extraction ratio (O_2ER)	%	$VO_2 \div DO_2$
Shunt fraction (Qs/Qt)	%	$100 \times (1.34 \times Hgb \div 0.0031) \times (PAO_2 - CaO_2)$
		$(1.34 \times Hgb \div 0.0031) \times PAO_2 - CvO_2)$
Alveolar-arterial oxygen difference ($AaDO_2$)	mmHg	$PAO_2 - PaO_2$

CO = cardiac output; Hgb = hemoglobin; PaO_2 = arterial oxygen tension; PAO_2 = alveolar oxygen tension; PvO_2 = venous oxygen tension; SaO_2 = arterial oxygen saturation; SvO_2 = mixed venous oxygen saturation.

these functions are presented in Table 5-5. A discussion of select parameters follows.

It should be recalled that oxygen delivery (DO_2), the total amount of oxygen made available to tissues per minute, is dependent on cardiac output (CO), arterial oxygen content (CaO_2, which consists of the concentration of hemoglobin), saturation of hemoglobin with oxygen in the arterial system (SaO_2), and, to a small degree, the amount of oxygen dissolved under pressure in the plasma (PaO_2). These concepts are discussed at length in Chapter 4.

Oxygen consumption (VO_2), the total amount of oxygen consumed globally by tissues per minute, is dependent on CO, venous oxygen content (CvO_2, which, similar to CaO_2, depends on the concentration of hemoglobin), saturation of hemoglobin with oxygen in the venous system (SvO_2), and the amount of oxygen dissolved under pressure in venous blood (PvO_2). The relationship between VO_2 and DO_2 is expressed in the oxygen extraction ratio (O_2ER). This helps to estimate oxygen reserve in the critically ill patient. Three additional hemodynamic parameters that are important to assess include shunt fraction (Qs/Qt), alveolar-arterial oxygen difference ($AaDO_2$), and the ratio of arterial oxygen pressure to fraction of inspired oxygen ($PaO_2:FiO_2$ ratio).

Shunt Fraction

This variable, the percent arteriovenous shunt, expresses the extent to which arterial blood is less than maximally oxygenated as it leaves the heart. A certain percentage of venous blood bypasses the pulmonary capillaries, even in healthy people. Some venous return from the bronchial arteries and the coronary circulation flows to the left side of the heart without being oxygenated. A shunt fraction (Qs/Qt) in a healthy person is usually between 3 and 5 percent. An elevated Qs/Qt is compatible

with a number of clinical conditions, including those where there is inadequate alveolar participation in gas exchange.

Alveolar-Arterial Oxygen Difference

The alveolar-arterial oxygen difference ($AaDO_2$) measures the difference in partial pressure of oxygen between the alveoli and the arteries. It characterizes the efficiency of oxygen exchange between the lung alveoli and the pulmonary capillaries. Normal values of $AaDO_2$ are from 10 to 15 mmHg for a patient breathing room air, and from 10 to 65 mmHg for a patient breathing 100 percent oxygen ($FiO_2 = 1.0$). The $AaDO_2$ gradient increases approximately 5 to 7 mmHg for every 10 percent increase in FiO_2. An abnormally large drop in oxygen partial pressure from alveoli to arteries may indicate impending respiratory failure.

Arterial PO_2 Fraction of Inspired Oxygen Ratio

The ratio between arterial oxygen pressure and the fraction of inspired oxygen ($PaO_2:FiO_2$) is a simple method that has been shown to correlate with changes in Qs/Qt. When this ratio is less than 200, the Qs/Qt may be estimated at greater than 20 percent. Conversely, when this ratio is greater than 200, the Qs/Qt may be estimated to be less than 20 percent.[19]

Ventilation calculations are most meaningful under the steady state of controlled ventilation when tidal volume can be unambiguously determined. The static nature of these formulae does not allow accurate determination of ventilatory parameters under SIMV ventilation. Thus, adjustments should be taken into consideration when applying clinical meaning to these parameters during SIMV.

Minute Volume

Minute volume is a measurement of the volume of gas exchanged in the lungs per minute. It is calculated as the product of the Vt, the volume of gas inspired or expired during each respiratory cycle, and the respiratory rate. Normal ranges of minute volume are approximately 2.5 to 7 liters per minute (L/min), with wide variations, especially during pregnancy. Because it is a measure of gas drawn into the lungs in a respiratory cycle, it includes both effective alveolar ventilation and the dead space ventilation. Thus, it is a good index of ventilation when used in conjunction with blood gas analysis.

Minute volume increases in response to hypoxemia, hypercarbia, and acidemia. It decreases in the presence of opposite clinical conditions. One clinical condition associated with decreased minute volume is pulmonary edema.

Compliance

Compliance may be expressed as either dynamic or static. Dynamic compliance is defined as the volume increase corresponding to each unit of pressure increase in the alveoli. It is calculated as the volume change during a breath divided by the change in transpulmonary pressure from end-inspiration. This pressure change is the difference in the peak inspiratory pressure and the positive end-expiratory pressure. The normal range of dynamic compliance is typically 25 to 35 mL/cmH$_2$O pressure. As compliance increases, the lung is less stiff and requires less pressure to produce a given tidal volume. A sudden decrease in compliance may indicate an airway obstruction.

Dead Space

Physiologic dead space (Vd) refers to the volume of the lungs that is ventilated but not perfused by pulmonary capillary blood flow. This does not contribute to gas exchange and may be considered wasted ventilation. Normal Vd in healthy people is usually 145 to 155 mL at rest. This is approximately 20 to 30 percent of each tidal volume. This amount may be increased in clinical conditions where blood flow is obstructed through pulmonary capillaries. It also may increase with over- or under-ventilation of normally perfused alveoli.

In addition to assessment of these derived calculations, clinical care should include assessment of the patient's hemodynamic and oxygenation status. These measures are outlined in the care guidelines in the last section of this text. Adjuncts useful in this assessment include pulse oximetry and end-tidal CO$_2$ monitoring via capnography.

Airway Care

Care of the airway of the mechanically ventilated patient includes provision of adequate humidification, measures to mobilize secretions, position changes, suctioning, and the use of bactericidal mouth swabs as outlined in the CDC VAP prevention guidelines. Humidification and warming of inspired gas are provided mechanically as adjuncts to the ventilator. Mobilization of secretions is most often accomplished by position change and chest physiotherapy.

Suctioning

Because it exposes the patient to risks including infection, hypoxemia, atelectasis, and aspiration, suctioning should be performed only when necessary. In general, suctioning is indicated when rhonchi are auscultated or secretions are heard during respiration. An increase in ventilator peak inspiratory pressures (PIP) may indicate the presence of a mucous plug or narrowing of the airways secondary to secretions.

Various strategies have been described to decrease the risk of suction-induced hypoxemia. In a nonobstetric population, a 25 to 30 percent drop in oxygen saturation has been reported, followed by a slow rise back to baseline over a 3-minute period, during endotracheal suctioning.[20] Recommendations based on this finding include the use of intermittent suction for less than 15 seconds. Prolonged, continuous suctioning causes microatelectasis and reduction of the oxygen concentration in the tracheobronchial tree. Additional methods of reducing hypoxemia include preoxygenation, hyperoxygenation, hyperinflation, and hyperventilation. A description of each of these practices is presented in Table 5-6.

TABLE 5-6

Methods of Reducing Suction-induced Hypoxemia

Technique	Description
Hyperinflation	Increasing the tidal volume to 1½ times the preset ventilation volume by the use of a resuscitation bag or the "sigh" function of the ventilator
Preoxygenation	Administration of oxygen before suctioning
Hyperoxygenation	Administration of oxygen at a greater FiO$_2$ than the preset ventilator level
Hyperventilation	Increasing the respiratory/ventilator rate without changing tidal volume or oxygen concentration

Box 5-2. FACTORS CONTRIBUTING TO DISTRESS DURING MECHANICAL VENTILATION

- Inability to speak
- Pain and discomfort from endotracheal tube
- Suctioning
- Inability to determine time of day, date, or nature of surroundings
- Noise
  - From other patients
  - Alarms
  - Water movement in ventilator tubing
  - Care providers talking
  - Telephone
- Concern for nearby patients
- Lack of sleep
- Bright lights
- Weaning
- Position and infrequent position change
- Pulling of ventilator tubing
- Inability to see doors or windows
- Being paralyzed while remaining alert
- Sight of unfamiliar equipment

PSYCHOSOCIAL SUPPORT

Use of mechanical ventilation subjects the patient to physical and emotional stress in the critical care environment. It is also a stressful time for the patient's family and support system. Factors that may contribute to emotional stress are presented in Box 5-2. Factors that are particularly stressful are related to the inability to speak and the pain and discomfort associated with the presence and manipulation of the endotracheal tube. Every possible effort should be made to relieve physical discomfort, minimize manipulation of the endotracheal tube, facilitate communication, and include family and support system in the provision of care. This is especially relevant when providing care to a patient who needs mechanical ventilation during pregnancy.

CONSIDERATIONS RELATED TO DELIVERY OF THE FETUS

For the undelivered obstetric patient requiring mechanical ventilation, an integral component of care is fetal surveillance. The method selected for surveillance and the frequency of assessment vary depending on the estimated gestational age of the fetus. Guidelines for fetal monitoring, including interpretation of data, are presented elsewhere in this text.

Limited data exist to guide decision making with respect to the timing and mode of delivery in this patient population. A small retrospective study conditionally suggested that delivery may improve maternal status in ventilated women, and some authors have suggested that elective delivery is indicated for women in late pregnancy who have ARDS and are clinically stable.[21,22] Other studies have not supported an improvement in maternal condition secondary to delivery of the fetus.[23,24]

Given the risk of inducing labor or performing a Cesarean delivery, the indications for delivery should be based on obstetric indications until more evidence is available.[25] Although vaginal delivery may not be well tolerated in a woman with ARDS due to increased oxygen consumption, Cesarean delivery results in fluid shifts and blood loss that are both larger and more rapid than occur with vaginal delivery and may thus present a greater physiologic stress.[16,26] Attempts should be made to optimize maternal oxygenation during labor and subsequent vaginal delivery. A more thorough discussion of induction of labor in the obstetric patient with complications may be found in Chapter 12.

SUMMARY

Caring for the obstetric patient requiring mechanical ventilation presents unique challenges to the health care team. Irrespective of the location in which care is provided, clinicians should enhance their knowledge base with respect to reasons pregnant women develop respiratory compromise sufficient to require intubation and ventilatory support. In addition, clinical care should be based on a framework that incorporates the significant physiologic alterations associated with pregnancy. The need for collaboration is essential in order to optimize maternal and fetal outcomes.

REFERENCES

1. Whitty, J. E. (2004). Airway management in critical illness. In G. A. Dildy, M. A. Belfort, G. R. Saade, J. P. Phelan, G. D. V. Hankins, & S. L. Clark, (Eds.), *Critical care obstetrics* (4th ed., pp. 43–59). Malden, MA: Blackwell Science.
2. Troiano, N. H., & Dorman, K. (1992). Mechanical ventilation during pregnancy. *NAACOGS Clinical Issues in Perinatal and Women's Health Nursing, 3*(3), 399–407.
3. Downs, J. B., Klein, E. F., Desautels, D., et al. (1973). IMV: A new approach to weaning patients from mechanical ventilators. *Chest, 87,* 612–618.
4. Marino, P. L. (1991). Modes of mechanical ventilation. In P. L. Marino (Ed.), *The ICU book.* Philadelphia: Lea & Febiger/Williams & Wilkins.
5. Marini, J. J., & Wheeler, A. P. (1989). Mechanical ventilation. In J. J. Marini & A. P. Wheeler (Eds.), *Critical care medicine: The essentials.* Baltimore: Williams & Wilkins.
6. Schaffer, T. H., Wolfson, M. R., & Clark, L. C., Jr. (1992). Liquid ventilation. *Pediatric Pulmonology, 14,* 102–109.

7. Greenspan, J. S., Wolfson, M. R., Rubenstein, D., & Shaffer, T. H. (1990). Liquid ventilation of human preterm neonates. *The Journal of Pediatrics, 117*(1), 106–111.

8. Tutuncu, H., Faithful, S., & Lachman, B. (1993). Intrathecal perfluorocarbon administration combined with mechanical ventilation in experimental respiratory distress syndrome. *Critical Care Medicine, 1*(7), 962–969.

9. Dirkes, S. (1996). Liquid ventilation: New frontiers in the treatment of ARDS. *Critical Care Nurse, 16,* 53–58.

10. Fuhrman, B. P., Paczan, P. R., & DeFrancis, M. (1991). Perfluorocarbon-associated gas exchange. *Critical Care Medicine, 19*(5), 712–722.

11. Rose, L. (2006). Advanced modes of mechanical ventilation. *AACN Advanced Critical Care, 17*(2), 145–160.

12. Schweiger, J. W., & Dresden, J. (1997). Monitoring during ventilatory support. In M. C. Stock & A. Perel (Eds.), *Handbook of mechanical ventilatory support* (2nd ed.). Philadelphia: Lippincott Williams & Wilkins.

13. Centers for Disease Control and Prevention. (2010). *Ventilator-associated pneumonia (VAP): Resources for patients and healthcare providers.* Retrieved from http://www.cdc.gov/HAI/vap/vap.html

14. Coffin, S. E., Klompas, M., Classen, D., Arias, K. M., Podgorny, K., Anderson, D. J., et al. (2008). Supplement article: SHEA/IDSA practice recommendation. Strategies to prevent ventilator-associated pneumonia in acute care hospitals. *Infection Control and Hospital Epidemiology, 29,* S31–S40.

15. Joint Commission. (2011). *National patient safety goals.* Retrieved from http://www.jointcommission.org/standards_information/npsgs.aspx

16. Jenkins, T. M., Troiano, N. H., Graves, C. R., Baird, S. M., & Boehm, F. H. (2003). Mechanical ventilation in an obstetric population: Characteristics and delivery rates. *American Journal of Obstetrics & Gynecology, 188*(2), 549–552.

17. Baird, S. M., & Troiano, N. H. (2010). Critical care obstetric nursing. In M. A. Belfort, G. R. Saade, M. R. Foley, J. P. Phelan, & G. A. Dildy, III. (Eds.), *Critical care obstetrics* (5th ed.). Hoboken, NJ: Wiley-Blackwell.

18. Clark, S. L., Cotton, D. B., Hankins, G. D. V., & Phelan, J. P. (1994). Adult respiratory distress syndrome. In *Handbook of critical care obstetrics.* Cambridge, MA: Blackwell Science.

19. Ahrens, T. S., Beattie, S., & Nienhaus, T. (1996). Experimental therapies to support the failing lung. *AACN Clinical Issues, 7*(4), 507–518.

20. Stone, K. S., & Turner, B. (1989). Endotracheal suctioning. *Annual Review of Nursing Research, 7,* 27–47.

21. Catanzarite, V., Willms, D., Wong, D., Landers, C., Cousins, L., & Schrimmer, D. (2001). Acute respiratory distress syndrome in pregnancy and the puerperium: Causes, courses, and outcomes. *Obstetrics & Gynecology, 97*(5 Pt 1), 760–764.

22. Tomlinson, M. W., Caruthers, T. J., Whitty, J. E., & Gonik, B. (1998). Does delivery improve maternal condition in the respiratory-compromised gravida? *Obstetrics & Gynecology, 91,* 108–111.

23. Mabie, W. C., Barton, J. R., & Sibai, B. M. (1992). Adult respiratory distress syndrome in pregnancy. *American Journal of Obstetrics & Gynecology, 167*(4 Pt 1), 950–957.

24. Collop, N. A., & Sahn, S. A. (1993). Critical illness in pregnancy: An analysis of 20 patients admitted to a medical intensive care unit. *Chest, 103,* 1548–1552.

25. Cole, D. E., Taylor, T. L., McCullough, D. M., Shoff, C. T., & Derdak, S. (2005). Acute respiratory distress syndrome in pregnancy. *Critical Care Medicine, 33*(Suppl. 10), 269–278.

26. Sauer, P. M. (1997). Maternal-fetal assessment of the critically ill parturient: Decisions related to delivery. *AACN Clinical Issues, 8,* 564–573.

CHAPTER 6

Pharmacologic Agents

Suzanne McMurtry Baird, Stephen D. Krau, and Michael A. Belfort

Women who become critically ill during pregnancy or birth generally require medications to stabilize their condition and optimize outcomes. The goals for medication administration vary according to the patient's specific clinical condition and assessment findings. The goals also seek to minimize potential undesirable side effects for the fetus and/or neonate. Because randomized clinical trials of medication administration to stabilize critically ill pregnant women are limited, most recommendations for dosage and administration are based on retrospective reviews, case reports, and expert opinion. This chapter discusses general principles of perinatal drug safety and examines the characteristics of select agents commonly used in critical care. It also presents select dosage recommendations specific to pregnancy, potential interactions with other medications, precautions for select drugs, and unknown maternal, fetal and/or neonatal effects.

DRUG SAFETY

Medication errors, including infusions, are one of the most common preventable causes of harm to patients in health care agencies. Such errors account for approximately 33 percent of incident reports electronically submitted, and are the seventh leading cause of Sentinel Events reported to the Joint Commission.[1,2] Reducing the risks of drug administration is a requirement for all areas of clinical practice. Data from reporting systems, published case reports, and surveys of more than 770 health care practitioners, were recently evaluated by the Institute for Safe Medication Practices, resulting in a published list of high-alert medications (Table 6-1). Medications on the list are more likely to cause significant patient harm when compared with other groups of medications and have more reported administration errors.[3] Frequently, medications on the

high-alert list are administered to high-risk and critically ill pregnant women. Therefore, in order to promote patient safety, a medication's mechanism of action, correct dose, recognized drug interactions, and precautions regarding administration should be known. Safe-practice strategies to decrease the inherent risk when prescribing, dispensing, and administering these medications should also be developed in clinical agencies.

FETAL AND NEWBORN EFFECTS

In the critically ill gravida, fetal and newborn outcomes are usually dependent upon timely maternal stabilization. Many of the medications administered for the purpose of maternal stabilization have a direct effect on uterine blood flow or uterine activity. Some cross the placental barrier and have varying effects on the fetal heart rate (FHR). Potential effects include baseline FHR changes, suppression or exaggeration of decelerations, frequency and amplitude of accelerations, and degree of variability.[4] Therefore, as a result, it is difficult for the health care provider to determine whether changes in fetal status are a result of a specific medication that has been administered, physiologic variation, or both. For example, if maternal oxygen delivery is impaired and leads to a decrease in uterine perfusion and fetal oxygenation, the electronic fetal monitor (EFM) may no longer show signs of fetal well-being. Although there are no predictive or diagnostic EFM tracings for fetal hypoxia, assessment parameters that have been associated with fetal stress include the combination of fetal tachycardia, absent or minimal baseline variability, and recurrent late decelerations. Specific information related to FHR assessment may be found in the *Guidelines for Fetal Heart Rate Monitoring,* which includes a description of the three-tiered classification system used to collectively interpret assessment findings. Sustained

TABLE 6-1

High-Alert Medications

Classes/Categories of Medications

adrenergic agonists, IV (e.g., epinephrine, phenylephrine, norepinephrine)

adrenergic antagonists, IV (e.g., propranolol, metoprolol, labetalol)

anesthesia agents, general, inhaled, and IV (e.g., propofol, ketamine)

antiarrhythmics, IV (e.g., lidocaine, amiodarone)

antithrombotic agents (anticoagulants), including warfarin, low-molecular-weight heparin, IV unfractionated heparin,
  Factor Xa inhibitors (fondaparinux), direct thrombin inhibitors (e.g., argatroban, lepirudin, bivalirudin),
  thrombolytics (e.g., alteplase, reteplase, tenecteplase), and glycoprotein IIb/IIIa inhibitors (e.g., eptifibatide)

cardioplegic solutions

chemotherapeutic agents, parenteral and oral

dextrose, hypertonic, 20% or greater

dialysis solutions, peritoneal and hemodialysis

epidural or intrathecal medications

hypoglycemics, oral

inotropic medications, IV (e.g., digoxin, milrinone)

liposomal forms of drugs (e.g., liposomal amphotericin B)

moderate sedation agents, IV (e.g., midazolam)

moderate sedation agents, oral, for children (e.g., chloral hydrate)

narcotics/opioids IV, transdermal, and oral (including liquid concentrates and immediate and sustained-release
  formulations)

neuromuscular blocking agents (e.g., succinylcholine, rocuronium, vecuronium)

radiocontrast agents, IV

total parenteral nutrition solutions

Specific Medications

colchicine injection

epoprostenol (Flolan), IV

insulin, subcutaneous and IV

magnesium sulfate for injection

methotrexate, oral, non-oncologic use

opium tincture

oxytocin, IV

nitroprusside sodium for injection

potassium chloride for injection concentrate

potassium phosphates injection

promethazine, IV

sodium chloride for injection (concentrate)

sterile water for injection, inhalation, and irrigation (excluding pour bottles) in containers of 100 mL or more

IV = intravenous

From Institute for Safe Medicine Practices. (2008). *ISMP's list of high-alert medications.* Horsham, PA: Author. Retrieved from http://www.ismp.org/Tools/highalertmedications.pdf

decreases in uterine perfusion may lead to further decreases in fetal oxygenation, a shift to anaerobic metabolism, accumulation of lactic acid, and metabolic acidosis. Specific EFM signs that indicate the possibility of fetal metabolic acidemia include absent baseline variability, absence of accelerations, an abnormal baseline rate (tachycardia and/or bradycardia), and recurrent late and/or prolonged decelerations.[4]

Early in pregnancy, teratogenic exposure is a concern with medication administration. A teratogen is any chemical, substance, or exposure that may cause birth defects, permanent abnormality of structure or function, in a developing fetus. Women may be reluctant to

take any medication during pregnancy due to the possibility or perceived possibility of fetal effects. In an attempt to prevent harmful medications from reaching the market, clinical drug trials to determine safety and efficacy are required for new drugs marketed and sold in the United States (U.S.) by the Food and Drug Administration (FDA). The FDA places medications into risk categories regarding use during pregnancy and potential effects on the developing fetus (Table 6-2). However, because medications are not tested on pregnant women, and animal studies do not always predict effects in humans, approximately 80 percent of marketed medications have unknown teratogenic risk in

TABLE 6-2

FDA Categories for Drug Use in Pregnancy

Category	Description
A	Adequate, well-controlled studies in pregnant women have not shown an increased risk of fetal abnormalities.
B	Animal studies have revealed no evidence of harm to the fetus; however, there are no adequate and well-controlled studies in pregnant women. OR Animal studies have shown an adverse effect, but adequate and well-controlled studies in pregnant women have failed to demonstrate a risk to the fetus.
C	Animal studies have shown an adverse effect and there are no adequate and well-controlled studies in pregnant women. OR No animal studies have been conducted and there are no adequate and well-controlled studies in pregnant women.
D	Adequate well-controlled or observational studies in pregnant women have demonstrated a risk to the fetus. However, the benefits of therapy may outweigh the potential risk.
X	Adequate well-controlled or observational studies in animals or pregnant women have demonstrated positive evidence of fetal abnormalities. Use of the product is contraindicated in women who are or may become pregnant.

From U. S. Food and Drug Administration. (1980). *Federal Register, 44,* 37434–37467.

Box 6-1. DRUGS OR SUBSTANCES SUSPECTED OR PROVEN TO BE HUMAN TERATOGENS

angiotensin-converting enzyme inhibitors
aminopterin
androgens
angiotensin-II receptor antagonists
busulfan
carbamazepine
chlorbiphenyls
cocaine
coumarin derivatives
cyclophosphamide
danazol
diethylstilbestrol (DES)
ethanol
etretinate
iodine, radioactive
isotretinoin
kanamycin
lithium
methimazole
methotrexate
misoprostol
penicillamine
phenytoin
streptomycin
tamoxifen
tetracycline
thalidomide
tretinoin
trimethadone
valproic acid

Adapted from Yaffe, S. J., & Briggs, G. G. (2003). Is this drug going to harm my baby? *Contemporary OB/GYN, 48,* 57.

pregnancy.[5] Box 6-1 lists the drugs or substances suspected or proven to be human teratogens.[6]

BREAST-FEEDING

Many drugs present in the bloodstream will be excreted in breast milk. The drug concentration in milk depends on many factors, such as the amount of drug in the maternal serum, the transfer of the drug across the placental barrier, its lipid solubility, its degree of ionization, its molecular size, and the extent to which it is excreted. Fetal accumulation of a drug that is transmitted in breast milk is contingent upon a variety of factors. Variations in the amount of milk formed in the breast may be altered due to decreased blood flow to breast tissue. Alterations in milk pH and composition also affect the concentrations of drugs found in breast milk.[7]

Drug exposure to the breast-feeding newborn is greatest when feeding or pumping occurs immediately following medication administration to the mother.[7] An effective strategy to decrease the drug concentration in breast milk is to pump or feed the infant when the maternal serum levels begin to decline. Women who desire to breast-feed their infants should be encouraged not to abandon this desire due to critical illness and current medications. Nurses and lactation consultants can assist the breast-feeding woman with pumping to promote breast milk production and to relieve engorgement. Discarding the milk is advised if drug toxicity and adverse pharmacologic actions of the drug are known, or if the drug transfer is unknown.[7]

NEUROHORMONAL RESPONSE TO CRITICAL ILLNESS

Neurotransmitters in the peripheral nervous system—epinephrine and norepinephrine—are synthesized and primarily stored in nerve terminals until released by a nerve impulse. Medications that mimic the actions of epinephrine and norepinephrine are called adrenomimetic drugs. Receptors for epinephrine and norepinephrine (adrenoceptors) are selective for their respective agonists and antagonists (medications that enhance or block epinephrine and/or norepinephrine at adrenoreceptors).[7]

Autonomic receptors include those for acetylcholine (cholinergic) and those for catecholamines (adrenergic). The actions of catecholamines are determined by their ability to bind to three major classes of receptors: alpha (α), beta (β), and dopaminergic (Δ) (Table 6-3). Alpha receptors mediate excitation of the effector cells, whereas beta receptors provoke relaxation.[7] A woman's neurohormonal response has an important effect on the pharmacodynamics of medications used during critical illness. Heart rate, contractility, peripheral vascular tone, and metabolic changes are regulated by these endogenous changes. Also, certain diseases causing critical illness can change the receptor density, alter affinity, and change the response to agents (Table 6-4). Therefore, the pharmacologic effect is not necessarily equivalent to plasma drug concentrations, and may lead to substantial variation.[8]

USING MEDICATIONS TO OPTIMIZE HEMODYNAMIC STABILITY

A thorough discussion of concepts related to hemodynamic function including oxygen transport physiology

TABLE 6-3
Physiologic Effects of Receptor Activity

Receptor	Effect
A	Vasoconstriction
	Increased cardiac contractility
	Decreased heart rate
β_1	Increased heart rate
	Increased cardiac contractility
β_2	Vasodilation
	Relaxed uterine, bronchial, and GI smooth muscle
Δ_1	Decreased Na+ reabsorption in proximal renal tubules
Δ_2	Decreased ventilatory response to hypoxia
	Decreased aldosterone synthesis and release

α = alpha, β = beta, Δ = dopaminergic.

TABLE 6-4
Receptor Alterations Based on Disease or Condition

Disease or Condition	Alteration in Receptor
Asthma	Decreased β (lung, leukocytes)
Congestive heart failure	Increased β (heart)
Glucocorticoid administration	Increased β (heart, leukocytes)
Hyperthyroidism	Increased β (heart)
Hypothyroidism	Decreased β (heart)
Myocardial ischemia	Increased α
	Decreased β (heart)
Sepsis	Decreased α (liver, vasculature)

α = alpha; β = beta.
From ACOG Practice Bulletin: Clinical Management. Guidelines for Obstetrician-Gynecologists. Number 6, October 2006.

is found in Chapter 4. Review of these concepts may be helpful as the reader considers select pharmacologic agents in context with the patient's complete physiologic condition.

Preload

Evaluation of the patient's intravascular volume is imperative prior to the administration of an agent that causes constriction or dilation of blood vessels. This may be accomplished using noninvasive methods; however, central hemodynamic monitoring provides more specific and reliable information regarding preload, afterload, and left ventricular contractility. Failure to ensure adequate preload prior to administration of vasoactive medication may result in circulatory insufficiency, inability to achieve effective oxygen extraction, distributive shock, and cardiovascular collapse. If hypovolemia is suspected, crystalloid solutions are used for initial volume resuscitation. Blood product replacement may also be necessary to augment volume status, replace clotting factors, and increase oxygen carrying capacity.[9]

The use of diuretics in obstetrics to reduce preload is typically reserved for patients with cardiogenic pulmonary edema from inadvertent fluid overload.[10] A thorough discussion of the types and etiologies of pulmonary edema may be found in Chapter 9. Because excessive preload is rarely seen in combination with common critical illnesses during pregnancy, these agents should be administered with caution, especially if invasive hemodynamic data are not available. For example, the use of some tocolytic agents has been associated with accumulation of volume leading to pulmonary vascular congestion and cardiogenic pulmonary edema. Diuretics would be indicated for use in this group of women when non-cardiogenic pulmonary edema can be ruled out as a probable cause.

Severe elevation of systemic afterload may decrease cardiac output and lead to a hypervolemic state in the pulmonary vasculature. Treatment for this etiology of "pulmonary volume overload" would be to lower the systemic resistance with an afterload-reducing agent and allow the intrapulmonary pressures/volume to decrease. Nitroglycerin can be used to decrease excessive preload in a patient who requires meticulous preload adjustments during labor or postpartum. Regional anesthesia may also accomplish this goal, albeit with less precision. Diuretics in this scenario would only be indicated if systemic hypervolemia is discovered following normalization of afterload values. Diuretics are not administered to patients with pulmonary edema from excessive intrapulmonary volumes or pressures when systemic intravascular volume and afterload are normal. This is due to the high probability of undiagnosed pulmonary hypertension, which may be a life-threatening cardiac complication.

Afterload – Systemic Vascular Resistance

Systemic blood pressure is the product of cardiac output and systemic vascular resistance. Significant increases of either parameter will increase blood pressure. Conversely, a dramatic decrease in one of the two components for which the other cannot compensate results in a decrease in systemic blood pressure.

Numerous options and combinations of vasoactive medications have been studied and safely used in critically ill patients. When choosing an agent, knowledge of the specific pathophysiology associated with the disease and the drug's pharmacologic actions should be applied. Vasoactive and inotropic medications are classified according to their capacity to activate adrenergic receptors that produce a range of physiologic actions (Table 6-5).

During stabilization, agents with a short half-life are selected for the pregnant woman due to the possibility of an immediate delivery and the desire to minimize fetal/newborn effects. Regardless of the medication or combination of medications used, the mother and fetus should be monitored frequently for desired and adverse effects. When rapid-acting vasoactive medications are administered by continuous infusion and titration, continuous, intra-arterial pressure monitoring is the preferred method for blood pressure measurement.[9] Intra-arterial pressure monitoring provides a real-time measurement of blood pressure and constantly displays blood pressure approximately every 1 to 3 seconds, depending on the specific manufacturer and model of monitor. This rapidity of blood pressure measurements is necessary when titrating vasoactive medications that have a half-life of seconds rather than minutes. Such rapid-acting agents make the use of external blood pressure monitoring with automated cuff inflation and deflation unsuitable. Evaluation of the systolic and diastolic blood pressures, pulse, and mean arterial pressures allows the provider to adjust the medication administration for optimal dosing and desired effects. Hemodynamic parameters may also be monitored with a pulmonary artery catheter to assess cardiac function (e.g., cardiac output, pulmonary capillary wedge pressure, central venous pressure, pulmonary arterial pressure, pulmonary and systemic vascular resistance, left and right ventricular stroke work [index], and other parameters) before and after the administration of a rapid-acting intravenous medication (e.g., dopamine, norepinephrine). Adequate preload should be ensured before administering these agents in order to prevent a decrease in maternal cardiac output.[9]

TABLE 6-5

Vasopressor and Inotropic Agent Effects on Adrenergic Receptors

Medication	Adrenergic Receptor Activation	Inotropic	Chronotropic	Vasoconstriction
Milrinone	α	+++	0	Vasodilation
Dobutamine	α, β_1, β_2	+++	+	Dose dependent
Dopamine	α, β_1, Δ	+++	++	Dose dependent
Epinephrine	α, β_1, β_2	+++	+++	++
Isoproterenol	β_1, β_2	++++	++++	Vasodilation
Methoxamine	α	0	0	++++
Norepinephrine	α, β_1	+++	+++	++++
Phenylephrine	α, β_1	+	0	++++
Vasopressin	0	+ or −	+ or −	+ to +++

α = alpha; β = beta; Δ = dopaminergic.

Adapted from Marini, J. J., & Wheeler, A. P. (2006). *Critical care medicine: the essentials* (3rd ed.). Philadelphia: Lippincott Williams & Wilkins.

Hypotension

Hypotension is usually progressive if untreated and may result in profound decreases in tissue perfusion and shock. The initial response to hypotension is the release of catecholamines, resulting in an increased rate and force of myocardial contractility. Peripheral vasoconstriction will also occur, resulting in a diversion of cardiac output and decreased perfusion of non-vital organs.[9] Because blood flow to the uterus is directly related to maternal blood pressure, rapid assessment and initiation of interventions as needed should be implemented to increase the woman's blood pressure and prevent decreased oxygen delivery to the fetus. Other compensatory mechanisms occur with hypotension, including an increase in secretion of aldosterone and antidiuretic hormone (ADH), which aids in maintaining circulating volume. Cortisol release also provides increased glucose for the tissues.[9]

Vasopressors are agents that cause the constriction of blood vessels (Table 6-6). The hemodynamic effects of vasopressors vary and are dependent upon adrenostimulation stimulation in the heart and vascular system. Blood vessel vasoconstriction is mediated by the stimulation of alpha receptors. However, some vasopressors may also stimulate beta receptors, resulting in positive inotropic, chronotropic, and vasodilatory effects.[7] The goal of vasopressor therapy is to optimize vital organ perfusion, not to obtain a particular blood pressure. A minimum mean arterial pressure of approximately 70 mmHg is generally required to perfuse the heart, brain, and kidneys. In order to achieve maximum vasopressor effects, correction of inadequate preload, severe electrolyte imbalances, and maternal acidemia should be a priority.[9]

Even though invasive hemodynamic monitoring may be in place when caring for pregnant women on vasopressors, noninvasive parameters of oxygenation and tissue perfusion should be frequently assessed. The use of a pulse oximeter may be unreliable in women being treated with vasopressor agents.[9] Therefore, other parameters of perfusion adequacy, such as urine output, capillary refill, peripheral pulses, and skin color and warmth should be assessed. Because vasoactive agents usually increase heart rate and have arrhythmogenic potential, continuous electrocardiogram (ECG) monitoring and interpretation are necessary. An indwelling urinary catheter should be placed to monitor urine output as a reflection of renal perfusion and oxygen delivery. Caution should be used to avoid rapidly induced blood pressure changes leading to hypertensive episodes with medication administration. Acute pulmonary edema, cerebral hemorrhage, and cardiac arrest have been reported with such changes.[9]

Vasopressors distribute well in extracellular fluid, but poorly in fat. When determining the initial dose, the woman's actual weight in kilograms is calculated in order to use the lowest effective dose. However, in the obese woman, ideal body weight is used. Central venous infusion with a volumetric pump is optimal, because peripheral infiltration can cause skin necrosis and ulceration. If peripheral infiltration occurs, phentolamine 5 to 10 mg in 10 to 15 mL normal saline solution should be injected directly into the site. All doses should be tapered when discontinuing a vasopressor infusion.[9]

Hypertension

Acute treatment of severe hypertension is initiated to prevent cerebrovascular or cardiovascular complications; however, recommendations as to when to initiate therapy differ greatly based on systolic and diastolic blood pressures, mean arterial pressure, or both (Table 6-7).[11] Antihypertensive therapy is consistently recommended for repeated diastolic pressures above 110 mmHg. Systolic pressures above 160 mmHg are treated by some health care providers, but others may delay treatment until the patient reaches consistent values of 180 mmHg. Mean arterial pressures may also be utilized as a measurement for treatment.[12,13]

The choice of an agent to lower blood pressure should depend on blood pressure values as well as the suspected cause of the elevation in order to match the desired effects of the drug (Table 6-8).[14,15] For example, many antihypertensives cause tachycardia. If an elevated heart rate is a causative factor for an increase in blood pressure, an agent without this effect should be considered (e.g., labetalol). Tachycardia may be a compensatory response to significant hypovolemia. In such situations, the central hypovolemia is the cause of the hypertension; thus, administration of intravenous fluids sufficient to optimize vascular volume and preload may effectively lower the blood pressure. If an elevated systemic vascular resistance is the causative factor, an agent that results in vasodilation should be administered (e.g., hydralazine).

Intravenous hydralazine, labetalol, and oral nifedipine are the most commonly used first-line medications for acute treatment of severe hypertension during pregnancy. In a meta-analysis done by Magee and colleagues, 21 clinical trials were analyzed comparing the use of hydralazine with other agents.[14] The comparison suggested that oral nifedipine and intravenous labetalol have fewer side effects and the same efficacy as intravenous hydralazine.[16] If the woman remains hypertensive after administration of one of these medications, rapid-acting second-line medications should be considered. Intravenous nitroglycerin or sodium nitroprusside are

(text continues on page 70)

TABLE 6-6

Vasopressors

Drug	Description	Dose	Contraindications
ephedrine sulphate	First-line medication in pregnancy to counteract hypotensive effects of epidural or spinal anesthesia Stimulates both alpha and beta receptors Peripheral actions due to release of norepinephrine Peripheral vasoconstriction with out reducing uterine blood flow ↑ glycogenolysis in liver ↑ oxygen consumption ↑ metabolic rate	10–25 mg slow IV push May repeat q 15 min prn × 3	Blood pressure >130/80 mmHg Angle closure glaucoma In conjunction with anesthesia agents that may sensitize the heart to arrhythmic action (e.g., cyclopropane or halothane)
metaraminol (Aramine)	Potent sympathomimetic amine that increases systolic and diastolic blood pressures from peripheral vasoconstriction. Positive inotropic effect on heart. ***Use only with severe maternal hypotension unresponsive to other agents.***	Initial dose of 0.1 mg/min Titrate to 2 mg/min after 10 min if needed Pressor effect begins in 1 to 2 min Effects last 20 min to 1 hr	Hypersensitivity to sulfites In conjunction with anesthesia agents (e.g., cyclopropane or halothane) that may sensitize heart to arrhythmic action such as VT/VF

Possible Maternal Side Effects	Possible Fetal/Neonatal Side Effects	Interactions	Precautions
Tachycardia, headache, anxiety, tremors, dizziness, respiratory difficulty	EFM: Observe for fetal tachycardia and decreased baseline variability following administration.	Diuretics may decrease vascular response. Medications that decrease norepinephrine in sympathetic nerve endings (e.g., methyldopa, reserpine) may reduce vascular response.	Correct blood volume depletion before administration to maintain coronary and cerebral perfusion. If administration is continued without blood volume replacement, severe peripheral and visceral vasoconstriction may occur, resulting in decreased urine output, renal perfusion, tissue hypoxia and lactic acidosis. Use cautiously in patients with hyperthyroidism, coronary heart disease, angina pectoris, cardiac arrhythmia, or diabetes.
May interact with oxytoxics and ergot medications to produce severe maternal hypertension Sinus or ventricular tachycardia	Potential for reduced uterine blood flow and fetal hypoxia	Use cautiously with digitalis—may cause ectopic arrhythmias MAOIs or tricyclic antidepressants may potentiate the pressor action of sympathomimetic amines.	Preferred infusion via central line. Peripheral infusion may cause abscess formation or tissue necrosis. Assess peripheral perfusion frequently. Correct blood volume depletion before administration to maintain coronary and cerebral perfusion. If administration is continued without blood volume replacement, severe peripheral and visceral vasoconstriction may occur, resulting in decreased urine output, renal perfusion, tissue hypoxia, and lactic acidosis. Give cautiously in patients with diabetes or heart or thyroid disease. May cause relapse in patients with a history of malaria.

(continued)

TABLE 6-6 (Continued)

Vasopressors

Drug	Description	Dose	Contraindications
norephinephrine (Levophed)	Peripheral vasoconstriction due to alpha-adrenergic action Inotropic stimulation of heart Dilates coronary arteries (β-adrenergic action) ***Use only with severe maternal hypotension unresponsive to other agents.*** **Indications** Hypotension from decreased systemic vascular resistance with normal cardiac output Examples: septic shock, spinal shock, narcotic overdose **Low Dose** ***β effect*** ↑ cardiac contractility (LVSWI) ↑ conduction velocity ↑ heart rate **Higher Dose** ***α and β effects*** ↑ cardiac contractility (further) ↑ stroke volume ↑ cardiac workload ↑ SVR	Initial dose of 0.05 mcg/kg/min Must be diluted in dextrose-containing solutions before administration to prevent oxidation. Titrate to maximum dose of 1 mcg/kg/min based on patient response Infusion should be decreased gradually. Central venous administration preferred. Peripheral infusion may result in extravasation and necrosis of the tissues.	Hypovolemia Hypotension from blood volume loss Use in patients with hypoxia and/or hypercarbia may result in cardiac arrhythmias. Mesenteric or peripheral thrombosis In conjunction with anesthesia agents (e.g. cyclopropane or halothane) that may sensitize the heart to arrhythmic action such as VT/VF. Hypersensitivity to sulfites
phenylephrine hydrochloride (Neo-synephrine)	Pure α agonist without cardiac stimulating properties ***Use only with severe maternal hypotension unresponsive to other agents.***	Initial dose of 0.1 mcg/kg/min Titrate up to 0.7 mcg/kg/min based on patient response	Hypovolemia, hypotension from blood loss, hypertension

Possible Maternal Side Effects	Possible Fetal/Neonatal Side Effects	Interactions	Precautions
Ischemic injury due to tissue hypoxia as a result of vasoconstriction Reflex bradycardia. Anxiety, transient headache, respiratory difficulty, palpitations, angina	May compromise uterine blood flow, causing fetal hypoxia and bradycardia	MAOIs or tricyclic antidepressants may potentiate the pressor action of sympathomimetic amines.	Arterial line placement is recommended to continuously monitor blood pressure response. Hemodynamic monitoring with a pulmonary artery catheter may be indicated. Correct blood volume depletion before administration to maintain coronary and cerebral perfusion. If administration is continued without blood volume replacement, severe peripheral and visceral vasoconstriction may occur, resulting in decreased urine output, renal perfusion, tissue hypoxia and lactic acidosis. Assess peripheral perfusion frequently.
Reflex bradycardia, headache, nausea, tingling in hands and feet	Potential for reduced uterine blood flow and fetal hypoxia Excreted in breast milk	May interact with uterine stimulant (e.g., oxytocics) and ergot medications to produce severe maternal hypertension	Use cautiously in patients with sulfite hypersensitivity. Arterial line placement is recommended to continuously monitor blood pressure response. Hemodynamic monitoring with a pulmonary artery catheter may be indicated. Correct blood volume depletion before administration to maintain coronary and cerebral perfusion. If administration is continued without blood volume replacement, severe peripheral and visceral vasoconstriction may occur, resulting in decreased urine output, renal perfusion, tissue hypoxia and lactic acidosis. Assess peripheral perfusion frequently.

(continued)

TABLE 6-6 (Continued)

Vasopressors

Drug	Description	Dose	Contraindications
vasopressin	Direct vasoconstrictor increasing mean arterial pressure and systemic vascular resistance Indicated in the early phases of vasodilatory shock states (e.g., severe septic shock) and may be considered for resuscitation during cardiopulmonary arrest May be combined with another vasopressor ↑ cerebral, coronary, and pulmonary perfusion (↓ PVR). May be superior to norepinephrine by not compromising profusion to other organ systems. Restores renal blood flow, improving urine output and creatinine clearance. ↑ serum cortisol levels	0.01–0.04 units/min IV (mimics physiologic doses) Pulseless VT/VF dose: 40 units IV or endotrachial—one dose Half-life approximately 10–35 min Effects last approximately 30–60 min if given IV Doses greater than 0.04 units/min may cause platelet aggregation; renal, mesenteric, pulmonary and coronary vasoconstriction; decreased cardiac output, cardiac arrest.	Hypovolemia, hypotension from blood loss, hypertension

EFM = electronic fetal monitoring, LVSWI = left ventricular stroke work index, MAOI = monoamine oxidase inhibitor, PVR, = pulmonary vascular resistance, SVR = systemic vascular resistance, VT/VF = ventricular tachycardia/ventricular fibrillation.

two medications that have been effective in lowering systemic afterload. Invasive hemodynamic monitoring with an arterial line and pulmonary artery catheter should be initiated with use of these potent vasodilating medications.[9,13]

Sodium nitroprusside is a rapid-acting arterial and venous dilator with a half-life of about 2 minutes. These qualities make it an attractive option in the treatment of hypertension resistant to first-line medications. The concern for use is that each nitroprusside molecule contains five cyanide molecules, which cross the placenta and may lead to elevated fetal concentrations.[13] Cyanide normally combines with methemoglobin for elimination or is metabolized into thiocyanate and excreted in urine. Infusion doses of greater than 2 mg/kg/min, prolonged use, renal insufficiency, or decreased metabolism by the liver may result in increased levels of cyanide and inhibit oxygen utilization by tissues. Thiocyanate toxicity may also occur with impaired renal function. Therefore, recommendations during pregnancy limit this medication to the postpartum period or if delivery is imminent.[13,15] Signs of cyanide and thiocyanate toxicity are listed in Table 6-9.[9,13,15]

General precautions should be taken when administering any antihypertensive during pregnancy. To maintain cardiac, renal, and uteroplacental perfusion, diastolic pressures should not be lowered too rapidly or drop below 90 mmHg.[12,15] Care should be taken to not lower the blood pressure too rapidly in women with chronic hypertension who have a right shift of the cerebral autoregulation curve as a result of medial hypertrophy of the cerebral vasculature. Rapidly lowering blood pressure in these women may result in decreased cerebral blood flow, ischemia, stroke, or coma.[13]

The woman's intravascular volume status should be assessed before administering any vasodilator. With relaxation of venous smooth muscle, the woman's preload and cardiac output will decrease if preload status is impaired.[16] If the woman's preload is not enhanced prior to vasodilation, cardiac output will fall.[9] For example, the majority of women with severe preeclampsia are hypovolemic due to increased capillary permeability. In this population, elevated systemic vascular resistance and blood pressures may be a compensatory result of a low preload and cardiac output. Prior to vasodilation, volume resuscitation should be undertaken to prevent

(text continues on page 74)

Possible Maternal Side Effects	Possible Fetal/Neonatal Side Effects	Interactions	Precautions
Decreased peripheral circulation with high doses	Potential for reduced uterine blood flow and fetal hypoxia		Arterial line placement is recommended to continuously monitor blood pressure response. Hemodynamic monitoring with a pulmonary artery catheter may be indicated. Correct blood volume depletion before administration to maintain coronary and cerebral perfusion. If administration is continued without blood volume replacement, severe peripheral and visceral vasoconstriction may occur, resulting in decreased urine output, renal perfusion, tissue hypoxia, and lactic acidosis. Monitor peripheral pulses, skin color and temperature—observe for signs of decreased tissue perfusion.

TABLE 6-7

Indications for Antihypertensive Therapy

Antepartum and Intrapartum Periods	
Persistent elevations for at least 1 hour	SBP ≥160 mmHg or DBP ≥110 mmHg or MAP ≥130 mmHg
Persistent elevations for at least 30 minutes	SBP ≥200 mmHg or DBP ≥120 mmHg or MAP ≥140 mmHg
Thrombocytopenia or congestive heart failure with persistent elevations for at least 30 minutes	SBP ≥155 mmHg or DBP ≥105 mmHg or MAP ≥125 mmHg
Postpartum Period	
Persistent elevations for at least 1 hour	SBP ≥155 mmHg or DBP ≥105 mmHg or MAP ≥125 mmHg

DBP = diastolic blood pressure, MAP = mean arterial blood pressure, mmHg = milliliters of mercury, SBP = systolic blood pressure.

From Sibai, B. M. (2010). Hypertensive emergencies. In M.R. Foley, T.H. Strong, & T.J. Garite (Eds.). *Obstetric intensive care manual* (3rd ed.). New York: McGraw-Hill.

TABLE 6-8

Vasodilators and Antihypertensive Agents

Drug	Description	Dose	Contraindications
hydralazine (Apresoline)	Decreases systemic resistance through direct dilation of arterioles	5–10 mg IV over 1–2 min May repeat q 20 min up to total cumulative dose of 30 mg	Mitral valve rheumatic heart disease
labetalol (Normodyne)	Blocks α-adrenergic, $β_1$-adrenergic, and $β_2$-adrenergic receptor sites Decreases SVR, HR, and myocardial oxygen consumption Onset of action within 5 minutes Peak effect at 10–20 min Duration of action is up to 6 hr Does not decrease cardiac output	20 mg IV; may follow with 40 mg IV and 80 mg IV every 10 min if needed to stabilize BP Cumulative maximum dose 300 mg Continuous infusion (1 mg/kg)	Reactive airway disease (asthma), congestive heart failure, cardiogenic shock, bradycardia, pulmonary edema, hypoglycemia, atrioventricular block, or with hepatic failure
nifedipine (Procardia, Adalat)	Oral calcium channel blocker Acts on arteriolar smooth muscle and induces vasodilation by blocking calcium entry into cells; minimal venous effect Indicated for treatment of hypertension and as a tocolytic for preterm labor	10 mg PO May repeat dose every 15–30 min to cumulative dose of 30 mg	Hypotension
nicardipine hydrochloride (Cardene IV)	Parenteral calcium channel blocker; inhibits transmembrane influx of calcium ions into cardiac and smooth muscle; does not change serum calcium levels Decreases SVR	Initial infusion of 5 mg/hr Titrate dose by 2.5 mg/hr every 15 min to maximum dose of 10 mg/hr Onset of action in 10 min Duration of action 4–6 hr Infusion should be decreased gradually	Aortic stenosis

Possible Maternal Side Effects	Possible Fetal/Neonatal Side Effects	Interactions	Precautions
Reflex tachycardia, dizziness, headache, palpitations, flushing, vomiting, numbness and tingling of extremities	EFM—Fetal tachycardia Thrombocytopenia and a lupus-like syndrome have been reported in neonate if mother is treated in 3rd trimester.	MAOIs and beta-blockers may increase hydralazine toxicity. Pharmacologic effects may be decreased by indomethacin.	Implicated in myocardial infarction; use with caution in suspected coronary artery disease.
May diminish reflex tachycardia, cause bradycardia, and increase intracranial pressure May increase transaminase and urea levels	Potential for IUGR Hypotension, hypoglycemia, hypothermia, and bradycardia in the neonate	Co-administration of a calcium channel blocker may increase cardiodepressant effects. Decreases effectiveness of diuretics and increases toxicity of methotrexate, lithium, and salicylates Cimetidine may increase labetalol blood levels.	Use cautiously in impaired hepatic function; discontinue therapy if patient develops signs of hepatic failure.
Tachycardia, palpitations, headache, facial flushing, ankle edema May increase ALT, AST, alkaline phosphatase, and LD levels	Potential for fetal tachycardia	Magnesium sulfate may potentiate action resulting in neuromuscular blockade, severe hypotension, and decreased uterine blood flow. Signs of neuromuscular blockade include weakness, involuntary muscle jerks, dysphagia, and decreased rate and depth of respirations.	Sublingual dosing associated with rapid decrease in BP, hypotension, acute myocardial ischemia, and death
Hypotension, headache, and tachycardia	Research conducted on rats has indicated high concentrations in breast milk.	Not compatible with sodium bicarbonate (5%) or lactated Ringer's solution	Infusion site should be changed every 12 hr if administered into peripheral vein. Use cautiously in patients with impaired liver or renal function.

(continued)

TABLE 6-8 (Continued)

Vasodilators and Antihypertensive Agents

Drug	Description	Dose	Contraindications
nitroglycerin (Nitrostat IV, Tridil, Nitro-Bid IV)	Organic nitrate that causes venous vascular smooth muscle relaxation; arterial smooth muscle relaxation is dose related ↓ preload (CVP and PCOP) ↓ SVR Dilates coronary arteries ↑ HR (slight) ↓ myocardial oxygen consumption	IV infusion 10 mcg/min; titrate up by 10–20 mcg/min prn 0.3–0.6 mg sublingual 1–2 inches of dermal paste	Early myocardial infarction, severe anemia, and increased intracranial pressure
sodium nitroprusside (Nitropress, Nipride)	Peripheral vasodilation by directly acting on venous and arteriolar smooth muscle, reducing peripheral vascular resistance	Initial dose 0.3 mcg/kg/min Titrate to 10 mcg/kg/min	Subaortic stenosis, idiopathic hypertrophic, atrial fibrillation or flutter

aPTT = activated partial thromboplastin times, BP = blood pressure, CVP = central venous pressure, EFM = electronic fetal monitoring, HR = heart rate, IUGR = intrauterine growth restriction, MAOI = monoamine oxidase inhibitor, PCOP = pulmonary capillary occlusive pressure, SVR = systemic vascular resistance.

Data from Report of the National High Blood Pressure Education Program Working Group on High Blood Pressure in Pregnancy: Summary report. (2000). *American Journal of Obstetrics & Gynecology, 183*(1):S1–S22; Sibai, B. M. (2007). Hypertension. In: S. G., Gabbe, J. R. Niebyl, & J. L. Simpson. (Eds.) Obstetrics: Normal and problem pregnancies (5th ed.) New York, Churchill Livingstone; Sibai, B. M. (2010). Hypertensive emergencies. In M. R. Foley, T. H. Strong, & T. J. Garite (Eds.). Obstetric intensive care manual (3rd ed.). New York: McGraw-Hill.

lowering of the systemic vascular resistance and blood pressure, causing a further decrease in cardiac output, organ, and uterine perfusion.[16]

Heart Rate

Variations in heart rate (bradycardia and tachycardia) have the potential for decreasing cardiac output. Tachycardia is more common in the conditions that cause critical illness and as a side effect of medications given during pregnancy. As a general rule, a heart rate greater than 220 beats per minute, minus the patient's age, produces decreased cardiac output and myocardial perfusion.[9] Beta blockers have been successfully utilized to decrease the maternal heart rate associated with tachyarrhythmias, myocardial contractility, and oxygen consumption while increasing end diastolic filling time and cardiac output.[17] However, prior to the use of any beta blocking agent, preload status should be assessed in order to prevent blocking the compensatory response of catecholamines due to hypovolemia.[9]

Beta-adrenergic blockers have different mechanisms of action and should be selected for the desired effect (Table 6-10). Beta blockers are classified into groups based on their receptor selectivity. Nonselective beta blockers produce blockade of both beta$_1$ and beta$_2$ receptors. The effect of selective beta blockers is dose dependent. For example, beta$_1$ selective medications have a higher affinity for beta$_1$ than beta$_2$ receptors.[18]

Beta-adrenergic blockers should be reserved for patients with myocardial ischemia, thyroid storm, or symptomatic tachyarrhythmias (e.g., supraventricular tachycardia). They are not the first-line choice for left ventricular dysfunction or congestive heart failure.[9] Patients with reactive airway diseases (e.g., asthma) should not be given a beta blocker unless it has only beta$_1$ cardiac selectivity. Beta$_2$ blockers may provoke a bronchial asthmatic attack due to the blockade of beta receptors in the lungs that provide for bronchodilation produced by endogenous and exogenous catecholamine stimulation. Beta blockers should be used cautiously in patients with diabetes because they may decrease tachycardia associated with hypoglycemia. If beta blockers are taken during times of physiologic stress (e.g., infection, sepsis, decreased cardiac output) compensatory mechanisms in patients with cardiovascular compromise may be blocked.[9]

Possible Maternal Side Effects	Possible Fetal/Neonatal Side Effects	Interactions	Precautions
Severe, persistent headache, dizziness, vertigo, weakness, palpitations, hypotension	None reported	Aspirin may augment vasodilation effect. Reduced anticoagulant effect of heparin Potential for orthostatic hypotension when used with calcium channel blocking agents	aPTT should be monitored if used in conjunction with heparin. Nitrate therapy may enhance angina caused by hypertrophic cardiomyopathy. Sublingual administration may cause a burning sensation.
In renal and hepatic insufficiency, levels may increase and cause cyanide toxicity.	Avoid prolonged use due to potential for fetal cyanide toxicity.	None reported	Use caution in increased intracranial pressure, hepatic failure, severe renal impairment, hypothyroidism

TABLE 6-9

Signs and Symptoms of Cyanide and Thiocyanate Toxicity

Cyanide Toxicity
- Increased heart rate
- Metabolic acidosis
- Increased lactate despite normal SaO_2
- Decreased response to drug
- Rapid progressive tolerance (an important early indication of toxicity)

Thiocyanate Toxicity
- Changes in level of consciousness: confusion, delirium
- Hallucinations
- Seizures
- Fatigue and weakness
- Papillary constriction
- Tinnitus
- Rash
- Hypothyroidism (blocks thyroid uptake and binding of iodine)

SaO_2 = saturation of arterial hemoglobin via pulse oximetry.

ANTIARRHYTHMICS

Use of antiarrhythmics should be limited to life-threatening situations or situations in which severe debilitation may occur without intervention. Clear diagnosis of the type and origin of the arrhythmia is needed prior to pharmaceutical intervention. Beta blockers are frequently used in the treatment of tachyarrhythmias (see Table 6-10). When a patient presents with a ventricular arrhythmia, primarily supraventricular tachycardia, pharmacologic intervention may be required. Conservative interventions such as vagal stimulation or valsalva maneuvers are first-line interventions. If these noninvasive maneuvers do not convert the arrhythmia, adenosine, digoxin, or calcium channel blockers may be administered (Tables 6-11 and 6-12; also see Table 6-10.)[10,17,19]

Contractility

Changes in preload and afterload greatly influence myocardial contractility. Other causes for a depressed myocardium are acute ischemia, extensive myocardial necrosis, myocardial depressant humoral mediators

(text continues on page 86)

TABLE 6-10

Beta-blocking Agents

Drug	Description	Dose	Contraindications
atenolol (Tenormin)	Synthetic, cardioselective β_1 adrenoreceptor blocking agent Early treatment in myocardial infarction	5 mg IV over 5 min; repeat dose in 10 min If tolerated, begin oral dose of 50 mg 10 min after last IV dose and then every 12 hr. Peak plasma levels within 5 min for IV administration Half-life if administered by mouth is approximately 6–7 hr β-blocking and antihypertensive effects continue for at least 24 hr.	Sinus bradycardia, heart block greater than 1st degree, cardiogenic shock
esmolol (Brevibloc)	Rapid acting, β_1 cardioselective adrenergic receptor blocking agent Indicated for short-term control ventricular rates in patients with atrial flutter or fibrillation or sinus tachycardia in order to optimize cardiac output. After stabilization of heart rate, transition to another agent such as propranolol, digoxin or verapamil. May be used to control BP during endotracheal intubation. Less likely to have withdrawal effects that may occur with other beta-blocking agents.	500 mcg/kg IV over 1 min Infusion rate of 50–200 mcg/kg/min Half-life is approximately 9 min with IV administration. Reduce dose by 50% 30 min after administration of alternative agent; if patient remains stable, esmolol can be discontinued following second dose of alternative agent.	Sinus bradycardia, heart block greater than 1st degree, cardiogenic shock
metoprolol tartrate (Lopressor)	Selective β_1 adrenoreceptor blocking agent Early treatment with myocardial infarction	Give 3 bolus doses of 5 mg IV every 2 min. If tolerated, give oral dose of 25–50 mg 15 min following last IV bolus and then every 6 hr.	Pheochromocytoma, sinus bradycardia, heart block greater than 1st degree, cardiogenic shock, sick sinus syndrome, severe peripheral arterial circulatory disorders

Possible Maternal Side Effects	Possible Fetal/Neonatal Side Effects	Interactions	Precautions
Hypotension, bradycardia	EFM: Observe for fetal bradycardia. May cause IUGR Potential for persistent β-blockade and hypoglycemia in newborn Excreted in breast milk	Calcium channel blockers may have an additive effect if given concurrently with Tenormin. Prostaglandin-inhibiting agents (indomethacin) may inhibit the hypotensive effects of beta-blockers.	Continuous monitoring of ECG and blood pressure Use cautiously in patients with depressed myocardial contractility. Use cautiously in patients on digitalis. Both agents slow A–V conduction. In the absence of hypersensitivity, Tenormin should not be stopped abruptly.
Hypotension, peripheral ischemia, dizziness, headache, agitation, fatigue, nausea, inflammation of infusion site	Fetal bradycardia Potential risks for decreased uterine blood flow, fetal hypoxia, and late decelerations	↑ serum levels of digoxin when given concurrently ↑ serum levels of esmolol when given concurrently with morphine ↑ neuromuscular effects of succinylcholine	Monitor ECG and BP. Use cautiously in patients with renal impairment.
Fatigue, dizziness, depression, headache, migraine headache, cold extremities, shortness of breath, bradycardia, wheezing, pruritus, diarrhea Animal studies have shown increased pregnancy loss and neonatal death rate.	Rapidly enters fetal circulation; fetal serum levels equal to maternal levels May cause persistent β-blockade in newborn	Concurrent use with digitalis may increase risk of bradycardia. Medications that inhibit the CYP2D6 enzyme (e.g., antidepressants, antipsychotics, quanidine, antifungals, cimetidine) may increase serum concentrations of Lopressor. Rebound hypertension may occur following cessation of clonidine. Excreted in breast milk in small amounts.	Monitor ECG and BP. Use cautiously in patients with hepatic impairment.

(continued)

TABLE 6-10 (Continued)

Beta-blocking Agents

Drug	Description	Dose	Contraindications
propranolol (Inderal)	Synthetic, β-adrenergic receptor blocking agent Used to control ventricular rate in patients with atrial fibrillation Reduces cardiovascular mortality if given during acute phase of myocardial infarction Improves NYHA functional classification levels in patients with hypertrophic subaortic stenosis Used in conjunction with alpha-adrenergic blocking agents to control hypertension associated with catecholamine-secreting tumors (e.g., pheochromocytoma) Prophylaxis for migraine headaches	1 mg IV every 2 min prn	Cardiogenic shock, sinus bradycardia, greater than 1st degree heart block, reactive airways disease (asthma)

EFM = electronic fetal monitoring, IUGR = intrauterine growth restriction.

Possible Maternal Side Effects	Possible Fetal/Neonatal Side Effects	Interactions	Precautions
Bradycardia, congestive heart failure, hypotension, paresthesia of hands, thrombocytopenia purpura, lightheadedness, depression, insomnia, fatigue, nausea, diarrhea, constipation, bronchospasm, agranulocytosis, systemic lupus erythematosus, Stevens-Johnson syndrome, toxic epidermal necrolysis	Potential for IUGR, small placenta size and congenital abnormalities Observe for fetal bradycardia, hypoglycemia and/or respiratory depression in the neonate. Excreted in breast milk	↑ serum concentrations when given concurrently with quinidine ↓ clearance of lidocaine resulting in potential for lidocaine toxicity Potential for severe bradycardia, asystole, and heart failure if given with disopyramine. Use cautiously if given with other medications that decrease A–V node conduction (e.g., calcium channel. blockers, lidocaine) Concurrent use with digitalis may increase risk of bradycardia. ↓ myocardial contractility if administered concurrently with methoxyflurane and trichloroethylene (anesthetic agents) ↑ warfarin concentrations (postpartum use only) Hypotension and cardiac arrest potential if administered with haloperidol Lower T_3 concentrations when used with thyroxine, which may increase symptoms of hyperthyroidism and cause thyroid storm	Associated with increased serum potassium, transaminases and alkaline phosphatase in hypertensive patients

TABLE 6-11

Antiarrhythmic Agents

Drug	Description	Dose	Contraindications
adenosine (Adenocard)	Endogenous Decreases conduction through A–V node and may interrupt reentry pathway through A-V node Used for conversion of paroxysmal supraventricular tachycardia (including SVT caused by Wolff-Parkinson-White syndrome) Vagal maneuvers should be attempted prior to administration. Increases minute ventilation Reduces arterial PCO_2	6 mg rapid IV bolus over 1–3 sec followed by 20 mL saline bolus May repeat with 12 mg in 1–2 min × 2 if needed Larger doses may cause hypotension by decreasing vascular resistance. Administration directly into closest proximal vein Half-life is less than 10 sec.	Asthma Obstructive lung disease not associated with bronchoconstriction (e.g., emphysema, bronchitis) Sinus node disease or 2nd or 3rd degree heart block without artificial pacemaker

Possible Maternal Side Effects	Possible Fetal/Neonatal Side Effects	Interactions	Precautions
May cause 1st, 2nd, or 3rd degree heart block. Transient or prolonged periods of asystole may occur. Transient arrhythmias may occur (e.g., premature atrial or ventricular contractions, sinus bradycardia or tachycardia). *Cardiovascular:* facial flushing (18%), headache (2%), sweating, palpitations, chest pain, hypotension (less than 1%) *Respiratory:* shortness of breath, dyspnea (12%), chest pressure (7%), hyperventilation *CNS:* light-headedness (2%), dizziness, tingling in arms, numbness (1%), apprehension, blurred vision, burning sensation, heaviness in arms, neck and back pain (less than 1%) *Gastrointestinal:* nausea (3%), metallic taste, tightness in throat, pressure in groin (less than 1%)	Category C. No fetal effects have been reported.	Use with verapamil and digoxin may be associated with ventricular fibrillation due to synergistic depressant effects of the SA and AV nodes. Effects are antagonized by methylxanthines (e.g., caffeine, theophylline). Effects are potentiated by dipyridamole.	Continuous ECG monitoring is necessary

(continued)

TABLE 6-11 (Continued)

Antiarrhythmic Agents

Drug	Description	Dose	Contraindications
amiodarone HCl/cord-arone (oral preparation)	Antiarrhythmic agent used to treat VF and hemodynamically unstable VT refractory to other agents Blocks sodium channels Slows conduction by blocking myocardial potassium channels Antisympathetic effect causing slowing of heart rate and conduction Lengthens cardiac action potential ↓ cardiac work load and myocardial oxygen consumption Combination of amiodarone with other antiarrhythmic agents should be reserved for unstable ventricular arrhythmias or refractory to other medications.	5 mg/kg IV over 3 min; then 10 mg/kg/day	Known hypersensitivity to iodine Cardiogenic shock, sinus bradycardia and 2nd/3rd degree AV blocks
bretylium tosylate	Used in treatment of VF and unstable VT that has failed other antiarrhythmic agents Mechanism of action not fully understood	5 mg/kg IV bolus If ventricular fibrillation persists, 10 mg/kg IV bolus may be given and repeated as necessary. Infusion of 1–2 mg/min for continuous suppression	Bradycardia

Possible Maternal Side Effects	Possible Fetal/Neonatal Side Effects	Interactions	Precautions
Hypotension, cardiac arrhythmias (e.g., bradycardia and ventricular rhythms)	EFM: Observe for fetal bradycardia. Potential for congenital goiter and hypothyroidism with oral administration May cause IUGR Observe for transient bradycardia and prolonged QT segment in newborn. Excreted in breast milk	IV use incompatible with aminophylline, cefamandole naftate, cefazolin, mezlocillin, heparin, and sodium bicarbonate ↑ serum digoxin levels. Digoxin dose should be reduced by 50% with concurrent use. Cimetidine inhibits metabolized form of amiodarone (CYP3A4) and may cause increased serum levels. Elevated cyclosporine levels with concurrent use Phenytoin decreases serum amiodarone levels ↑ serum quinidine levels Rifampin effects decreased if given with oral amiodarone Use with fentanyl may cause hypotension, bradycardia, and decreased cardiac output. Sinus bradycardia may be caused by concurrent use with local lidocaine administration.	Continuous ECG monitoring with observation for prolonged QT Administration via central line with an in-line filter is recommended. Use with caution in patients receiving β-receptor blocking agents (e.g. propranolol) or calcium channel blocking agents (e.g., verapamil). This may cause bradycardia, sinus arrest and A–V block. Correct electrolyte imbalances prior to administration. Hypokalemia and hypomagnesemia may prolong QT interval. Check baseline liver enzymes prior to administration. High doses and rapid administration have been associated with acute hepatic necrosis, hepatic coma, renal failure, and death. May cause or exacerbate ARDS May cause development of pulmonary fibrosis Close monitoring needed for myocardial depression if used with halogenated inhalation anesthetics Consumption of grapefruit juice with oral administration may increase plasma levels.
Hypotension, cardiac arrhythmias (e.g., bradycardia, increased PVCs), hyperthermia, transient hypertension, angina, renal dysfunction, diarrhea, abdominal pain, macular rash, confusion, paranoid psychosis, anxiety, diaphoresis, mild conjunctivitis	Potential risks for decreased uterine blood flow, fetal hypoxia, late decelerations, and bradycardia	Pressor effects of catecholamines (e.g., dopamine and norepinephrine) are increased by bretylium.	ECG monitoring BP monitoring with an arterial line Monitor maternal temperature. Keep patient supine during administration to prevent postural hypotension. Caution when administered with digitalis—may enhance symptoms of digitalis toxicity In patients with fixed cardiac output (e.g., severe aortic stenosis, pulmonary hypertension), hypotension may cause further decrease in cardiac output.

(continued)

TABLE 6-11 (Continued)

Antiarrhythmic Agents

Drug	Description	Dose	Contraindications
lidocaine	Indicated for treatment of wide-complex tachycardia, stable ventricular tachycardia, and control of PVCs Requires multiple doses to achieve adequate serum concentrations	1 mg/kg bolus IV; ETT bolus 2–4 mg/kg Repeat ½ bolus at 10 min to a total cumulative dose of 3 mg/kg. Infusion at 2–4 mg/min Decrease dose after 24 hr (half-life increases after 24 hr)	Hypersensitivity to local anesthetics of the amide type
procainamide (Pronestyl)	Used in treatment of life-threatening ventricular rhythms (e.g., VT) and arrhythmia suppression Increases refractory period of the atria Slows conduction	Dilute procainamide (100 mg/mL or 500 mg/mL) 100 mg every 5 min until arrhythmia suppression (cumulative dose of) 500 mg has been given **or** Loading infusion of 500–600 mg Maintenance infusion of 2–6 mg/min	Hypersensitivity to sulfite medications Complete heart block Lupus erythematosus Torsades de pointes—ventricular arrhythmia
quinidine gluconate (Quinidex po)	Used to convert or suppress symptomatic atrial fibrillation and flutter or ventricular tachycardia. Prolongs the QT interval	5–10 mg/kg IV (maximum infusion rate of 1 mL/kg/hr) Maintenance infusion 0.02 mg/kg/min	Patients with junctional or ideoventricular pacemakers Myasthenia gravis

ANA = antinuclear antibody, ARDS = acute respiratory distress syndrome, AV = atrioventricular, BP = blood pressure, BUN = blood urea nitrogen, CBC = complete blood count, CNS = central nervous system, ECG = electrocardiogram, ETT = endotracheal tube, IUGR = intrauterine growth restriction, PVC = premature ventricular contraction, SVT = supraventricular tachycardia, VF = ventricular fibrillation, VT = ventricular tachycardia.

Possible Maternal Side Effects	Possible Fetal/Neonatal Side Effects	Interactions	Precautions
Neurologic toxicity with serum levels >5 mg/mL	Rapidly crosses placenta; potential for fetal bradycardia Associated with neonatal muscular weakness, decreased tone, and altered neurologic behavior in the newborn	May exacerbate neuromuscular blocking effects of paralytic agents	Monitor serum levels (normal 1–4 mg/L). Continuous ECG monitoring and 6–12 hours following administration
Hypotension, ventricular rhythms (e.g., fibrillation) Lupus symptoms (arthralgia, pleural or abdominal pain) *Hematologic:* neutropenia, thrombocytopenia, hemolytic anemia, agranulocytosis *Other:* anorexia, nausea, vomiting, skin lesions (urticaria, pruritus), elevated transaminase, dizziness, mental depression, and psychosis	Excreted in breast milk	None known	Administer with patient in supine position. Monitor vital signs and ECG. Discontinue infusion with drop in blood pressure of 15 mmHg. CBC, serum creatinine, and BUN before administration If used for conversion of atrial fibrillation, dislodgment of thrombi may occur. Prolonged administration may lead to development of a positive ANA test and lupus-like syndrome. Atrial flutter or fibrillation should be treated before administration of procainamide. May cause rapid AV node conduction. Use cautiously with congestive heart failure, acute ischemic heart disease or cardiomyopathy. May cause decrease in myocardial contractility. Concurrent use with other antiarrhythmic agents may prolong conduction and decrease cardiac output. May enhance symptoms of myasthenia gravis
Potential oxytocic properties with high doses Widened QRS complex Nausea, vomiting, diarrhea, heartburn, headache, fatigue, angina-like discomfort	Potential for 8th cranial nerve damage and thrombocytopenia. Serum levels in neonate may equal maternal levels Levels in amniotic fluid are 3 times higher than the serum level Excreted in breast milk	↑ serum levels if given concurrently with amiodarone or cimetidine ↓ serum levels with concurrent administration of nifedipine ↑ hepatic elimination with concurrent use of phenobarbital, phenytoin, rifampin Potentiates action of warfarin ↑ serum levels of haloperidol with concurrent administration	Continuous ECG monitoring. Continuous blood pressure monitoring. Discontinue if QRS complex widens to 130% of pretreatment time. Absorbed in polyvinyl chloride tubing. Use short IV tubing (less than 12 inches) on an infusion pump.

TABLE 6-12

Calcium Channel Blocking Agents

Drug	Description	Dose	Contraindications
diltiazem (Cardizem)	Calcium ion influx inhibitor (calcium antagonist) during membrane depolarization in cardiac and vascular smooth muscle Relaxes smooth muscle and decreases vascular resistance Prolongs AV node refractory periods slowing the HR Decreases myocardial oxygen demand Dilates coronary blood vessels	20 mg IV bolus over 2 min; repeat in 15 min 180–240 mg daily for initial oral dosing; maximum oral dose is 540 mg daily	Sick sinus syndrome, 2nd or 3rd degree heart block, hypotension, acute myocardial infarction, pulmonary edema
verapamil (Calan)	Calcium ion influx inhibitor Indicated to treat hypertension, atrial flutter and fibrillation or prophylaxis treatment of SVT Maternal administration to treat fetal SVT Negative inotropic effects Decreases systemic vascular resistance	2.5–5 mg IV bolus over 2 min May repeat in 5 min and then every 30 min prn to maximum cumulative dose of 20 mg	Decreased myocardial contractility, hypotension, sick sinus syndrome, 2nd or 3rd degree heart block, Wolff-Parkinson-White or Lown-Ganong-Levine syndrome

AV = atrioventricular, ECG = electrocardiogram, HR = heart rate, SVT = supraventricular tachycardia.

released during the inflammatory response, and trauma (e.g., tumor necrosis factor). Medications such as beta blockers, calcium channel blockers, and antiarrhythmics may also depress contractility. Because contractility is decreased in hypovolemic states, the initial management to improve myocardial force should be volume resuscitation. Augmentation of myocardial contractility with positive inotropic agents should be considered if contractility remains low (Table 6-13).[9]

ANTICOAGULANTS

Pregnancy is a procoagulant state, and women may require therapeutic-dose anticoagulation for a variety of reasons. Women who have a history of thromboemboli or are being anticoagulated for such issues as heart valve disease or a history of antiphospholipid antibody syndrome, and women who present with other risk factors for thromboemboli are all candidates for anticoagulation therapy during pregnancy and postpartum.

Possible Maternal Side Effects	Possible Fetal/Neonatal Side Effects	Interactions	Precautions
Edema of lower extremities, sinus congestion, rash, dizziness, fatigue, bradycardia, 1st degree AV block, cough, flushing, headache, nausea, hypotension	Possible teratogenic effects of the skeleton, heart, retina, and tongue Excreted in breast milk and may approximate serum levels	Prolonged AV conduction with concurrent use of digitalis or beta blockers ↑ effects and toxicity of quinidine and buspirone when used concurrently ↑ serum levels of propranolol, carbamazepine, and lovastatin when used concurrently Concurrent use with cimetidine causes increased serum levels of dilitiazem. Myocardial contractility, conductivity, and vascular dilation may be enhanced with concurrent use of anesthetics. ↓ serum levels of dilitiazem if used concurrently with rifampin.	Oral doses should be taken at the same time each day. Monitor digitalis levels if used concurrently. May elevate liver enzymes following initial therapy Use cautiously in patients with liver and renal impairment.
Hypotension (5%–10% of patients), dizziness, nausea, headache, pulmonary edema	Potential for reduced uterine blood flow and fetal hypoxia Excreted in breast milk	↑ serum digoxin, carbamazepine and theophylline levels Counteracts effects of quinidine on AV conduction Rifampin decreases availability ↑ effects of lithium May potentiate neuromuscular blocking agents	ECG monitoring Monitor liver enzymes; may elevate transaminases. Use cautiously in patients with impaired hepatic or renal function.

Warfarin, which is often used to manage issues relating to hypercoagulability in a non-pregnant state, crosses the placenta and can have adverse fetal effects during the first trimester of pregnancy.[20]

Once a decision has been made to provide therapeutic anticoagulation, unfractionated heparin (UH) and low-molecular-weight heparin (LMWH) are the two commonly used anticoagulants in the U.S. (Table 6-14). Of these, LMWH is generally considered the preferable option for long-term anticoagulation therapy. Low-molecular-weight heparins were developed because of a greater separation between antithrombic and hemorrhage dose ranges, which results in a greater margin of safety than other heparins.[21] LMWH vitamin K antagonists are used in many places in the world, but not in the U.S., because there have been reports of teratogenic effects during the 6th and 9th weeks of pregnancy, and they cause an increased risk for fetal complications.[21]

A woman in a critical care setting with newly diagnosed deep vein thrombosis or pulmonary embolism

(text continues on page 96)

TABLE 6-13

Positive Inotropic Agents

Drug	Description	Dose	Contraindications
dobutamine	Rapid acting, synthetic catecholamine Positive inotropic support used to enhance myocardial contractility and cardiac output. Stimulates β-receptors in the heart Increases AV node conduction May cause decrease in systemic vascular resistance Increases myocardial oxygen demand	Initial dose of 0.5–1 mcg/kg/min Titrate every few minutes to 20 mcg/kg/min based on patient response. Central line administration due to potential for phlebitis and necrosis of skin tissue Onset of action within 1–2 min; peak effect may take 10 min Half-life is approximately 2 min	Idiopathic hypertrophic sub-aortic stenosis (IHSS) Use with caution in patients with known hypersensitivity to sulfite medications.
digoxin (Lanoxin)	Positive inotropic agent used to treat mild to moderate heart failure. Increases myocardial contractility Slows conduction in the SA and AV nodes Increases myocardial oxygen demand.	Loading dose 0.5 mg IV over 5 minutes; then 0.25 IV q 6 hr × 2 Maintenance dose 0.125–0.375 mg PO daily Initial effects within 5–30 minutes and peak effect within 1–4 hr if administered IV Dosing may be based on the following: • Body weight • Renal function (creatinine clearance) • Serum levels (normal range 0.8–2.0 ng/mL) • Other medications concurrently administered Due to increased maternal blood volume and elimination, increased doses are required to obtain therapeutic levels.	Ventricular fibrillation

Possible Maternal Side Effects	Possible Fetal/Neonatal Side Effects	Interactions	Precautions
Ventricular ectopy, tachycardia, hypertension (especially systolic pressure increase)	Not known if excreted in breast milk	Enhanced cardiac output and lowers left preload (PCOP) when used concurrently with nitroprusside Recent administration of beta blockers may decrease effectiveness of dobutamine.	Continuous ECG and SaO_2 monitoring Arterial line placement to continuously monitor blood pressure Hemodynamic monitoring with a pulmonary artery catheter Monitor left ventricular stroke work index (LVSWI), pulmonary capillary occlusion pressure (PCOP), and cardiac output every hour until stabilization. Monitor potassium levels (may decrease potassium levels).
Heart block, nausea/vomiting, diarrhea, headache, blurred vision, dizziness, mental disturbances	Fetal toxicity and neonatal death have been reported. Excreted in breast milk	↑ serum levels with concurrent use of quinidine, verapamil, amiodarone, propafenone, indomethacin, itraconazole, alprazolam, and spironolactone Macrolide antibiotics (e.g., erythromycin, clarithromycin) may increase absorption of digoxin and cause toxicity. ↓ absorption and serum levels with concurrent use of antacids, rifampin, kaolinpectin, neomycin, cholestyramine, sulfasalazine, and metoclopraminde. Concurrent use with succinylcholine may result in increased potassium levels and result in cardiac arrhythmias.	ECG monitoring—prolongs PR interval and depresses ST segment Serum levels should be done prior to the next scheduled dose. Assessment of response should be done prior to next scheduled dose. Monitor serum electrolytes. Hypokalemia, hypomagnesemia, and hypercalcemia may result in digoxin toxicity. Administration of potassium depleting diuretics may cause toxicity. Rapid intravenous administration of calcium may cause life-threatening arrhythmias. Monitor renal function labs. Use with caution in patients with hyperthyroidism. Decreased doses are usually required for this population. Use with caution in patients with suspected or diagnosed acute myocardial infarction. Use may increase myocardial oxygen demand and ischemia.

(continued)

TABLE 6-13 (Continued)

Positive Inotropic Agents

Drug	Description	Dose	Contraindications
dopamine hydrochloride	Naturally occurring catechol-amine Directly stimulates α, β_1, and dopaminergic (DA) recep-tors **Indications** • Oliguria • Shock accompanied by hypotension **unresponsive to fluid resuscitation** • Congestive heart failure Hemodynamic effect related to dosage Increases pulmonary blood flow with minimal changes in PAP or PCOP (*Exception*: patients with septic shock and underlying pulmonary hypertension) Increases myocardial work and O_2 demand without a compensatory increase in coronary blood flow (*Risk* of myocardial ischemia) Decreases aldosterone secre-tion Inhibits insulin secretion from pancreatic islet cells Inhibits prolactin and TSH release	Central line administration is preferred due to potential for tissue extravasation **Infusion rate:** 0.5–2.0 mcg/kg/ min *Receptor stimulated:* DA *Clinical effect:* Increase urine output No change in HR and BP **Infusion rate:** 2.0–5.0 mcg/kg/ min *Receptors stimulated:* α, β_1 *Clinical effect:* Increases car-diac contractility and CO Minimal change in HR, BP, SVR **Infusion rate:** 5.0–10 mcg/kg/ min *Receptors stimulated:* α, β_1 *Clinical effect:* Further increase in CO Mild increase in HR, BP **Infusion rate:** >10 mcg/kg/min *Receptor stimulated:* α *Clinical effect:* Increased SVR and MAP Increased preload	Pheochromocytoma, uncor-rected tachyarrhythmias or ventricular fibrillation
epinephrine (Adrenalin)	Stimulates α and β receptor sites of sympathetic effector cells Increases blood pressure, myocardial contractility, heart rate, cardiac output Vasoconstriction of arterioles in skin, mucosa, and splanchnic tissue Relaxes smooth muscle in the bronchi Antagonizes histamine released from mast cells during an allergic reaction **Indications** • Anaphylactic hypersensitiv-ity reactions • Relief of bronchospasm with acute asthma attack • Treatment and prophylaxis of cardiac arrest	**Hypersensitivity reactions or relief of bronchospasm:** • 0.1 to 0.25 mg slow IV push Cardiac arrest • Initial bolus 0.5 mg to 1 mg IV • Repeat dose of 0.5 mg IV every 5 min • Follow with 2–10 mcg/kg/ minute infusion • Endotracheal dose 0.5–1 mg every 5 min	Shock (not related to anaphy-laxis), angle closure glaucoma

Possible Maternal Side Effects	Possible Fetal/Neonatal Side Effects	Interactions	Precautions
May interact with uterine stimulant (e.g., oxytocics) and ergot medications to produce severe maternal hypertension Cardiac arrhythmias, palpitations, changes in blood pressure (hypotension or hypertension), dyspnea, nausea, azotemia, headache, anxiety, gangrene of extremities with high doses	None noted at this time Category C: Risk cannot be ruled out.	Potential for ventricular arrhythmias with concurrent use of anesthetic agents (e.g., cyclopropane or halogenated cydrocarbon) MAO inhibitors prolong and increases the effects of dopamine. Concurrent use with phenytoin may result in bradycardia and hypotension. Inactive in alkaline solutions	Correct intravascular volume prior to administration. Avoid hypovolemia. Hemodynamic monitoring may be helpful to determine preload values. Monitor urine output every hour. Monitor blood pressure—observe for a decreased pulse pressure (due to elevation of diastolic pressure); discontinue with hypotension. Monitor cardiac output. Continuous ECG monitoring— observe for ectopic beats and ventricular rhythms. Hypoxia, hypercapnia, and acidosis may decrease the effectiveness of dopamine. Use with caution in patients with hypersensitivity to sulfites. Monitor peripheral pulses, skin color. and temperature—observe for signs of decreased tissue perfusion.
Transient anxiety, headache, palpitations, cardiac arrhythmias, hypertension, cerebral or subarachnoid hemorrhage, hemiplegia, angina, tremor, dizziness, dyspnea	Fetal tachycardia	Potential for ventricular arrhythmias with concurrent use of anesthetic agents (e.g., cyclopropane or halogenated cydrocarbon) Caution if used with other sympathomimetic medications Diuretics may decrease vascular response.	Continuous ECG monitoring Monitor urine output—may cause vasoconstriction in renal blood vessels. Use with caution in patients with hyperthyroidism or hypersensitivity reactions to sulfite medications.

TABLE 6-14

Anticoagulant and Thrombolytic Agents

Drug	Description	Dose	Contraindications
enoxaparin sodium (Lovenox)	Low-molecular-weight heparin Indicated for the prevention or treatment of deep vein thrombosis Fragments of unfractionated heparin (UFH) When compared with unfractionated heparin • ↑ bioavailability • ↑ half-life • ↑ anticoagulant activity • Predicable dose-response ratio • Less lab monitoring needed • ↓ risk of thrombocytopenia, bleeding and osteoporosis • allows outpatient management of most DVT	30 mg SQ twice a day	Active bleeding, thrombocytopenia, known hypersensitivity to heparin, benzyl alcohol or pork products
recombinant Activated Factor VIIa (NovoSeven)	Vitamin K–dependent glycoprotein similar to human plasma-derived Factor VIIa Indicated for the treatment and prevention of bleeding episodes in hemophilia A or B patients with inhibitors to Factor VIII or Factor IX, in patients with acquired hemophilia and in patients with congenital FVII deficiency Indicated for the control of hemorrhage by activating the extrinsic pathway of the coagulation cascade and promoting hemostasis OFF-LABEL USE—reported in trauma, military combat and obstetric literature for control of massive hemorrhage when traditional treatment is unsuccessful at stopping bleeding. Controversial, no randomized studies in obstetrics.	90 mcg/kg IV bolus q 2 hr until hemostasis is achieved	Hypersensitivity to bovine, hamster, or mouse proteins

Possible Maternal Side Effects	Possible Fetal/Neonatal Side Effects	Interactions	Precautions
Potential for bleeding is low Thrombocytopenia	No placental transfer Breast-feeding is safe.	None reported	Risk of epidural or spinal hematoma Monitor coagulation lab trends.
Thrombotic events, pyrexia, hemorrhage, injection site reaction, arthralgia, headache, blood pressure changes, nausea, vomiting, pain, edema, rash Hypersensitivity reactions: hives, urticaria, tightness of the chest, wheezing, hypotension, and anaphylaxis	Category C: Risk cannot be ruled out. Human studies are lacking. Not known if excreted in breast milk	Concomitant treatment with prothrombin complex concentrates should be avoided.	Increased risk of thrombotic event if used in patients with disseminated intravascular coagulopathy (DIC), sepsis, or concomitant treatment with prothrombin complex concentrates Do not mix with infusion solutions. Monitor coagulation lab trends.

(continued)

TABLE 6-14 (Continued)

Anticoagulant and Thrombolytic Agents

Drug	Description	Dose	Contraindications
recombinant tissue plasminogen activator (alteplase [Activase])	Thrombolytic agent **Indications:** • Acute myocardial infarction to improve myocardial function and reduce mortality • Acute ischemic stroke to improve neurologic recovery and decrease potential disability • Pulmonary embolism with hemodynamic instability—for lysis of emboli Reports of use in pregnancy and outcomes are very limited	**Acute myocardial infarction:** 15 mg IV bolus followed by an infusion of 50 mg over the next 30 min, and then 35 mg over the next 60 min (dose for patients weighing >67 kg) **Ischemic stroke:** 0.9 mg/kg (not to exceed 90 mg total dose) infused over 60 min; initial bolus of 10% of the total dose may be given over 1 min **Pulmonary embolism:** 100 mg IV over 2 hr; heparin therapy should be instituted immediately following infusion	**Acute myocardial infarction and pulmonary embolus:** Evidence of internal bleeding, history of cerebrovascular accident, recent intracranial or intraspinal surgery or trauma, intracranial neoplasm, arteriovenous malformation, aneurysm, known diathesis, severe, uncontrolled hypertension **Acute ischemic stroke:** Evidence of intracranial or subarachnoid hemorrhage; intracranial or intraspinal surgery within previous 3 months; head trauma or previous stroke; severe, uncontrolled hypertension (systolic >185 mmHg or diastolic >110 mmHg); seizure following stroke; active internal bleeding; intracranial neoplasm, arteriovenous malformation, aneurysm; INR >1.7; PT >15 seconds; platelet count <100,000/mm^3; heparin administration within previous 48 hr in conjunction with an elevated aPTT
streptokinase (Streptase)	Thrombolytic: causes lysis of fibrin clots Prolongs clotting cascade times Contains albumin **Indications** • Acute myocardial infarction (lysis of intracoronary thrombi) • Pulmonary embolus • Deep vein thrombosis • Arterial thrombosis or embolus	**Myocardial infarction** *Initial loading dose:* 1,500,000 units IV *Maintenance infusion duration:* Within 60 min **Pulmonary embolus** *Initial loading dose:* 250,000 units IV every 30 min *Maintenance infusion duration:* 100,000 units/hr × 24 hr **Deep vein thrombosis** *Initial loading dose:* 250,000 units IV every 30 min *Maintenance infusion duration:* 100,000 units/hr × 72 hr **Arterial thrombosis or embolism** *Initial loading dose:* 250,000 units IV over 30 min *Maintenance infusion duration:* 100,000 units/hr × 24–72 hr	Active internal bleeding, cerebrovascular accident within 2 months, intracranial or intraspinal surgery, intracranial neoplasm, severe hypertension

Possible Maternal Side Effects	Possible Fetal/Neonatal Side Effects	Interactions	Precautions
Hemorrhage, cardiac arrhythmias, pulmonary embolus, pulmonary edema, cerebral edema, seizure, hypotension	Category C: Risk cannot be ruled out. Human studies are lacking.	↑ effects with concurrent use of medications that decrease platelet function	Monitor for signs/symptoms of bleeding. Monitor vital sign and coagulation trends. Other recommended treatments for myocardial infarction and pulmonary embolus should be done with concurrent use of Activase. Internal jugular and subclavian arterial punctures should be avoided because these sites cannot be compressed to minimize bleeding. Risk of epidural or spinal hematoma
Bleeding or hemorrhage, respiratory depression, transient elevations of serum transaminases, reperfusion arrhythmias, hypotension, recurrent pulmonary embolus	Small amounts transferred to fetus—fetal antibodies formed	Concurrent use with other anticoagulants or antiplatelet medications may increase bleeding risk.	Monitor coagulation lab trends. ↓ fibrinogen and plasminogen ↑ TT, aPTT, PT No intramuscular injections Limit venipunctures. Risk of epidural or spinal hematoma
May cause onset of preterm labor			

(continued)

TABLE 6-14 (Continued)

Anticoagulant and Thrombolytic Agents

Drug	Description	Dose	Contraindications
unfractionated heparin	Large molecular weight Interferes with fibrin formation	*Initial treatment of deep vein thrombosis:* 100 units/kg bolus—loading dose; minimum of 5000 units *Initial treatment of pulmonary embolus:* 150 units/kg bolus—loading dose *Infusion rate DVT or PE:* 15–25 units/kg/hr IV; IV treatment × 5 days; then transition to SQ or low-molecular-weight heparin	Risk of hemorrhage
urokinase (Kinlytic)	Thrombolytic: acts on the fibrinolytic system Indicated for pulmonary embolus Made from human neonatal kidney cells—an enzyme produced by the kidneys and found in urine Formulated in 5% albumin	*Loading dose:* 4,400 international units/kg over 10 min *Maintenance infusion:* 4,400 IU/kg for 12 hr	Active internal bleeding, cerebrovascular accident within 2 months, intracranial or intraspinal surgery, intracranial neoplasm, severe hypertension, trauma or recent cardiopulmonary resuscitation

aPTT = activated partial thromboplastin time, DVT = deep vein thrombosis, INR = international normalized ratio, PT = prothrombin time, TT = thrombin time.

will often have therapy started with a continuous infusion of UH. The goal of the therapy is to maintain the activated partial thromboplastin time (aPPT) within the range of 1.5 to 2.5 times the upper limit of normal.[22] After several days of intravenous therapy, treatment should be transitioned to subcutaneous UH or LMWH. It has been clearly demonstrated that two doses provide the best anticoagulation due to the short half-lives of both UH and LMWH.[22]

Continuation of anticoagulant therapy at either therapeutic or prophlylactic dosages may inhibit the use of epidural or spinal anesthesia due to the risk for hematoma formation at the site of injection. Before regional anesthesia, it is currently recommended that prophylactic-dose anticoagulation be discontinued for at least 12 hours and therapeutic anticoagulation be discontinued for at least 24 hours before delivery.[23] It is also recommended that these patients be switched from subcutaneous anticoagulation to intravenous anticoagulation. The variability of absorption and effects are minimized with a more controlled and regulated intravenous administration of these drugs.[23]

When anticoagulation use warrants continuation during the postpartum period, current recommendations include the administration of LMWH and the initiation

of warfarin. Therapeutic blood levels of warfarin rise over a minimum of 4 to 5 days; therefore, both agents should be used. The parameters of effectiveness are determined by the aPPT and international normalized ratio (INR). The overall goal is to discontinue the heparin and achieve an INR between 2.0 and 3.0 on the warfarin alone. Warfarin is not secreted in breast milk and is considered safe for use in postpartum breast-feeding mothers.[24]

Lepridium is a hirudin that has recently been approved by the FDA for the treatment of heparin-induced thrombocytopenia and thrombosis syndrome. It acts as a direct thrombin inhibitor, requires parenteral administration, has a short half-life, but has a narrow therapeutic margin. There are several case reports in which lipridium has been used without fetal complications.[25]

Thrombolytic Therapy in Pregnancy

Thrombolytics are used in cases of ischemic stroke, myocardial infarction, pulmonary embolism, and thrombosed cardiac valve prostheses; however, reported use in pregnancy is rare (Table 6-14). A comprehensive review by Leonhardt and colleagues looked at 28 case

Possible Maternal Side Effects	Possible Fetal/Neonatal Side Effects	Interactions	Precautions
Hemorrhage (5%–10% incidence), thrombocytopenia (5%–10% incidence), osteoporosis (2%–7% incidence with >15,000 units/day for >6 months), hypotension, alopecia, pain at injection site	Does not cross placenta or cause teratogenic effects Breast-feeding is safe.	Protamine sulfate counteracts effects of heparin. • 1 mg neutralizes 100 units of heparin • Should not exceed 50 mg in a single dose	aPTT 4 hours after initiation and after dose change Goal with heparin therapy: aPTT: 1.5–2.5 × control (60–80 seconds) Monitor coagulation lab trends. Risk of epidural or spinal hematoma
Bleeding or hemorrhage, recurrent pulmonary embolus, pulmonary edema, reperfusion cardiac arrhythmias	Not teratogenic	Concurrent use with other anticoagulants or antiplatelet medications may increase bleeding risk.	Monitor coagulation lab trends. No intramuscular injections Limit venipuncture. Risk of epidural or spinal hematoma

reports of recombinant tissue plasminogen activator (rt-PA) use in pregnancy (stroke, n = 10; thrombosis of cardiac valve prosthesis, n = 7; pulmonary embolism, n = 7; deep venous thrombosis, n = 3; myocardial infarction, n = 1).[26] The report showed comparable complication rates in non-pregnant, randomized control trials. Complications were noted in women changing from warfarin to heparin in order to prevent teratogenic complications early in pregnancy. Even though rt-PA (alteplase) is an approved thrombolytic agent, guidelines are not well established for use in pregnancy. However, treatment should not be withheld in pregnant women with potentially high morbidity or life-threatening thromboembolic disease. Streptokinase and urokinase are rarely used in most developed countries.[26]

SEDATIVES

Benzodiazepines are a broad category of medications having sedative, amnesic, anti-anxiety, muscle relaxant, and anticonvulsant properties (Tables 6-15 and 6-16). Benzodiazepines also reduce cerebral blood flow, oxygen consumption, and intracranial pressure. Even though benzodiazepines provide sedation and may induce an unconscious state, psychiatric and paradoxical symptoms may occur in some patients. In the mechanically ventilated patient, benzodiazepines may be combined with propofol or neuromuscular blockers with minimal cardiovascular effects, such as mild tachycardia and decreased blood pressure.[9] Benzodiazepines cross the placental barrier with similar effects in the fetus. To minimize risks to the mother, fetus, or nursing newborn, benzodiazepine use is recommended with established safety records, the smallest possible dose for the shortest period of time while avoiding multiple drug regimes, and use in the first trimester.[27] Obtaining fetal reassurance with electronic fetal monitoring is difficult due to decreased baseline variability. Biophysical profile parameters may also be decreased (e.g., fetal movement and tone).

OTHER MEDICATIONS USED IN CRITICAL CARE OBSTETRICS

Other medications include drotrecogin alfa (Xigris), which is used for adults with severe sepsis (associated with acute organ dysfunction) who have a high risk of death (Table 6-17). To date, no studies have been done

(text continues on page 104)

TABLE 6-15

Sedatives

Drug	Description	Dose	Contraindications
diazepam (Valium)	Benzodiazepine derivative that has long-acting sedative, muscle relaxant, anticonvulsant, and amnestic effects. Increases the actions of GABA, an inhibitory neurotransmitter Depresses all levels of the CNS	2–10 mg IV every 5–10 min to initiate therapy Repeat 2–4 hr as needed Cumulative maximum dose not to exceed 30 mg in 8 hr Phlebitis common with IV use	Myasthenia gravis, respiratory depression or insufficiency, hepatic insufficiency, sleep apnea patients, narrow-angle glaucoma
lorazepam (Ativan)	Benzodiazepine used for sedation and relief of anxiety Slow onset, long acting	1–2 mg IV repeated every few min until desired effect	Acute, narrow-angle glaucoma
midazolam (Versed)	Short, rapid-acting (2–3 min) benzodiazepine causing CNS depression. Indicated for sedation and amnesia for mechanically ventilated patients High lipid solubility; after days of use may result in prolonged effects due to accumulation in adipose tissue	Rapid initiation of sedation for intubated patients: Loading dose 0.05–0.2 mg/kg given over several min Maintenance infusion 0.06–0.12 mg/kg/hr; infusion may be titrated to desired effect	Acute, narrow-angle glaucoma

Possible Maternal Side Effects	Possible Fetal/Neonatal Side Effects	Interactions	Precautions
Drowsiness, muscle weakness, ataxia, dizziness, hypotension, elevated transaminases and alkaline phosphatase Potential for withdrawal symptoms with abrupt cessation	*Potential teratogen:* cleft lip, inguinal hernia, cardiac defects, nerve palsies, and pyloric stenosis High doses may cause mental retardation Decreased baseline variability and biophysical profile scores Depressed Apgar scores Potential for feeding difficulties (poor sucking), and hypothermia in the newborn Withdrawal symptoms in the newborn with prolonged maternal use Excreted in breast milk	Increases toxicity of benzodiazepines in CNS with co-administration of phenothiazines, barbiturates, alcohols, and MAOIs ↓ serum levels with concurrent use of antacids	Use with caution if patient has decreased level of consciousness. Respiratory depression may occur following administration. Position patient in side-lying position to decrease risk of aspiration. Use with caution if given concurrently with other CNS depressants, low albumin levels, or hepatic disease. Psychiatric and paradoxical reactions may occur with administration.
Sedation, dizziness, weakness, fatigue, unsteadiness	Possible teratogenic effects Decreased baseline variability Depressed Apgar scores with respiratory depression and hypotonia Observe for hypothermia, apnea, feeding problems, and impaired metabolic response to cold stress in the newborn. Withdrawal symptoms in the newborn if used in the mother for prolonged time Excreted in breast milk	Use with clozapine may produce marked sedation, increased salivation, hypotension, ataxia, delirium, and respiratory arrest. ↑ serum levels if used concurrently with valproate. ↑ half-life with concurrent use of probenecid.	Use cautiously in patients with sleep apnea. Dose should be adjusted with hepatic impairment.
Hypotension, respiratory depression (e.g., decreased rate and tidal volume), bradycardia, amnesia Withdrawal symptoms may occur.	Crosses the placenta Increased risk of congenital malformations Decreased baseline variability Neonatal depression Excreted in breast milk	Sedation increased with concurrent use of other CNS depressants or opioids Decreased elimination with concurrent use of cimetidine, erythromycin, diltiazem, or verapamil	Continuous monitoring of respiratory and cardiac function is required. Monitor vital sign and SaO$_2$ trends. Assess sedation frequently. Elimination may be decreased in patients with hepatic dysfunction or decreased cardiac output requiring positive inotropic agents.

(continued)

TABLE 6-15 (Continued)

Sedatives

Drug	Description	Dose	Contraindications
propofol (Diprivan)	Hypnotic-sedative used for intubated and mechanically ventilated patients Provides continuous sedation	Initiation of sedation with 5 mcg/kg/min IV over 5 min; repeat with 5–10 mcg/kg/min until desired effect Maintenance infusion 5–50 mcg/kg/min Administer in a large vein or central line. Recommended that lidocaine be administered before diprivan or added to diprivan immediately before administration due to localized pain and burning at infusion site Dose adjusted to desired level of sedation Wean dosage to prevent anxiety, agitation, and resistance to mechanical ventilation. Continue infusion for light sedation and discontinue 10–15 min before extubation.	Hypersensitivity to eggs, soybeans, or soy products
remifentanil (Ultiva)	μ–opioid agonist Used as an analgesic	0.05–0.1 mcg/kg/min infusion Use most proximal port of IV. Clear tubing when discontinuing medication. Blood concentrations decrease by 50% within 3–6 min after infusion	None reported

CNS = central nervous system, GABA = gamma aminobutyric acid, MAOI = monoamine oxidase inhibitor.

TABLE 6-16

Observer's Assessment of Alertness/Sedation (OAA/S)

Responsiveness	Speech
Responds readily to name spoken in normal tone	Normal
Lethargic response to name spoken in normal tone	Mild slowing or thickening
Responds only after slurring or name is called loudly and/or repeatedly	Slurring or prominent slowing
Responds only after mild prodding or shaking	Few recognized words
Does not respond to mild prodding or shaking	

Possible Maternal Side Effects	Possible Fetal/Neonatal Side Effects	Interactions	Precautions
Bradycardia, cardiac arrhythmias, decreased cardiac output, hypotension, hyperlipidemia, decreased lung function, green urine, intracranial hypertension Potential blood gas changes—respiratory acidosis during weaning May increase lab values—liver enzymes, BUN, creatinine, hyperglycemia, osmolality Propofol infusion syndrome (associated with doses >5 mg/kg/hr for more than 48 hr) and characterized by: • severe metabolic acidosis • hyperkalemia • hyperlipidemia • rhabdomyolysis • hepatomegaly • cardiac and renal failure	Crosses the placenta Neonatal depression Excreted in breast milk	↓ sedative effects with concurrent use of opioids (e.g., morphine, meperidine, fentanyl) or sedatives (e.g., benzodiazepines, barbiturates, droperidol)	Maintain strict aseptic technique when handling Diprivan. Contamination can cause fever, infection, sepsis and death. Change and discard IV tubing and any unused portions of Diprivan every 12 hr. Monitor for cardiac depression and hypotension. Supplemental zinc may be required.
Respiratory depression, bradycardia, hypotension, skeletal muscle rigidity, nausea, pruritus, headache, sweating, dizziness, pain at infusion site	Placental transfer Newborn depression if given shortly before delivery May be excreted in breast milk	Antagonized by naloxone	Resuscitation and intubation equipment should be readily available. Continuous monitoring of vital signs and SaO$_2$ Effects clear rapidly when medication is discontinued (usually within 5–10 min).

Facial Expression	Eyes	Composite Score
Normal	Clear, no ptosis	5 (Alert)
Mild relaxation	Glazed or mild ptosis (less than half the eye)	4
Marked relaxation (Slack jaw)	Glazed and marked ptosis (half the eye or more)	3
		2
		1 (Deep sleep)

TABLE 6-17

Other Medications Used in Critical Care Obstetrics

Drug	Description	Dose	Contraindications
activated protein C—drotrecogin alfa (Xigris)	Antithrombotic effect by inhibiting clotting Factors Va and VIIIa Indicated to reduce the mortality associated with severe sepsis	24 mcg/kg/min IV (based on actual body weight) Total duration of infusion is 96 hours	Active internal bleeding, previous hemorrhagic stroke, intracranial or intra-spinal surgery, head trauma, presence of epidural catheter, intracranial neoplasm
furosemide (Lasix)	Diuretic used to decrease preload Should not be used for management of hypertension during pregnancy unless hypervolemia is the causative factor	10–20 mg IV (dose should be based upon the amount of hypervolemia)	Anuria
magnesium sulfate	**Indications** • To treat and prevent seizures in women with pre-eclampsia or eclampsia • Also used as a tocolytic in preterm labor patients	6 gm bolus IV Infusion rate of 2 grams/hr Dose may be adjusted to 4-gram bolus and 1 gram/hr with decreased urine output or renal impairment.	Heart block, Addison disease, severe hepatitis

Possible Maternal Side Effects	Possible Fetal/Neonatal Side Effects	Interactions	Precautions
Hemorrhage	Category C: Risk cannot be ruled out. Human studies are lacking	Caution if used with other agents that interfere with hemostasis (e.g., heparin)	Monitor coagulation lab trends. aPTT and PT may be prolonged with Xigris use and cannot be used to guide therapy. Discontinue 2 hr before surgery or invasive procedures. Increased risk of hemorrhage: • platelet count <30,000 • PT—INR >3.0 • Gastrointestinal bleeding within 6 weeks • Thromboembolic therapy within 3 days • Ischemic stroke within 3 months • Intracranial arteriovenous malformation or aneurysm • Bleeding tendencies • Chronic, severe liver disease • Any condition that predisposes patient to hemorrhage
Excessive volume loss, electrolyte imbalance (e.g., hypokalemia, hyponatremia, hypocalcemia, hypomagnesemia), tachycardia, hypotension May increase blood glucose levels	Placental transfer with fetal serum levels similar to maternal levels after 8 hr of use Increased fetal urine production—may cause alterations in amniotic fluid volume Monitor for serum electrolyte imbalances in the newborn. Excreted in breast milk	↑ potential for ototoxic reactions to aminoglycoside antibiotics ↓ arterial response of norepinephrine Concurrent use with indomethacin may decrease natriuetic and antihypertensive effects.	Monitor serum electrolytes (potassium) and correct as needed. Observe for signs of electrolyte changes. Monitor hemodynamics. Monitor intake and output. Caution with use in women with preeclampsia—potential for severe hypovolemia, decreased cardiac output, tissue perfusion, and fetal compromise.
Respiratory and neuromuscular depression, cardiac arrhythmias	With increased serum magnesium levels in the mother, the fetus and/or newborn may have: • decreased baseline variability • depressed Apgar scores with respiratory depression, loss of reflexes, and lack of muscle tone • Hypocalcemia and hypermagnesemia in the newborn	May alter cardiac conduction, leading to heart block in patients taking digitalis ↑ neuromuscular blockade with concurrent use of calcium channel blockers (e.g., nifedipine)	Monitor DTRs, respiratory rate, and urine output trends. Calcium gluconate 10–20 mL IV of 10% solution can be given as an antidote for clinically significant hypermagnesemia. Discontinue with absent DTRs or magnesium serum levels of >8 mEq/L.

(continued)

TABLE 6-17 (Continued)

Other Medications Used in Critical Care Obstetrics

Drug	Description	Dose	Contraindications
mannitol	**Indications** • promote diuresis for prevention and treatment of acute renal failure • ↓ intracranial pressure	Initial test dose for patients with impaired renal function: 0.2 g/kg IV over 3–5 min; check for urine flow of 30–50 mL/hr; second dose may be given with less than 30–50 mL urine output Reduction of intracranial pressure: 0.25–2 g/kg Administer in large vein	Hypovolemia, increased oliguria and azotemia, pulmonary edema, intracranial bleeding

aPTT = activated partial thromboplastin time, DTR = deep tendon reflexes, GFR = glomerular filtration rate, INR = international normalized ratio, I&O = input and output, PT = prothrombin time.

to demonstrate fetal harm or reproduction capacity.[28] Although no case reports indicate major malformations or adverse effects with drotrecogin alfa use, the limitation of studies do not reliably estimate the frequency of adverse outcomes.

REFERENCES

1. Milch, C. E., Salem, D. N., Pauker, S. G., Lundquist, T. G., Kumar S., & Chen J. (2006). Voluntary electronic reporting of medical errors and adverse events. *Journal of General Internal Medicine, 21,* 165–170.
2. Joint Commission. (2011). *Sentinel event statistics.* Washington, DC: Author. Retrieved from http://www.joint-commission.org/sentinel_event_statistics_quarterly/
3. Institute for Safe Medicine Practices. (2008). *ISMP's list of high-alert medications.* Horsham, PA: Author. Retrieved from http://www.ismp.org/Tools/highalertmedications.pdf
4. Tucker, S. M., Miller, L. A., & Miller, D. A. (2008). *Fetal monitoring: A multidisciplinary approach* (6th ed.). St. Louis, MO: Mosby.
5. Lo, W. Y., & Friedman, J. M. (2002). Teratogenicity of recently introduced medication in human pregnancy. *Obstetrics & Gynecology, 100*(3), 465–473.
6. Yaffe, S. J., & Briggs, G. G. (2003). Is this drug going to harm my baby? *Contemporary OB/GYN, 48,* 57.
7. Lehn, M. C. E., Salem, D. N., Pauker, S. G., Lundquist, T. G., Kumar, S., & Chen, J. (2006). Voluntary electronic reporting of medical errors and adverse events. *Journal of General Internal Medicine, 21,* 165–170.
8. ACOG Practice Bulletin: Clinical Management Guidelines for Obstetrician-Gynecologists. Number 6, October 2006.
9. Marini, J. J., & Wheeler, A. P. (2006). *Critical care medicine: The essentials* (3rd ed.). Philadelphia: Lippincott Williams & Wilkins.
10. Cunningham, F. G., Leveno, K. J., Bloom, S. L., Hauth, J. C., Gilstrap II, L. C., & Wenstrom, K. D. (2005). *Williams obstetrics* (23rd ed., pp. 341–364). New York: McGraw-Hill.
11. Sibai, B. M. (2010). Hypertensive emergencies. In M. R. Foley, T. H. Strong, & T. J. Garite (Eds.), *Obstetric intensive care manual* (3rd ed.). New York: McGraw-Hill.
12. Report of the National High Blood Pressure Education Program Working Group on High Blood Pressure in Pregnancy: Summary report. (2000). *American Journal of Obstetrics & Gynecology, 183*(1), S1–S22.
13. Sibai, B. M. (2007). Hypertension. In S. G. Gabbe, J. R. Niebyl, & J. L. Simpson (Eds.), *Obstetrics: Normal and problem pregnancies* (5th ed.). New York: Churchill Livingstone.
14. Magee, L. A., Cham, C., Waterman, E. J., Ohlsson, A., & Von Dadelszen, P. (2003). Hydralazine for treatment of severe hypertension in pregnancy: Meta-analysis. *BMJ, 327,* 1–10.
15. Vidaeff, A. C., Carroll, M. A., & Ramin, S. M. (2005). Acute hypertensive emergencies in pregnancy. *Critical Care Medicine, 33*(10), S307–S312.
16. Gonik, B. G., & Foley, M. R. (2004). Intensive care monitoring of the critically ill pregnant patient. In R. K. Creasy, R. Resnik, & J. D. Iams (Eds.), *Maternal-fetal medicine* (5th ed., pp. 925–951). Philadelphia: W.B. Saunders Company.
17. Blanchard, D. G., & Shabetai, R. (2004). Cardiac diseases. In R. K. Creasy, R. Resnik, & J. D. Iams (Eds.), *Maternal-fetal medicine* (5th ed., pp. 815–843). Philadelphia: W.B. Saunders Company.
18. López-Sendó, J., Swedberg, K., McMurray, J., Tamargo, J., Maggioni, A. P., Dargie, H., et al. Task Force on Beta-Blockers of the European Society of Cardiology. (2004). Expert consensus document on β-adrenergic receptor blockers. *European Heart Journal, 25*(15), 1341–1362.
19. Kron, J., & Conti, J. (2007). Arrhythmias in the pregnant patient: Current concepts in evaluation and management. *Journal of Interventional Cardiology and Electrophysiology, 19,* 95–107.
20. Briggs, G. G., Freeman, R. F., & Yaffe, S. J. (2008). *Drugs in pregnancy and lactation* (8th ed.). Philadelphia: Lippincott Williams & Wilkins.

Possible Maternal Side Effects	Possible Fetal/Neonatal Side Effects	Interactions	Precautions
Hypovolemia, electrolyte imbalance, pulmonary edema, headache, blurred vision	Maternal hypovolemia may impair uterine perfusion, resulting in fetal hypoxia and acidosis.	None noted	Assess intravascular volume status before administration. Use with caution for acute renal failure in pregnancy, because most cases are a result of hypovolemia. Monitor I&O every hour. Monitor renal function labs—GFR. Monitor serum electrolyte trends. Assess for venous thrombosis, phlebitis and extravasation of tissue at infusion site.

21. Casele, H. L. (2006). The use of unfractionated heparin and low molecular weight heparins in pregnancy. *Clinical Obstetrics and Gynecology, 49*(4), 895–905.
22. American Academy of Pediatrics and American College of Obstetrics and Gynecologists. (2007). *Guidelines for perinatal care* (6th ed.). Elk Grove Village, IL: American Academy of Pediatrics.
23. Horlocker, T. T., Wedel, D. J., Benzon, H., Brown D. L., Enneking, F.K., Heit, J.A., et al. (2003). Regional anesthesia in the anticoagulated patient: Defining the risks (The second ARSA Consensus Conference on Neuraxial Anesthesia and Anticoagulation). *Regional Anesthesia and Pain Medicine, 28*(3), 172–197.
24. Marks, P. W. (2007). Management of thromboembolism in pregnancy. *Seminars in Perinatology, 31,* 227–231.
25. Silver, R. M. (2008). New anticoagulants and pregnancy. *Obstetrics & Gynecology, 112*(2), 419–420.
26. Leonhardt, G., Gaul, C., Nietsch, H., Buerke, M., & Schleussner, E. (2006). Thrombolytic therapy in pregnancy. *Journal of Thrombosis and Thrombolysis, 21*(3), 271–276.
27. Iqbal, M. M., Sobhan, T., & Ryals, T. (2002). Effects of commonly used benzodiazepines on the fetus, the neonate, and the nursing infant. *Psychiatric Services, 53,* 39–49.
28. Eli Lilly and Company (2008). *Xigris: Full prescribing information.* Indianapolis, IN: Author. Retrieved from http://pi.lilly.com/us/xigris.pdf

PART III

Clinical Application

CHAPTER 7

Hypertension in Pregnancy

Carol J. Harvey and Baha M. Sibai

According to the Centers for Disease Control and Prevention (CDC), 29 percent of adults in the United States (U.S.) who are 18 years of age or older have hypertension. Approximately 25 to 30 percent of them are unaware of their disease or may be receiving ineffective treatment.[1,2] Therefore, it should be no surprise that many women are initially diagnosed with chronic hypertension during pregnancy, because they may not have had their blood pressure assessed by a health care provider prior to conception. Hypertension in the U.S. and other countries strongly correlates to obesity, which is now endemic in most regions of North America. Thus, identification of hypertension in a pregnant woman must be followed by an in-depth evaluation to determine the type of hypertension and its potential etiology. To differentiate preexisting hypertension (e.g., chronic hypertension) from the diagnostic subsets of hypertension that occur during pregnancy (e.g., preeclampsia-eclampsia, gestational) is challenging, and frequently can only be definitively accomplished after the 12th postpartum week.

Hypertension affects 12 to 22 percent of all pregnancies in the U.S. and is one of the top three causes of maternal mortality.[3,4] Preeclampsia affects 5 to 8 percent of pregnant women in the U.S. and Canada, and approximately 3 to 14 percent of pregnant women in other countries.[5]

This chapter addresses the current nomenclature used to describe hypertensive disorders in pregnancy, pathophysiologic principles of hypertensive disorders, treatment of severe preeclampsia and eclampsia, identification of HELLP syndrome, the use of magnesium sulfate and antihypertensive agents as pharmacotherapy, and hemodynamic findings associated with preeclampsia-eclampsia.

BLOOD PRESSURE MEASUREMENT DURING PREGNANCY

The accurate, reproducible measurement of blood pressure in any patient is integral to making the diagnosis of hypertension and to determining when treatment is indicated. However, this core component of medical and nursing practice is frequently assigned to the least trained care provider and, even when done by the most experienced authors and researchers, is rarely performed correctly.[6,7] Training of all levels of clinicians to improve noninvasive blood pressure assessment skills is critical to avoid misdiagnosis of hypertension and to prevent over- or undertreatment.

Blood pressure assessment using an inflatable bladder placed over the brachial artery and listening for characteristics of sounds audible above the artery has been the mainstay of blood pressure measurements for over a century. In 1905, Nikolai Korotkoff described a procedure to auscultate the sounds emitted near the artery when it is occluded and subsequently allowed to slowly fill. He then correlated these findings with the associated readings on the sphygmomanometer. He termed the sounds "Korotkoff" sounds and identified five distinct characteristics or phases (Table 7-1). That the procedure has remained essentially unchanged for decades is a tribute to the simplicity of manual blood pressure measurement using mercury, but also may reflect the fallibility of even a simple technology to produce accurate results.

The mercury sphygmomanometer is considered the gold standard in noninvasive blood pressure technology and is superior to aneroid, digital, and/or oscillometric machines. Sphygmomanometers include an inflatable cuffed bladder, a bulb for inflating the bladder, a valve to control the amount of air in the bladder,

TABLE 7-1

Korotkoff Phases and Sounds

Phase	Description of Sound
First*	First sound heard after inflation of the cuff and gradual release of the air from the bladder or cuff. May be "snapping," "clicking," or a deep thudding. Used for systolic pressure.
Second	Murmurs heard between the systolic and diastolic pressures
Third	Distinct, loud crisp tapping sound
Fourth	Thumping or "muffle" of sounds
Fifth**	Disappearance of the sounds. Used for diastolic pressure.

*First sound used to measure *systolic* pressure

**Diastolic pressure is recorded as 2 mmHg above the last sound heard. The second and third Korotkoff sounds have no clinical value at this time.

From Pickering, T.G., Hall, J.E., Appel, L.J., et al. (2005). Recommendations for blood pressure measurement in humans and experimental animals. Part 1: Blood pressure measurement in humans: A statement for professionals from the Subcommittee of Professional and Public Education of the American Heart Association Council on High Blood Pressure Research. *Circulation, 111,* 697–716.

and a gauge from which blood pressure can be read and recorded. The inflated cuff occludes arterial blood flow and allows auscultation of the artery via stethoscope.[8] The mercury sphygmomanometer is made by placing liquid mercury in a glass cylinder to create a vertical column. Mercury is displaced into the column when pressure is placed on the opposite side. The pressure required to move liquid mercury up the glass column against the force of gravity is measured in "millimeters of mercury" (mmHg), the internationally recognized standard unit of pressure employed when assessing and recording blood pressures.

Mercury is a stable metal at room temperature and when sealed from the atmosphere. It requires little maintenance as long as it remains encased in the glass cylinder and the cylinder has no damage or leaks. Because it is a heavy metal, mercury is toxic to the environment and can cause devastating neurologic damage in infants, children, and adults. Therefore, state and federal agencies have implemented programs to educate industries that use mercury to consider replacement alternatives. There is also a national movement to sequester existing mercury manometers and thermometers and to remove them from the environment to prevent toxic spills in patient care areas.

TABLE 7-2

Common Errors in Blood Pressure Measurement

Cuff too small	Falsely increases both SBP and DBP
Cuff too large	Falsely decreases both SBP and DBP
Bias	Clinicians have terminal number bias, whereby the last sound heard (diastolic) frequently ends in a zero.
Patient arm not supported	Falsely elevated pressures
Patient's arm and brachial artery are above the heart	Falsely low pressures
Patient's arm is hanging at her side while in high Fowler's or sitting position	Falsely elevated pressures
Talking	Increases BP
Patient sitting but back not supported (e.g., on exam table, sitting for epidural placement)	Diastolic blood pressure may increase 6 mmHg
Patient's legs are crossed	SBP may increase 2–8 mmHg
Not familiar with more accurate device	Oscillatory machines measure BP as the cuff is inflated *or* deflated. In pregnancy, machines that measure during inflation may be more accurate.
Use of oscillatory instead of invasive arterial line pressures	Compared to intra-arterial pressure catheters, oscillatory BP machines have lower systolic values and higher diastolic values.
Device not approved in pregnancy	Only BP machines specifically approved for use in pregnancy and validated as accurate in preeclampsia should be used.
Device not tested for accuracy	BP devices should be tested for accuracy annually.

BP = blood pressure, DBP = diastolic blood pressure, mmHg = millimeters of mercury, SBP = systolic blood pressure.

The down side of the replacement campaign is the removal of one of the most accurate methods for measuring blood pressure.

To replace mercury manometers, facilities may select from a number of available devices such as manual "dial" aneroid pressure manometers or automated oscillometric devices that inflate the cuff, deflate the cuff, and calculate pressures based on data derived from arterial pulsations and proprietary algorithms. Both substitutes are known for inherent inaccuracies, with aneroid devices more likely to have greater margins of error than automated blood pressure devices.[9,10] However, it is not possible to determine the exact range of pressure variance based on monitor type, because almost all classes of non-mercury devices have sources of error. The result is erroneous blood pressure values that may be significantly inaccurate.[11] Thus, when measuring blood pressure on a patient who is hypertensive or may require antihypertensive medications, the method for monitoring should be standardized in order to optimize the quality of the results. Common errors in blood pressure measurement can be found in Table 7-2. To reduce the contribution of human error and faulty technique to blood pressure assessment, a list of recommendations for practice can be found in Box 7-1. Further, it is not unreasonable to validate the competence of medical, nursing, and allied professional staff in measuring blood pressure using a variety of devices.

Systolic blood pressure is measured at the first Korotkoff sound, where the first beat of the heart is heard. Diastolic blood pressure is measured at the value point where the sound disappears, which is the fifth Korotkoff sound. In rare patients, the fifth Korotkoff sound may be zero due to the hyperdynamic state of pregnancy. In those cases, the fourth Korotkoff sound (muffling of the sounds) should be used as the diastolic

Box 7-1. METHODS FOR IMPROVED ACCURACY IN BLOOD PRESSURE MEASUREMENTS

- Place the patient in a comfortable chair in the sitting position, feet flat on the floor (supported), and body relaxed. Allow at least 10 minutes for the patient to relax. Neither the patient nor clinician should talk during the procedure.
- Position the patient's arm on a table so that it is relaxed and completely supported. Place the arm on a folded sheet or small pillow to elevate the brachial artery (where the stethoscope is placed) at the level of the patient's phlebostatic axis* (mid to upper-mid sternum in pregnant patients).
- Select the correct-sized BP cuff. Confirm the appropriate cuff size by following the manufacturer's sizing guide, usually found on the inside of the cuff.
- An appropriately sized cuff is at least 1.5 times the circumference of the arm. This allows the cuff to wrap around the arm to secure the device during inflation.
- The *bladder,* located inside the cuff, should at least be 80 percent of the circumference of the arm. The bladder width should be half the size of the bladder length—or 40 percent of the circumference of the arm.
- Place the cuff on the patient's arm, with the center of the bladder (lengthwise) 2 to 3 cm above the artery to prevent the stethoscope from touching the cuff.

- While palpating the radial artery, inflate the cuff until the pulsations are no longer felt. Note the pressure reading.
- Using a high-quality stethoscope with short tubing, place the bell over the brachial artery and inflate the cuff 30 mmHg higher than the pressure at which radial pulsations became absent.
- Deflate the cuff at no more than 2 to 3 mmHg per second, or per heartbeat if the rate is slow. Read the pressures to the nearest 2 mmHg.
- Note the first (Korotkoff Phase 1) and last (Korotkoff Phase 5) audible sounds for systolic and diastolic pressures. Completely deflate the cuff. Accurately record the values.
- Allow at least 1 minute of rest and measure the blood pressure again in the same arm. If you find more than a 5 percent difference in the first pressure, omit the first pressure (usually the highest) and take one to two more readings and average them.
- Repeat the procedure in the opposite arm. Record and use the highest pressure. If blood pressure is significantly higher in one arm, use the arm with the higher values.

*The phlebostatic axis is a landmark at approximately the level of the right atrium of the heart. It is at the 4th intercostal space where it crosses the mid-axillary line. The location where BP is measured (brachial artery for most measurements) should be placed at the level of this landmark.
BP = blood pressure.
Data from Magee, L., Helewa, M., Moutquin, J., et al. (2008). Diagnosis, evaluation, and management of the hypertension disorders of pregnancy. *Journal of Obstetrics and Gynaecology Canada, 30,* S1–S48; and Pickering, T.G., Hall, J.E., Appel, L.J., et al. (2005). Recommendations for blood pressure measurement in humans and experimental animals: part 1: blood pressure measurement in humans: A statement for professionals from the Subcommittee of Professional and Public Education of the American Heart Association Council on High Blood Pressure Research. *Circulation, 111,* 697–716.

value and should be documented as the source of the diastolic reading.[7]

The parturient should be in a sitting position with her legs uncrossed and feet flat on the floor or supported by a footrest. The arm used for blood pressure measurement should be completely supported by a table or pad, with the brachial artery of the arm positioned at the level of the patient's right atrium. This landmark is known as the *phlebostatic axis* and is located at the intersection of the fourth intercostal space at the mid-axillary line. It approximates the level of the aorta and is the same reference point used to zero-reference invasive hemodynamic pressure tubing. The patient is allowed time (minimum, 10 minutes) to sit quietly without talking or moving to try to achieve a relaxed state prior to evaluation. Blood pressure evaluation then begins with location of the maximal impulse of the brachial artery by palpation. A blood pressure cuff of the correct size is placed above the brachial artery according to the artery placement marks on the inside of the cuff. The correct size for the bladder (not the cuff) is at least 80 percent of the circumference of the arm. The ratio of length to width should be 1.5 to 1; in other words, the length should be 1.5 times the width of the bladder.[7,12] Ideally, the clinician assessing blood pressure is sitting so that his or her eyes are at the level of the mercury meniscus of a sphygmomanometer or the numbers and dial of an aneroid manometer.

The radial artery is palpated at the point of maximal impulse, and the blood pressure cuff is inflated to 70 mmHg. The cuff is then quickly inflated in increments of 10 mmHg until the pulse is no longer palpable. It is important to note the pressure reading at which this occurs and the reading at which arterial pulsations return during deflation of the cuff. The bell of the stethoscope is placed over the strongest pulsation of the artery. The cuff is rapidly inflated 20 to 30 mmHg above the level where the pulse was no longer felt. The cuff is then deflated at a rate of 2 mmHg/sec until the first Korotkoff sound is heard (systole). Deflation of the cuff at 2 mmHg/sec continues until the Korotkoff sounds disappear (Korotkoff 5), which is diastole.[12] After the last sound is identified, the clinician continues to listen for additional sounds as pressure decreases at least another 10 mmHg. If no sounds are audible, rapid and complete deflation of the cuff is the endpoint. Systolic and diastolic pressures should be recorded to the nearest 2 mmHg.[12] Wait at least 1 minute between blood pressure measurements to allow venous emptying from the limb.

Initially, blood pressure should be measured in both arms to assess for differences between them. The arm with the highest pressure should be used for the duration of care. When patients are in a recumbent position in a hospital bed, it is important to follow the same procedure as outlined for patients in a sitting position. It is critical that the artery where blood pressure is measured be positioned at the level of the heart.

CLASSIFICATIONS OF HYPERTENSION IN PREGNANCY

The study of hypertension in pregnancy has been hindered by a lack of agreement on a set of definitions to define subsets of the disease. It is difficult to interpret research findings when investigators use different criteria to identify preeclampsia and other hypertensive disorders. In an attempt to standardize terminology, professional organizations develop and publish independent classification systems for hypertension in pregnancy. The World Health Organization (WHO), the United Kingdom's Royal College of Obstetricians and Gynaecologists (RCOG), the Society of Obstetricians and Gynaecologists of Canada (SOGC), and the U.S. National High Blood Pressure Education Program Work Group on High Blood Pressure in Pregnancy (NHBPEPWG, commonly called the NHBP Group) are examples of professional organizations that have developed terminology to use in the diagnosis and management of hypertension in pregnancy. There is, however, no universal agreement among professional groups regarding terminology, which may perpetuate the lack of meaningful data to further the study of hypertension in pregnancy. This chapter uses terms recommended by the NHBP Group, which are also used by the American College of Obstetricians and Gynecologists (ACOG), as defined in Table 7-3.

Hypertension is defined as a systolic pressure of 140 mmHg or higher or a diastolic pressure of 90 mmHg or higher, measured on at least two occasions at least 6 hours but not more than 7 days apart. Only one pressure (systolic *or* diastolic) needs to be elevated to meet the definition of hypertension. The NHBP Group's terms for hypertensive conditions of pregnancy are chronic hypertension, preeclampsia-eclampsia, chronic hypertension with superimposed preeclampsia, and gestational hypertension.[13] In part, the definitions imply the time of onset of the disease state. For example, chronic hypertension is elevated blood pressure that occurs prior to pregnancy or before the 20th week of pregnancy. Hypertension that develops during pregnancy and does not resolve by the 12th postpartum week is also classified as chronic hypertension.[13]

Preeclampsia-eclampsia is diagnosed when hypertension develops after the 20th week of pregnancy and is accompanied by proteinuria. Superimposed preeclampsia-eclampsia on chronic hypertension is considered when new onset proteinuria is present. In patients who have proteinuria prior to pregnancy, worsening of the proteinuria or hypertension is considered

TABLE 7-3

Categories of Hypertension In Pregnancy

Chronic Hypertension	Hypertension (≥140 mmHg systolic or ≥90 mmHg diastolic), measured on at least two occasions 4–6 hours apart *before* the 20th week of pregnancy
Preeclampsia	Hypertension measured on at least two occasions at least 4–6 hours apart *after* the 20th week of gestation, in a woman without a history of hypertension prior to pregnancy *and* proteinuria of 300 mg (0.3 grams) or more in a 24-hour urine collection
Eclampsia	The progression of preeclampsia to the seizure state. The occurrence of grand mal seizure(s) or coma in a patient with preeclampsia, or, in a patient *after* the 20th week of gestation when all other causes have been ruled out.
Gestational Hypertension	Hypertension diagnosed *after* the 20th week of pregnancy, *without* proteinuria.
Superimposed Preeclampsia-eclampsia	Preeclampsia and/or eclampsia diagnosed in a patient with chronic hypertension[3]

Data from the American College of Obstetricians and Gynecologists. (2002). Diagnosis and management of preeclampsia and eclampsia. ACOG Practice Bulletin No. 33. *Obstet Gynecol, 99,* 159–67; and National High Blood Pressure Education Program Working Group on High Blood Pressure in Pregnancy. (2000) Report of the National High Blood Pressure Education Program Working Group on High Blood Pressure in Pregnancy. *Am J Obstet Gynecol,* 183, S1-S22.

a marker for superimposed preeclampsia. Gestational hypertension is diagnosed when blood pressure is elevated after the 20th week of pregnancy, but proteinuria does not develop.

The NHBP Group recommends that the term *pregnancy-induced hypertension* no longer be used. Rather, terms should be used that more accurately describe the patient's hypertensive state.

CHRONIC HYPERTENSION

Chronic hypertension in pregnancy is defined as hypertension (systolic 140 mmHg or higher, diastolic 90 mmHg or higher) that occurs prior to pregnancy, before the 20th week of pregnancy, or more than 12 weeks after delivery.[13] The rate of chronic hypertension in pregnancy has increased in part due to the number of women

who delay childbirth until their 30s, 40s, and 50s, a time when many non-pregnant women will first be diagnosed. The rate is further elevated in African-American women, women with type 2 diabetes mellitus, and obese women (body mass index 30 or above).[14]

Chronic hypertension is classified as mild or severe based on systolic or diastolic blood pressure thresholds. Mild chronic hypertension is a systolic blood pressure of 140 to less than 160 mmHg or a diastolic pressure of 90 to less than 100 mmHg.[15] Severe chronic hypertension is a systolic pressure of 180 mmHg or higher or a diastolic pressure of 110 mmHg or higher.

For counseling purposes for the parturient and family, chronic hypertension is based on the blood pressure and the presence of organ system involvement. Patients are considered at lower risk if their blood pressure is in the mild chronic hypertension range and there is no organ involvement or injury.[14] Most women with mild chronic hypertension are counseled to discontinue antihypertensive medications prior to pregnancy. This reduces the risk of fetal exposure to potential teratogenic effects of some antihypertensive drugs (e.g., angiotensin-converting enzyme inhibitors, angiotensin II receptor blockers) and decreases the risk of fetal compromise from hypoperfusion pressures.[14]

Chronic hypertension is also categorized as primary or secondary, based on the causative factor.[2] Primary (essential) hypertension is the presence of elevated blood pressure in the absence of a causative disease or condition. Primary hypertension accounts for more than 90 percent of chronic hypertension in pregnancy. Risk factors for primary hypertension include:

- age 35 or older
- insulin resistance or diabetes
- obesity
- family history
- smoking
- stress
- limited physical activity
- a diet high in sodium, processed foods, and/or saturated fats.[15]

Secondary hypertension, in contrast, is elevated blood pressure caused by another condition, such as kidney disease, endocrine disorders, adrenal gland tumors, collagen vascular diseases, arteriosclerosis, coarctation of the aorta, and some medications (Box 7-2).

Patients with chronic hypertension who are pregnant are at increased risk for perinatal morbidity and mortality when compared with women without hypertension. Chronic hypertension diagnosed before pregnancy begins has worse perinatal and maternal outcomes than chronic hypertension diagnosed during pregnancy.[14,15] This finding may be related to preexisting vascular injury and compromised end-organ function in this

Box 7-2. CAUSES OF SECONDARY HYPERTENSION

Adrenal gland tumor
Arteriosclerosis
Coarctation of the aorta
Cushing syndrome
Hyperaldosteronism
Kidney disease
• glomerulonephritis
• renal failure
• renal artery stenosis
• renal vascular obstruction
Medications
• appetite suppressants
• cold medications
• corticosteroids
• migraine headache medications
• oral contraceptives
Sleep apnea

population. Women with chronic hypertension also are at increased risk for superimposed preeclampsia and placental abruption.

PREECLAMPSIA

Preeclampsia is diagnosed when hypertension and significant proteinuria appear after the 20th week of gestation in a parturient with no history of either complication. Significant proteinuria is defined as more than 0.3 g/L (i.e., 300 mg), which typically corresponds to 1+ proteinuria or greater on a random dipstick urine sample. However, dipstick urine samples are notorious for having high false-positive and false-negative results in preeclamptic and non-preeclamptic women. Also, the level of protein in the urine of a preeclamptic patient will fluctuate throughout the day and may lead to a false-negative result. A more specific test for proteinuria is a 24-hour urine collection for direct measurement of the total amount of protein in the urine, as well as other blood and urine markers of renal function. Although alternative methods have been proposed to identify significant proteinuria in patients with hypertension (e.g., 12-hour, 8-hour, and 4-hour urine samples, and creatinine to protein ratios), there are limited data to support these tests at this time.

It is important to point out that the laboratory markers for preeclampsia are not necessarily specific for the degree of illness or end-organ compromise, and abnormal test results do not help in predicting which patient will have an eclamptic seizure. Rather, the historical markers for preeclampsia were selected for their relative

ease of use and low cost compared with other more sensitive and potentially accurate tests.

In the past, the presence of edema was an element of the diagnostic triad for preeclampsia, which included elevated blood pressure, proteinuria, and edema. However, this finding is no longer required for diagnosing the disease because many pregnant women have some degree of dependent edema. More importantly, the presence, absence, or degree of edema does not directly correlate with maternal or fetal outcomes.

Similarly, an absolute elevation of blood pressure from the patient's baseline values to a 30 mmHg or greater increase in systolic pressure or a 15 mmHg or greater increase in diastolic pressure was considered relative "hypertension" in pregnancy, even if the patient's blood pressure was less than 140/90 mmHg. Recent studies have shown that such relative increases in baseline blood pressures do not increase the patient's risk of eclampsia; development of the syndrome of hemolysis, elevated liver enzymes, and low platelets (HELLP); or increased maternal or neonatal morbidity.[16] Thus, the current definition of preeclampsia no longer includes relative increases in systolic or diastolic blood pressures, but rather is based on pressures that reach the threshold of 140 mmHg or greater (systolic) or 90 mmHg or greater (diastolic). Of course, when a pregnant woman develops elevated blood pressure, it is reasonable to monitor her for the development of preeclampsia.

Etiology of Preeclampsia-Eclampsia

Preeclampsia is a multisystem disorder unique to humans and therefore difficult to study in laboratory animals—a formidable obstacle to discovering its exact etiology. Historically, there have been several theories on causative factors and potential markers of the disease, but no hypothesis has survived scientific scrutiny over time. The recent past has seen renewed interest and activity toward identifying factors that predispose a patient to development of preeclampsia, fueled in part by the potential role that abnormal trophoblast invasion may have in its genesis.[17]

Current hypotheses on the pathology of preeclampsia target five general areas:

• the effect of abnormal trophoblastic invasion of uterine blood vessels on the maternal blood supply to the placenta
• the response and potential intolerance of the mother's immune system to partially foreign genetic placental and fetal tissue
• stimulation of the maternal inflammatory system by cardiovascular changes of pregnancy
• various dietary deficiencies

- genetic abnormalities that may predispose the patient to the disease.[18]

The pathologic hallmark of preeclampsia may be the early failure of trophoblasts to invade the maternal spiral arteries to accomplish the large and dilated low-pressure arteries associated with a normal pregnancy.[17] In parturients with preeclampsia, the invasion is shallow, which prohibits the spiral arteries from dilating and obstructs them so that normal adjustment to increased blood flow does not occur. The local vasculature develops into a high-resistance state and contributes to a dysfunctional placenta unable to adequately perfuse and sustain a normal pregnancy.[17]

The incidence of preeclampsia may be modified, in part, by familial traits. Women whose mothers or sisters had preeclampsia in pregnancy are more likely to have the disease compared with women in the general population. Interestingly, there is evidence to suggest that these factors are not unique to women, because a man who fathers a child with a woman diagnosed with preeclampsia may also contribute to an increased risk of preeclampsia; if he fathers a child with another woman, she too is at increased risk for preeclampsia. As a result, some data suggest that preeclampsia is a consequence of maternal intolerance to paternal antigenic material. Evidence that supports this theory emphasizes the activation of inflammatory mediators and altered cytokine function in women with preeclampsia. For example, women who become pregnant after limited sexual encounters with the father of the child are more likely to develop preeclampsia compared with women who have more sexual contact (maternal exposure to paternal semen) with their partners. A similar observation is the increased rate of preeclampsia compared with the general population in women who use condoms as a form of birth control in contrast to non-barrier methods. It has been theorized that condoms limit the mother's exposure to paternal antigens, thereby increasing the risk of a novel antigen–antibody response.[17,20]

These and other abnormalities known to occur in parturients with preeclampsia support the list of theoretical etiologies of preeclampsia presented in Box 7-3. As a group, the data show promise that researchers are closer to identifying etiologic factors of hypertension in pregnancy. When this historic milestone is accomplished, methods to predict and ultimately prevent the devastating consequences of the disease may become a reality.[21,23]

Risk Factors and Complications

Factors that may predispose a patient to preeclampsia reflect the potentially complex etiology of the disease and are described in Table 7-4.

Box 7-3. PATHOPHYSIOLOGIC ABNORMALITIES IN WOMEN WITH PREECLAMPSIA

- Placenta ischemia[5]
- Generalized vasospasm
- Abnormal hemostasis with activation of the coagulation system
- Vascular endothelial dysfunction
- Abnormal nitrous oxide and lipid metabolism
- Leukocyte activation
- Changes in cytokines
- Changes in insulin resistance

From Sibai, B.M. (2003). Diagnosis and management of gestational hypertension and preeclampsia. *Obstet Gynecol, 102,* 181–92.

When trophoblasts fail to penetrate deeply into the maternal spiral arteries, the result is tortuous vessels with high resistance.[17,21,24] Vasospasm and endothelial damage occur, but organ system involvement or damage from preeclampsia does not necessarily follow a single path of progression and cannot be predicted based on a patient's demographic factors. Individual patients present with the disease in myriad ways. As an example, one group of women who develop preeclampsia may have severe hypertension and renal arterial spasm that decreases renal arterial blood flow, prevents the normal increase in creatinine clearance, and produces severe vascular injury to the kidneys. Pathophysiologic consequences may include maternal oliguria, severe proteinuria, and intrauterine fetal growth restriction (IUGR). As a second example, another group of parturients with preeclampsia may have injury to the vascular endothelium from increased cardiac output or increased vascular resistance, where both stimulate inflammation, trigger cytokine release, alter leukocyte production, and create a syndrome similar to sepsis and septic shock. A third group of pregnant women with preeclampsia may show dramatic changes in cardiac output, arterial afterload, ventricular performance, and oxygen transport that produces injury of end-organs, such as the maternal liver, via turbulent blood flow, vasospasm, or both. These patients may develop hepatic ischemic insult, increased production of liver enzymes, and hepatic subcapsular hematomas. These three clinical scenarios represent a small sample of the numerous pathologic courses that preeclampsia may take in individual patients. Thus, clinicians must be alert for multiple complications of the disease and understand that there are no absolute patterns of deterioration that all patients will take.[17]

Severe Preeclampsia

Severe preeclampsia is diagnosed when one or more of the conditions in Box 7-4 is identified in patients with

TABLE 7-4

Risk Factors for Preeclampsia-Eclampsia

Demographics	• Maternal age 35 years or older (40 years or older doubles the risk for preeclampsia) • African American race • Non-smoker
Co-morbidities	• Vascular/thrombotic/inflammation • Chronic hypertension • Elevated BP in current pregnancy, DBP >80 mmHg • Renal disease • Androgen excess • Obesity; increased BMI • Insulin resistance/pregestational diabetes • Dyslipidemia • Vascular disease • Connective tissue disease (e.g., lupus erythematosus, rheumatoid arthritis, scleroderma) • Antiphospholipid antibody syndrome • Thrombophilias (i.e., anti-phospholipid, protein C or S deficiency, antithrombin deficiency, factor V Leiden mutation, MTHFR mutation) • Maternal infection/inflammation in current pregnancy (UTI, periodontal disease)
Pregnancy-Fetus	• Twin/triplet pregnancy (multi-fetal) • Molar pregnancy
Family History/Genetics	• Personal history—preeclampsia in a previous pregnancy • Family history—mother/sister had disease • Paternal history—preeclampsia in a previous partner pregnancy
Maternal Immunity	• History of condom use • Fertilization with donor sperm • Donor sperm and egg • New sexual partner

BMI = body mass index, DBP = diastolic blood pressure, MTHRF = Methylenetetrahydrofolate reductase, UTI = urinary tract infection.

From Duckitt, K.& Harrington, D. (2005). Risk factors for pre-eclampsia at antenatal booking: Systematic review of controlled studies. *BMJ, 330,* 565.

Box 7-4. CRITERIA FOR SEVERE PREECLAMPSIA

Preeclampsia* plus one of the following:
• BP of 160 mmHg systolic or above, or 110 mmHg diastolic or greater, on two occasions at least 6 hours apart
• Proteinuria of 5 grams or more in a 24-hour urine collection, or 3+ or greater on two random urine samples collected at least 4 hours apart
• Cerebral or visual disturbances
• Cyanosis
• Epigastric pain, or right upper quadrant pain
• Fetal growth restriction
• Headache, severe
• Impaired liver function (elevated liver enzymes)
• Oliguria (less than 500 mL/24 hours)
• Pulmonary edema
• Thrombocytopenia

*Preeclampsia is BP of 140 mmHg systolic or greater, or 90 mmHg diastolic or greater, measured on at least two occasions at least 4–6 hours apart <u>after</u> the 20th week of gestation, in a woman without a history of hypertension prior to pregnancy AND proteinuria of 300 mg (0.3 grams) or greater in a 24-hour urine collection, or 1+ or greater on two random urine samples collected at least 4–6 hours apart.
From the American College of Obstetricians and Gynecologists. (2002). ACOG practice bulletin no. 33. Diagnosis and management of preeclampsia and eclampsia. *Obstet Gynecol, 99,* 159–67.

agents. Abruption and fetal compromise also are more likely in patients with severe preeclampsia. Table 7-5 lists the complications of severe preeclampsia.

PREECLAMPSIA SUPERIMPOSED ON CHRONIC HYPERTENSION

The approximately 10 to 25 percent of women with chronic hypertension who develop superimposed preeclampsia have almost three times the risk of acquiring severe preeclampsia compared with women who are normotensive at the beginning of pregnancy. The risk of developing preeclampsia further increases in women with cardiovascular or renal disease prior to pregnancy.[14,15]

Development of preeclampsia in women with chronic hypertension may be difficult to detect early in the disease. However, patients with pre-existing hypertension who have an increase in blood pressure midtrimester (when most patients decrease or sustain earlier reduced blood pressures), and women who need new or increased antihypertensive therapy, should be closely monitored for gestational hypertension and preeclampsia. Clinicians should be particularly alert to possible superimposed preeclampsia in parturients

preeclampsia. Parturients with severe preeclampsia are more likely to progress to eclampsia, develop morbid conditions, require longer hospitalizations, and experience neurologic injury or death. Blood pressure elevations in severe preeclampsia are frequently in the range that may require treatment with antihypertensive

TABLE 7-5

Complications of Severe Preeclampsia

Neurologic	• Cerebral edema
	• Eclampsia
	• Intracranial hemorrhage
	• Blindness (one or both eyes, usually temporary)
	• Papilledema
Cardio-pulmonary	• Severe hypertension
	• Myocardial ischemia
	• Pulmonary edema
	• Exacerbation of congestive heart failure
Renal	• Oliguria
	• Acute kidney injury (acute tubular necrosis)
	• Azotemia, severe
Hepatic	• Hepatic failure
	• Hepatic rupture
Hematologic	• Hemolysis
	• Anemia, severe
	• Thrombocytopenia
	• Disseminated intravascular coagulation
	• Hemorrhage
Uteroplacental	• Intrauterine growth restriction
	• Fetal hypoxia
	• Fetal death
	• Placental abruption

with chronic hypertension and proteinuria before pregnancy or before the 20th week of pregnancy who develop double or triple the amount of protein in a typical 24-hour urine sample.[14]

The goal of caring for a patient with chronic hypertension in pregnancy is to maintain acceptable maternal blood pressure to protect her from end-organ damage, prevent endothelial damage, and maintain cardiac output/oxygen delivery (DO_2), while also ensuring adequate cardiac output and perfusion pressure for placental gas exchange.

GESTATIONAL HYPERTENSION

Gestational hypertension is diagnosed when hypertension (systolic pressure 140 mmHg or greater or diastolic pressure 90 mmHg or greater on at least two occasions at least 6 hours apart) appears after the 20th week of gestation in a woman who does not have proteinuria. Gestational hypertension does not persist beyond 12 weeks postpartum and resolves more rapidly than preeclampsia, typically by the first postpartum week.[13] As many as 20 percent of patients with gestational hypertension develop

preeclampsia at some time in the pregnancy. Thus, close monitoring and follow-up are important to identify the disease early and prevent potential complications.

ECLAMPSIA

Eclampsia is the presence of tonic–clonic (grand mal) seizures or coma in a patient diagnosed with preeclampsia, when other causes of the seizure have been ruled out. The origin of the word eclampsia is Greek: the preposition *ek* means "out," and the verb *lampein* means "to shine forth" or "to flash." The two words describe a state of "flashing out" or, more literally, "a bolt from the blue," and the sudden onset of eclampsia's tonic-clonic seizures clearly fits this description.

The seizures of eclampsia are almost always tonic-clonic in nature, and are typically self-limited. Although a presumptive diagnosis of eclampsia can be made, it is prudent to search for other causes of the seizure(s) to avoid misdiagnosis and delay in treating the underlying disease. Alternative causes of seizures in women of childbearing age include:

- intracranial bleeding (e.g., ruptured aneurysm, arteriovenous malformation),
- encephalitis or meningitis
- severe hypoglycemia
- severe electrolyte imbalance
- head injury
- use of or withdrawal from drugs or alcohol
- brain tumors.

The presence or absence of such neurologic complications may be investigated after a seizure occurs. A patient who may have eclampsia should receive magnesium sulfate and blood pressure control (as indicated) until diagnosis of a different disease is confirmed. In most patients with preeclampsia, an alternative cause for the seizure is not found, and eclampsia is diagnosed.

Eclampsia may occur during the antepartum, intrapartum, or postpartum period. Table 7-6 shows the

TABLE 7-6

Timing of Eclamptic Seizures

Onset of Seizures	Percent of Patients
Antepartum	38–53
Intrapartum	18–36
Postpartum	11–44

From Sibai, B.M. (2005). Diagnosis, prevention, and management of eclampsia. *Obstet Gynecol, 105,* 402–10.

percentage of patients with ecalmpsia who have seizure activity in each stage of labor. There are no accurate methods to prospectively identify patients who will present with eclampsia. In most industrialized nations that integrate patient safety initiatives into obstetric care, most cases of eclampsia are considered unpreventable.[25]

In the past, it was thought that preeclampsia progressed in an orderly manner from mild preeclampsia to severe preeclampsia and ended with eclampsia. Interestingly, the disease does not necessarily progress in such a pattern. Eclampsia may occur in patients with severe preeclampsia, but it also appears in patients without severe preeclampsia.[17] Approximately 20 percent of eclamptic women in the U.S. and Europe have no signs or symptoms of severe disease prior to seizure activity.[25]

The etiology of eclamptic seizures remains uncertain. Proposed mechanisms or causes include progressive cerebral vasospasm, edema, and ischemia; hypertensive encephalopathy; and endothelial damage that produces vascular leaks and increased intracranial pressure. Eclampsia is responsible for an estimated 50,000 maternal deaths each year worldwide and is responsible for 15 percent of all maternal deaths in the U.S.[17]

Magnesium Sulfate Therapy

Magnesium sulfate is the drug of choice to prevent and abate eclamptic seizures and to prevent repeated seizure activity. Recent large clinical trials have shown that magnesium sulfate is effective at preventing eclamptic seizures and controlling seizure activity once it has occurred.[26] Magnesium sulfate is superior to phenytoin sodium (Dilantin), diazepam (Valium), and nimodipine (Nimotop) in preventing and treating eclamptic seizures. One of the advantages of magnesium sulfate is its ability to protect the parturient from seizures but not depress the gag reflex. Thus, compared with other medications used in seizure prophylaxis, magnesium sulfate works to reduce the risk for maternal aspiration, acute respiratory distress syndrome, hypoxic brain injury, and death.[26]

It is unclear how magnesium sulfate works to prevent and treat the seizures of eclampsia. Proposed actions include the possibility that the drug causes vasodilation in the peripheral and cerebral circulation, that it protects the blood–brain barrier to prevent or decrease cerebral edema, and that it functions as a central anticonvulsant.[27]

Guidelines for Magnesium Sulfate Administration

Magnesium sulfate is administered in two steps: first, as a loading dose (bolus) to rapidly increase maternal serum magnesium levels, followed by a maintenance infusion to maintain the level. The bolus dose usually is 4 or 6 grams of magnesium sulfate diluted in an isotonic solution. It is delivered via infusion pump and administered over 20 to 30 minutes. When the bolus dose is complete, a maintenance infusion of 1 to 3 grams magnesium sulfate per hour is administered via infusion pump. Clinical assessment parameters and recommendations for fetal surveillance during the magnesium sulfate infusion can be found in the *Guidelines for Care of the Patient with Preeclampsia-Eclampsia* in the guidelines section of this text.

In low-resource settings, magnesium sulfate may be administered intramuscularly (IM). Like the IV method, there is a loading dose followed by a maintenance dose. The IM loading dose of magnesium sulfate is 10 grams divided and administered as two separate 5-gram injections, one into each buttock. The maintenance dose is 5 grams of magnesium sulfate administered IM every 4 hours into alternating buttocks.

Treatment of Eclamptic Seizures

For the parturient who has an eclamptic seizure and has not received a magnesium sulfate loading dose, the interventional dose is a 4- to 6-gram loading dose (diluted in approximately 100 mL of isotonic intravenous solution) and administered by infusion pump over 15 to 20 minutes. The loading dose is followed by a maintenance dose of 2 grams magnesium sulfate per hour by infusion pump. Approximately 10 percent of women who have an eclamptic seizure will have a second seizure that can be treated with an additional 2 grams of magnesium sulfate IV by slow push over 3 to 5 minutes. For the rare patient who has recurrent seizures despite magnesium sulfate treatment, a short-acting barbiturate may be administered, such as sodium amobarbital 250 mg IV over 3 to 5 minutes. Patients who do not respond to magnesium sulfate therapy and continue to have seizures may have an undiagnosed neurologic complication. Box 7-5 lists non-eclamptic conditions that may cause maternal seizures. When patients have "atypical" eclampsia, or eclampsia that manifests late postpartum, comprehensive neurologic evaluation may be helpful to identify or exclude medical causes of the seizures.

Magnesium Sulfate Toxicity

Magnesium sulfate is labeled as a "High Alert" drug by the Institute for Safe Medication Practices (ISMP). A high-alert medication is one that may cause significant harm when used incorrectly. Magnesium sulfate is in this category due to the risk of maternal respiratory arrest, hypoxic injury, cardiopulmonary arrest, and death if an overdose occurs. The Agency for Healthcare

Box 7-5. NON-ECLAMPTIC CAUSES OF MATERNAL SEIZURES

Cerebrovascular accidents
- Hemorrhage
- Ruptured aneurysm
- Ruptured A-V malformation

Hypertensive encephalopathy

Brain tumor

Metastatic gestational trophoblastic disease

Metabolic diseases/electrolyte abnormalities
- Severe hypoglycemia
- Severe hyponatremia

Thrombophilia

Thrombotic thrombocytopenia purpura

Postdural puncture syndrome

Cerebral vasculitis

Encephalitis/meningitis (infection)

From Sibai, B.M. (2005). Diagnosis, prevention, and management of eclampsia. *Obstet Gynecol, 105,* 402–10.

Research and Quality encourages all providers to establish institutional mechanisms and guidelines to prevent accidental magnesium sulfate overdose.

Clinical signs and symptoms of magnesium toxicity are, in general, those that would develop if calcium could no longer enter the calcium channels to effect muscle contractions. The movement of calcium into and out of muscle cells creates contraction and relaxation of muscle fibers. Magnesium, which displaces calcium, cannot enter the calcium channels and indirectly causes ineffective muscle movement and contractions. Many of the signs and symptoms of magnesium toxicity are physical markers of abnormal muscle function (Box 7-6). The diaphragm and myocardium are muscles that require adequate levels of calcium to function. In extreme cases of magnesium overdose, the diaphragm loses its ability to contract, and respiratory arrest ensues. Also, cardiac arrest may occur if magnesium levels continue to increase. Clearly, clinicians must assess the patient for evidence of magnesium toxicity during magnesium sulfate infusion. It also is important to observe for early signs of toxicity prior to

Box 7-6. SIGNS AND SYMPTOMS OF MAGNESIUM TOXICITY

- Absent deep-tendon reflexes
- Respiratory depression
- Blurred vision
- Slurred speech
- Severe muscle weakness
- Cardiac arrest

respiratory or cardiac compromise. Screening the patient for markers of toxicity should occur every 1 to 2 hours during magnesium sulfate infusion.

HELLP SYNDROME

Hemolysis, microangiopathic anemia, and/or thrombocytopenia have long been known to occur in select patients with preeclampsia-eclampsia. Medical journals at the turn of the 20th century described women who had eclampsia and co-existent anemia, jaundice, and bleeding complications. By the 1960s, articles appeared in the world literature describing individual cases and series of cases of parturients who acquired hematologic failure or compromise that, with the diagnosis of preeclampsia, was associated with significant morbidity and mortality.

The HELLP syndrome, named by Weinstein in 1982, is an acronym for one such variant of severe preeclampsia. The letters represent the words Hemolysis, Elevated Liver enzymes, and Low Platelets. HELLP syndrome is a severe manifestation of preeclampsia that has a maternal mortality rate in industrialized nations of approximately 1 percent. The syndrome occurs in 0.5 to 0.9 percent of all pregnancies and in 10 to 20 percent of parturients with severe preeclmapsia.[23] Although there is no standard set of symptoms in all patients with HELLP, general observations regarding the characteristics of the disease are presented in Table 7-7.

Most women who develop HELLP syndrome do so in the antepartum period and commonly present with nonspecific complaints such as malaise and viral-like symptoms.[22,23] There is a tendency for the disease to worsen at night and improve during daylight hours.[23] HELLP syndrome can progress rapidly, making delivery of the fetus and placenta (to resolve the disease) an urgent priority.

Specific laboratory findings are needed to confirm HELLP syndrome or distinguish it from other diseases with similar physical and laboratory findings. Two classification systems for HELLP are the Tennessee Classification System and the Mississippi-Triple Class System. A comparison of these two classification systems is presented in Table 7-8.[23,28] Historically, HELLP syndrome was diagnosed only when all three findings were present (sometimes referred to as complete HELLP syndrome). Recently, there has been an increased interest in measuring outcomes and risk factors for patients who do not have all three criteria, but who have one or two of the triad of test results (conditions variously called incomplete HELLP, partial HELLP, or ELLP syndrome).[23]

Because several serious diseases share the identical signs and symptoms of HELLP syndrome, the differential diagnoses for alternative causes is routinely explored. Included in this group of diagnoses is acute fatty liver of pregnancy, thrombotic thrombocytopenia purpura,

TABLE 7-7

Patient Characteristics in HELLP Syndrome

Characteristics	Occurrence In Patients With HELLP (%)
Right upper quadrant pain	80
Hypertension and proteinuria present	>70
Develops prior to labor or delivery	70
Excessive weight gain and generalized edema in this pregnancy	>50
Develops subcapsular hematoma, rupture	30
Maximum blood pressure less than 140/90 mmHg	20
Diagnosed after 37 weeks	20
Post Cesarean-section hematoma formation	20
Hypertension and proteinuria absent	10–20
Diagnosed before 27 weeks	10
Develops renal failure	7.3
No significant proteinuria at diagnosis	6

Data from Sibai, B.M. (2004) Diagnosis, controversies, and management of the syndrome of hemolysis, elevated liver enzymes, and low platelet count. *Obstet Gynecol, 103,* 981–91; and Martin, J.N., Jr., Rose, C.H.& Briery, C.M. (2006) Understanding and managing HELLP syndrome: The integral role of aggressive glucocorticoids for mother and child. *Am J Obstet Gynecol, 195,* 914–34.

hemolytic uremic syndrome, immune thrombocytopenia purpura, and others (Box 7-7).[22]

HELLP syndrome carries an overall increased risk for severe morbidity and mortality from multiple organ system derangements that may now allow a complete

Box 7-7. DIFFERENTIAL DIAGNOSIS IN WOMEN WITH HELLP SYNDROME

- Acute fatty liver of pregnancy
- Antiphospholipid syndrome
- Cholecystitis
- Disseminated herpes simplex
- Disseminated intravascular coagulation
- Hemolytic uremic syndrome
- Hepatitis (acute viral)
- Immune thrombocytopenic purpura
- Pancreatitis, acute
- Shock, hemorrhagic or septic
- Systemic inflammatory response syndrome
- Systemic lupus erythematosus
- Thrombotic thrombocytopenic purpura

From Sibai, B.M. (2004). Diagnosis, controversies, and management of the syndrome of hemolysis, elevated liver enzymes, and low platelet count. *Obstet Gynecol, 103,* 981–91.

recovery. One percent of parturients with HELLP syndrome die from the disease.

The only known treatment for HELLP syndrome is to empty the uterus of the fetus and placenta. Vaginal delivery is preferred, with Cesarean section reserved for the customary obstetric indications.[22,23]

HYPERTENSIVE CRISIS AND ANTIHYPERTENSIVE THERAPY

The goal of antihypetensive therapy in severe preeclampsia, eclampsia, chronic hypertension, or HELLP syndrome is to safely reduce the maternal blood pressure below the level that may cause a stroke or placental abruption, but sufficient to maintain adequate arterial perfusion to vital organs.[17]

The threshold for administering antihypertensive medications to women with preeclampsia has decreased over time because there are current reports of patients having intracranial hemorrhage at systolic pressures near and above 160 mmHg. Therefore, primary providers should be alerted when a patient's systolic pressure is approximately 160 mmHg.[29] Elevations of diastolic pressure above 110 mmHg remain a concern, and antihypertensive therapy may be indicated.

Drugs used most often to treat hypertensive crisis in patients with preeclampsia are labetalol hydrochloride (Trandate), hydralazine hydrochloride (Apresoline), and nifedipine (Procardia). Table 7-9 presents information about these and other drugs; however, a detailed discussion of the pharmacokinetics of these drugs is beyond the scope of this chapter.

Severe hypertension is defined as a blood pressure of 180/110 mmHg or greater and is associated with an increased risk of morbidity and mortality for both mother and fetus.[13,14] When maternal systolic pressure reaches 180 mmHg or greater, it should be reduced gradually to a level that reduces the risk of intracranial hemorrhage and abruption. Mean arterial pressure should not be reduced suddenly. Rapid blood pressure reduction in patients with pressures in the severe range may result in seizures, coma, neurologic injury, and death.

Invasive Hemodynamic Monitoring in Preeclampsia-Eclampsia

Invasive hemodynamic monitoring is reserved for patients who have preeclampsia-eclampsia, chronic hypertension, superimposed preeclampsia, gestational hypertension, or HELLP syndrome and who have co-morbidities or critical complications of these diseases. There are no randomized trials that support or refute the benefits of routine invasive hemodynamic monitoring in patients with preeclampsia. However, ACOG identifies preeclamptic women who

TABLE 7-8

Tennessee and Mississippi Classification Systems for HELLP Syndrome

Category	Tennessee Classification System		Mississippi Triple-class HELLP System		
	Complete	**Incomplete**	**Class 1**	**Class 2**	**Class 3**
	Based on presence of all three findings	*Based on one or two of the three findings*	*Based on the nadir of the platelet count*		
Hemolysis	Micro-angiopathic hemolytic anemia		Micro-angiopathic hemolytic anemia		
Bilibrubin	≥20.5 µmol/L, or, ≥1.2 mg/dL		—		
LDH (*U/L*)	>600		>600		
AST (*U/L*)	≥70		>70		>40
Platelets ($\times 10^9$/L)	<100,000		≤50,000	>50,000 to ≤100,000	>100,000 to ≤150,000
Notes	"Complete" HELLP is: platelets ≤100,000 • LDH >600 • AST >70 • Evidence of hemolysis	"Incomplete" HELLP is one or two of the laboratory findings.	"Hemolysis + Hepatic Dysfunction" All must be present to qualify for Class 1.	"Hemolysis + Hepatic Dysfunction"	"Hemolysis + Hepatic Dysfunction"

AST = aspartate aminotransferase; HELLP = hemolysis, elevated liver enzymes, low platelets count; LDH = lactate dehydrogenase; umol/L = micromole per liter; µmol/L = micromoles per liter.

Data from Haram, K., Svendsen, E.& Abildgaard, U. (2009). The HELLP syndrome: Clinical issues and management. A Review. *BMC Pregnancy Childbirth*, 9, 8; Martin, J.N., Jr., Rose, C.H. & Briery, C.M. (2006). Understanding and managing HELLP syndrome: The integral role of aggressive glucocorticoids for mother and child. *Am J Obstet Gynecol*, 195, 914–34; and Sibai, B.M. (2004). Diagnosis, controversies, and management of the syndrome of hemolysis, elevated liver enzymes, and low platelet count. *Obstet Gynecol,* 103, 981–91.

may benefit from invasive hemodynamic monitoring as those with severe cardiac disease, severe renal disease, refractory hypertension, oliguria, or pulmonary edema. Other indications for invasive monitoring exist and should be considered on an individual basis.

For women with severe preeclampsia or HELLP syndrome, who have the most critical hypertensive states of pregnancy, there is evidence of abnormal oxygen transport. Such patients are at risk for fixed states of oxygen consumption and an inability to increase consumption in hypoxic or acidemic states. The cause of the abnormality remains unknown, but it is strikingly similar to oxygen utilization characteristics of patients with sepsis, systemic inflammatory response syndrome, and other diseases that result in maladaptive inflammatory mediator stimulation.[30]

Future Ideas on the Hemodynamic Parameters in Preeclampsia

Investigators have reported on hemodynamic and oxygen transport findings in women with preeclampsia using invasive and non-invasive technology. Thus far,

study results demonstrate large variability in the manifestation of preeclampsia in individual women. As an example, there are conflicting data on the hemodynamic profiles of severe preeclampsia versus mild preeclampsia, on cardiopulmonary findings in women who have eclamptic seizures, and on patients who develop oliguria. Of interest is the recent report that early and late preeclampsia may have differing pathophysiologic bases and may develop from two distinct hemodynamic states.[31,32] Valensise and colleagues followed 1688 women with abnormal bilateral notching of uterine arteries beginning at 20 to 22 weeks gestation.[32] (The identification of bilateral arching of uterine arteries in the second trimester is a potential screening test for increased vascular resistance that may predict the later development of preeclampsia and IUGR.) The women had uterine artery Doppler studies and maternal echocardiograms to estimate vascular resistance. One hundred and seven of the subjects had preeclampsia, 119 had other pregnancy complications, and the remaining 1119 had normal outcomes. In the preeclampsia group, 75 women had early onset of preeclampsia and 32 had late onset. Women who had

TABLE 7-9

Antihypertensive Medications Used in Pregnancy

Drug	Dosage	Maximum Dose	Caution	Special Monitoring Requirements
labetalol	20–40 mg IV Escalating dosing protocol (in mg) every 10–15 min: 20–40–80–80— move to alternative drug	220 mg*	Do not use in asthma, heart failure. Do not exceed 80 mg in a single dose.	ECG if patient has chronic hypertension, cardiovascular disease, bundle branch block, or other longstanding disease that increases the risk for myocardial ischemia or dysrhythmias.
nifedipine	10–20 mg orally every 30 min	50 mg*	Do not give sublingually.	Invasive BP and ECG not required.
hydralazine	5–10 mg IV every 20 min	30 mg*	Avoid hypotension that reduces placental perfusion.	Invasive BP and ECG not required.
nitroprusside	IV titration as a diluted continuous drip Initial dose is 0.25–0.5 mcg/kg/min. Increase by 0.5 mcg/kg/min	5 mcg/kg/min	Fetal cyanide poisoning may occur if used for more than 2-4 hours. Arterial line necessary due to short half-life of drug. Agent of last resort. Maternal cyanide toxicity possible.	Side effect – increased intracranial pressure Requires arterial line Should be used by those with experience administering the drug.
nitroglycerin	5 mcg/min IV continuous infusion. May increase every 5 min until desired effect.	100 mcg/min	Contraindicated in hypertensive encephalopathy, increased cerebral blood flow, and increased intracranial pressure.	Requires arterial line Should be used by those with experience administering the drug.

ECG = electrocardiogram, IV = intravenous.
*Dosage may not be the pharmacologic maximum dose, but is the point to consider an alternative drug.

preeclampsia early were significantly older, had greater uterine artery notching, and delivered at lower gestational ages compared with the women who had late onset preeclampsia.[32] Important in the discussion on hemodynamic monitoring in preeclampsia is the high resistance index values in the early onset group compared with the group with late onset. The increased resistance measured in the early onset preeclampsia group suggests earlier disease onset, higher systemic vascular resistance, and lower cardiac output—a familiar subset of cardiac performance described in patients with complex complications of preeclampsia. Before meaningful use can occur from any investigation, further studies are needed.

SUMMARY

This chapter presents current information on ongoing discoveries into the genesis of one of the most enigmatic diseases in modern medicine. Recent theories to

find common linkage among the many faces of hypertension in pregnancy have advanced the investigation of preeclampsia-eclampsia.

It is ironic, however, that the diagnosis of hypertensive states in pregnancy, one of the most serious and potentially lethal complications of pregnancy, is completely dependent on the identification of elevated blood pressure; yet current methods to measure blood pressure are no better than methods used more than 20 years ago. Additionally, it has been demonstrated that all levels of care providers have some degree of observational bias when manually acquiring blood pressure. Actions that may improve accuracy in the detection of hypertension can be implemented in the clinical environment with no or little increase in cost.

Use of a standardized nomenclature system to identify the categories of hypertension during pregnancy may improve communication and increase opportunities for collaboration in the care of complex and critically ill patients. Also addressed in the chapter are results of large studies that have shown magnesium sulfate to not only be the drug of choice for preventing eclamptic seizures but also superior to phenytoin sodium, diazepam, and nimodipine in the prevention and abatement of eclamptic seizures.

Hypertension that occurs in pregnancy is responsible for the deaths of tens of thousands of women each year in developed and developing nations. In the U.S. and Canada, hypertension in pregnancy is one of the top causes of maternal morbidity and mortality. It is estimated that for every maternal death recorded, there are at least 50 women who experience severe morbidity during pregnancy, which may result in permanent disability. Although researchers have proposed and continue to investigate hypotheses of abnormal trophoblastic invasion, endothelial dysfunction, maternal immune response to the pregnancy, and overexpression of inflammatory mediators, the etiology of preeclampsia remains unknown.[33]

Current treatment is based on early identification of the disease, close monitoring of disease progression, control of severe elevations of blood pressure to prevent intracranial hemorrhage and placental abruption, seizure prophylaxis with magnesium sulfate, fetal surveillance for adequate growth, and early treatment of severe complications when they occur.[33] The investigation for select biomarkers that may prospectively signal and identify individual women who will develop hypertension in pregnancy offers an exciting area of study and future possibility to improve the lives of women around the world.

REFERENCES

1. Ostchega, Y., Yoon, S. S., Hughes, J., & Louis, T. (2008). Hypertension awareness, treatment, and control—continued disparities in adults: United States, 2005–2006. *NCHS Data Brief.* National Center for Health Statistics: Hyattsville, MD, pp. 1–8.
2. Herman, A. (2010). Hypertension: The pressure's on. *Nursing Made Incredibly Easy, 8*(4), 40–52.
3. American College of Obstetricians and Gynecologists. (2002). Diagnosis and management of preeclampsia and eclampsia. ACOG Practice Bulletin No. 33. *Obstetrics & Gynecology, 99,* 159–167.
4. Berg, C. J., Mackay, A. P., Qin, C., & Callaghan, W. M. (2009). Overview of maternal morbidity during hospitalization for labor and delivery in the United States: 1993–1997 and 2001–2005. *Obstetrics & Gynecology, 113,* 1075–1081.
5. Cudihy, D., & Lee, R. V. (2009). The pathophysiology of preeclampsia: Current clinical concepts. *Journal of Obstetrics & Gynaecology, 29,* 576–582.
6. Millay, J. M. (2010). *Accurately measuring blood pressure.* Retrieved from http://accuratebloodpressure.com/blood_pressure.html
7. Pickering, T. G., Hall, J. E., Appel, L. J., Falkner, B. E., Graves J., Hill M. N., et al. (2005). Recommendations for blood pressure measurement in humans and experimental animals: Part 1: Blood pressure measurement in humans: A statement for professionals from the Subcommittee of Professional and Public Education of the American Heart Association Council on High Blood Pressure Research. *Circulation, 111,* 697–716.
8. Beevers, G., Lip, G. Y., & O'Brien, E. (2001). ABC of hypertension: Blood pressure measurement. Part II-conventional sphygmomanometry: Technique of auscultatory blood pressure measurement. *BMJ, 322,* 1043–1047.
9. Nelson, D., Kennedy, B., Regnerus, C., & Schweinle, A. (2008). Accuracy of automated blood pressure monitors. *Journal of Dental Hygiene, 82,* 35.
10. Coleman, A. J., Steel, S. D., Ashworth, M., Vowler, S. L., & Shennan, A. (2005). Accuracy of the pressure scale of sphygmomanometers in clinical use within primary care. *Blood Pressure Monitoring, 10,* 181–188.
11. Pickering, T. (2003). What will replace the mercury sphygmomanometer? *Blood Pressure Monitoring, 8,* 23–25.
12. Mcalister, F. A. & Straus, S. E. (2001). Evidence based treatment of hypertension: Measurement of blood pressure: An evidence based review. *BMJ, 322,* 908–911.
13. National High Blood Pressure Education Program Working Group on High Blood Pressure in Pregnancy. (2000). Report of the National High Blood Pressure Education Program Working Group on High Blood Pressure in Pregnancy. *American Journal of Obstetrics and Gynecology, 183,* S1–S22.
14. Sibai, B. M. (2002). Chronic hypertension in pregnancy. *Obstetrics & Gynecology, 100,* 369–377.
15. Jim, B., Sharma, S., Kebede, T., & Acharya, A. (2010). Hypertension in pregnancy: A comprehensive update. *Cardiology in Review, 18,* 178–189.
16. Levine, R. J., Ewell, M. G., Hauth, J. C., Curet, L. B., Catalano, P. M., Morris, C. D., et al. (2000). Should the definition of preeclampsia include a rise in diastolic blood pressure of >/ = 15 mm Hg to a level <90 mm Hg in association with proteinuria? *American Journal of Obstetrics & Gynecology, 183,* 787–792.
17. Norwitz, E. R., Hsu, C. D., & Repke, J. T. (2002). Acute complications of preeclampsia. *Clinical Obstetrics & Gynecology, 45,* 308–329.
18. Sibai, B. M. (2003). Diagnosis and management of gestational hypertension and preeclampsia. *Obstetrics & Gynecology, 102,* 181–192.
19. Sibai, B. M. (2007). Caring for women with hypertension in pregnancy. *JAMA, 298,* 1566–1568.
20. Sibai, B. M., Caritis, S., Hauth, J., & National Institute of Child Health and Human Development Maternal-Fetal Medicine Units Network. (2003). What we have learned about preeclampsia. *Seminars in Perinatology, 27,* 239–246.
21. ACOG Committee on Obstetric Practice. (2002). Diagnosis and management of preeclampsia and eclampsia. *ACOG practice bulletin.* No. 33. Washington, DC: American College of Obstetricians and Gynecologists.
22. Sibai, B. M. (2004). Diagnosis, controversies, and management of the syndrome of hemolysis, elevated liver enzymes, and low platelet count. *Obstetrics & Gynecology, 103,* 981–991.
23. Haram, K., Svendsen, E. & Abildgaard, U. (2009). The HELLP syndrome: Clinical issues and management. A Review. *BMC Pregnancy and Childbirth, 9,* 8.
24. Barton, J. R., & Sibai, B. M. (2008). Prediction and prevention of recurrent preeclampsia. *Obstetrics & Gynecology, 112,* 359–372.
25. Sibai, B. M. (2005). Diagnosis, prevention, and management of eclampsia. *Obstetrics & Gynecology, 105,* 402–410.
26. Sibai, B. M. (2004). Magnesium sulfate prophylaxis in preeclampsia: Lessons learned from recent trials. *American Journal of Obstetrics & Gynecology, 190,* 1520–1526.

27. Euser, A. G., & Cipolla, M. J. (2009). Magnesium sulfate for the treatment of eclampsia: A brief review. *Stroke, 40,* 1169–1175.

28. Martin, J. N., Jr., Rose, C. H., & Briery, C. M. (2006). Understanding and managing HELLP syndrome: The integral role of aggressive glucocorticoids for mother and child. *American Journal of Obstetrics & Gynecology, 195,* 914–934.

29. Martin, J. N., Jr., Thigpen, B. D., Moore, R. C., Rose, C. H., Cushman, J., & May, W. (2005). Stroke and severe pre-eclampsia and eclampsia: A paradigm shift focusing on systolic blood pressure. *Obstetrics & Gynecology, 105,* 246–254.

30. Vanhook, J., & Harvey, C. (1994). Oxygen delivery and consumption in severe preeclampsia: Observations in patients with HELLP syndrome. *Critical Care Medicine, 22,* A06.

31. Sibai, B. M. (2008). Maternal and uteroplacental hemodynamics for the classification and prediction of preeclampsia. *Hypertension, 52,* 805–806.

32. Valensise, H., Vasapollo, B., Gagliardi, G., & Novelli, G.P. (2008). Early and late preeclampsia: Two different maternal hemodynamic states in the latent phase of the disease. *Hypertension, 52,* 873–880.

33. Sibai, B. M. (2008). Hypertensive disorders of pregnancy: The United States perspective. *Current Opinion in Obstetrics and Gynecology, 20,* 102–106.

CHAPTER 8

Cardiac Disorders in Pregnancy

Sreedhar Gaddipati and Nan H. Troiano

The physiologic changes associated with pregnancy are significant, yet the healthy gravida is able to accommodate these changes without difficulty. In the presence of a cardiac disorder, however, the pregnant woman may face significant risks for morbidity or mortality.

Cardiac disorders have been reported to occur in 0.5 to 4.0 percent of all pregnancies and represent one of the most important nonobstetric causes of maternal death.[1–5] In the United States, the maternal death rate has risen from 7.2 deaths per 100,000 live births in 1987 to 13 deaths per 100,000 live births in 2004.[6] While the leading causes of maternal death in the U.S. are embolism, hemorrhage, hypertension, and infection, cardiac disease, specifically cardiomyopathy, has increased.[7] Another factor is the increasing population of women with underlying congenital heart disease (CHD). It is estimated that the adult population with CHD is increasing by 5 percent per year.[8] As the increased number of women with successfully managed CHD reach childbearing age, the need for appropriate collaborative care across the specialty practice of women's health is crucial.

This chapter describes the classification of cardiac disorders in pregnancy, presents information regarding specific cardiac lesions, and illustrates how selected lesions impact the woman during pregnancy. The necessity for collaborative management throughout pregnancy is emphasized, and data from clinical case studies are presented to illustrate significant concepts.

CLASSIFICATION

Cardiac disease during pregnancy may generally be categorized as congenital, acquired, or ischemic in nature. The utility of a classification system is to facilitate prediction of risk with respect to how pregnancy will be tolerated by both the pregnant woman with a cardiac disorder and her fetus, and to enhance the quality of patient counseling. It is preferable that women with a known cardiac disorder be counseled *prior* to conception so that they have a more thorough understanding of their specific risk for morbidity and mortality should they become pregnant. However, since 49 percent of pregnancies are unplanned, and the presence of a cardiac disorder may not be known, or may be diagnosed after the pregnancy has progressed, all obstetric health care providers should be familiar with signs and symptoms of cardiac dysfunction and the risks associated with pregnancy.[9]

The risk of perinatal morbidity and mortality for the pregnant woman with preexisting cardiac disease is dependent on three factors: (1) the specific cardiac lesion, (2) the functional abnormality produced by the lesion, and (3) the development of complications such as hemorrhage, infection, and pregnancy-induced hypertension.[10] A classification system that identifies the risk of mortality associated with specific cardiac lesions during pregnancy has been described and is presented in Table 8-1.[11,12] In addition, risk factors predictive of congestive heart failure, stroke, or arrhythmias during the pregnancy of a woman with cardiac disease have been described and are presented in Tables 8-2A and 8-2B.[13,14]

Functional ability also influences pregnancy outcome. Prior to 1973, the Criteria Committee of the New York Heart Association (NYHA) recommended a classification system of cardiac disease based on clinical function. This system is currently utilized as part of a thorough assessment of the pregnant woman with cardiac disease. A description of the NYHA functional classification system is found in Table 8-3. Patients classified as NYHA class I or II prior to pregnancy generally do well during pregnancy. Those with functional classification III or IV have a significantly increased risk of morbidity and mortality during pregnancy. Although this system is useful in caring for the pregnant patient with cardiac disease, it has distinct limitations with respect to its ability to predict successful pregnancy outcome. As many as 40 percent of women who develop congestive heart failure

TABLE 8-1

Mortality Risk Associated with Pregnancy and Cardiac Disorders

Mortality (%)	Disorder
<1	Atrial septal defect*
	Ventricular septal defect (uncomplicated)*
	Patent ductus arteriosus*
	Pulmonic and tricuspid disease
	Corrected tetralogy of Fallot
	Biosynthetic valve prosthesis (porcine and human allograft)
	Mitral stenosis, NYHA classes I and II
5–15	Mitral stenosis with atrial fibrillation[†]
	Mechanical valve prosthesis[†]
	Mitral stenosis, NYHA class III or IV
	Aortic stenosis
	Coarctation of the aorta (uncomplicated)
	Uncorrected tetralogy of Fallot
	Previous myocardial infarction
	Marfan syndrome with normal aorta
25–50	Pulmonary hypertension
	Coarctation of the aorta (complicated)
	Marfan syndrome with aortic involvement

*If not associated with pulmonary hypertension
[†]If anticoagulated with heparin rather than coumadin

TABLE 8-2A

Predictors of Congestive Heart Failure, Stroke, or Arrhythmia

- NYHA classes III–IV, or cyanosis
- Left outflow obstruction (mitral valve area <2 cm^2, aortic valve area <1.5 cm^2, or peak left-ventricular outflow tract gradient >30 mmHg by echocardiography)
- Systemic ventricular dysfunction (ejection fraction <40 percent)
- Arrhythmia or prior cardiac event (heart failure, transient ischemic attack, or stroke before pregnancy)

TABLE 8-2B

Risk of Congestive Heart Failure, Stroke, or Arrhythmia During Pregnancy by Number of Risk Factors

Number of Risk Factors	Rate of Cardiac Event (%)
0	5
1	27
More than 1	75

TABLE 8-3

NYHA Functional Classification System

Class	Description
I	Asymptomatic
	No limitation of physical activity
II	Asymptomatic at rest
	Symptomatic with heavy physical activity
	Slight limitation of physical activity
III	Asymptomatic at rest
	Symptomatic with minimal physical activity
	Considerable limitation of physical activity
IV	Symptomatic with any physical activity
	May be symptomatic at rest
	Severe limitation of physical activity

and pulmonary edema during pregnancy are functional class I prior to pregnancy.[15] Therefore, it is imperative that pregnant women with cardiac disorders be assessed at each prenatal visit, hospital presentation, or admission, and reclassified incorporating any adverse change in functional ability.

CONGENITAL CARDIAC DISORDERS

Incidence

The incidence of congenital heart disease (CHD) is 9 per 1,000 liveborn infants. The incidence is higher if infants are included who have bicuspid aortic valves (incidence of 13.7 per 1,000 adults), or if the approximately 5 percent of all infants who are born with small ventriculoseptal defects that spontaneously close are included.[16,17] The frequency of congenital as opposed to acquired cardiac disease has increased.[8] Two factors have contributed to this change.[18,19] First, advances in neonatal intensive care and pediatric cardiac surgery have allowed children with CHD to reach reproductive age. Second, the incidence of rheumatic fever in the U.S. as well as worldwide has decreased significantly over time. The ratio of rheumatic heart disease to CHD seen during pregnancy decreased from approximately 20:1 in the early 1950s to 3:1 by the late 1970s. Currently this ratio has approached unity, and in some populations the ratio has reversed.[20]

Etiology

Based on earlier studies regarding the risk of recurrence and transmission, a hypothesis of multifactorial etiology was proposed for CHD, which attributed these defects to *interactions* between genetic predisposition and environmental influences.[21] However, more recent studies suggest *separate* genetic and environmental causes.[19] As cytogenetic testing techniques have advanced, high-resolution karyotypic analysis has more precisely revealed chromosome deletions, duplication, and translocations, some of which are very subtle. Analysis of the telomeric and subtelomeric regions has led to discovery of such variants; one of the most recognizable is 22q11 deletion. This deletion has been estimated to occur in 1 per 5,950 live births, and has been associated with DiGeorge syndrome and velocardiofacial syndrome. Similarly, Williams-Beuren syndrome has been found, as a result of analysis by both fluorescence in situ hybridization (FISH) and DNA mutation, to have a microdeletion at chromosome 7q11.23. Linkage analysis and polymerase chain reaction (PCR) are techniques that have helped identify single genes that may be linked to both syndromic (e.g., Noonan syndrome, Holt-Oram syndrome) and nonsyndromic CHD.

Similarly, CHD has been associated with non-inheritable risk factors. Wilson, et al., estimated that up to 30 percent of these factors may be modifiable, thus suggesting that the incidence may potentially be decreased.[22,23] Examples of maternal diseases that increase the risk of fetal congenital cardiac disorders include diabetes mellitus, lupus erythematosus, and phenylketonuria. Systemic lupus erythematosus, while not associated with structural disease, has been associated with heart block via ssA and ssB antibodies, which damage the conduction pathways within the fetal heart. Another example is maternal exposure to environmental factors. This category includes viral illness, drug exposure, and factors within the home or workplace. Febrile illness, influenza, and rubella viral infection have been associated with CHD. Similarly, exposure to drugs such as vitamin A, other retinoids, and anticonvulsants has been linked to CHD. Lithium, once linked to increased incidence of Ebstein's anomaly, is no longer thought to be a cardiac teratogen. While there are no data to support a causative association between caffeine and CHD, alcohol ingestion remains of concern.[23]

It is clear that further research is needed to identify both genetic and environmental causes in order to provide effective prenatal counseling, and to potentially modify risk.

Of equal concern in pregnant women with CHD is the risk of fetal congenital cardiac anomalies. The risk of fetal cardiac anomalies is approximately 5 percent, although the actual incidence may be higher in women whose congenital lesion involves ventricular outflow obstruction. During the antepartum period, serial ultrasonography should be performed in order to assess the fetus for appropriate interval growth. Fetal echocardiography is indicated for prenatal diagnosis of congenital cardiac defects. Of special interest is that affected fetuses appear to be concordant for the maternal lesion in approximately 50 percent of cases.[12] Figure 8-1 depicts an echocardiographic image of a fetus at 32 weeks and 5 days gestational age in a pregnant woman with a ventricular septal defect (VSD). A similar VSD is demonstrated in this fetus.

Left-to-Right Shunts

Atrial Septal Defect

Atrial septal defect (ASD) is one of the most common congenital cardiac lesions found during pregnancy, and

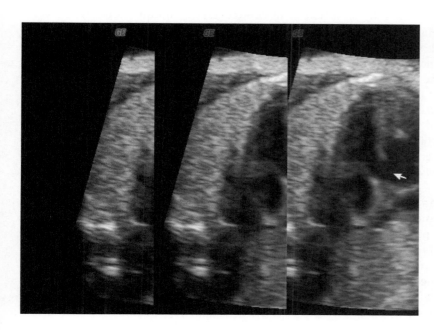

FIGURE 8-1 Echocardiographic image of a fetus at 32 weeks and 5 days' gestation in a pregnant woman with a VSD. A similar VSD is demonstrated in this fetus. (The defect is noted by the arrow.)

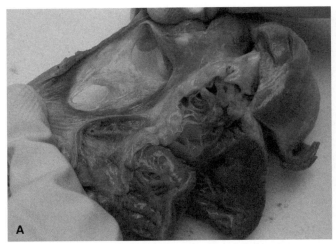

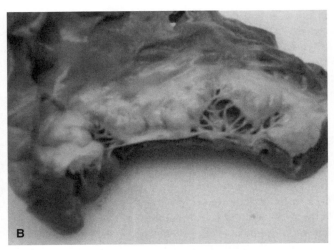

FIGURE 8-2 (**A**) The right atrium is significantly thin, almost transparent. A two-part ASD is visible with a trabeculated area. The ASD is significantly large, measuring 4 centimeters. (**B**) The presence of a thickened, myxomatous mitral valve, in addition to the ASD, is visible in this image.

is the third most common in adults.[1] In a study of a series of 113 women with a known ASD, one death was noted in 219 pregnancies.[24] Three important potential complications seen with ASDs are arrhythmias, paradoxical embolism, and congestive heart failure (CHF). Figures 8-2A and 8-2B depict cardiac abnormalities documented following the death of a pregnant woman from complications of an ASD. Figure 8-2A demonstrates the right atrium to be significantly thin, almost transparent. A two-part ASD is visible with a trabeculated area. The ASD is significantly large, measuring 4 centimeters. Figure 8-2B reveals the presence of a thickened, myxomatous mitral valve, in addition to the ASD. Myxomatous mitral valve disease is a disorder characterized by enlarged, thickened, floppy, gelatinous leaflets, and elongated chordae tendineae. The myxomatous valve as a whole is often moderately to severely regurgitant, which means that blood may leak back through the valve into the left atrium. A summary of the autopsy findings in this case included: a fenestrated ASD measuring 4 centimeters, significant myxomatous changes of the mitral valve consistent with severe mitral valve prolapse, dilation of the right heart chambers, and absence of evidence of a pulmonary embolism. The likely cause of death was noted to be cardiac arrhythmia.

The presence of a large ASD allows for an increased risk for paradoxical emboli, and consideration should be paid to venous thromboembolic (VTE) prophylaxis during labor and the postpartum period, either by application of venous compression devices or administration of prophylactic heparin. Hypervolemia associated with pregnancy results in an increased left-to-right shunt of blood through the ASD, which inflicts a significant

burden on the right ventricle.[25] Although the subsequent additional right preload is tolerated well by most patients, CHF and death have been reported.[26] ASD is usually characterized by normal to low pulmonary artery pressures. Therefore, the development of pulmonary hypertension is uncommon. Although the majority of pregnant women with an ASD tolerate pregnancy, labor, and delivery well, significant morbidity and mortality may occur as a result of complications from an ASD during pregnancy.

Ventricular Septal Defect

Ventricular septal defect (VSD) may occur as a single lesion or in combination with other congenital cardiac anomalies, such as tetralogy of Fallot or transposition of the great vessels. Many VSDs are diagnosed by ultrasound in utero and corrected soon after birth. The majority of VSDs are diagnosed and repaired before the woman reaches childbearing age. In women with an uncorrected VSD, the size of the defect is the most important variable when one evaluates the risk of development of complications during pregnancy. Risk is associated primarily with fluid overload. In patients with a small defect, labor, delivery, and postpartum are usually tolerated without difficulty. Larger defects are associated more commonly with CHF or the development of pulmonary hypertension, as filling pressures increase within chambers on the right side of the heart. A large VSD may also be associated with aortic regurgitation, which can increase the risk of CHF. As with ASD, there are more consequences from embolus formation; thus, prophylaxis should be considered. A significant risk associated with a large VSD is development of right-to-left shunting of blood, thereby bypassing the oxygenation process and exchange of gases that normally occur in the lungs. This condition, referred to as *shunting,* causes a significant percentage of blood pumped from the left ventricle to leave the heart without oxygen. Although cardiac output may remain normal, oxygen transport is severely impaired and can lead to multiple organ system dysfunction or failure, and maternal death.

Patent Ductus Arteriosus

Although a common congenital cardiac anomaly, patent ductus arteriosus (PDA) is generally detected and closed during the newborn period. Therefore, it is an unusual finding during pregnancy. Patients who present with a PDA during pregnancy usually tolerate the hemodynamic stress of pregnancy, labor, and delivery without difficulty. However, the high-pressure, high-flow, left-to-right shunt associated with a large uncorrected PDA can result in the development of pulmonary hypertension or CHF.[25]

Other Congenital Lesions

Tetralogy of Fallot

Tetralogy of Fallot refers to the complex of four cardiac lesions: ventricular septal defect, overriding aorta, pulmonary stenosis, and right ventricular hypertrophy. It is the most common cyanotic heart defect in individuals who survive to adulthood, and accounts for approximately 10 percent of all CHD.[27] The major physiologic risk posed by tetralogy of Fallot is the potential shunting of blood past the lungs without being oxygenated. As much as 75 percent of the venous blood that returns to the heart may pass directly from the right ventricle into the aorta without becoming oxygenated. Most cases are surgically corrected in early childhood. The procedure involves reduction of the pulmonary stenosis, closure of the septal defect, and reconstruction of the flow pathway into the aorta. Although there are late sequelae of this surgery, long-term survival is 86 percent at 32 years.[28,29] The majority of patients with corrected tetralogy of Fallot experience good outcomes in pregnancy. Meijer and colleagues reviewed the cases of 29 women with tetralogy of Fallot who underwent 63 pregnancies.[30] Thirteen of these resulted in abortion, twelve of which were spontaneous. Of the remaining 50 successful pregnancies, statistics were available on 46 deliveries. Five delivered between 16 and 36 weeks, and the remaining were >37 weeks. Of the 26 women who had successful pregnancies, five experienced cardiac events in six pregnancies. Each of these patients experienced either ventricular tachycardia (VT) or supraventricular tachycardia (SVT), and two experienced right-sided cardiac failure.[30] It should be noted that all of these women were NYHA class I prior to pregnancy,

further emphasizing the importance of reassessing patients at each visit to determine if NYHA reclassification is necessary. Patients with an uncorrected VSD may experience worsening of the right-to-left shunt related to the decrease in systemic vascular resistance (SVR) that accompanies pregnancy. Poor prognosis has been associated with patients who have a prepregnancy hematocrit greater than 65 percent, a history of syncopal episodes, CHF, oxygen saturation less than 90 percent, high right-ventricular pressures, or cardiomegaly.[1] Death may occur following surgical repair secondary to arrhythmias, sudden coronary death (6 to 9 percent risk after 30 years), CHF, and complications from subsequent surgery. Thus, while corrected tetralogy of Fallot is usually well tolerated in pregnancy, a good outcome should not be presumed. Cardiac consultation and evaluation should be included as part of prepregnancy counseling of women with corrected tetralogy of Fallot.

Coarctation of the Aorta

The most common site of coarctation is distal to the left subclavian artery.[1] This condition is most commonly seen with a bicuspid aortic valve but also may be associated with aortic stenosis or regurgitation, thoracic aortopathy, aneurysm of the circle of Willis, and the cardiac and systemic results of long-standing arterial hypertension.[24] If left untreated, patients with coarctation of the aorta are at increased risk for the development of arterial hypertension, CHF, infectious aortitis or endocarditis, myocardial infarction, cerebrovascular accidents, aortic aneurysms, and dissection or rupture complicating aortopathy.[25]

Historically, pregnancy in women with coarctation of the aorta was discouraged. In a review of 200 pregnant women with coarctation of the aorta before 1940, Mendelson reported 14 maternal deaths and thus concluded that pregnancy, labor, and delivery posed significant risk to patients with this disorder.[31] Consequently, contraception, therapeutic abortion, Cesarean section, and sterilization were among the therapeutic options recommended for women with this disorder. Similar recommendations were reported in the literature 20 years later.[32] Deal and Wooley reported the outcomes of 28 women with uncorrected coarctation of the aorta who had 83 pregnancies.[33] All were classified as NYHA class I or II prior to pregnancy. In this group of women, no maternal deaths or permanent cardiovascular complications occurred. More recently, Beauchesne and colleagues reported the pregnancy outcomes in a study that included 10 pregnant women with uncorrected coarctation of the aorta and 30 pregnant women who had successfully repaired coarctation of the aorta.[34] Hypertension was noted in 30 percent of the total pregnancies. One maternal death occurred in the study population. That patient also had Turner syndrome and underwent surgery at age 4 to repair coarctation of her aorta. Aortic dissection occurred during her subsequent pregnancy at 36 weeks gestation, from which complications developed that resulted in her death. Vriend and colleagues reported on the outcomes of 54 women from the Netherlands who experienced 126 pregnancies.[35] Results included 98 live births; six were preterm and the gestational age at delivery ranged from 28 to 43 weeks. Twenty-eight spontaneous pregnancy losses were reported. Twenty-six (22 percent) of the pregnancies were complicated by hypertension.

Assessment of the aortic gradient may also be useful in predicting pregnancy outcome in patients with coarctation of the aorta. In general, aortic gradients across the site of coarctation that are less than 20 mmHg are associated with good maternal and fetal outcomes. Thus, with close monitoring and treatment of blood pressure, this lesion is usually associated with a good outcome during pregnancy.[1,27] However, for those with additional manifestations of this defect, pregnancy may pose increased risk. For example, patients with an untreated aortic aneurysm or aneurysm in the circle of Willis may have a mortality rate as high as 15 percent. Thus, pregnancy termination for such patients may be considered.[25]

Eisenmenger Syndrome

Eisenmenger syndrome refers to a condition in which progressive pulmonary hypertension leads to a shunt reversal. The subsequent right-to-left shunting of blood creates a condition whereby an increased percentage of blood is ejected from the left ventricle into the systemic circulation without being oxygenated. This phenomenon, assessed via measurement of shunt fraction, refers to the percentage of blood that leaves the heart without being oxygenated. A normal shunt fraction in a healthy individual is approximately 3 to 5 percent. In the presence of a condition that causes the shunt fraction to rise above approximately 20 percent, serious sequelae may ensue. This syndrome is more likely to occur with a VSD or a PDA because of the high pressure and high flow associated with these defects. Poor prognosis associated with patients with Eisenmenger syndrome is associated with arterial oxygen saturation (SaO_2) levels less than 85 percent, history of syncope, early onset of clinical deterioration, complexity of CHD, and ventricular dysfunction. Death secondary to Eisenmenger syndrome generally occurs in patients in their 30s and 40s and can be attributed to heart failure, hemoptysis, complications from surgery, and consequences of exercise and pregnancy.[36] Decreased SVR associated with normal pregnancy increases the occurrence of right-to-left shunting of blood, resulting in decreased pulmonary perfusion and hypoxemia, thus causing adverse effects for the mother and fetus. Continued pulmonary hypertension may lead to systemic hypotension and decreased right heart filling pressures that may be inadequate to perfuse the pulmonary arterial system. This insufficiency may subsequently result in sudden severe hypoxemia and death.

Women with Eisenmenger syndrome should be counseled with respect to the significant risks that accompany pregnancy. Despite improvements in clinical management, maternal mortality associated with this syndrome has not declined, and is reported to be between 30 and 50 percent.[32,37] Termination of pregnancy is generally strongly considered as an option for women with this cardiac disorder. However, there have been reports that note the possibility of improved pregnancy outcome. One such report by Gleicher and colleagues described 13 pregnancies in 12 women with this syndrome who desired to continue their pregnancies, despite recommendations for therapeutic abortion.[38] Three maternal deaths occurred, and eight infants were born alive. In this group of women, successful outcomes were attributed to prolonged bed rest and the use of heparin and oxygen therapy. Saha and colleagues noted 1 postpartum death in a group of 26 pregnant women with Eisenmenger syndrome.[39] Smedstad and colleagues reported on the outcomes of a series of eight patients with Eisenmenger syndrome.[40] Seven women survived following vaginal deliveries, with follow-up ranging from 3 months to 4 years. The one death occurred in a woman with undiagnosed disease who underwent operative delivery, following the onset of progressive hypoxia and cardiovascular decompensation with concomitant fetal compromise.

Despite these series, which may suggest the potential for a better prognosis during pregnancy, it is clear that the risk of maternal mortality remains significant. The ability to predict who will survive is imprecise, and prior successful pregnancy does not assure the absence of complications in a future pregnancy. This remains a disease for which pregnancy termination should be a subject of discussion between the patient and her health care provider. Information presented in Chapter 3 of this text may be useful to the health care team when addressing this ethical challenge.

ACQUIRED CARDIAC DISORDERS

Mitral Stenosis

Mitral stenosis is the most common rheumatic lesion of pregnancy. Rheumatic fever is caused by group A streptococci and occurs most often after infections such as scarlet fever, middle ear infections, or sore throat. Antibodies formed in response to the infection can also target the mitral valve, causing immunologic or inflammatory damage. Scar tissue involving the valve leaflets and chordae tendineae result in valvular stenosis which, in turn, impedes forward flow of blood through the heart. The normal valve area for the mitral valve is greater than 2.5 cm^2, but when it is less than 1.5 cm^2, flow restriction may become clinically significant. If the orifice is reduced to less than one-half of normal, blood can flow to the left ventricle only with abnormally elevated atrial-to-ventricular pressure gradients. Thus, adequate time for left-ventricular filling is essential to maintain cardiac output. Morbidity has been documented in several recent studies. Hameed and colleagues reported outcomes from a series of 46 pregnancies in 44 women with mild, moderate, or severe mitral stenosis.[41] Although all were either NYHA class I or II, 74 percent experienced a change in classification during pregnancy. Morbidity was most closely associated with women who had moderate or severe mitral stenosis. Those patients experienced heart failure, arrhythmias, and required hospitalization. Similar outcomes were reported by Silversides in a series of 80 pregnancies in 74 women with mitral stenosis.[42] In that series, 35 percent of women experienced cardiac events that included arrhythmias and pulmonary edema.

Labor, delivery, and the immediate postpartum period pose significant stress for patients with mitral stenosis. The normal high cardiac output and low systemic vascular resistance associated with pregnancy, including marked fluctuations in cardiac output that occur during labor and delivery, dynamic fluid shifts, and peripartum blood loss may not be tolerated well by these patients.[43] The normal fluctuations in cardiac output that occur throughout the intrapartum and postpartum period are presented in Table 8-4. The autotransfusion from the utero-placental circulation that occurs at the time of delivery may produce acute pulmonary edema during the postpartum period. Pulmonary artery

catheterization may be utilized in patients with NYHA class III or IV disease as well as other select patients. Because of the need to avoid central volume overload yet maintain sufficient volume to support adequate cardiac output, it is especially important to assess the patient's fluid status. It is important to note, however, that in patients with mitral stenosis, the pulmonary capillary wedge pressure (PCWP) may not represent an accurate appraisal of left-ventricular diastolic filling pressure. Frequent assessment of cardiac output and other invasive hemodynamic parameters is beneficial in the evaluation of left-ventricular function in pregnant women with this cardiac disorder, especially if the patient has received diuretics to reduce preload.[25]

Atrial fibrillation is often associated with mitral stenosis and may have serious implications. The stenotic valve does not allow complete emptying of blood from the left atrium into the left ventricle; therefore, pooling of blood occurs around the valve. As pregnancy is a hypercoagulable state, thrombi can rapidly form and fibrillation can dislodge the thrombi and cause arterial embolism. Thus, prophylactic anticoagulation should be considered in this subset of women.[44]

Aortic Stenosis

Aortic stenosis, though occasionally congenital in nature, is most commonly of rheumatic origin. It generally does not become hemodynamically significant until the orifice has diminished to one-third or less of its normal size. The major difficulty associated with this lesion is maintenance of adequate cardiac output. Because of the increased plasma volume, most patients tolerate early pregnancy well and have an improved cardiac output. However, patients may experience a relatively *fixed* cardiac output which, during periods of exertion, may be insufficient to sustain cardiac or cerebral perfusion. Long-standing disease eventually leads to left-ventricular hypertrophy, a less compliant ventricle, and possible left-ventricular failure.

Arias and Pineda reported a review of aortic stenosis and pregnancy, citing a 17 percent maternal mortality rate in cases of severe stenosis.[45] More recent data reflect improvement in pregnancy outcome. Lao and colleagues reviewed 25 pregnancies in 13 women with varying degrees of aortic stenosis.[46] Five underwent termination of pregnancy, two because of cardiac decompensation. Of the remaining pregnancies, 20 percent had deterioration in functional status; none of the women in the series died. Hameed and colleagues reviewed the outcomes of 12 pregnancies in 12 women with moderate and severe aortic stenosis.[41] Such conditions are significant, as higher rates of complications have been reported compared to matched controls. Forty-four percent of patients experienced heart failure,

TABLE 8-4

Cardiac Output During Normal Labor, Delivery, and Postpartum

Stage of Labor	Cardiac Output
Early first	↑ 15% (plus an additional 15% with each uterine contraction)
Late first	↑ 30% (plus an additional 15% with each uterine contraction)
Second	↑ 45% (plus an additional 15% with each uterine contraction)
Postpartum—5 minutes	↑ 65%
Postpartum—60 minutes	↑ 40%

25 percent had arrhythmias, and 33 percent required hospitalization. One of the 12 women died during aortic valve replacement 10 days after operative delivery.[40] Silversides and colleagues reported on the outcomes of 49 pregnancies in 39 women with congenital aortic stenosis.[42] Fifty-nine percent of the women (29) had severe stenosis, yet 90 percent (44) of the women were NYHA class I prior to labor, the other five were class II. Adverse maternal events were seen only in the 29 women with severe stenosis; two developed pulmonary edema and one developed atrial arrhythmias. No maternal deaths were noted in the series.

The maintenance of adequate cardiac output and oxygen transport is vital in the clinical management of pregnant women with aortic stenosis. Invasive hemodynamic monitoring permits more thorough evaluation of all variables that affect hemodynamic function. Because hypovolemia is a much greater risk than pulmonary edema caused by hypervolemia, the PCWP should be maintained at a slightly higher than normal value in order to provide a margin of safety against unexpected blood loss during delivery or immediately postpartum.[25] Autotransfusion which accompanies the immediate postpartum period subsequently increases intravascular volume and preload; thus, pulmonary edema may develop, especially during the first 24 hours following delivery. For this reason, the PCWP should be assessed more frequently during this period of time. Significantly elevated values should be appreciated by clinicians and consideration given to administration of furosemide. If invasive hemodynamic monitoring is not being utilized in a pregnant woman with aortic stenosis during the peripartum period, the patient should be frequently and thoroughly assessed for evidence of signs and symptoms of pulmonary edema. Abnormal assessment findings should be documented and discussed, and a collaborative plan of clinical management determined.

In general, pregnancy is well tolerated. Women who are symptomatic prior to pregnancy should consider delaying pregnancy until the stenosis is surgically addressed. However, as noted above, even asymptomatic women with aortic stenosis are not without risks of complications during pregnancy. Pregnant women with moderate to severe valve stenosis are at higher risk for adverse events, which can be surgically addressed during pregnancy either by balloon valvuloplasty or valve replacement if indicated. The necessity of collaboration between health care professionals in such cases cannot be stressed enough. Overall, the risk for mortality is low.[47]

Peripartum Cardiomyopathy

Peripartum cardiomyopathy (PPCM) is defined as cardiomyopathy that develops in the last month of pregnancy or in the first 5 months postpartum in a patient with no previous history of cardiac disease and after elimination of *all other causes of cardiac failure.*[48] The incidence of PPCM in the U.S. is reported to be between 1 in 1,300 and 1 in 15,000 pregnancies.[49,50] Risk factors include advanced maternal age (greater than 30 years of age), multiparity, black race, obesity, tocolytic use, preeclampsia, and chronic hypertension. [49,50] It should be recalled, however, that the definition of peripartum cardiomyopathy excludes pregnant women who may have developed cardiomyopathy secondary to other disease processes known to cause cardiovascular changes commensurate with those of cardiomyopathy. Such conditions include sepsis, hypertension, preeclampsia, cardiac disease that predates the pregnancy, side effects of medications, and the presence of autoimmune disorders. Thus, a thorough history with careful attention to other potential causes of cardiomyopathy is important prior to concluding that the patient indeed has peripartum cardiomyopathy. Although black race had previously been thought to account for a significant percentage of the patient population with PPCM in the U.S., Elkayam and colleagues published a survey and review of 123 women with PPCM in which 67 percent of women with PPCM were white.[51]

The exact etiology is unknown; however, several mechanisms have been proposed including autoimmune mechanisms, apoptosis, infectious agents, and nutritional deficiencies. However, none of these has been shown to be conclusive.[49] The survey by Elkayam and colleagues of 123 women with PPCM represents the largest summary in the U.S. that reflects recent therapeutic modalities. While the mortality rate was noted to be lower than in other reports (9 percent mortality rate at 2 years compared to a 32 percent mortality rate reported by Sliwa and colleagues), this may have been influenced by reporting bias.[52] This may not be an unreasonable estimate, as differences in management of heart failure have contributed to a reduction in mortality.[53]

The clinical presentation of pregnant women with PPCM includes the presence of dyspnea, fatigue, and peripheral or pulmonary edema. Cardiomegaly and pulmonary edema are noted on chest radiograph. General clinical management includes sodium and fluid restriction, decreased physical activity, inotropic support, and diuretic therapy. Over 60 percent of patients will recover and return to normal cardiac function; however, a notable feature of peripartum cardiomyopathy is its tendency to recur with subsequent pregnancies.[10,25] In a survey published by Elkayam and colleagues, women who had PPCM were divided into two groups, and outcomes of subsequent pregnancies were analyzed.[51] One group consisted of 28 women who had achieved normalization of left-ventricular function; defined as an increase in left-ventricular ejection fraction of 50 percent or greater. The second group consisted of 16 women whose left-ventricular ejection fraction was less than 50 percent. Within the group of women with normalization of left-ventricular ejection fraction, 21 percent developed symptoms of CHF in their subsequent pregnancy. In the group of women with persistently decreased left-ventricular ejection fraction, 44 percent developed CHF in their subsequent pregnancy. There were no maternal deaths in the first group, but 19 percent of women in the second group died. Because of the inability to adequately predict the risk of cardiac decompensation, and continued uncertainty regarding etiology of the disease, future pregnancy is generally not advisable for women with a history of PPCM.

Marfan Syndrome

Marfan syndrome is an autosomal dominant connective tissue disorder which primarily results in skeletal, ocular, and cardiovascular abnormalities. It has an estimated prevalence of 2 to 3 cases per 10,000 people.[54] A mutation in the *FBN1* gene, which codes for the glycoprotein fibrillin-1, a major component of the extracellular microfibril, results in the classic presentation. The increased risk of maternal mortality during pregnancy relates to aortic root and wall involvement, which may result in aneurysm formation, rupture, or aortic dissection. Figure 8-3 illustrates an aortic dissection that resulted in the death of a pregnant woman with undiagnosed Marfan syndrome.

Prior to medical advances, life expectancy for individuals with Marfan syndrome was 45 years. Currently, with appropriate clinical surveillance, surgical therapy, β-adrenergic receptor antagonist therapy, and exercise

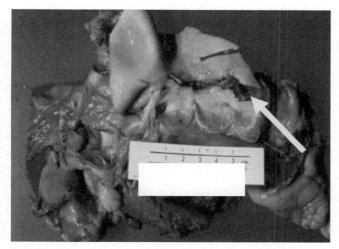

FIGURE 8-3 Aortic dissection (indicated by arrow) which occurred during the pregnancy of a woman with undiagnosed Marfan syndrome.

modification, the average life expectancy for these individuals is 70 years.[55]

In a review of the literature prior to 1981, Pyeritz reported 32 women with Marfan syndrome who had experienced at least one pregnancy.[56] Acute aortic dissection occurred in 20 of these women. Sixteen women died during or shortly after pregnancy, and four died during the postpartum period secondary to aortic rupture or regurgitation. Pyeritz also reported that women with an abnormal aortic valve or aortic dilation may have up to a 50 percent risk of pregnancy-associated mortality; women without these changes and who have an aortic root diameter of less than 40 mm have a risk of mortality of less than 5 percent.[56]

More recent reports note more favorable outcomes. Rossiter and colleagues reviewed 45 pregnancies in 21 women with Marfan syndrome. Two women with aortic root diameter measurements greater than 40 mm suffered aortic dissection, but no deaths occurred. Pregnancy did not appear to affect the rate of aortic root dilation following pregnancy when compared to other women with Marfan syndrome who did not become pregnant.[57] Lind and Wallenburg evaluated 44 women with Marfan syndrome who had 78 pregnancies beyond 24 weeks gestation, and compared outcomes with 51 non-affected women.[58] Obstetric outcomes were similar, and pregnancy was generally well tolerated. Five women with Marfan syndrome experienced aortic dissection, three of whom had aortic root dilation of less than 40 mm. No maternal deaths were noted in the series.

Recommendations, based on existing data regarding pregnancy and Marfan syndrome, have been developed by a number of professional organizations. The American Heart Association stated in 1998 that pregnancy should be discouraged in women with Marfan syndrome who have an aortic root diameter greater than 40 mm.[59] Similarly, the 2003 European Society of Cardiology Task Force pointed to a 10 percent risk of aortic rupture in pregnant women with Marfan syndrome and an aortic root diameter greater than 40 mm.[60] In contrast, the 2001 Consensus Conference of the Canadian Cardiovascular Society recommended that pregnancy be discouraged in women with Marfan syndrome with an aortic root diameter greater than 45 mm, based on a study that included nine women with aortic root diameter measurements between 40 and 45 mm.[61] None had complications during pregnancy, but over a follow-up period of 20 years demonstrated progression in aortic root dilation. Meijboom and colleagues reported a review of 47 pregnancies in 23 women with Marfan syndrome, nine of whom had aortic root diameters between 40 and 45 mm.[62] No aortic dissections occurred in patients without previous aortic dissection and an aortic root diameter of 45 mm or less.

In a follow-up article that reviewed obstetric complications, Meijboom and colleagues reviewed 111 completed pregnancies, and noted a 15 percent preterm delivery rate, somewhat higher than previously reported in a smaller series.[63]

For pregnant women with Marfan syndrome, clinical care during labor includes positioning to maintain adequate cardiac output, use of regional anesthesia, and avoidance of valsalva by shortening the second stage of labor. Assisted operative vaginal delivery reduces the stress on the aorta and thus reduces the risk of cardiovascular complications. Delivery by Cesarean section is recommended if there is evidence of aortic dissection, or, from a more conservative standpoint, if the aortic root diameter is greater than 40 mm. If Cesarean section is performed, retention sutures should be considered because of generalized connective tissue weakness in this patient population.[12]

In summary, women with Marfan syndrome should receive counseling prior to pregnancy regarding the risk for potential pregnancy-related complications and a 50 percent risk for transmission of the syndrome to the baby.

ISCHEMIC CARDIAC DISEASE

Pregnancy complicated by acute myocardial infarction (MI) is relatively rare. It has been estimated that MI occurs in 1 out of every 10,000 pregnancies.[64] In a review by Hankins and colleagues, 70 well-documented cases in the world literature were analyzed.[64] Of those patients, only 13 percent had known coronary artery disease antedating their pregnancy. Two-thirds had an infarct in the third trimester with a mortality rate of 45 percent. When delivery occurred within 14 days of the infarction, the mortality rate was 50 percent. In the most recent comprehensive review of acute MI associated with pregnancy, 125 well-documented cases of MI in 123 pregnancies were identified.[65] This retrospective review revealed that MI most often occurred during the third trimester in multigravidas older than 33 years of age. The most common anatomic location of the infarct was the anterior wall.[66] The left anterior descending artery is the most commonly identified on angiographic study as the site of infarction. However, up to 47 percent of affected women will have normal angiograms, meaning coronary artery spasm is the most common cause of MI in pregnancy.[65] The overall maternal mortality rate was 21 percent, with death occurring either acutely or within 2 weeks of delivery. Neonatal mortality in pregnancies complicated by MI is closely associated with maternal death, and ranges from 13 to 17 percent.[65] Of the women studied, 54 percent underwent cardiac catheterization. Coronary atherosclerosis with or without intracoronary thrombus was found in 43 percent of patients, coronary thrombus without atherosclerotic disease was noted in 21 percent, and coronary dissection was present in 16 percent. Although the majority displayed pathology, 29 percent of this subgroup had normal coronary arteries. Atherosclerotic disease was most often associated with MI in the antepartum period, whereas coronary dissection was seen most frequently in the postpartum period. In a concurrent review of MI during pregnancy and the puerperium, the overall findings were remarkably similar in a study by Bandui et al.[67] Thus, it appears that the increased hemodynamic burden imposed on the maternal cardiovascular system in late pregnancy may unmask latent coronary artery disease in some women and worsen the prognosis for patients suffering infarction.[12]

While coronary artery disease and MI in women of childbearing age occur infrequently, the increased number of women delaying pregnancy to later in life may contribute to an increased incidence of MI in pregnancy and postpartum. In addition, more women with preexisting cardiovascular risk factors such as chronic hypertension and diabetes become pregnant. Lastly, even women with a history of an MI may become pregnant. It is readily apparent that these issues necessitate a heightened awareness of the significance of cardiac disorders in pregnancy on the part of all professionals who provide health care to women.

When MI occurs, the extent and significance of damage to the heart muscle depends upon several factors: (1) the number of vessels and branches involved, (2) disease within the vessels, (3) the area(s) of myocardium supplied by the affected vessel(s), (4) the amount of collateral circulation to provide alternative perfusion to the affected region, and (5) the oxygen demands on the heart during and after the infarction. Typically, coronary oxygen delivery exceeds oxygen demand by 75 percent. Myocardial oxygenation is maintained through physiologic mechanisms that ensure appropriate coronary perfusion pressure, adequate volumes of oxygenated blood, and unobstructed coronary flow. Myocardial ischemia may occur when one or all of these mechanisms are challenged. However, a substantial deficit must exist before symptoms are present. In fact, a major coronary vessel has typically lost 70 percent in diameter before angina occurs.[68]

Under normal conditions, oxygen consumption is determined by the metabolic rate. However, vascular diseases can compromise the ability to deliver an adequate amount of oxygen for cellular metabolism. Oxygen delivery is not only dependent upon cardiac output, but also on the oxygen-carrying capacity of the blood and the ability of the lungs to exchange respiratory gases. A more thorough presentation of concepts related to hemodynamic and oxygenation dynamics and assessment

TABLE 8-5

Review of the Coronary Artery Blood Supply

Artery	Branches	Areas Supplied
Left main coronary artery	Left anterior descending	Anterior two thirds of ventricular septum
		Anterior left ventricle
		Entire apex
	Left circumflex	Posterior left ventricle
		Left atrium
		Entire posterior wall
Right coronary artery		Posterosuperior ventricular septum
		Part of left atrium
		Right atrium
		Sinoatrial node
		Arterioventricular node
		Right ventricle
		Posterior left ventricle
		Diaphragmatic left ventricle

parameters may be found in Chapter 4 of this text. When oxygen delivery is reduced, the tissues increase the rate of oxygen extraction. When the limits of extraction are reached, tissues rely on anaerobic glycolysis for energy and release lactate as a metabolic by-product. During periods of prolonged oxygen deprivation, metabolic acidosis is followed by permanent tissue damage.

Coronary arteries perfuse the myocardial tissue during ventricular diastole and are dependent on vascular distensability and left-ventricular function to maintain adequate perfusion pressure. A review of the coronary artery blood supply is presented in Table 8-5.

Diagnosis of MI is based on serial electrocardiographic findings and evaluation of fractionated cardiac enzymes. Criteria for diagnosis of MI, now classified as an acute coronary syndrome, typically include at least two of the following symptoms of MI: elevation of cardiac enzyme concentrations in the blood, and electrocardiographic changes involving the development of Q waves or persistent T wave changes. Cardiac enzymes typically evaluated include lactic dehydrogenase (LDH), aspartate aminotransferase (AST), total serum creatine kinase and MB fractions (CK-MB$_{mass}$).[69] In the nonobstetric patient population, CK-MB levels are assessed every 8 hours, and three negative CK-MB levels are used to rule out an acute MI. CK-MB levels greater than 3 percent of total CK levels are used to make a diagnosis of an acute MI. However, since uterine contractions also cause significant increase in cardiac markers such as myoglobin and serum CK-MB$_{mass}$, recent literature endorses the use of the biochemical markers troponin I and T for the diagnosis of MI in pregnant women.[70] These are sensitive and specific biochemical markers released from injured cardiac muscle. Blood levels of

these proteins rise 3 to 6 hours after myocardial injury and peak at 20 hours. Unlike other laboratory values, troponin I and T are not increased above the upper normal limits in healthy pregnant women, even in the immediate postpartum period. However, troponin levels are increased in pregnant women with preeclampsia and gestational hypertension.[71] The reason for this alteration is currently unclear, though perhaps the incidence of myocardial ischemia in preeclampsia is higher than previously suspected.

Clinical management of the pregnant woman with an acute MI is dependent on the etiology and complications of the infarction. Early goals of collaborative clinical therapy include: (1) relief of pain and anxiety, (2) reperfusion of affected vessels, (3) improvement of the balance between myocardial oxygen supply and demand, (4) initiation of antithrombotic therapy to prevent the formation of a secondary thrombus, (5) improvement of ventricular function, and (6) limitation of the size of the infarction.[72]

Utilization of invasive modalities to assess hemodynamic and oxygen transport status may be useful. The ability to detect specific abnormal values facilitates identification of interventions to correct abnormalities and optimize hemodynamic function. Pulmonary artery catheterization is also beneficial during administration of vasoactive drugs and evaluation of the patient's response to therapy.

Pharmacotherapy is an integral component of the clinical management for a pregnant woman with an acute MI. Medications may be indicated for pain management, reduction of oxygen demand, optimization of oxygen delivery, treatment of congestive heart failure, relief of ischemic chest pain, reduction of coronary vasospasm and ventricular preload, limitation of the area of damaged cardiac tissue, correction of arrhythmias, and for anticoagulation. A thorough discussion of the numerous medications that may be utilized in this population is beyond the scope of this chapter. However, more detailed information regarding pharmacotherapy, including medications specifically utilized for patients with an MI or acute coronary syndrome, is presented in Chapter 6 of this text.

Thrombolysis is a classic therapeutic procedure used in non-pregnant patients with MI to revascularize blocked or constricted arteries and minimize permanent myocardial tissue damage. Thrombolytic agents such as urokinase, streptokinase, and tissue plasminogen activator (tPA) do not appear to cross the placenta. However, they have been considered relatively contraindicated in pregnancy secondary to the risk for hemorrhage to both the pregnant woman and her fetus. Use of these agents has also been associated with reports of first trimester pregnancy loss, preterm labor, placental abruption, and fetal death.[73] The risk for maternal hemorrhage following administration of thrombolytic agents may be as high as 8 percent, with a fetal mortality risk of nearly 6 percent. The greatest risk for hemorrhage is present if thrombolytics are given at the time of birth.[65] Successful use of tPA to treat MI in the second trimester of pregnancy has been reported and may be an effective treatment alternative.[74] Women who have received thrombolytics should not undergo any operative procedure for 10 days after their administration. This brings up ethical issues which may complicate decision-making with respect to obstetric management if the fetus is viable at or near the time of thrombolytic therapy. Refer to Chapter 3 in this text for presentation of an ethical framework from which clinicians may glean strategies to address and resolve such management decisions. Additional concerns about the use of thrombolytics include allergic reactions, fibrinolytic effects on placental implantation, activation of circulating plasminogen as a trigger for preterm labor, and the development of reperfusion arrhythmias.[65,74]

Percutaneous transluminal coronary angioplasty (PTCA) is now commonly used to improve the patency of blocked arteries.[73] Stent placement increases the diameter of the vessel and decreases the rate of restenosis, thereby improving clinical outcomes. Complications of PTCA with stent placement include arterial embolization, contrast toxicity, arrhythmias, and vascular injury. The timing of birth after PTCA with stent placement can become an issue because of the subsequent anticoagulation requirements. Because of the increased risk for hemorrhage from anticoagulation, decisions about the use of regional anesthesia and operative delivery may be difficult.

Most maternal deaths occur at the time of infarction or within 2 weeks following the infarction.[64,65] Thus, delivery should be postponed for at least 2 weeks after acute MI to allow for adequate cardiac healing. If tocolysis is used to delay delivery, magnesium sulfate or indocin are preferred. Sympathomimetics are contraindicated as they increase heart rate and myocardial oxygen demand, and have been associated with ischemia, even in otherwise healthy women.[75]

In general, vaginal delivery holds many advantages over Cesarean section. While operative delivery allows for control of timing, vaginal delivery is preferred because it eliminates surgical morbidity risks, decreases hemodynamic fluctuations during the intraoperative period, and most often results in less blood loss. In a hemodynamically stable woman, obstetric factors should dictate the mode of delivery.[65]

GENERAL CLINICAL MANAGEMENT PRINCIPLES

Initial clinical assessment of the pregnant woman with cardiac disease begins with a thorough history. The patient's chief complaint should be determined and documented. History of her present cardiac disease should be elicited and include review of the specific lesion or disorder, functional classification, and current medications. The patient should be questioned regarding the presence of symptoms such as chest pain, dyspnea, cyanosis, fatigue, palpitations, or skin changes. Complaints of pain require further evaluation including onset, duration, character, location, radiation, alleviating factors, aggravating factors, and accompanying signs or symptoms. Past medical history should also be reviewed including previous illnesses, surgical procedures, or hospitalizations. Family history should be evaluated including hereditary, familial diseases that pertain to the cardiovascular system. Assessment of social history includes use of alcohol or tobacco, chemical dependence, occupation, educational level, and support system.

General physical assessment involves use of inspection, palpation, percussion, and auscultation to determine the presence or absence of signs and symptoms associated with cardiac disease. Additional noninvasive assessment parameters include level of consciousness, blood pressure, arterial oxygen saturation, urinary output, and electrocardiographic findings.

Hemodynamic Assessment

Cardiac output, the amount of blood ejected from the left ventricle, is determined by four variables: preload, afterload, contractility, and heart rate. Cardiac output may be adjusted by manipulating any of these four variables. The intense cardiovascular demands of pregnancy actuate a challenge in the management of the pregnant woman with a cardiac disorder. The labor, delivery, and immediate postpartum period provide a time of increased risk secondary to the rapid volume changes that occur. For the patient with valvular disease, the major management considerations during the intrapartum period are preload optimization, control of heart rate, alterations in afterload, and prevention of hypotension or other events that result in fluid imbalance.

Invasive hemodynamic monitoring may be indicated for certain patients with a cardiac disorder to more accurately evaluate hemodynamic function and adequacy of cardiac output. Use of a pulmonary artery catheter with the ability to continuously monitor mixed-venous oxygen saturation (SvO_2) as well as other oxygen transport parameters may be particularly beneficial in this patient population. Invasive hemodynamic monitoring provides more accurate information that may either reinforce or dispute clinical impressions based on noninvasive evaluation.

Epidural Anesthesia

Epidural anesthesia is appropriate for most patients with cardiac disease during labor. By eliminating pain, associated changes in heart rate and cardiac output may be avoided. Epidural anesthesia also decreases preload secondary to peripheral vasodilation. Hypotension, a frequent side effect of epidural anesthesia, should be avoided, especially in the pregnant woman with cardiac disease. Repositioning of the patient and administration of intravenous fluids are useful interventions to correct abnormalities in preload. Administration of ephedrine to correct hypotension following epidural administration in a pregnant woman with cardiac disease should be done with extreme caution. Because maintenance of adequate preload is vital to maintaining adequate cardiac output in the presence of many cardiac lesions during pregnancy, care should be taken to assure that preload is adequate prior to administration of vasoactive drugs to correct hypotension.

Route of Delivery

Vaginal delivery is advisable for most patients with cardiac disease, with Cesarean delivery retained for obstetric indications, such as cephalopelvic disproportion, failure to progress, and nonreassuring fetal heart rate responses that do not respond to interventions. Continuous invasive hemodynamic monitoring is advantageous because of the autotransfusion that occurs immediately following birth and placental expulsion. It is thus possible to more accurately evaluate rapid changes in the pulmonary capillary wedge pressure (PCWP), cardiac output, and heart rate.

Antibiotic Prophylaxis

Antibiotic prophylaxis is indicated for select patients with cardiac disease because of their predisposition to developing endocarditis during invasive procedures. While the incidence of bacteremia is between 1 and 5 percent of women who have an uncomplicated delivery, bacteremia may occur more frequently following Cesarean delivery, depending on specific circumstances and indications for operative intervention. Despite the American Heart Association's opinion that prophylaxis is optional for high-risk patients and not necessary for patients with moderate lesions undergoing uncomplicated vaginal delivery, many physicians prefer to administer prophylaxis to select high-risk patients based on the risk-benefit ratio, specifically the unpredictability of the timing of vaginal delivery, and the inability to predict complications.[76] Current American Heart Association and American College of Obstetricians and Gynecologists (ACOG) recommendations for prophylaxis are presented in Tables 8-6A and B.[77]

Anticoagulation

Anticoagulation in the pregnant woman with an artificial heart valve and/or atrial fibrillation remains somewhat controversial. The key issue involves the lack of an ideal agent for anticoagulation during pregnancy. Warfarin (Coumadin) is relatively contraindicated at all stages of gestation because of its association with fetal warfarin syndrome in weeks 6 to 9 and its relationship to fetal intracranial hemorrhage and secondary scarring at later stages.[12] Known teratogenic effects of oral anticoagulants must be weighed against the potential increased risk of thrombosis and thromboembolism incurred by using heparin rather than warfarin. Nevertheless, use of heparin rather than warfarin is advocated by most experts in the United States.

Any patient with cardiac disease who requires anticoagulation when not pregnant should be treated during pregnancy, although the medication used may be different. Pregnant women with prosthetic heart valves should be treated with adjusted dose subcutaneous heparin from conception until delivery.[78] Coumadin may be reinstituted during the postpartum period. The adjusted dose regimen is heparin given subcutaneously every 12 hours in a dose sufficient to prolong the activated partial thromboplastin time (aPTT) obtained 6 hours after the dose to 1.5 to 2.0 times the normal control. Plasma heparin levels should be 0.2 to 0.4 units/mL if measured by heparin assay.

Heparin is withheld during labor. Epidural anesthesia may be administered, if appropriate, 12 hours or more after the last dose of heparin or when the patient is no longer anticoagulated. Heparin is resumed 6 hours

TABLE 8-6A

American Heart Association and American College of Obstetricians and Gynecologists: Risk Classification of Cardiac Lesions for Infective Endocarditis

Risk Level	
High	Prosthetic cardiac valves
	Prior bacterial endocarditis
	Complex cyanotic congenital malformations
	Surgically corrected systemic pulmonary shunts
Moderate	Congenital cardiac malformations (except repaired atrial septal defect, ventricular septal defect, patent ductus arteriosus, or isolated secundum atrial septal defect)
	Acquired valvular dysfunction
	Hypertrophic cardiomyopathy
	Mitral valve prolapse with regurgitation and/or thickened leaflets
Negligible	Surgical repair of atrial septal defect, ventricular septal defect, patent ductus arteriosus
	Isolated secundum atrial septal defect
	Prior coronary artery bypass graft
	Mitral valve prolapse without regurgitation
	Physiologic, functional, or innocent heart murmurs
	Previous Kawasaki disease without valve dysfunction
	Previous rheumatic fever without valvular dysfunction
	Cardiac pacemakers and implanted defibrillators

postpartum following vaginal delivery. The incidence of serious bleeding complications following Cesarean delivery is rare if therapy is resumed in 18 to 24 hours. Heparin is administered intravenously during the initial postpartum period. Postpartum anticoagulation is then continued with warfarin.

Intrapartum Recommendations: Select Disorders

Specific recommendations for intrapartum collaborative care of patients with select cardiac lesions are reviewed in Table 8-7. Additional issues may be identified when providing care for intrapartum patients with cardiac disease. These include the following: (1) single-room care if possible, (2) sufficient space to accommodate specialized personnel, procedures, and equipment, (3) proper positioning of the patient to achieve desired hemodynamic goals, (4) administration of drugs to optimize hemodynamic function, (5) regulation of all intravenous fluids with an infusion pump, with frequent assessment of intake and output, (6) avoidance of hypotension, (7) investigation of cause of tachycardia, (8) anticipation of autotransfusion following delivery, and (9) avoidance of the lithotomy position during the second stage of labor.

As is the case with any pregnant woman in labor, fetal surveillance is required. Continuous electronic fetal heart rate monitoring is particularly beneficial in the patient with cardiac disease. A less than optimal cardiac output in the mother is often reflected in adverse fetal heart rate changes. Proper maternal positioning and maintenance of hemodynamic values within the desired range will facilitate adequate placental perfusion and therefore optimize oxygen delivery to the fetus.

TABLE 8-6B

American Heart Association and American College of Obstetricians and Gynecologists: Recommended Antibiotic Regimens for High and Moderate Risk Cardiac Lesions for Infective Endocarditis Prophylaxis

Category	Antibiotic Regimen
High Risk	Ampicillin (2 grams IV or IM) plus gentamicin (1.5 mg/kg IV up to a maximal dose of 120 mg) shortly before delivery (within 30 minutes), followed by ampicillin (1 gram IV or IM) or amoxicillin (1 gram orally) 6 hours later
	Women who are allergic to penicillin should receive the same dose of gentamicin plus vancomycin (1 gram IV) infused over 1 to 2 hours
Moderate Risk	Ampicillin only (2 grams IV or IM) shortly before delivery
	Women who are allergic to penicillin can be treated with only vancomycin (1 gram IV) infused over 1 to 2 hours

TABLE 8-7

Intrapartum Management of Selected Cardiac Lesions

Mitral Stenosis	Aortic Stenosis	Pulmonary Hypertension
Left atrial outflow obstruction with decreased left ventricular diastolic filling rate and a "fixed" cardiac output.	Left ventricular outflow obstruction with "fixed" cardiac output and left ventricular hypertrophy.	Often the result of an uncorrected congenital left-to-right shunt (PDA, ASD, VSD) and ultimately leading to reversal of the shunt.
• SBE prophylaxis	• SBE prophylaxis	• SBE prophylaxis
• Continuous pulse oximetry	• Continuous pulse oximetry	• Continuous pulse oximetry
• Maintain PCWP at 12–14 mmHg	• Maintain PCWP at 16–18 mmHg	• Maintain PCWP at 16–18 mmHg
• Epidural anesthesia	• Epidural anesthesia	• Epidural with caution
• Avoid hypotension	• Avoid hypotension	• Avoid hypotension
		• Must maintain adequate right preload
• Maintain HR <100 bpm	• Avoid tachycardia	
• May use propranolol or esmolol to treat tachycardia		
• Vaginal delivery preferred	• Vaginal delivery preferred	• Vaginal delivery preferred
• Decrease PCWP prior to delivery		
• Anticoagulation with atrial fibrillation		• Anticoagulation
	• Treat blood loss promptly	• Oxygen administration—helps to keep pulmonary vasculature maximally dilated

CASE EXAMPLE

These concepts are represented in the following excerpt from an intrapartum clinical case study of a pregnant woman with aortic stenosis. The case involved a 32-year-old gravida 2 with a history of one prior preterm delivery whose pregnancy was complicated by the presence of aortic stenosis. With respect to functional status, she had remained NYHA class I to II throughout her prenatal course. At 36 weeks gestation, she presented to the hospital because of the onset of regular uterine contractions, chest pain, shortness of breath, and extreme fatigue. She was initially assessed in the Obstetric Triage Unit and then admitted to the Labor and Delivery Unit. A Critical Care Obstetric (CCOB) team of nurses and physicians had been identified, oriented, and mentored in order to provide care to critically ill pregnant women within the Labor and Delivery Unit of the hospital. Assessment findings by the CCOB nurse revealed the presence of a sustained elevated blood pressure, tachycardia, tachypnea, and low arterial oxygen saturation. Electrocardiographic findings included a sinus tachycardia with no other abnormalities. Continuous electronic monitoring was initiated to assess uterine activity and fetal heart rate responses.

It should be recalled that aortic stenosis is a Group II lesion with respect to pregnancy and is associated with a risk of mortality between 5 and 15 percent. For these women it is important to maintain a margin of safety in left-ventricular end-diastolic volume. The principal risks during pregnancy are decreased cardiac output and oxygen delivery associated with central hypovolemia. It is important therefore to avoid supine hypotension and to maintain a maternal heart rate less than 100 beats per minute to allow for adequate ventricular filling time.

Following collaboration with the CCOB physician, the decision was made to insert a pulmonary artery catheter with continuous SvO_2 monitoring capability. Initial vital signs and hemodynamic data are presented in Table 8-8. The fetal heart rate (FHR) tracing obtained at the time initial hemodynamic data were obtained is depicted in Figure 8-4.

These initial data indicated the patient was centrally hypovolemic (PCWP = 5 mmHg), her left-ventricular function was depressed (LVSWI = 33), and her cardiac output was significantly decreased (4.1 L/minute). Oxygen delivery was consequently significantly low (DO_2 = 451 mL/min). Compensatory responses to these abnormal findings included maternal tachycardia and systemic vasoconstriction (SVR = 2360). Clinical indications of inadequate oxygen perfusion included the symptoms noted at the time of admission as well as the FHR tachycardia. Regular uterine contractions were

TABLE 8-8

Case Study Excerpt: Initial Vital Signs and Hemodynamic Data

	Parameter	Value Before Intervention	Value After Intervention
Vital Signs	Blood pressure	160/108 mmHg	130/72 mmHg
	Heart rate	130	88
	Respiratory rate	36	22
	SaO_2	92% (on O_2 at 10 L/min)	98% (room air)
	SvO_2	55%	82%
Laboratory Data	Hemoglobin	9.2 g/dL	12 g/dL
Hemodynamic Data	CVP	4 mmHg	4 mmHg
	PAP	14/5 mmHg	24/18 mmHg
	PCWP	5 mmHg	18 mmHg
	Cardiac output	4.1 L/min	9.2 L/min
	Cardiac index (BSA = 1.6 m²)	2.5 L/min	5.7 L/min
	SVR	2360 dynes/sec/cm⁵	756 dynes/sec/cm⁵
	PVR	58 dynes/sec/cm⁵	17 dynes/sec/cm⁵
	LVSWI	33 gm/M/M²	104 gm/M/M²
Oxygen Transport	CaO_2	11 mL/dL	16 mL/dL
	DO_2	451 mL/min	1472 mL/min
	CvO_2	7 mL/min	13 mL/min
	$avDO_2$	4 mL/dL	3 mL/dL
	VO_2	164 mL/min	276 mL/min
	O_2ER	36%	19 %

$avDO_2$ = arteriovenous oxygen difference, CaO_2 = arterial oxygen content, CvO_2 = venous oxygen content, CVP = central venous pressure, DO_2 = oxygen delivery, LVSWI = left-ventricular stroke work index, O_2ER = oxygen extraction ratio, PAP = pulmonary artery pressure, PCWP = pulmonary capillary wedge pressure, PVR = pulmonary vascular resistance, SVR = systemic vascular resistance, VO_2 = oxygen consumption.

noted at the time of admission, and cervical change was noted between the first and second assessments.

Interventions included lateral positioning of the patient with elevation of the lower extremities, volume resuscitation with crystalloid, and administration of packed red blood cells to improve arterial oxygen content. Subsequent patient assessment findings are presented in Table 8-8. Assessment of the subsequent FHR tracing was reassuring and included a normal baseline rate, absence of decelerations, and the presence of

FIGURE 8-4   FHR tracing at the time initial hemodynamic data were obtained

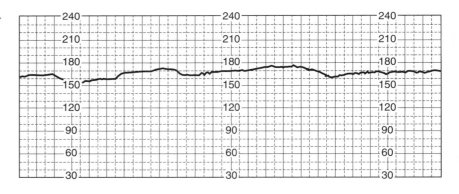
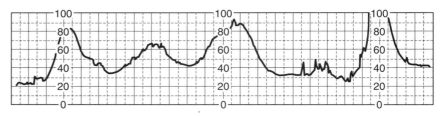

occasional accelerations. With the presence of a favorable cervix and spontaneous regular uterine contractions, augmentation of labor with oxytocin was initiated the following day. Hemodynamic and oxygen transport data were obtained and interpreted throughout the intrapartum period. The patient's family members remained with her throughout labor. She subsequently had a spontaneous vaginal delivery of a female infant with Apgar scores of 6 and 7. Arterial cord blood gases were obtained and were normal. Following initial assessment by the Neonatal Intensive Care Unit (NICU) personnel at the time of birth, and a brief period of observation in the Transitional Nursery, the baby was brought to the Labor and Delivery unit and remained with the patient and her family until the time of discharge.

SUMMARY

Care of the pregnant woman with known cardiac disease presents a unique clinical challenge. Knowledge of the disease process as well as astute assessment of hemodynamic function during pregnancy is essential. Collaborative care should focus on assessment, early detection of abnormalities, initiation of appropriate interventions, and prevention of complications.

REFERENCES

1. Hameed, A. B., & Sklansky, M. S. (2007). Pregnancy: Maternal and fetal heart Disease. *Current Problems in Cardiology, 32,* 419–494.
2. Cunningham, F. G., Hauth, J. C., Leveno, K. J., Hauth, J. C., Leveno, K. J., & Wenstrom, K. D. (2005). Cardiovascular disease. In F. G. Cunningham, J. C. Hauth, K. J. Leveno, J. C. Hauth, K. J. Leveno, & K. D. Wenstrom (Eds.), *Williams obstetrics* (22nd ed., pp. 1017–1043). New York: McGraw-Hill Companies, Inc.
3. van Mook, W. N., & Peeters, L. (2005). Severe cardiac disease in pregnancy, part II: Impact of congenital and acquired cardiac diseases during pregnancy. *Current Opinion in Critical Care, 11,* 435–448.
4. Oakley, C. M. (1989). Pregnancy and heart disease: Pre-existing heart disease. *Cardiovascular Clinics, 19,* 57–80.
5. McFaul, P. B., Dornan, J. C., Lamki, H., & Boyle, D. (1988). Pregnancy complicated by maternal heart disease. A review of 519 women. *British Journal of Obstetrics & Gynaecology, 95,* 861–867.
6. Centers for Disease Control and Prevention. National Center for Health Statistics. (2010). *Deaths: Final data for 2007.* Retrieved from http://www.cdc.gov/nchs/data/nvsr/nvsr58/nvsr58_19.pdf
7. Berg, C. J., Callaghan, W. M., Syverson, C. & Henderson, Z. (2010). Pregnancy-related mortality in the United States: 1998–2005. *Obstetrics & Gynecology, 116,* 1302–1309.
8. Brickner, M. E., Hillis, L. D., & Lang, R. A. (2000). Congenital heart disease in adults. First of two parts. *The New England Journal of Medicine, 342,* 256–263.
9. National Center for Health Statistics. (n.d.) *Healthy People 2010 Midcourse Review.* Retrieved from http://www.healthy people.gov/2010/Data/midcourse/default.htm
10. Gianopoulos, J. G. (1989). Cardiac disease in pregnancy. *The Medical Clinics of North America, 73*(3), 639–651.
11. Clark, S. L. (1987). Structural cardiac disease in pregnancy. In S. L. Clark and J. P. Phelan (Eds.), *Critical care obstetrics* (pp. 92–113). Oradell, NJ: Medical Economics Books.
12. Foley, M. R. (2004). Cardiac disease. In G. A. Dildy, M. A. Belfort, G. R. Saade, et al. *Critical care obstetrics* (4th ed., pp. 252–274). Malden, MA: Blackwell Publishing.
13. Siu, S. C., Sermer, M., Harrison, D. A., Grigoriadis, E., Liu, G., Sorensen, S., et al. (1997). Risk and predictors for pregnancy related complications in women with heart disease. *Circulation, 96,* 2789–2794.
14. Siu, S. C., Sermer, M., Colman, J. M., Alvarez A. N., Mercier, L. A., Morton B. C., et al. Cardiac Disease in Pregnancy (CARPREG) Investigators. (2001). Prospective multicenter study of pregnancy outcomes in women with heart disease. *Circulation, 104,* 515–521.
15. Shime, J., Mocarski, E. J. M., Hastings, D., Webb C. D., & McLaughlin, P. R. (1990). Congenital heart disease and pregnancy. In U. Elkayam & N. Gleicher (Eds.), *Cardiac problems in pregnancy: Diagnosis and management of maternal and fetal disease* (2nd ed., p. 73). New York: Alan Liss.
16. Hoffman, J. I., & Kaplan, S. (2002). The incidence of congenital heart disease. *Journal of the American College of Cardiology, 39,* 1890–1900.
17. Thom, T., Haase, N., Rosamond, W., Rumsfeld, J., Manolio, T., Zheng Z. J., et al. American Heart Association Statistics Committee and Stroke Statistics Subcommittee. (2006). American Heart Association Statistics Committee and Stroke Statistics Subcommittee. Heart disease and stroke statistics-2006 update: A report from the American Heart Association Statistics Committee and Stroke Statistics Subcommittee. *Circulation, 113,* e85–151.
18. Cooper, D. S., & Nichter, M. A. (2006). Advanced in cardiac intensive care. *Current Opinion in Pediatrics, 18,* 503–511.
19. Pierpont, M. E., Basson, C. T., Benson, D. W., Gelb, B. D., Giglia, T. M., Goldmuntz, E., et al. (2007). Genetic basis for congenital heart defects: Current knowledge. *Circulation. American Heart Association Scientific Statement, 115,* 3015–3038.
20. Hsieh, T. T., Chen, K. C., & Soong, J. H. (1993). Outcome of pregnancy in patients with organic heart disease in Taiwan. *Asia-Oceania Journal of Obstetrics & Gynaecology, 19,* 21–27.
21. Ramin, S. M., Maberry, M. C., & Gilstrap, L. C. (1989). Congenital heart disease. *Clinical Obstetrics & Gynecology, 32,* 41–47.
22. Wilson, P. D., Loffredo, C. A., Correa-Villasenor, A., & Ferencz, C. (1998). Attributable fraction for cardiac malformations. *American Journal of Epidemiology, 148,* 414–423.
23. Jenkins, K. J., Correa, A., Feinstein, J. A., Botto, L., Britt, A. E., Daniels, S. R., et al. American Heart Association Council on Cardiovascular Disease in the Young. (2007). Noninherited risk factors and congenital cardiovascular defects: Current knowledge. American Heart Association Scientific Statement. *Circulation, 115,* 2995–3014.
24. Warnes, C. A., & Elkayam, U. (1998). In U. Elkayam & N. Gleicher (Eds.), *Cardiac problems in pregnancy* (3rd ed., pp. 39–53). New York: Wiley-Liss, Inc..
25. Clark, S. L. (1991). Structural cardiac disease in pregnancy. In S. L. Clark, G. D. V. Hankins, D. B. Cotton, & J. P. Phelan (Eds.). *Critical care obstetrics* (2nd ed.). Boston: Blackwell Science.

26. Hibbard, L. T. (1975). Maternal mortality due to cardiac disease. *Clinical Obstetrics & Gynecology, 18,* 27–36.

27. Bashore, T. M. (2007). Adult congenital heart disease: Right ventricular outflow tract lesions. *Circulation, 115,* 1933–1947.

28. Murphy, J. G., Gersh, B. J., Mair, D. D., Fuster, V., McGoon, M. D., Ilstrup, D. M., et al. (1993). Long-term outcome in patients undergoing surgical repair of tetralogy of Fallot. *The New England Journal of Medicine, 329,* 593–599.

29. Williams, R. G., Pearson, G. D., Barst, R. J., Child, J. S., del Nido, P., Gersony, W. M., et al. National Heart, Lung, and Blood Institute Working Group on research in adult congenital heart disease. (2006). Report of the National Heart, Lung, and Blood Institute Working Group on research in adult congenital heart disease. *Journal of the American College of Cardiology, 47,* 701–707.

30. Meijer, J. M., Pieper, P. G., Drenthen, W., Voors, A. A., Roos-Hesselink, J. W., van Dijk, A. P., et al. (2005). Pregnancy, fertility, and recurrence risk in corrected tetralogy of Fallot. *Heart, 91,* 801–805.

31. Mendelson, C. L. (1940). Pregnancy and coarctation of the aorta. *American Journal of Obstetrics & Gynecology, 39,* 1014–1021.

32. Mendelson, C. L. (1960). Cardiac disease in pregnancy: Medical care, cardiovascular surgery and obstetric management as related to maternal and fetal welfare. In C. E. Heaton (Ed.), *Obstetrics and gynecology monographs* (pp. 124–132). Philadelphia: Davis.

33. Deal, K., & Wooley, C. F. (1973). Coarctation of the aorta and pregnancy. *Annals of Internal Medicine, 78,* 706–710.

34. Beauchesne, L. M., Connolly, H. M., Ammash, N. M., & Warnes, C. A. (2001). Coarctation of the aorta: Outcome of pregnancy. *Journal of the American College of Cardiology, 38,* 1728–1733.

35. Vriend, J. W., Drenthen, W., Pieper, P. G., Roos-Hesselink, J. W., Zwinderman, A. H., van Veldhuisen D. J., et al. (2005). Outcome of pregnancy in patients after repair of aortic coarctation. *European Heart Journal, 26,* 2173–2178.

36. Weiss, B. M., & Hess, O. M. (2000). Pulmonary vascular disease and pregnancy: Current controversies, management strategies, and perspectives. *European Heart Journal, 21*(2), 104–115.

37. Weiss, B. M., Zemp, L., Seifert, B., & Hess, O. M. (1998). Outcome of pulmonary vascular disease in pregnancy: A systematic overview from 1978 through 1996. *Journal of the American College of Cardiology, 31*(7), 1650–1657.

38. Gleicher, N., Midwall, J., Hochberger, D., & Jaffin, H. (1979). Eisenmenger's syndrome and pregnancy. *Obstetrics & Gynecology, 34,* 721–741.

39. Saha, A., Balakrishnan, K. G., Jaiswal, P. K., Venkitachalam, C. G, Tharakan, J., Titus, T., et al. (1994). Prognosis for patients with Eisenmenger syndrome of various etiology. *International Journal of Cardiology, 45*(3), 199–207.

40. Smedstad, K. G., Cramb, R., & Morison, D. H. (1994). Pulmonary hypertension and pregnancy: A series of 8 cases. *Canadian Journal of Anaesthesia, 41,* 502–512.

41. Hameed, A., Karaalp, I. S., Tummala, P. P., Wani, O. R., Canetti, M., Akhter, M. W., et al. (2001). The effect of valvular heart disease on maternal and fetal outcome of pregnancy. *Journal of the American College of Cardiology, 37,* 893–899.

42. Silversides, C. K., Colman, J. M., Sermer, M., & Siu, S. C. (2003). Cardiac risk in pregnant women with rheumatic mitral stenosis. *American Journal of Cardiology, 91,* 1382–1385.

43. Kennedy, B. (1995). Mitral stenosis: Implications for critical care nursing. *Journal of Obstetrics, Gynecology, and Neonatal Nursing, 24*(5), 406–412.

44. Elkayam, U., & Bitar, F. (2005). Valvular heart disease and pregnancy part I: Native valves. *Journal of American College of Cardiology, 46*(2), 223–230.

45. Arias, F., & Pineda, J. (1978). Aortic stenosis and pregnancy. *The Journal of Reproductive Medicine, 20,* 229–232.

46. Lao, T. T., Adelman, A. G., Sermer, M., & Colman, J. M. (1993). Balloon valvuloplasty for congenital aortic stenosis in pregnancy. *British Journal of Obstetrics & Gynaecology, 100,* 1141–1142.

47. Siu, S., & Colman, J. M. (2004). Cardiovascular problems and pregnancy: An approach to management. *Cleveland Clinical Journal of Medicine, 71,* 977–985.

48. Demakis, J. G., & Rahimtoola, S. H. (1971). Peripartum cardiomyopathy. *Circulation, 44,* 964–968.

49. Abboud, J., Murad, Y., Chen-Scarabelli, C., Saravolatz, L., & Searabelli, T. M. (2007). Peripartum cardiomyopathy: A comprehensive review. *International Journal of Cardiology, 118*(3), 295–303.

50. Sliwa, K., Fett, J., & Elkayam, U. (2006). Peripartum cardiomyopathy. *Lancet, 368,* 687–693.

51. Elkayam, U., Tummala, P. P., Rao, K., Akhter, M. W., Karaalp, I. S., Wani, O. R., et al. (2001). Maternal and fetal outcomes of subsequent pregnancies in women with peripartum cardiomyopathy. [Erratum appears in *The New England Journal of Medicine,* 2001, August 16; 345(7), 552]. *The New England Journal of Medicine, 344*(21), 1567–1571.

52. Sliwa, K., Skudicky, D., Bergemann, A., Candy, G., Puren, A., & Sareli, P. (2000). Peripartum cardiomyopathy: Analysis of clinical outcome, left ventricular function, plasma levels of cytokines and Fas/APO-1. *Journal of the American College of Cardiology, 35,* 701–705.

53. Felker, G. M., Thompson, R. E., Hare, J. M., Hruban, R. H., Clemetson, D. E., Howard, D. L., et al. (2000). Underlying causes and long-term survival in patients with initially unexplained cardiomyopathy. *The New England Journal of Medicine, 342,* 1077–1084.

54. Pyeritz, R. E. (2000). The Marfan syndrome. *Annual Review of Medicine, 51,* 481–510.

55. Milewicz, D. M., Dietz, H. C., & Miller, D. C. (2005). Treatment of aortic disease in patients with Marfan syndrome. *Circulation, 111,* e150–157.

56. Pyeritz, R. E. (1984). Maternal and fetal complications of pregnancy in the Marfan syndrome. *American Journal of Medicine, 71,* 784–790.

57. Rossiter, J. P., Repke, J. T., Morales, A. J., Murphy, E. A., & Pyeritz, R. E. (1995). A prospective longitudinal evaluation of pregnancy in the Marfan syndrome. *American Journal of Obstetrics Gynecology, 173,* 1599–1606.

58. Lind, J., & Wallenburg, H. C. (2001). The Marfan syndrome and pregnancy: A retrospective study in a Dutch population. *European Journal of Obstetrics & Gynecology and Reproductive Biology, 98,* 28–35.

59. Bonow, R. O., Carabello, B., de Leon, A. C., Edmunds, L. H. Jr., Fedderly, B. J., Freed, M. D., et al. (1998). ACC/AHA guidelines for the management of patients with valvular heart disease. Executive summary. A report of the American College of Cardiology/American Heart Association Task Force on Practice Guidelines (Committee on Management of Patients with Valvular Heart Disease). *The Journal of Heart Valve Disease, 7,* 672–707.

60. Task Force on the Management of Cardiovascular Diseases During Pregnancy of the European Society of Cardiology.

(2003). Expert consensus document on management of cardiovascular diseases during pregnancy. *European Heart Journal, 24,* 761–781.

61. Therrien, J., Gatzoulis, M., Graham, T., Bink-Boelkens, M., Connelly, M., Niwa, K, et al. (2001). Canadian Cardiovascular Society Consensus Conference 2001 update: Recommendations for the management of adults with congenital heart disease–part II. *The Canadian Journal of Cardiology, 17,* 1029–1050.

62. Meijboom, L. J., Vos, F. E., Timmermans, J., Boers, G. H., Zwinderman, A. H., & Mulder, B. J. (2005). Pregnancy and aortic root growth in the Marfan syndrome: A prospective study. *European Heart Journal, 26,* 914–920.

63. Meijboom, L. J., Drenthen, W., Pieper, P. G., Groenink, M., van der Post, J. A., Timmermans, J., et al. ZAHARA investigators (2006). Obstetric complications in Marfan syndrome. *International Journal of Cardiology, 110,* 53–59.

64. Hankins, G. D. V., Wendel, G. D., Leveno, K. J., & Stoneham J. (1985). Myocardial infarction in pregnancy: A review. *Obstetrics & Gynecology, 65,* 139–146.

65. Roth, A., & Elkayam, U. (1996). Acute myocardial infarction associated with pregnancy. *Annals of Internal Medicine, 125*(9), 751–762.

66. James, A. H., Jamison, M. G., Biswas, M. S., Brancazio, L. R., Swamy G. K., Myers E. R. (2006). Acute myocardial infarction in pregnancy: A United States population based study. *Circulation, 133*(12), 1564–1571.

67. Bandui, E., Rangel, A., & Enciso, R. (1996). Acute myocardial infarction during pregnancy and puerperium review. *Angiology, 47*(8), 739–756.

68. Graber, E. A. (1989). When an ob patient has coronary disease. *Contemporary Obstetrics & Gynecology, 6,* 56–62.

69. Shivvers, S. A., Wians, F. H., Keffer, J. H., & Ramin, S. M. (1999). Maternal cardiac troponin I levels during normal labor and delivery. *American Journal of Obstetrics & Gynecology, 180*(1), 122–127.

70. Shade, G. H., Ross, G., Bever, F. N., Uddin, Z., Devireddy, L., & Gardin, J. M. (2002). Troponin I in the diagnosis of acute myocardial infarction in pregnancy, labor and postpartum. *American Journal of Obstetrics & Gynecology, 187*(6), 1719–1720.

71. Nabatian, S., Quinn, P., Brookfield, I., & Lakier, J. (2005). Acute coronary syndrome and preeclampsia. *Obstetrics & Gynecology, 106*(5), 1204–1206.

72. Baird, S. M., & Kennedy, B. (2006). Myocardial infarction in pregnancy. *The Journal of Perinatal & Neonatal Nursing, 20*(4), 311–321.

73. Dwyer, B. K., Taylor, I., Guller, A., Brummel, C., & Lyell, D. J. (2005). Percutaneous transluminal coronary angioplasty and stent placement in pregnancy. *Obstetrics & Gynecology, 106*(5), 1163–1164.

74. Schumacher, B., Belfort, M. A., & Card, R. J. (1997). Successful treatment of acute myocardial infarction during pregnancy with tissue plasminogen activator. *American Journal of Obstetrics & Gynecology, 176*(3), 716–719.

75. Sheikh, A. U., & Harper, M. A. (1993). Myocardial infarction during pregnancy: Management and outcome of two pregnancies. *American Journal of Obstetrics & Gynecology, 169,* 279–284.

76. Dajani, A. S., Taubert, K. A., Wilson, W., Bolger, A. F., Bayer, A., Ferrieri, P., et al. (1997). Prevention of bacterial endocarditis. *JAMA, 277*(22), 1794–1801.

77. American College of Obstetricians and Gynecologists. (2003). ACOG practice bulletin number 47. Prophylactic antibiotics in labor and delivery. *Obstetrics & Gynecology, 102*(4), 875–882.

78. Clark, S. L. (1994). Arrhythmias, artificial valves and anticoagulation in pregnancy. In S. L. Clark (Ed.), *Handbook of critical care obstetrics.* Boston: Blackwell Scientific.

CHAPTER 9

Pulmonary Disorders in Pregnancy

Brian A. Mason and Karen Dorman

Pregnancy causes profound changes in the physiology of respiration such that the physiologic adaptations of pregnancy may cause respiratory sequelae in any pregnant woman. Beyond the normal respiratory changes, there are certain pathologic pulmonary complications which are unique to pregnancy and are explored at length in this chapter. In addition to the pulmonary conditions unique to pregnancy, pregnant women may be subject to the entire host of respiratory complications which occur in the non-pregnant population as well. The pathophysiology and treatment of these conditions can be altered by pregnancy, and a number of these conditions and their treatments are outlined in this chapter.

MATERNAL CARDIOPULMONARY CHANGES IN PREGNANCY

It is impossible to speak of respiratory changes in pregnancy in isolation from the cardiovascular changes. The maternal cardiovascular system undergoes changes to allow it to support the increased oxygen and nutrient delivery demands of the growing fetus. During an average singleton pregnancy, maternal blood volume increases by at least 40 percent.[1,2] While red cell mass rises as well, it increases less than 30 percent above baseline, which causes a 10 percent apparent drop in hematocrit values. This is sometimes referred to as a *physiologic anemia* of pregnancy.[2,3] As a result, the oxygen carrying capacity of an individual milliliter of maternal blood is slightly less than that of her non-pregnant counterpart. Furthermore, as intravascular volume expands, plasma protein density decreases, which leads to a decrease in plasma colloid osmotic pressure (COP).

With the advent of membrane transducer systems developed in the 1960s, measurement of COP became a reality. A number of commercial devices are available for the determination of plasma COP. A schematic of such a device is represented in Figure 9-1. A semipermeable membrane, usually selectively permeable to proteins with 30,000 particle weight, separates two chambers. A sensitive pressure transducer which incorporates a Wheatstone bridge is located in the membrane. The chamber below the membrane is the reference chamber, and that above the membrane is the sample chamber. First, both chambers are filled with isotonic saline and the device is zeroed. In addition, daily (or more frequent) calibration of various COP values is performed through the use of a water manometer connected to the sample chamber or through the use of a standard solution with a known COP value. The sample to be processed is placed in the upper chamber and the solutions equilibrated for a short time. From the reference chamber, saline is drawn across the semipermeable membrane and into the sample chamber. This movement is a result of the presence of the colloid protein molecules. The net movement of fluid results in a negative pressure in the reference chamber. After amplification of the electronic signal, a value for the oncotic pressure of the sample is displayed. Several determinations are then made and the results averaged. A comparison of COP values in non-pregnant and pregnant women is presented in Table 9-1. In addition to measurement via a commercial device, COP may be estimated based on a calculation from an equation. Equations for this calculation are presented in Box 9-1.

Interest in the clinical application of COP resulted in multiple studies which have demonstrated the role of COP in the development of pulmonary edema. The alterations in COP associated with pregnancy greatly increase the patient's risk for pulmonary edema, even at lower intravascular hydrostatic pressures. There is an additional fall in COP in the first 24 hours after delivery, which is likely due to blood loss and mobilization of extravascular fluid. This makes the first 24 hours after parturition potentially hazardous for a woman predisposed to pulmonary edema.

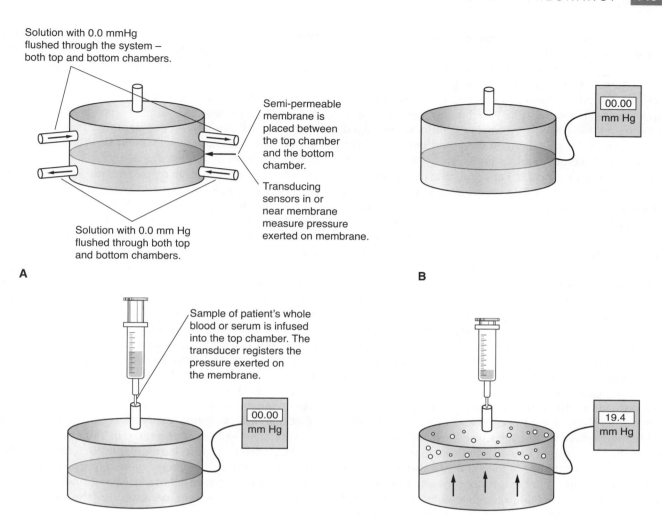

FIGURE 9-1 **A–D.** Schematic of device to directly measure colloid oncotic pressure. (**A**) Most oncometers have two chambers or compartments that are initially flushed with saline or water. Between the two compartments is a semipermeable membrane attached to a pressure manometer. (**B**) When the same solution is placed on each side of the membrane, the pressure is zero. (**C**) Next, a patient's blood or serum (that contains proteins) is injected into one of the chambers. (**D**) The movement of water towards the chamber with the higher concentration of proteins results in a measured pressure in the oncometer. In this illustration the small circles represent proteins in the patient's blood that pull fluid toward the top chamber. The colloid oncotic pressure of the fluid moving into the top chamber in this example is 19.4 mmHg.

TABLE 9-1	
Colloid Osmotic Pressure Values	
Non-pregnant	25.4 ± 2.3 mmHg
Pregnant—antepartum	22.4 ± 0.54 mmHg
Pregnant—postpartum	15.4 ± 2.1 mmHg
Preeclampsia—antepartum	17.9 ± 0.68 mmHg
Preeclampsia—postpartum	13.7 ± 0.46 mmHg

Box 9-1. FORMULAS FOR CALCULATING COLLOID ONCOTIC PRESSURE

These formulae can be used to calculate colloid osmotic pressure (COP) within ± 10%. The top formula has a 75% correlation, and the bottom formula has an 80% correlation/

$$COP = 5.21 \times total\ serum\ protein - 11.4$$
$$COP = 8.1 \times serum\ albumin - 8.2$$

The hemodynamic alterations that occur during pregnancy, specifically the increased intravascular volume, are largely accommodated by an increase in vascular capacitance. This increased capacitance, coupled with an increase in left ventricular compliance, allows the central venous pressure (CVP) and pulmonary capillary wedge pressure (PCWP) to remain essentially unchanged in pregnancy. This leads to an increased left ventricular end-diastolic volume and an increase in stroke volume. The increase in vascular capacitance causes systemic vascular resistance (SVR) to decrease. Despite the fact that the cardiac ejection fraction is essentially unchanged in pregnancy, the increased stroke volume and decreased SVR, in addition to the physiologic increase in heart rate, lead to a significant increase in cardiac output. Cardiac output at rest increases by at least 45 percent by 32 weeks of gestational age.

Oxygen delivery to tissues is determined by cardiac output and arterial oxygen content. In pregnancy, despite a slight decrease in oxygen-carrying capacity related to hemodilution, arterial oxygen content actually increases. The net effect of these normal physiologic changes is a significant increase in cardiac output with a consequent increase in oxygen delivery. This is largely accomplished through changes in cardiorespiratory physiology during pregnancy.[3,4] Concepts related to hemodynamic and oxygen transport physiology are described in depth in Chapter 4 of this text.

There are a number of mechanical as well as physiologic alterations in the respiratory system during pregnancy. Although the diaphragm becomes elevated by at least 5 centimeters near term, its excursion does not decrease. Further, there is a 50 percent increase in the average costal angle resulting in an increase in the circumference of the lower chest wall.[5] The net effect of these changes is a slight decrease in total lung capacity. However, vital capacity does not change secondary to intrapulmonary dilation, possibly related to the influence of progesterone and its resultant slight decrease in airway resistance. The intrinsic increase in pulmonic volume leads to a 35 percent increase in tidal volume, which in turn leads to an increase in minute ventilation, despite a minimal increase in respiratory rate (less than 10 percent) late in pregnancy. This large increase in tidal volume, in the face of a relatively fixed or slightly decreased total lung volume, causes the gravida to utilize respiratory reserves. This results in a significant decrease in functional residual capacity (FRC). During normal pregnancy, the 30 percent increase in oxygen consumption related to maternal and fetal metabolic requirements is well balanced with the increase in minute ventilation, cardiac output, and oxygen delivery. However, should oxygen demand increase or respiratory function be compromised, there is extremely limited respiratory reserve in the pregnant woman. There

is an even greater loss of FRC near term when the patient is recumbent. The reduction in FRC results in a loss of the "oxygen reservoir" function of end-expiratory lung volume and causes a much more rapid hemoglobin desaturation during periods of respiratory compromise. This makes maintaining oxygenation during endotracheal intubation considerably more difficult in the pregnant woman, especially in the supine position and at advanced fetal gestational age.

There are dramatic changes in minute ventilation and respiratory drive in pregnancy. Central respiratory drive is increased as early as 13 weeks gestation and continues to increase until approximately 37 weeks gestation. It does not fully return to normal until approximately 4 months postpartum. These changes in respiratory drive are believed to be related to increased sensitivity of the respiratory center to the partial pressure of carbon dioxide (CO_2) in the blood or because of the direct respiratory stimulation effect of progesterone.[6,7] Minute ventilation increases so dramatically that a respiratory alkalemia develops, despite the increased CO_2 production in pregnancy. The respiratory alkalemia is partially compensated by renal bicarbonate wasting; therefore, a normal arterial blood gas in a pregnant woman reflects a partially compensated respiratory alkalemia. A comparison of normal arterial blood gases during pregnancy and in non-pregnant women is presented in Table 9-2.

As a result of these cardiorespiratory changes, the pregnant woman has very limited cardiopulmonary reserve. It is therefore relatively easy for her to demonstrate pulmonary decompensation in the presence of any respiratory compromise.

Although the etiologies of various pulmonary disorders differ, the clinical signs and symptoms of pulmonary compromise are similar. Thus, it is extremely important for the care provider to understand potential etiologies and predisposing factors of these complications in order to facilitate correct diagnosis and treatment modalities. Early detection and resolution of the disease process is important for optimizing maternal and fetal outcomes.

TABLE 9-2

Arterial Blood Gas Values During Pregnancy

Value	Pregnant	Not Pregnant
pH	7.40–7.45	7.35–7.45
PaO$_2$	104–108	90–100
PaCO$_2$	27–32	35–45
HCO$_3$	18–22	22–26

Note: PaO$_2$ decreases approximately 3.12% or 7.5 mmHg for every 1,000 feet above sea level.

PHYSIOLOGIC PULMONARY COMPLICATIONS

Dyspnea of Pregnancy

Dyspnea, synonymous with shortness of breath or air hunger, is a common feature of normal pregnancy affecting up to 70 percent of gravidas. Patients may experience dyspnea as early as the first trimester, although symptoms typically peak between 28 and 32 weeks of gestation. This occurs independent of exertion and may occur spontaneously at rest. As common as this finding is, its etiology is not fully understood. It does not correlate well to increasing abdominal girth, as has been previously suggested. However, some studies have demonstrated that women who have a higher baseline pre-pregnancy arterial partial pressure of carbon dioxide ($PaCO_2$) have a higher tendency toward dyspnea. In addition, there appears to be a correlation between falling $PaCO_2$ in pregnancy and symptoms of shortness of breath or air hunger. This is likely a manifestation of rising levels of progesterone on oxygen chemoreceptors in the carotid body which increase the physiologic set point of oxygen tension.

In a pregnant woman who presents with a chief complaint of shortness of breath or air hunger, absent any identified history or evidence of a concomitant cardiac or respiratory complication, and in the presence of an arterial oxygen saturation (SaO_2) of 95 percent or greater via pulse oximetry on room air or a normal arterial PaO_2 for pregnancy, it is reasonable to reassure her that this may be a normal effect of pregnancy. It represents a normal physiologic adaptation to increased partial oxygen tension, thus increasing the O_2 diffusion gradient. This facilitates oxygenation of the developing fetus. If no adverse change in maternal or fetal status is evident, no additional evaluation or treatment is necessary.[8,9] It may be difficult, however, to differentiate benign dyspnea of pregnancy from other pathologic causes of shortness of breath or air hunger. Pulmonary edema, pulmonary embolism, cardiomyopathy, and even asthma may present similarly. As always, proper evaluation begins with a meticulous history and physical examination. The inherent need for effective collaboration between health care providers cannot be overemphasized.

Special attention should be paid to ascertaining if there is a history of asthma or other chronic airway disease as well as preexisting cardiac disease. These chronic conditions may be exacerbated by the increased cardiorespiratory work of pregnancy. A sudden onset of shortness of breath or air hunger with or without chest pain might suggest the possibility of pulmonary embolism as a cause for the adverse symptoms. Wheezing and coughing, especially with a history suggestive of a restrictive airways disease such as asthma, would make this a likely cause. Physical findings such as an abnormal chest X-ray, adventitious breath sounds such as respiratory crackles on auscultation, the presence of a cardiac murmur, tachycardia, elevated jugular venous distention (JVD) with tachypnea, suggest a possible cardiac etiology.

Pulmonary function testing may assist in the confirmation of a diagnosis of asthma because an obstructive pattern will most likely be evident. Echocardiography should be performed if findings from the history and physical examination suggest a potential cardiac etiology. Other adjuncts to facilitate diagnosis include an evaluation of hemoglobin to rule out the presence of anemia. The assessment of SaO_2 with a pulse oximeter at rest and with moderate exertion is an easy non-invasive method to differentiate benign dyspnea from more worrisome pathophysiology. If the patient is able to maintain a SaO_2 of 95 percent or greater with moderate exertion, the probability of major cardiorespiratory compromise is greatly reduced. If the patient is unable to meet this standard or if results are equivocal, the measurement of arterial blood gas values may be helpful but is rarely essential in the initial evaluation.

Radiographic studies such as chest X-ray, spiral computed tomography (CT), ventilation/perfusion (V/Q) scanning, or angiography should not be withheld simply because the patient is pregnant. The relative risk of ionizing radiation is minimal, compared to the potentially life-threatening conditions which these techniques may reveal.[10]

PATHOLOGIC PULMONARY COMPLICATIONS

Pulmonary Edema

Etiology

Pulmonary edema results when the normal homeostasis of fluid between the pulmonary capillaries and alveoli is disrupted. The net effect is an increase in the amount of fluid in the alveoli. A distinction is often made between hydrostatic (cardiogenic) and osmotic (non-cardiogenic) causes of pulmonary edema. The two primary mechanisms for development of pulmonary edema are *increased hydrostatic pressure*, and *increased capillary permeability* caused by endothelial damage or lowered COP. A comparison of these two mechanisms is presented in Table 9-3. Hydrostatic pulmonary edema results when there is a net increase in hydrostatic pressure within the capillary. This is reflected by a high pulmonary capillary wedge pressure (PCWP). Fluid is forced across the semipermeable membrane of the capillary secondary to increased intracapillary hydrostatic

TABLE 9-3

Comparison of Hydrostatic and Nonhydrostatic Pulmonary Edema

	Hydrostatic	*Nonhydrostatic*
Other terms	Cardiogenic	Noncardiogenic Osmotic/oncotic
Etiology	Increased hydrostatic pressure	Increased capillary permeability or low COP
Basis	Net increase in hydrostatic pressure within capillaries	Protein concentrations greater in interstitial space are responsible for the net flux of protein and fluid across the capillary; net decrease in hydrostatic pressure in capillary
PCWP values	High PCWP	Normal or low normal PCWP
Osmotic/oncotic effect	Fluid forced/"pushed" across semipermeable membrane of capillary secondary to increased hydrostatic pressure	Fluid "leaked" out across semipermeable membrane due to increased permeability or "pulled" across membrane secondary to higher protein concentration in interstitial space
Results	Congestive heart failure Decreased cardiac output and decreased oxygen delivery	Net filtration of fluid out of the vessel across the capillary membrane Decreased cardiac output and decreased oxygen delivery
Hemodynamic category	Intravascular: "centrally wet"	Intravascular: "centrally dry"
Treatment	Treatment: reduce PCWP, optimize left ventricular contractility, improve cardiac output	Treatment: resolve/treat condition causing capillary permeability and subsequent osmotic movement of fluid from capillaries

PCWP = pulmonary capillary wedge pressure; COP = colloid osmotic pressure.

pressure. This phenomenon is sometimes referred to as *congestive heart failure*. Osmotic pulmonary edema, also referred to as *noncardiogenic* or *nonhydrostatic* pulmonary edema, results when factors other than elevated intravascular pressure are responsible for the net flux of protein and fluid across the capillary wall into the alveolus. In order to make the diagnosis of osmotic pulmonary edema, hydrostatic contribution must be ruled out. This means there should be no evidence of a cardiac causative factor and that the PCWP should be normal or low for pregnancy.[11] Reasonable efforts should be made to distinguish between these two types of pulmonary edema because treatment may be significantly different, depending on the underlying mechanism. Unfortunately, it is often difficult to distinguish between the two types based strictly on chest X-ray or the presence of clinical signs and symptoms. Compounding this dilemma is the fact that the two may exist concomitantly.

There are a number of physiologic changes in pregnancy that predispose the gravida to the development of pulmonary edema. The progressive increase in blood volume and cardiac output, in combination with other factors such as pain, multiple gestations, etc., may significantly increase cardiac work and lead to a rise in pulmonary arterial pressure (PAP), even though abso-

lute values may remain within the normal limits for pregnancy. The subsequent increase in hydrostatic pressure within the vessel, in the setting of other pregnancy-associated changes, may predispose the pregnant woman to pulmonary edema. As previously described, there is a significant drop in plasma COP in pregnancy secondary to the increase in plasma free water, which decreases the concentration of plasma proteins. This can be seen when serum albumin levels are measured. A progressive decrease is also evident with advancing gestation. Without the pull of plasma COP, there tends to be a net filtration of fluid out of the vessel across the capillary membrane. Although the drop in plasma COP is progressive throughout pregnancy, there is an additional, significant decrease immediately after delivery. This is believed to be attributed in part to normal blood loss that occurs with delivery. This drop in COP may be as much as 20 percent below baseline values. Predisposition alone does not cause pulmonary edema. There are a number of inciting events that may lead to osmotic pulmonary edema in pregnancy. Some of these are naturally occurring and others are iatrogenic.

Up to 3 percent of patients with preeclampsia will develop pulmonary edema at some point during their illness, with roughly 70 percent occurring within the first 72 hours following delivery. This may lead to a maternal mortality rate as high as 10 percent. There are several mechanisms at play in pulmonary edema caused by preeclampsia. The endothelial damage characteristic of severe preeclampsia disrupts the normal endothelial barrier and may lead to a leaky capillary syndrome. The intense vasospasm caused by preeclampsia leads to increased afterload or SVR. Although rare, this in turn may lead to significant diastolic dysfunction with a decrease in myocardial contractility.[12–17] This may add a significant hydrostatic component to pulmonary edema that develops in women with preeclampsia. Furthermore, there is an additional decrease in plasma COP in preeclampsia greater than that in normal pregnancy. This combination of factors can easily increase the risk that the woman with preeclampsia may develop fulminant pulmonary edema. A detailed presentation of hypertensive disorders and associated secondary complications during pregnancy is presented in Chapter 7 of this text.

Tocolysis has also been cited as a possible cause of pulmonary edema. The practice of volume loading patients as the first-line treatment of preterm uterine contractions is of dubious benefit, yet is widely practiced. In addition, tocolytic agents such as magnesium sulfate and beta-andrenergic agents such as terbutaline are also associated with an increased risk of pulmonary edema. The major side effects of the beta-sympathomimetic tocolytic agents fall into two broad categories:

- metabolic—including glucose, sodium, potassium, and water homeostasis
- cardiopulmonary—including cardiac arrhythmias, pulmonary edema, and myocardial ischemia.

Increased myocardial work related to the beta-agonist–induced increase in cardiac output may also lead to myocardial depression and a resultant hydrostatic component to pulmonary edema. These effects are generally not seen when beta-agonists are used in non-pregnant individuals.[18–25] A detailed presentation of pharmacologic agents used in the care of pregnant women with complications or critical illness is found in Chapter 6 of this text.

Aspiration syndrome and aspiration pneumonia are both of great concern in pregnancy and may cause pulmonary edema. There is significantly decreased lower esophageal sphincter pressure in pregnant women as well as delayed gastric emptying. Chemical pneumonitis and bacterial pneumonias may ensue and result in significant endothelial damage and disruption of normal lung water homeostasis resulting in pulmonary edema. Maternal hemorrhage, especially when associated with a need for massive red blood cell transfusion, may lead to pulmonary edema through a variety of mechanisms.

Colloid osmotic pressure is decreased by replacement of whole blood loss with packed red blood cells and crystalloids, which lack the osmotically active proteins present in normal serum. There is also a tendency to exceed actual volume deficit with resultant volume overload and increased hydrostatic pressure. In addition, there is a systemic inflammatory response to massive hemorrhage which may be associated with endothelial damage, making the lung more permeable to the influx of fluid from the capillary. This may lead to an osmotic pulmonary edema. Transfusion-related acute lung injury (TRALI), thought to be caused by a reaction to leukocyte antibodies present in the plasma of blood products, causes fluid to rapidly leak into the lungs, producing acute pulmonary edema. It has become the number one cause of transfusion reaction mortality, and is further discussed in Chapter 15. Rare but potentially catastrophic causes of pulmonary edema include amniotic fluid embolism, also referred to as anaphylactoid syndrome of pregnancy, as well as sepsis. Detailed discussions of these complications are found in Chapters 19 and 18, respectively. Acute lung injury or pneumonia may progress to acute respiratory distress syndrome. In addition, bacterial infections outside the lung which are systemic may lead to pulmonary edema. There is a strong increased tendency for development of sepsis-related pulmonary edema in pregnant women, which is most likely related to an increased sensitivity of pregnant women to endotoxins as well as altered capillary permeability and the natural decrease in plasma COP. This is often seen in cases of pyelonephritis in which up to 10 percent of pregnant women subsequently develop pulmonary edema.[26–30]

Clinical Signs and Symptoms

The initial signs and symptoms of pulmonary edema may be very subtle. Frequently, the diagnosis of pulmonary edema is delayed because of the tendency of pregnant women to maintain cardiorespiratory stability better than the average non-pregnant patient with pulmonary edema. This is secondary to their relative youth and overall good health. This often will cause the health care provider to attribute clinical signs and symptoms of pulmonary edema to less significant causes such as dyspnea of pregnancy, asthma, or lower respiratory tract infections. An important presenting symptom is dyspnea, especially if it is associated with a degree of anxiety or tachypnea. As the alveoli progressively fill with fluid, the patient will display the classic signs of a cough, wheeze, or diffuse crackles upon auscultation of the lungs. However, early in the course of the process, chest auscultation may reveal clear breath sounds. Although pregnant women have an elevated resting heart rate, a pulse greater than 100 beats per minute (tachycardia) is a common symptom associated with pulmonary edema.

Non-invasive assessment of oxygen saturation via pulse oximetry is increasingly available in obstetric units. This is an extremely useful adjunct to diagnosis and treatment, but acquired data should be interpreted with caution. In normal pregnancy, SaO_2 ranges from 98 to 100 percent saturation. A SaO_2 of 90 percent reflects a PaO_2 of 60 mmHg. A PaO_2 of 70 mmHg is consistent with early ventilatory failure in a pregnant woman. Should it be necessary to obtain arterial blood gases in a patient with pulmonary edema, these will generally reflect a decreased PaO_2 as well as $PaCO_2$ secondary to initial hyperventilation. However, as the pulmonary edema progresses, $PaCO_2$ increases as the patient is no longer able to maintain adequate minute ventilation. PaO_2 will also continue to decrease. A $PaCO_2$ greater than 40 mmHg in a pregnant woman is strongly suggestive of ventilatory insufficiency and indicative of impending respiratory failure.

The chest X-ray is another important adjunct to the diagnosis of pulmonary edema in pregnant women and should not be withheld because of concerns of radiation exposure to the mother or fetus. The amount of radiation used in a standard posterior to anterior projection chest X-ray is well below levels considered safe in pregnancy. Unfortunately, chest X-ray findings in pulmonary edema often lag behind the onset of clinical symptoms. It may take hours from the onset of symptoms before pulmonary infiltrates, pleural effusions, and other typical findings are visualized on a radiograph.

In all suspected cases of pulmonary edema, a complete blood count with differential and platelets should be obtained, in order to rule out anemia or systemic infection as a possible underlying cause. In addition, if preeclampsia is suspected, laboratory studies to rule out HELLP syndrome (hemolysis, elevated liver enzymes, and low platelets) and distinguish the hypertension of preeclampsia from chronic hypertension should be conducted. This includes analysis of uric acid, urinalysis for protein, aspartate aminotransferase analysis, and complete blood count.

Clinical Management

Treatment for pulmonary edema in pregnancy should be initiated promptly, even if the underlying etiology has not yet been determined. Certain principles apply in treating this condition in pregnancy regardless of the underlying cause. The first goal is to maintain adequate maternal oxygenation with a PaO_2 of 70 mmHg or greater. This may be reasonably approximated by keeping the maternal SaO_2 above 95 percent. This is initially accomplished by maternal positioning in an upright posture with lateral uterine displacement as well as the addition of supplemental oxygen as needed. Next, provided there is no contraindication, intravenous morphine sulfate is generally safe and effective in improving patient comfort,

decreasing maternal anxiety, and decreasing pulmonary congestion by relaxing pulmonary vasculature. Fluid volume should be carefully monitored and recorded using intake and output balance sheets. Most pregnant women with pulmonary edema are not intravascularly volume overloaded; however, administration of low-dose diuretics (e.g.,10 mg of intravenous furosemide) should lower the PCWP and decrease the hydrostatic component of pulmonary edema. Furosemide may be safely administered, provided a normal blood pressure is maintained, in most patients with pulmonary edema regardless of the underlying etiology. Caution should be employed if cardiac lesions such as mitral stenosis, aortic stenosis, and/or idiopathic hypertrophic subaortic stenosis (IHSS) exist with the pulmonary edema. Judicious use of diuretics in pregnant women is highly advisable, since aggressive diuresis of these patients, in the absence of invasive hemodynamic confirmatory data, can lead to significant intravascular hypovolemia, impaired placental perfusion, and fetal compromise. This is especially true of the patient with preeclampsia who, in spite of having extensive peripheral edema and an elevated total body water, may be intravascularly contracted. Pregnant women without underlying renal disease and who have not been exposed to loop diuretics may be extremely sensitive to these agents and may have a brisk response to even small amounts of furosemide.[31–33]

Once these initial measures have been implemented, a review of the differential diagnosis of pulmonary edema and the search for its underlying cause should be undertaken to further direct therapy. In addition, other causes of respiratory failure should be ruled out. For example, unknown valvular heart disease, peripartum cardiomyopathy, or in rare instances ischemic heart disease may all present in a similar fashion to osmotic pulmonary edema. In addition to history and physical examination, including auscultation of heart sounds, an electrocardiogram should be performed. As many as half of all pregnant women with pulmonary edema have an unsuspected cardiac abnormality, and, for this reason, echocardiography may be routinely performed in any pregnant woman presenting with pulmonary edema. If there is any question as to the underlying cause of pulmonary edema in the gravida, such readily available and non-invasive testing should be performed.

Acute cocaine intoxication can lead to cocaine-associated pulmonary edema and should be suspected in a patient presenting with pulmonary edema and severe hypertension. Likewise, heroin intoxication may also lead to pulmonary edema. Both these etiologies can be ruled out through evaluation of a drug screen. Even prescription medications such as nitrofurantoin may lead to an acute pulmonary reaction and respiratory failure. This underscores the need for a careful drug history in any patient with pulmonary edema. History and physical examination should help to differentiate a possible acute pneumonia from pulmonary edema. Patients who present with a history of chills and rigors or who are found to have fever and purulent sputum in addition to pulmonary edema likely suffer from infectious pneumonia. In these patients, in addition to the initial therapies for pulmonary edema, empiric antibiotic therapy should be initiated.

Once the underlying etiology of pulmonary edema is identified, further therapy should be initiated. For example, if preeclampsia is present, delivery of the fetus may be considered. Afterload should be reduced to optimize cardiac output with blood pressure maintained at or below 160/100 mmHg with a vasodilating antihypertensive agent (e.g., hydralazine). Unfortunately, seizure prophylaxis with magnesium sulfate (MgSO$_4$) may exacerbate pulmonary edema secondary to the tendency of MgSO$_4$ to lower COP and because of the high volume of fluid often administered with the medication. For this reason MgSO$_4$ should be concentrated as much as possible with careful attention to limiting extraneous intravenous fluid administration. As with all cases of pulmonary edema, close attention to fluid balance should be observed, particularly at the time of labor and delivery and in the immediate postpartum period.

If pulmonary edema is believed to be related to tocolytic agents, then these should be discontinued even if the patient is at an unfavorably early gestation and is having preterm contractions. Tocolytics are of limited proven efficacy for long-term prolongation of pregnancy and should not be continued when there is a clear contraindication to them on the basis of a potentially dangerous side effect. Additionally, hypoxemia can severely exacerbate uterine contractility, and proper oxygenation is essential to uterine quiescence. Finally, fetal status is dependent upon maternal status; therefore, every effort should be made to appropriately treat the mother.

If the pulmonary edema appears to be related to an infectious cause, then the site of infection should be discerned. Abdominal pain and tenderness may suggest intra-abdominal infection such as appendicitis. Uterine tenderness and contractions may indicate chorioamnionitis or endometritis. Pyelonephritis is particularly important to rule out and should be evaluated by assessing for flank tenderness with percussion and performing a urinalysis and urine culture. If pneumonia is suspected, initial empiric treatment with broad-spectrum antibiotics is advisable. Antibiotic regimens may be adjusted and tailored to individual organisms identified. If a source is not immediately found and sepsis is suspected, empiric treatment with broad-spectrum antibiotics should be initiated.

If pulmonary embolism is suspected, anticoagulation should be begun as soon as possible. The basic treatment for pulmonary edema should also be implemented as the patient is anticoagulated and the diagnosis of embolism should be confirmed with ventilation perfusion studies or CT studies.

Pleural Effusion

Pleural effusion may complicate 45 to 65 percent of normal pregnancies.[34] Physiologic pleural effusions of this type are generally asymptomatic and small, and are generally discovered as an incidental finding. Most occur within 24 hours of delivery. The increased blood volume and decreased COP of pregnancy may contribute to the development of a pleural effusion. In addition, the increased systemic venous pressure, related to Valsalva maneuvers during the second stage of labor, impairs lymphatic drainage and may further contribute to the development of a pleural effusion. While most are benign, a variety of pathologic conditions may also be associated with this finding. The presence of a pleural effusion, particularly a large effusion or one which is symptomatic, should alert the health care provider to the possibility of another underlying pathology such as preeclampsia, profound pulmonary edema, pulmonary embolism, or amniotic fluid embolism.[35]

Pulmonary Embolism

Pulmonary embolism remains a leading cause of maternal mortality and accounts for 20 percent of pregnancy-related deaths.[36–44] It usually results from deep venous thrombosis (DVT), occurs most often in the postpartum period, and has an incidence of approximately 40 per 100,000 pregnancies. Venous thromboembolism (VTE) during pregnancy is discussed at length in Chapter 17 of this text.

Unfortunately, physiologic changes associated with pregnancy may obscure the diagnosis of VTE during pregnancy. For example, air hunger may be misattributed to the benign physiologic dyspnea of pregnancy. The prompt diagnosis of VTE may be further inhibited by the reluctance of patients and practitioners to utilize appropriate diagnostic techniques which involve ionizing radiation such as ventilation perfusion scanning, chest X-ray, or spiral CT.

Pulmonary Hypertension

Four to eight percent of all cases of primary pulmonary hypertension are associated with pregnancy.[45] Primary pulmonary hypertension may occur in pregnancy in the absence of any other identifiable cause. Pulmonary hypertension increases hydrostatic pressure within the vessels of the lungs and leads to an increased risk of pulmonary edema. The underlying mechanism for the increased incidence of pulmonary hypertension in pregnancy remains unknown. Although it is a relatively rare cause of pulmonary edema in pregnancy, it should be kept in the differential diagnosis when other causes have been ruled out. Pulmonary hypertension is discussed at length in Chapter 8 of this text.

Pneumothorax and Pneumomediastinum

Pneumothorax or pneumomediastinum may occur spontaneously during pregnancy.[46] The most common cause of these in pregnancy is repeated, deep Valsalva maneuvers, but they may occur in the absence of such stimuli. Such cases of spontaneous pneumothorax are likely related to underlying maternal disease which has been previously undiagnosed, such as pleural blebs. Pneumomediastinum is considerably less common in pregnancy than pneumothorax and usually occurs following delivery. Both pneumothorax and pneumomediastinum may be incidental findings on a chest X-ray obtained for other indications. In these cases, expectant management is the preferred treatment. However, if a patient is symptomatic, especially in the presence of a tension pneumothorax, then conventional decompression measures with a chest tube or thoracic vent are indicated. Pneumothorax and pneumomediastinum are potential complications of positive-pressure ventilation, especially in cases of decreased lung compliance such as adult respiratory distress syndrome (ARDS) or severe pulmonary edema. This is likely related to high pressures required to adequately ventilate the non-compliant lung. Concepts related to mechanical ventilation during pregnancy are presented in Chapter 5 of this text.

Amniotic Fluid Embolism

A potentially catastrophic complication involving cardiopulmonary collapse in the pregnant woman is amniotic fluid embolism (AFE), also known as anaphylactoid syndrome of pregnancy. It has been reported to affect as many as 1 in 8,000 pregnancies but carries a mortality rate of up to 60 percent.[47–52] Therefore, although rare, it may be responsible for nearly 10 percent of the maternal deaths in the United States. A patient with AFE may present with a sudden onset of agitation and dyspnea, followed by symptomatic hypoxia, hypotension, and later disseminated intravascular coagulation (DIC) which may lead to massive obstetric hemorrhage. Other symptoms include seizures, fetal bradycardia, and cardiac arrest or severe dysrhythmia. The definitive diagnosis of AFE is difficult to make prospectively. However, it should be considered in any gravida, particularly one who is near term and in labor and presents with a

sudden onset of cardiorespiratory failure. A thorough discussion of AFE is presented in Chapter 19 of this text.

Aspiration Pneumonitis

Aspiration pneumonitis is not exclusive to pregnancy; however, it continues to be a major cause of maternal morbidity secondary to unique physiologic changes in pregnancy. There is a significant decrease in the tone of the lower esophageal sphincter related to the effect of progesterone as well as increased abdominal pressure caused by the gravid uterus. Furthermore, there is a significant delay in gastric emptying secondary to smooth muscle relaxation, which causes increased bowel transit time. In addition to these intrinsic changes, certain clinical practices implemented during labor and delivery, such as placing patients in a supine position for delivery, may contribute to the risk of aspiration. Consequently nearly two-thirds of cases of aspiration in pregnant women occur around the time of delivery. Unfortunately, the trachea can be difficult to intubate in a pregnant woman.[53,54] Failed intubation in a laboring patient has been estimated to occur at a rate eight times that of the general population. When highly acidic gastric contents (pH below 2.5) are aspirated into the airway, a severe chemical pneumonitis can result. This can lead to enhanced capillary permeability with an osmotic-type pulmonary edema, which can further lead to ARDS. In order to reduce this risk, patients may be discouraged from eating during labor and elective surgery may be delayed for 8 hours after oral intake.[55] When this is not possible, a regimen of metoclopramide, a non-particulate oral antacid such as sodium citrate, and an intravenous histamine-2 blocker may be administered. This is designed to facilitate gastric emptying and decrease the acidity of the gastric contents. In addition, the airway should be carefully assessed prior to the procedure and appropriate adjuncts to intubation made available.

NON-PREGNANCY–INDUCED PULMONARY COMPLICATIONS IN PREGNANCY

Asthma

Asthma is an increasingly common chronic pulmonary complication in reproductive age patients. Optimal control of asthma requires a combination of intensive patient education as well as a rational stepwise approach to pharmacotherapy. Fortunately, these management strategies do not differ significantly in the asthmatic pregnant population from non-pregnant individuals. These guidelines have been codified in publications from the National Institutes of Health (NIH).[56,57] Patient education related to asthma and pharmacotherapy is best optimized prior to pregnancy; however, patients should be educated and therapy optimized whenever the patient first presents for medical care, even if this occurs in the intrapartum period. Most pharmacologic agents and their doses are identical to what would be used in non-pregnant individuals.[58-60]

Currently, asthma is believed to be a chronic inflammatory airway disease with episodes of acute exacerbation. Treatment should focus on the avoidance of "triggers" and the use of agents that decrease underlying airway inflammation such as inhaled corticosteroids. All too often bronchodilators are used by patients as a cornerstone of asthma management; however, these agents should be viewed primarily as rescue medications that provide acute symptomatic relief rather than as agents of chronic control. Systemic side effects in the mother as well as hypothetical adverse effects on the fetus may be reduced by relying primarily on inhaled rather than oral or parenteral agents.[61] Patients should be educated regarding the proper use of inhalers including the use of spacers, which optimize delivery of the medication to the lung, minimize systemic absorption through the oral mucosa, and minimize systemic as well as local side effects such as oral thrush from inhaled steroids. In addition, patients should be educated about the use of specialized pillows and mattress covers which minimize the inhalation of dust mites. The patient should also avoid smoke, especially from cigarettes, and should be advised to remove carpeting and pets from the home if feasible, or at least from the area in which she sleeps. In order to track pulmonary performance and detect asthma exacerbations in their nascent phase when they are easiest to treat, the patient needs to measure peak expiratory flow rates (PEFR) in the morning and approximately 12 hours later.[62] Inexpensive hand-held meters are readily available, and no pregnant asthmatic should be without one. Patients obtain a baseline of best PEFR and clinical management responses based on changes in this "personal best." Benign conditions such as dyspnea of pregnancy will not significantly affect PEFR; however, if the patient experiences a 20 percent or greater drop from her personal best, then initiation of a medication and/or dose adjustment is warranted. Furthermore, if PEFR drops by more than 50 percent from the patient's personal best, then immediate therapy in an emergent care center should be sought. More elaborate pulmonary function testing is rarely needed in patients with an established diagnosis of asthma.

Patients may be fearful of the effect of asthma medications on pregnancy outcome, but should be reassured that, while poorly controlled asthma greatly increases pregnancy risk, well-controlled asthma does not appear to affect pregnancy adversely. They should be strongly encouraged not to discontinue necessary medications simply because they are pregnant.[63,64]

Pharmacologic Management of Asthma

Contemporary practice calls for the administration of asthma pharmacotherapy in a "step-wise" manner. Incremental increases or decreases in dose or the addition of agents are made based on the patient's asthma symptoms at any given time. For clinical convenience, asthma has been divided into four separate severity classifications and treatment determined dependent on the patient's classification. This approach has been widely endorsed.[65-69] When asthma symptoms worsen or are poorly controlled, treatment is stepped up to the next level. When control is maintained for at least 1 month, a step down in therapy to the next lower regimen level may be considered. Regardless of classification, occasional acute exacerbations may occur, often secondary to viral rhinitis. In these cases a short rescue course of oral prednisone (7 to 10 days) may be used to regain control regardless of the patient's asthma classification. For patients in whom control is especially difficult to achieve, other factors such as unrecognized environmental triggers, patient non-compliance with medication, chronic post-nasal discharge, and even gastroesophageal reflux disease should be considered.

Pharmacologic agents used to treat asthma in pregnancy fall into two principle categories: maintenance agents and rescue agents. Maintenance agents are those used to reduce the reactivity of the airway and target the underlying inflammation that leads to bronchospasm. The most commonly used agents in this category are the inhaled steroids; however, systemic steroids, mast cell stabilizers, methylxanthines, leukotriene antagonists, and desensitizing agents may all be used in pregnancy. Rescue agents by contrast are used to provide immediate symptomatic relief by reducing acute bronchospasm. Agents in this class include the inhaled beta agonists and inhaled anticholinergics. It is important to emphasize that these medications do not address the underlying inflammation that ultimately leads to bronchospasm and should not be relied upon as monotherapy for patients with ongoing asthma symptoms.[70-77]

Maintenance Medications

Mast Cell Stabilizers. These inhaled agents (e.g., cromolyn) decrease mast cell degranulation. These agents are poorly absorbed and are considered non-teratogenic. They may be used in mild cases of asthma that do not require administration of an inhaled steroid.

Inhaled Corticosteroids. These agents (e.g., beclomethasone) are well studied and widely prescribed in pregnancy. There has been no observed teratogenic effect from these agents related in part to the fact that only a minimal amount of corticosteroid is absorbed when administered by inhalation. In addition to being considered safe, they are also effective at minimizing acute attacks of asthma during pregnancy, with a greater than four-fold reduction in the incidence of acute attacks when compared with controls who did not receive these agents.

Systemic Corticosteroids. These agents (e.g., hydrocortisone or methylprednisolone) and oral prednisone are often used in more severe cases of asthma. Apart from beclomethasone and dexamethasone, these agents tend not to cross the placenta at doses less than the equivalent of 25 milligrams per day (mg/day) of prednisone. This is related to rapid placental metabolism.[78] While these agents are considered generally non-teratogenic, at least one case-control study found a significant association with first trimester exposure and oral clefts in the fetus.[79] Even if this effect proves to be causal, the use of these agents, even in the first trimester, may be justified given the life-threatening nature of the disease which they are being used to treat.

Long-Acting Methylxanthines. These agents (e.g., theophylline) were used extensively in pregnant women in the past. They were largely replaced by the inhaled corticosteroids under the erroneous belief that inhaled corticosteroids were safer and more efficacious. While these agents are safe and efficacious, they are generally considered to be second- or third-line agents because of their side effect profile, such as tachycardia, nausea, and challenges with dosing in pregnant women related to variable clearance in pregnancy.[80–83]

Leukotriene Antagonists. These agents (e.g., montelukast), unlike other agents in this category, are generally avoided in pregnancy. This is largely related to the lack of safety data in human pregnancy. As a result, these agents are generally limited to those cases in which a patient had significant improvement in asthma control that was not achieved with other methods before becoming pregnant. They are rarely added to a regimen during pregnancy.

Desensitization Therapy. Desensitization by giving increasing quantities of an allergen to a patient who is allergic to that allergen, in order to down-regulate the allergic response, is rarely initiated during pregnancy because of fear of provoking an anaphylactic response. However, data from human subjects suggest that continuing desensitization therapy in pregnancy does not present a risk.[74,85,86]

Rescue Agents

Inhaled Beta-Mimetics. These agents (e.g., albuterol) are frequently used as first-line therapy to acutely dilate constricted bronchioles. These agents have been extensively studied in both animals and humans and do not appear to increase the teratogenic risk to the fetus.[87] It must be emphasized that these are for short-term symptomatic relief and should be used in concert with a maintenance agent.

Long-Acting Inhaled Beta Agonists. These agents (e.g., salmeterol) are generally felt to be safe in humans when administered by inhalation; however, animal data using intravenously administered salmeterol have been concerning. This agent is widely used in non-pregnant individuals in combination inhalers with lyophilized corticosteroid powders. It is generally reserved for patients who do not respond to inhaled steroids alone or in combination with cromolyn and inhaled short-acting beta-mimetics.

Inhaled Anticholinergics. These agents (e.g., ipratropium) have been shown to be effective in the treatment of acute asthma exacerbations. Because they are poorly absorbed from the mucosa, teratogenic risk is most likely minimal; however, there are limited published human data on these drugs. Their efficacy, especially in combination with inhaled short-acting beta-mimetics, makes them useful for treating acute asthma exacerbations in an emergency care center. Their anticholinergic effect also limits hypersecretion in patients with bronchitis, pneumonia, and chronic obstructive pulmonary disease.

Agents of Concern

In addition to drugs that should be avoided in the general asthmatic population, such as beta blockers and nonsteroidal anti-inflammatories, there are a number of agents commonly employed in pregnancy which should be used with caution or avoided in the pregnant asthmatic. For example, 15-methyl prostaglandin F_2 alpha should be avoided in asthmatic patients because of its tendency to cause bronchoconstriction. On the other hand, uterotonics (e.g., oxytocin and prostaglandin E_2) may be safely used.[19,88] Likewise, the ergot alkaloids may cause severe bronchospasm, particularly when used in conjunction with general anesthesia, and should be avoided in the pregnant patient with asthma. In clinical practice, opioids such as morphine are used routinely without complications. They may theoretically cause histamine release, which may lead to bronchoconstriction. For this reason, agents without this effect, such as fentanyl or nalbuphine are often substituted when parenteral analgesia is required. Because of its profound cardiovascular effect, subcutaneous epinephrine is generally avoided in pregnancy.

Acute Asthma Exacerbation

In its most fulminant form, acute severe asthma exacerbation, also referred to as status asthmaticus, is a potentially life-threatening complication. It requires urgent medical attention in a health care facility with appropriate resources. Patients usually demonstrate progressive worsening of their asthma prior to status asthmaticus; thus, careful monitoring using the stepwise approach described previously should significantly reduce the incidence of this critical complication.

When a patient has a resting respiratory rate greater than 22 breaths/minute or a resting heart rate greater than 120 beats/minute, particularly if she has had a greater than 40 percent decrease in baseline PEFR, hospital admission should be considered. An arterial blood gas will help confirm the diagnosis and is of concern if the PaO_2 is less than 70 mmHg or the $PaCO_2$ is greater than 35 mmHg on room air. In the gravida, a normal $PaCO_2$ is approximately 30 mmHg; a $PaCO_2$ greater than 40 mmHg (which is considered normal in a general patient population) may signal impending respiratory failure in a pregnant woman.

Secondary to the lack of pulmonary reserve, the pregnant patient with severe acute asthma exacerbation tends to deteriorate very quickly. When the pregnant asthmatic presents to an emergency center with an acute exacerbation, she should immediately receive supplemental oxygen to keep her SaO_2 at 95 percent or above. Oxygen should not be withheld in order to obtain a room air arterial blood gas during an acute exacerbation. Inhaled beta-mimetics should be started immediately, preferably via a nebulizer, and should be repeated every 10 to 20 minutes as symptoms and side effects dictate. Early in the course of treatment, 1 milligram per kilogram (mg/kg) of methylprednisolone should be given intravenously and repeated every 6 hours until significant clinical improvement is noted. At that time, oral prednisone at an equivalent dosage (generally 40 to 60 mg daily) may be substituted. In refractory cases or when bronchial secretions appear to be complicating the situation, ipratropium 62.5 mL may be administered by hand-held nebulizer every 6 hours in addition to an inhaled beta-adrenergic agent. Subcutaneous terbutaline 0.25 mg is sometimes used, but its marginal efficacy and tendency to promote tachycardia limit its utility. Subcutaneous epinephrine on the other hand should be avoided in pregnant women. Delivery of the fetus is rarely indicated in the treatment of acute asthma exacerbations; however, delivery should not be withheld if obstetrically indicated. In addition, the patient may require steroid support of her hypothalamic pituitary adrenal axis if she has been on systemic steroids. The patient may be observed for signs of renal insufficiency such as nausea, vomiting, hypotension, weakness, anorexia, and laboratory anomalies such as hyponatremia and hyperkalemia. However, since these are common findings in normal pregnancy, many clinicians choose to give empiric

stress doses of steroids. One commonly employed regimen calls for administration of 100 mg of hydrocortisone intravenously every 8 hours the day of delivery, followed by 50 mg intravenously every 8 hours on postpartum day 1. On postpartum day 2, the patient is restored to her baseline dose of systemic steroids. Short-course parenteral steroid therapy is generally well tolerated and should be considered in any woman who, in the preceding 12 months, has received a course of steroids for longer than 2 weeks. If the patient requires Cesarean delivery, the optimal anesthesia is a regional block such as an epidural or spinal using a combination of local anesthetic and fentanyl. If the patient requires a general anesthetic or intubation secondary to respiratory failure, a bronchodilator such as the halogenated inhalational agents or ketamine should be used. After resolution of the acute asthma exacerbation, the patient should be maintained on a metered-dose inhaler (MDI) agent equivalent to those she received via nebulizer. In addition, her oral prednisone should be tapered gradually over a period of weeks, and the taper should be held at the last effective dose if the patient shows signs of deterioration as identified by the step therapy guidelines.

Pneumonia

Although relatively uncommon in pregnancy, pneumonia is a leading cause of infectious death in the U.S. Pneumonia remains a leading cause of maternal and fetal morbidity and mortality, with maternal mortality rates as high as 4 percent in some series.[89–91] With an incidence as high as 1 in 3,000 deliveries in a series published in 1992, compared to 1 in 3,800 deliveries in 1988, the incidence of pneumonia may actually be increasing. Some authors have speculated that this may reflect an increasing prevalence of chronic disease and human immunodeficiency virus (HIV), which are major risk factors for pneumonia.[92,93] Other risk factors for development of pneumonia include drug abuse and anemia. Pregnancy itself appears to be an independent risk factor for major complications of pneumonia. Of pregnant women suffering from pneumonia, up to 40 percent may suffer major complications such as empyema, or pneumothorax. In addition to maternal risk, the fetus of an infected mother is also at risk for complications. Growth restriction leading to small for gestational age neonates occurs in approximately 12 percent of cases.[90] Preterm labor may affect up to 40 percent of pregnancies complicated by pneumonia, and intrauterine and neonatal death rates have been reported to be as high as 12 percent.[90–92] In general, the most significant predictor of adverse outcome for the mother and fetus is the underlying disease process.

As is the case with most community-acquired pneumonias, the underlying organism is identified only about

50 percent of the time. It is believed that bacteria lead to most cases of pneumonia in pregnancy, with *Streptococcus pneumoniae* responsible for approximately half of community-acquired pneumonias. The second most common causative organism is *Hemophilus influenzae*. Like other community-acquired pneumonias, *Mycoplasma* and *Chlamydia* may account for a substantial number of cases and should be considered when selecting empiric treatment. Delays in diagnosis or failure to differentiate other potentially life-threatening disease processes place the gravida with suspected pneumonia at increased risk. Clinicians may be reluctant to obtain chest X-rays; however, the hazard to both mother and fetus of delaying the diagnosis is far greater than the small dose (approximately 300 microrads) to the fetus from a standard single view chest X-ray. Likewise, an inappropriate choice of antibiotic or administration of an inadequate dosage for fear of fetal effects can be equally damaging. In general, antibacterial therapy in pregnant patients is similar to the general population. However, quinolones and tetracyclines should generally be avoided. Misdiagnosis can be equally problematic. Pulmonary edema, chemical pneumonitis from aspiration, and life-threatening conditions such as AFE may initially present a clinical picture similar to pneumonia. Pulmonary embolism may cause dyspnea, chest pain, cough, fever, and infiltrates on chest X-rays; it is the leading cause of maternal death in the U.S., and its successful treatment requires an immediate and very different therapy from pneumonia. For this reason, if there is ambiguity in diagnosis, even in a patient with indeterminate physical and radiologic signs, therapy for pulmonary infection as well as pulmonary embolism may be started simultaneously, provided there are no contraindications to either therapy in an individual patient. Effort should be made to further delineate the diagnosis with more definitive tests such as CT angiography. In patients with uncomplicated pneumonia who do not require hospitalization, standard therapy is erythromycin 250 to 500 mg four times daily orally for 10 to 14 days. If the patient does not tolerate erythromycin because of allergy or GI side effects, then azithromycin 500 mg orally on day 1 followed by 250 mg daily for 4 additional days may be substituted. For patients with uncomplicated pneumonia but who require hospitalization, erythromycin is given at a dosage of 500 mg intravenously every 6 hours. In addition, 2 grams of ceftriaxone are given intravenously daily. Again, azithromycin 500 mg IV daily may be substituted if erythromycin is contraindicated or not tolerated by the patient. An alternative to ceftriaxone is cefuroxime, which may be given at a dose of 750 to 1,500 mg IV every 8 hours. When the patient is stable and without fever, intravenous antibiotics may be discontinued and she may be started on oral agents such as a cephalosporin and erythromycin for a total course (including intravenous therapy) of 14 days.

Viral pneumonia is a potentially serious complication of pregnancy. Pregnant women may be uniquely susceptible to viral infection secondary to the reduction in cell-mediated immunity that is associated with pregnancy. The maternal mortality rate from pneumonia was approximately 27 percent during the great influenza pandemic of 1918, and nearly 20 percent of all maternal deaths in Minnesota during the 1957 pandemic were due to complications of influenza.[94,95] The proportion of flu-related deaths in healthy pregnant women, while less than in prior pandemics, was disproportionate (13 percent) during the 2009 pandemic.[96] Although influenza does not cross the placenta and is unlikely to be teratogenic to the fetus, concomitant maternal morbidity may affect the fetus indirectly. Prevention through an active vaccination program is the most desirable means of dealing with this potential threat. However, once infection occurs with either influenza A or B, the neuraminidase inhibitor zanamivir may be given by inhalation, or oseltamivir (Tamiflu) may be given orally. Although both are pregnancy category "C" drugs, zanamivir is considered a drug of choice since the proportion of active drug that reaches the systemic circulation—and therefore the fetus—is much lower than oseltamivir (12 to 17 percent versus 80 percent).[97]

Pneumonia caused by rubeola does not appear to affect the fetus directly; however, spontaneous abortion, perinatal mortality, and preterm labor have been associated with this infection, with obvious adverse fetal consequences.[98] While varicella pneumonia may be dangerous in non-pregnant patients, it can be particularly lethal to the gravida, with a mortality rate as high as 35 percent.[99,100] Furthermore, unlike in most of the other viral pneumonias, the fetus may also be directly affected through the congenital varicella syndrome. While administration of varicella immune globulin to the mother does not completely eliminate the risk of fetal infection, it should be considered in any susceptible pregnant woman who is exposed to varicella within 72 hours of exposure. If varicella pneumonia should become established in the gravida, she should be treated with acyclovir in addition to supportive care.[100]

The corona virus responsible for severe acute respiratory syndrome (SARS) is extremely morbid and appears to be more so in the gravida than in her non-pregnant counterpart, with a mortality rate approaching 30 percent. SARS may progress from pneumonia to ARDS and lead to fetal compromise and intrauterine fetal death. This is most likely the result of profound hypoxia which accompanies this condition.[101,102]

An unfortunate sequela of most of the viral pneumonias is a tendency to develop secondary superinfection with staphylococci or gram-negative bacilli leading to severe bacterial pneumonia.

Fungi such as *Histoplasma* (histoplasmosis) and *Coccidioides* (coccidiomycosis) may cause fungal pneumonia and are endemic in certain regions of the U.S. Fortunately, they are relatively uncommon in pregnancy, although their course seems to be more severe in pregnant women. They also seem more likely to disseminate in the pregnant woman than in non-pregnant patients.[103,104] Coccidiomycosis affects approximately 1 in 5,000 pregnancies in the southwestern U.S. and has a strong tendency to disseminate in the pregnant woman. This unique predilection to disseminate in the gravida may be related to a stimulatory effect on fungal proliferation of progesterone and estrogen as well as a mild impairment of cell-mediated immunity. As a result, up to 50 percent of pregnant women who become infected with coccidiomycosis show dissemination. This is particularly prevalent if the infection was contracted during the second or third trimester. As in the non-pregnant patient, amphotericin B remains the drug of choice in disseminated coccidiomycosis. It poses minimal risk to the fetus and is no more dangerous to the gravida than it is to a non-pregnant patient.[104]

Tuberculosis

Most tuberculosis in pregnancy is pulmonary.[105] As in non-pregnant women, common signs and symptoms include cough, weight loss, fever, malaise, fatigue, and hemoptysis. Unfortunately, normal changes of pregnancy can mask or mimic many of these findings, and up to 20 percent of pregnant women with pulmonary tuberculosis are asymptomatic. Although tuberculosis does not appear to be more common or severe in pregnancy, the risk of maternal–fetal transmission or newborn transmission is a significant concern. Theoretically, the tubercle bacilli may pass from mother to fetus either by hematogenous or lymphogenous spread, transmission through the placenta or through the amniotic membrane or tuberculous endometritis in the pregnant woman. However, it is believed that in utero transmission is quite rare and that the greater risk of the newborn acquiring tuberculosis is after delivery, particularly if the mother is sputum-positive for tuberculosis and is undiagnosed and untreated. It is therefore prudent to screen every pregnant woman with a tuberculin skin test.

In those with a positive tuberculin skin test, active pulmonary disease can be reliably ruled out with a chest X-ray after the twelfth week of gestation.[106] If the patient has symptoms of active pulmonary tuberculosis, however, a shielded chest X-ray may be obtained immediately regardless of gestational age. Serially obtained gastric washings or sputum samples may be obtained and can be useful in confirming the diagnosis. When active pulmonary tuberculosis is diagnosed during pregnancy, immediate combination therapy should begin. This generally includes isoniazid, rifampin, and ethambutol as outlined in the Centers for Disease Control and Prevention's standard treatment regimen.[106] These drugs are considered to have an acceptable safety profile in pregnancy and are part of the standard treatment regimen. In cases where active disease and radiographic findings are absent, standard prophylaxis with isoniazid is recommended. Streptomycin is clearly associated with congenital deafness and is contraindicated during pregnancy. Pyrazinamide is approved for use in pregnancy by the World Health Organization and may be an important additional drug in treating the emerging multidrug-resistant tuberculosis cases.[106] Pharmacotherapy for tuberculosis is not contraindicated in breast-feeding. The diagnosis of tuberculosis is not an indication for routine therapeutic interruption of pregnancy; neither is route and timing of delivery generally affected by the diagnosis. General tuberculosis precautions (such as contact studies, preventive therapy for the infant and other close household contacts, and isolation precautions) apply in the pregnant woman as they do in the general patient population.

Sarcoidosis

Sarcoidosis is a granulomatous condition affecting the lung. Etiology and pathogenesis remain unknown. It is thought that infectious agents may produce the condition in individuals who are genetically predisposed. It is usually seen in reproductive-age women and tends to regress spontaneously, although in some cases it becomes progressive. Many cases of sarcoidosis remain undetected, and over half are detected incidentally on a chest X-ray obtained for other purposes. Sarcoidosis may present much like tuberculosis with cough, dyspnea, chest pain, fatigue, weakness, fever, and weight loss. The classic chest X-ray finding is bilateral hilar adenopathy and interstitital infiltrates. Other organs may be involved, such as the eyes, lymphatic system, liver, skin, kidneys, and joints.[107–109] The normal homeostasis of calcium may also be affected, and hypercalcemia, especially in patients receiving vitamin D supplementation, may lead to nephrolithiasis. Sarcoidosis does not appear to have any adverse effects on the course of pregnancy and in fact pregnancy may, in some cases, lead to improvement in the symptoms of sarcoidosis. This is believed to be related to the natural increase in maternal cortisol during pregnancy.[109] If sarcoidosis is complicated by pulmonary hypertension, the prognosis for pregnancy is extremely poor with a significant risk of maternal mortality. These patients should be carefully counseled and discouraged from proceeding with pregnancy. The fetus by contrast is generally unaffected by sarcoidosis except as it relates to maternal complications. The granulomas of sarcoidosis have not been found in the fetus although they have been noted in the placenta.[110]

In general, patients with sarcoidosis should avoid vitamin D and calcium supplementation, and these should be eliminated from prenatal vitamins. Should the patient become symptomatic, standard therapy includes administration of systemic steroids. Other agents such as chloroquine and cyclosporine should be used only if the benefits clearly exceed the risks. Some therapies for sarcoidosis, such as methotrexate and thalidomide, are strictly contraindicated in pregnancy.[111,112] Unfortunately, many patients, particularly those who have experienced some relief of their symptoms during pregnancy, will have significant exacerbation of their sarcoidosis within 3 to 6 months after delivery.[113]

Cystic Fibrosis

Improvements in cystic fibrosis management have led to increasing numbers of women with cystic fibrosis surviving to reproductive age.[114] Cystic fibrosis can lead to viscous secretions in the lungs, pancreas, liver, intestine, and reproductive tract; but pulmonary disease is the leading cause of morbidity and mortality in these patients. They often present with recurrent pneumonia and chronic bronchitis and develop an obstructive type pulmonary dysfunction.[115] Treatment centers on antibiotic therapy for infection and aerosolized beta agonists to promote bronchodilation, as well as the administration of nebulized endonuclease DNase I. This cleaves long strands of DNA and decreases the viscosity of the sputum. Inhaled corticosteroids are also used in some cases. Patients often require oral supplementation of pancreatic enzymes and these patients are at substantial risk for the development of diabetes mellitus, biliary cirrhosis and cholelithiasis.

Historically, mothers with cystic fibrosis have poor pregnancy outcomes. However, more recent reports suggest that in women with milder disease, pregnancy outcome can be favorable. If pre-pregnancy forced expiratory volume in 1 second (FEV_1) exceeds 60 percent of predicted value, there is no evidence of pulmonary hypertension, the patient has not been colonized by *Burkholderia cepacia,* and her body mass index (BMI) is greater than 19, then she is likely to have a good pregnancy outcome. Additionally the patient should receive genetic counseling regarding the risk of her children being affected by cystic fibrosis.[116-119]

The treatment of the pregnant patient with cystic fibrosis is sufficiently complex to warrant a multidisciplinary approach with pulmonologists, obstetricians, and nutritionists involved in the care. In general, therapy is similar to that in the non-pregnant patient.[120,121] If, despite optimal medical therapy, the patient has a progressive decline in respiratory function, intrauterine growth restriction or decreasing maternal weight, consideration should be given to delivery of the fetus. Care should be taken to limit maternal oxygen requirements as much as possible through the use of appropriate pain control and assisted delivery in the second stage of labor.

SUMMARY

The physiologic alterations associated with pregnancy have a profound effect on each of the major organ systems. These alterations are critical for maintaining homeostasis in the mother as well as providing an adequate environment for the fetus during pregnancy. The respiratory system is one of the most critical to maintain during a healthy pregnancy. It is also a system from which a variety of problems can arise that affects the outcome for the mother and fetus. Clinicians should be aware of the normal alterations in function and be astute regarding abnormal changes and actions required to treat these changes.

REFERENCES

1. Pritchard, J. A., Baldwin, R. M., Dickey, J. C., et al. (1962). Blood volume changes in pregnancy and the puerperium. *American Journal of Obstetrics and Gynecology, 84,* 1271–1281.
2. Silver, H. M., Seebeck, M., & Carlson, R. (1998). Comparison of total blood volume in normal, preeclamptic and nonproteinuric gestational hypertensive pregnancy by simultaneous measurement of red blood cell and plasma volumes. *American Journal of Obstetrics and Gynecology, 179,* 87–93.
3. Crapo, R. O. (1996). Normal cardiopulmonary physiology during pregnancy. *Clinical Obstetrics and Gynecology, 39,* 3–16.
4. Clark, S. L., Cotton, D. B., Lee, W., Bishop, C., Hill, T., Southwick, J. (1989). Central hemodynamic assessment of normal term pregnancy. *American Journal of Obstetrics and Gynecology, 161,* 1439–1442.
5. Weinberger, S. E., Weiss, S. T., Cohen, W. R., Weiss, J. W., & Johnson, T. S. (1980). Pregnancy and the lung: State of the art. *The American Review of Respiratory Disease, 121,* 559–581.
6. Contreras, G., Gutierrez, M., Berioza, T., Fantín, A., Oddó, H., Villarroel, L., et al. (1991). Ventilatory drive and respiratory function in pregnancy. *American Review of Respiratory Disease, 144,* 837–841.
7. Skatrud, J. B., Bempsey, J. A., & Kaiser, D. G. (1978). Ventilatory response to medroxyprogesterone acetate in normal subjects: Time course and mechanism. *Journal of Applied Physiology, 44,* 939.
8. Prowse, C. M., & Gaensler, E. A. (1965). Respiratory and acid-base changes during pregnancy. *Anesthesiology, 26,* 381–392.
9. Simon, P. M., Schwartzstein, R. M., Weiss, J. W., Fencl, V., Teghtsoonian, M., & Weinberger, S. E. (1990). Distinguishable

types of dyspnea in patients with shortness of breath. *The American Review of Respiratory Disease, 142,* 1009–1014.

10. Ponto, J. A. (1986). Fetal dosimetry from pulmonary imaging in pregnancy: Revised estimates. *Clinical Nuclear Medicine, 11,* 108–109.

11. Kollef, M. H., & Schuster, D. P. (1995). The acute respiratory distress syndrome. *The New England Journal of Medicine, 332,* 27–44.

12. Zinaman, M., Rubin, J., & Lindheimer, M. D. (1985). Serial plasma oncotic pressure levels and echoencephalography during and after delivery in severe pre-eclampsia. *Lancet, 325*(8440), 1245–1247.

13. Sibai, B. M., Mabie, W. C., Harvey, C. J., & Gonzalez, A. R. (1987). Pulmonary edema in severe pre-eclampsia–eclampsia: Analysis of thirty-seven consecutive cases. *American Journal of Obstetrics and Gynecology, 156,* 1174–1179.

14. Mabie, W. C., Hackman, B. B., & Sibai, B. M. (1993). Acute pulmonary edema associated with pregnancy: Echocardiographic insights and implications for treatment. *Obstetrics & Gynecology, 81,* 227–234.

15. Benedetti, T. J., Kates, R., & Williams, V. (1985). Hemodynamic observations in severe pre-eclampsia complicated by pulmonary edema. *American Journal of Obstetrics and Gynecology, 152,* 330–334.

16. Mabie, W. C., Ratts, T. E., Ramanathan, K. B., & Sibai, B. M. (1988). Circulatory congestion in obese hypertensive women: A subset of pulmonary edema in pregnancy. *Obstetrics & Gynecology, 72,* 553–558.

17. Gottlieb, J. E., Darby, M. J., Gee, M. H., & Fish, J. E. (1991). Recurrent noncardiac pulmonary edema accompanying pregnancy-induced hypertension. *Chest, 100,* 1730–1732.

18. Bienrarz, J., Ivankovich, A., & Scommegma, A. (1974). Cardiac output during ritodrine treatment in preterm labor. *American Journal of Obstetrics and Gynecology, 118*(7), 910–920.

19. Pisani, R. J., & Rosenow, E. C. III. (1989). Pulmonary edema associated with tocolytic therapy. *Annals of Internal Medicine, 110,* 714–718.

20. Benedetti, T. J., Hargrove, J. C., & Rosen, K. A. (1982). Maternal pulmonary edema during premature labor inhibition. *Obstetrics & Gynecology, 59*(Suppl. 6), 335–375.

21. Ingemarsson, I., Arulkomoran, S., & Kottegoda, S. R. (1985). Complications of beta mimetic therapy in preterm labour. *Australian and New Zealand Journal of Obstetrics and Gynaecology, 25*(3), 182–189.

22. Yeast, J. D., Halberstadt, C., Meyer, B. A., Cohen, G. R., & Thorp, J. A. (1993). The risk of pulmonary edema and colloid osmotic pressure changes during magnesium sulfate infusion. *American Journal of Obstetrics and Gynecology, 169*(6), 1566–1571.

23. Kirkpatrick, C., Quenon, M., & Desir, D. (1980). Blood anions and electrolytes during ritodrine infusion in preterm labor. *American Journal of Obstetrics and Gynecology, 139,* 523–527.

24. Hatjis, C. G., & Swain, M. (1988). Systemic tocolysis for premature labor is associated with an increased incidence of pulmonary edema in the presence of maternal infection. *American Journal of Obstetrics and Gynecology, 159,* 723–728.

25. Nimrod, C. A., Beresford, P., Frais, M., Belenkie, I., Tyberg, J., Fremit, A., et al. (1984). Hemodynamic observations on pulmonary edema associated with a B-mimetic agent. *The Journal of Reproductive Medicine, 29*(5), 341–344.

26. Goodrun, L. A. (1997). Pneumonia in pregnancy. *Seminars in Perinatology, 21,* 276–283.

27. Cunningham, F. G., Lucas, M. J., & Hankins, G. D. V. (1987). Pulmonary injury complicating antepartum pyelonephritis. *American Journal of Obstetrics and Gynecology, 156,* 797–807.

28. Pruett, K., & Faro, S. (1987). Pyelonephritis associated with respiratory distress. *Obstetrics and Gynecology, 69,* 444–446.

29. Elkington, K. W., & Greb, L. C. (1986). Adult respiratory distress syndrome as a complication of acute pyelonephritis during pregnancy: Case report and discussion. *Obstetrics and Gynecology, 67,* 18S–20S.

30. de Veciana, M., Towers, C. V., Major, C. A., Lien, J. M., & Toohey, J. S. (1994). Pulmonary injury associated with appendicitis in pregnancy: who is at risk? *American Journal of Obstetrics and Gynecology, 171*(4), 1008–1013.

31. Metcalfe, J. (1985). Oxygen supply and fetal growth. *Journal of Reproductive Medicine, 30*(4), 301–307.

32. Meschia, G. (1985). Safety margin of fetal oxygenation. *Journal of Reproductive Medicine, 30*(4), 308–311.

33. Meschia, G. (1979). Supply of oxygen to the fetus. *Journal of Reproductive Medicine, 23*(4), 160–165.

34. Hughson, W. G., Friedman, P. J., Feigin, D. S., Resnik, R., & Moser, K. M. (1982). Postpartum pleural effusion: A common radiologic finding. *Annals of Internal Medicine, 97,* 856–858.

35. Heffner, J. E., & Sahn, S. A. (1992). Pleural disease in pregnancy. *Clinics in Chest Medicine, 13,* 667–678.

36. Rochat, R. W., Koonin, L. M., Atrash, H. K., & Jewett, J. F. (1988). Maternal mortality in the United States: Report from the Maternal Mortality Collaborative. *Obstetrics & Gynecology, 72,* 91–97.

37. Schwartz, D. R., Malhotra, A., & Weinberger, S. E. (2010). *Deep vein thrombosis and pulmonary embolism in pregnancy: Epidemiology, pathogenesis, and diagnosis.* Retrieved from http://www.uptodate.com/contents/deep-vein-thrombosis-and-pulmonary-embolism-in-pregnancy-epidemiology-pathogenesis-and-diagnosis

38. Ginsberg, J. S., Brill-Edwards, P., Burrows, R. F., Bona, R., Prandoni, P., Büller, H. R., et al. (1992). Venous thrombosis during pregnancy: Leg and trimester of presentation. *Thrombosis and Haemostasis, 67,* 519–520.

39. Cockett, F., Thomas, M., & Negus, D. (1967). Iliac vein compression: Its relation to iliofemoral thrombosis and the post-thrombotic syndrome. *British Medical Journal, 2,* 14–19.

40. Branch, D. W., Silver, R. M., Blackwell, J. L., Reading, J. C., & Scott, J. R. (1992). Outcome of treated pregnancies in women with antiphospholipid syndrome: An update of the Utah experience. *Obstetrics and Gynecology, 80,* 614–620.

41. Silver, R. M., Draper, M. L., Scott, J. R., et al. (1994). Clinical consequences of antiphospholipid antibodies: An historic cohort study. *Obstetrics and Gynecology, 83,* 373–377.

42. Grandone, E., Margaglione, M., Colaizzo, D., D'Andrea, G., Cappucci, G., Brancaccio, V., et al. (1998). Genetic susceptibility to pregnancy-related venous thromboembolism: Roles of factor V Leiden, prothrombin G2021A and methylenetetrahydrofolate reductase C677T mutations. *American Journal of Obstetrics and Gynecology, 179,* 1324–1328.

43. Gerhardt, A., Scharf, R. E., Beckmann, M. W., Struve, S., Bender, H. G., Pillny, M., et al. (2000). Prothrombin and factor V Mutations in women with a history of thrombosis during pregnancy and the puerperium. *The New England Journal of Medicine, 342,* 374–380.

44. Hirsch, D. R., Mikkola, K. M., Marks, P. W., Fox, E. A., Dorfman, D. M., Ewenstein, B. M., ... Goldhaber, S. Z. (1996). Pulmonary embolism and deep venous thrombosis during pregnancy or oral contraceptive use: Prevalence of factor V Leiden. *American Heart Journal, 131,* 1145–1148.

45. Dawkins, K. D., Burke, C. M., Billingham, M. E., & Jamieson, S. W. (1986). Primary pulmonary hypertension and pregnancy. *Chest, 89,* 383–388.

46. VanWinter, J. T., Nichols, F. C. III, Pairolero, P. C., Ney, J. A., & Ogburn, P. L. Jr. (1996). Management of spontaneous pneumothorax during pregnancy: Case report and review of the literature. *Mayo Clinic Proceedings, 71,* 249–252.

47. Clark, S. L., Hankins, G. D. V., Dudley, D. A., Dildy, G. A., & Porter, T. F. (1995). Amniotic fluid embolism: Analysis of the national registry. *American Journal of Obstetrics and Gynecology, 172,* 1158–1169.

48. Martin, R. W. (1996). Amniotic fluid embolism. *Clinical Obstetrics and Gynecology, 39,* 101–106.

49. Burrows, A., & Khoo, S. K. (1995). The amniotic fluid embolism syndrome: 10 years experience at a major teaching hospital. *Australian and New Zealand Journal of Obstetrics and Gynaecology, 35*(3), 245–250.

50. Killam, A. (1985). Amniotic fluid embolus. *Clinical Obstetrics and Gynecology, 28,* 32–36.

51. Courtney, L. D. (1974). Amniotic fluid embolus. *Obstetrical and Gynecological Survey, 29,* 169–177.

52. Morgan, M. (1979). Amniotic fluid embolism. *Anesthesia, 34,* 20–32.

53. Rasmussen, G. E., & Malinow, A. M. (1999). Toward reducing maternal mortality: The problem airway in obstetrics. *International Anesthesiology Clinics, 32,* 83–101.

54. King, T. A., & Adams, A. P. (1999). Failed tracheal intubation. *British Journal of Anaesthesia, 65,* 400–414.

55. Scrutton, M. J., Metcalfe, G. A., Lowry, C., Seed, P. T., & O'Sullivan, G. (1999). Eating in labor: A randomized controlled trial assessing the risks and benefits. *Anesthesia, 54,* 529–534.

56. National Heart, Lung, and Blood Institute. (2007). *Guidelines for the diagnosis and management of asthma (EPR-3).* Bethesda, MD: National Institutes of Health (NIH Publication No. 08-4051). Retrieved from http://www.nhlbi.nih.gov/guidelines/asthma/asthgdln.htm

57. Busse, W. W., Cloutier, M., Dombrowski, M., et al. (2005). Working group report on managing asthma during pregnancy: recommendations for pharmacologic treatment. Update 2004. National Asthma Education and Prevention Program. National Institutes of Health and National Heart, Lung and Blood Institute. NIH Publication No. 05-5236.

58. Dombrowski, M. P., Schatz, M., Wise, R., Momirova, V., Landon, M., Mabie, W., et al. National Institute of Child Health and Human Development Maternal-Fetal Medicine Units Network and the National Heart, Lung, and Blood Institute (2004). Asthma during pregnancy. *Obstetrics and Gynecology, 103,* 5–12.

59. Schatz, M., & Dombrowski, M. (2000). Outcomes of pregnancy in asthmatic women. *Immunology and Allergy Clinics of North America, 20,* 715–727.

60. Alexander, S., Dodds, L., & Armson, B. A. (1998). Perinatal outcomes in women with asthma during pregnancy. *Obstetrics and Gynecology, 92,* 435–440.

61. Namazy, J. A., & Schatz, M. (2005). Pregnancy and asthma: Recent developments. *Current Opinion in Pulmonary Medicine, 11,* 56–60.

62. Tata, L. J., Lewis, S. A., McKeever, T. M., Smith, C. J., Doyle, P., Smeeth, L., et al. (2008). Effect of maternal asthma, exacerbations and asthma medication use on congenital malformations in offspring: A UK population-based study. *Thorax, 63,* 981–987.

63. Schatz, M., Dombrowski, M. P., Wise, R., Momirova, V., Landon, M., Mabie, W., et al. National Heart, Lung and Blood Institute. (2004). The relationship of asthma medication use to perinatal outcomes. *The Journal of Allergy and Clinical Immunology, 113,* 1040–1045.

64. British Thoracic Society, Scottish Intercollegiate Guidelines Network (SIGN). (2003). British guidelines on the management of asthma. *Thorax, 58*(Suppl. 1), 31–94.

65. Theodoropoulos, D. S., Lockey, R. F., Boyce, H. W. Jr, Bukantz, S. C. (1999). Gastroesophageal reflux and asthma: A review of pathogenesis, diagnosis, and therapy. *Allergy, 54,* 651–661.

66. Samuelson, W. M., & Kopita, J. M. (1995). Management of the difficult asthmatic. Gastroesophageal reflux, sinusitis and pregnancy. *Respiratory Care Clinics of North America, 1,* 287–308.

67. National Heart, Lung, and Blood Institute, National Asthma Education and Prevention Program Asthma and Pregnancy Working Group. NAEPP expert panel report. (2005). Managing asthma during pregnancy: Recommendations for pharmacologic treatment. 2004 update. *The Journal of Allergy and Clinical Immunology, 115,* 34–46.

68. Nelson-Piercy, C. (2001). Asthma in pregnancy. *Thorax, 56,* 325–328.

69. Schatz, M., Zeiger, R. S., Harden, K., Hoffman, C. C., Chilingar, L., & Petitti, D. (1997). The safety of asthma and allergy medications during pregnancy. *The Journal of Allergy and Clinical Immunology, 100,* 301–306.

70. Briggs, G. C., Freeman, R. J. K., & Yaffe, S. J. (2008). *Drugs in pregnancy and lactation: A reference guide to fetal and neonatal risk* (8th ed.). Baltimore, MD: Lippincott Williams & Wilkins.

71. Wilson, J. (1982). Use of sodium cromoglycate during pregnancy. *Acta Therapeutica, 8,* S45–S51.

72. Norjaara, E., & de Verdier, M. G. (2003). Normal pregnancy outcomes in a population-based study including 2,968 pregnant women exposed to budesonide. *Journal of Allergy and Clinical Immunology, 111,* 736–742.

73. Morrow-Brown, H., & Storey, G. (1975). Treatment of allergy of the respiratory tract with beclomethasone dipropionate steroid aerosol. *Postgraduate Medical Journal, 51*(Suppl. 4), 59–94.

74. Kemp, J. P., Schatz, M., Sander, N., & Olsen, C. (2003). *Breathing for two: A guide to asthma during pregnancy.* Fairfax, VA: Asthma & Allergy Network Mothers of Asthmatics.

75. Polifka, J. E., & Jones, K. L. (2000). General considerations regarding the use of asthma and allergy medications during pregnancy. *Immunology and Allergy Clinics of North America, 20*(4), 687–697.

76. Stenius-Aarniala, B., Hedman, J., & Terama, K. (1996). Acute asthma during pregnancy. *Thorax, 51,* 411–414.

77. Ballard, P. L., Granverg, P., & Ballard, R. A. (1975). Glucocorticoid levels in maternal and cord serum after prenatal beclomethasone therapy in pregnancy near term. *Journal of Pediatrics, 56,* 1548–1554.

78. Beitins, I. Z., Baynoard, F., Anaes, I. G., Kowarski, A., & Migeon, C. J. (1972). The transplacental passage of

prednisone and prednisolone in pregnancy near term. *The Journal of Pediatrics, 81,* 936–945.

79. Rodriguez-Pinilla, E., & Martinez-Frias, M. L. (1998). Corticosteroids during pregnancy and oral clefts: A case-control study. *Teratology, 58,* 2–5.

80. Schatz, M. (2001). The efficacy and safety of asthma medications during pregnancy. *Seminars in Perinatology, 25,* 145–152.

81. Liccardi, G., Cazzola, M., Canonica, G. W., D'Amato, M., D'Amato, G., & Passalacqua, G. (2003). General strategy for the management of bronchial asthma in pregnancy. *Respiratory Medicine, 97*(7), 778–789.

82. ACOG Committee on Practice Bulletins-Obstetrics. (2008). ACOG practice bulletin. Clinical management guidelines for obstetrician-gynecologists, number 90: Asthma in pregnancy. *Obstetrics & Gynecology, 111,* 457–464.

83. Bousquet, J., Khaltaev, N., Cruz, A. A., Denburg, J., Fokkens, W. J., Togias A, et al. (2008). Allergic rhinitis and its impact on asthma (ARIA) 2008 update. *Allergy, 63*(Suppl. 86), 8–160.

84. Gotzsche, P. C., Hammarquist, C., & Burr, M. (1998). House dust mite control measures in the management of asthma: Meta-analysis. *BMJ, 317,* 1105–1110.

85. Greenberger, P. S. (1996). Management of asthma in pregnancy. *Clinical Immunotherapeutics, 6,* 97–107.

86. Smith, A. P. (1973). The effects of intravenous infusion of graded doses of prostaglandins F2 alpha and E2 on lung resistance in patients undergoing termination of pregnancy. *Clinical Science, 44,* 17–25.

87. Weiner, C. P., & Buhimschi, C. (Eds.). (2009). *Drugs for pregnant and lactating women* (2nd ed.). Philadelphia: W.B. Saunders Company.

88. Gordon, M., Niswander, K. R., Berendes, H., & Kantor, A. G. (1970). Fetal morbidity following potentially anoxigenic obstetric conditions. VII. Bronchial asthma. *Obstetrics and Gynecology, 106,* 421–429.

89. Berkowitz, K., & LaSala, A. (1990). Risk factors associated with the increasing prevalence of pneumonia during pregnancy. *American Journal of Obstetrics and Gynecology, 163,* 981–985.

90. Madinger, N. E., Greenspoon, J. S., & Ellrodt, A. G. (1989). Pneumonia during pregnancy: Has modern technology improved maternal and fetal outcome? *American Journal of Obstetrics and Gynecology, 161,* 657–662.

91. Benedetti, T. J., Valle, R., & Ledger, W. J. (1982). Antepartum pneumonia in pregnancy. *American Journal of Obstetrics and Gynecology, 144,* 413–417.

92. Lim, W. S., Macfarlane, J. T., & Colthorpe, C. L. (2001). Pneumonia and pregnancy. *Thorax, 56,* 398–405.

93. McKinney, P., Volkert, P., & Kaufman, J. (1990). Fatal swine influenza pneumonia occurring during late pregnancy. *Archives of Internal Medicine, 150,* 213–215.

94. Harris, J. W. (1919). Influenza occurring in pregnant women. *JAMA, 72,* 978–980.

95. Freeman, D. W., & Barno, A. (1959). Deaths from Asian influenza associated with pregnancy. *American Journal of Obstetrics and Gynecology, 78,* 1172–1175.

96. Jamieson, D. J., Honein, M. A., Rasmussen, S. A., Williams, J. L., Swerdlow, D. L., Biggerstaff, M. S., et al. Novel Influenza A (H1N1) Pregnancy Working Group (2009). H1N1 2009 influenza virus infection during pregnancy in the USA. *Lancet, 374,* 451–458.

97. U.S. Department of Health and Human Services. (2005). *HHS pandemic influenza plan.* Retrieved from http://www.hhs.gov/pandemicflu/plan/pdf/hhspandemicinfluenzaplan.pdf

98. Rosa, C. (1998). Rubella and rubeola. *Seminars in Perinatology, 22,* 318–322.

99. Haake, D. A., Zakokwski, P. C., Haake, D. L., & Bryson, Y. J. (1990). Early treatment with acyclovir varicella pneumonia in otherwise healthy adults: Retrospective controlled study and review. *Reviews of Infectious Diseases, 12,* 788–798.

100. Broussard, R. C., Payne, K., & George, R. B. (1991). Treatment with acyclovir of varicella pneumonia in pregnancy. *Chest, 99,* 1045–1047.

101. Fowler, R., Lapinsky, S. E., & Hallett, D., Detsky, A. S., Sibbald, W. J., Slutsky, A. S., et al. Toronto SARS Critical Care Group. (2003). Critically ill patients with severe acute respiratory syndrome (SARS). *JAMA, 290,* 367–373.

102. Wong, S. F., Chow, K. M., & de Swiet, M. (2003). Severe acute respiratory syndrome and pregnancy. *British Journal of Obstetrics and Gynaecology, 110,* 641–642.

103. Stevens, D. A. (1995). Coccidiomycosis. *The New England Journal of Medicine, 332,* 1077–1082.

104. Peterson, C. M., Schuppert, K., Kelly, P. C., & Pappagianis, D. (1993). Coccidiomycosis and pregnancy. *Obstetrical and Gynecological Survey, 48,* 149–156.

105. Good, J. T. Jr., Iseman, M. D., Davidson, P. T., Lakshminarayan, S., & Sahn, S. A. (1981). Tuberculosis in association with pregnancy. *American Journal of Obstetrics and Gynecology, 140,* 492–498.

106. Blumberg, H. M., Burman, W. J., Chaisson, R. E., Daley, C. L., Etkind, S. C., Friedman, L. N., et al. American Thoracic Society, Centers for Disease Control and Prevention and the Infectious Diseases Society. (2003). American Thoracic Society/Centers for Disease Control and Prevention/Infection Diseases Society of America. Treatment of tuberculosis. *American Journal of Respiratory and Critical Care Medicine, 167,* 603–662.

107. Baughman, R. P., Teirstein, A. S., Judson, M. A., Rossman, M. D., Yeager, H. Jr, Bresnitz, E. A., et al. Case Control Etiologic Study of Sarcoidosis (ACCESS) research group. (2001). Case control etiologic study of sarcoidosis (ACCESS) research group. Clinical characteristics of patients in a case control study of sarcoidosis. *American Journal of Respiratory and Critical Care Medicine, 164,* 1885–1889.

108. Baughman, R. P., Lower, E. E., & du Bois, R. M. (2003). Sarcoidosis. *Lancet, 361,* 1111–1118.

109. Agha, F. P., Vade, A., Amendola, M. A., & Cooper, R. F. (1982). Effects of pregnancy on sarcoidosis. *Surgery, Gynecology and Obstetrics, 155,* 817–822.

110. Keleman, J. T., & Mandl, L. (1969). Sarcoidose in der placenta. *Zentrablatt fur Allgemeine Pathologie und Pathologische Anatomie, 281,* 520–522.

111. King, T. E. Jr. (2010). *Clinical manifestations and diagnosis of sarcoidosis.* Retrieved from http://www.uptodate.com/contents/clinical-manifestations-and-diagnosis-of-sarcoidosis?source=search_result&selectedTitle=1-150.

112. Haynes deRegt, R. (1987). Sarcoidosis and pregnancy. *Obstetrics and Gynecology, 70,* 369–373.

113. Selroos, O. (1990). Sarcoidosis and pregnancy: A review with results of a retrospective survey. *Journal of Internal Medicine, 227,* 221–224.

114. Matthews, L. W., & Drotar, D. (1984). Cystic fibrosis—a challenging long term chronic disease. *Pediatric Clinics of North America, 31,* 133–152.

115. Katkin, J. P. (2010). *Cystic fibrosis: Clinical manifestations and diagnosis*. Retrieved from http://www.uptodate.com/contents/cystic-fibrosis-clinical-manifestations-and-diagnosis?source=search_result&selectedTitle=1–150

116. Edenborough, F. P., Stableforth, D. E., Webb, A. K., Mackenzie, W. E., & Smith, D. L. (1995). Outcome of pregnancy in women with cystic fibrosis. *Thorax, 50,* 170–174.

117. Kent, N. E., & Farquaharson, D. F. (1993). Cystic fibrosis in pregnancy. *Canadian Medical Association Journal, 149,* 809–813.

118. Frangolias, D. D., Nakielna, E. M., & Wilcox, P. G. (1997). Pregnancy and cystic fibrosis. *Chest, 111,* 963–969.

119. Jankelson, D., Robinson, M., Parsons, S., Torzillo, P., Peat, B., & Bye, P. (1998). Cystic fibrosis and pregnancy. *Australian and New Zealand Journal of Obstetrics and Gynaecology, 38,* 180–184.

120. Liaschko, A., & Koren, G. (2002). Cystic fibrosis during pregnancy. *Canadian Family Physician, 48,* 463–467.

121. Koren, G., Pastuszak, A., & Ito, S. (1998). Drugs in pregnancy. *New England Journal of Medicine, 338,* 1128–1137.

CHAPTER 10

Diabetic Ketoacidosis and Continuous Insulin Infusion Management in Pregnancy

Maribeth Inturrisi, Nancy C. Lintner, and Kimberlee Sorem

It has been estimated that approximately 2 million women of reproductive age (18 to 44 years) have diabetes; about one-third of these women do not know they have the disease.[1] Diabetes is the most common metabolic disorder complicating pregnancy. In the United States, the incidence of diabetes in pregnancy is estimated to be 7 to 14 percent.[1] The type of diabetes most often diagnosed during pregnancy is gestational diabetes mellitus (GDM), which accounts for 95 percent of cases. Pre-gestational diabetes, type 1 or type 2, accounts for approximately 5 percent of diabetes cases seen in pregnancy. Both pre-gestational and gestational diabetes increase the risk for adverse maternal, fetal, and newborn outcomes and future metabolic abnormalities.

Identification and careful management of hyperglycemia during pregnancy can reduce adverse maternal and infant outcomes.[2,3] The risk for severe hyperglycemia during pregnancy increases:

- as gestation advances
- in association with rapid weight gain or obesity
- when infection is present
- during tocolysis with beta-mimetics and/or high-dose steroid administration to advance fetal lung maturation.

These situations increase the risk of diabetic ketoacidosis (DKA), an acute, life-threatening metabolic complication of diabetes associated with increased risk of maternal and fetal morbidity and mortality. Management of DKA or attentuation of its occurrence often requires continuous insulin infusion. Depending on the urgency of the clinical situation, an intravenous insulin infusion (continuous intravenous insulin infusion, or CIII) or a continuous subcutaneous insulin pump infusion (continuous subcutaneous insulin infusion, or CSII) will be utilized.

A comprehensive discussion of diabetes in pregnancy, including management of diabetes in preterm labor or specific infections is beyond the scope of this chapter. This chapter will focus on the pathophysiology of glucose metabolism related to DKA and factors and events that predispose a patient to the development of DKA. Clinical management strategies for patients with DKA in pregnancy are reviewed in detail. In addition, the clinical management of continuous insulin infusions, both intravenous and subcutaneous, will be briefly discussed.

DIABETIC KETOACIDOSIS

The incidence of DKA in pregnancy is approximately 1 to 3 percent.[4,5] The fetal mortality rate in cases of maternal DKA is approximately 9 percent.[4] The risk of maternal death has been estimated at less than 1 percent.[6] Although more prevalent in patients with type 1 diabetes, there are case reports of DKA in patients with GDM and in patients with type 2 diabetes who have a concomitant illness (e.g., infection) or following administration of medications (e.g., corticosteroid or β_2 agonist). Between 78 and 90 percent of cases of DKA during pregnancy occur in the second and third trimesters, typically as a result of increased insulin resistance associated with advancing gestation.[4,5] DKA with blood glucose (BG) levels of less than 200 mg/dL does occur during pregnancy and necessitates prompt recognition and treatment.[7,8]

DKA during pregnancy fortunately has become a relatively uncommon event.[9] Kilvert and colleagues reported 11 cases of ketoacidosis in 635 insulin-treated pregnancies between 1971 and 1990.[4] One fetal loss and one spontaneous miscarriage occurred in this study. Advances in clinical management and BG monitoring

FIGURE 10-1 Pathophysiology of diabetic ketoacidosis. Adapted from Carroll, M.A., & Yeomans, E. R. (2005). Diabetic ketoacidosis in pregnancy. *Critical Care Medicine, 33*(Suppl. 10), S347–S353.

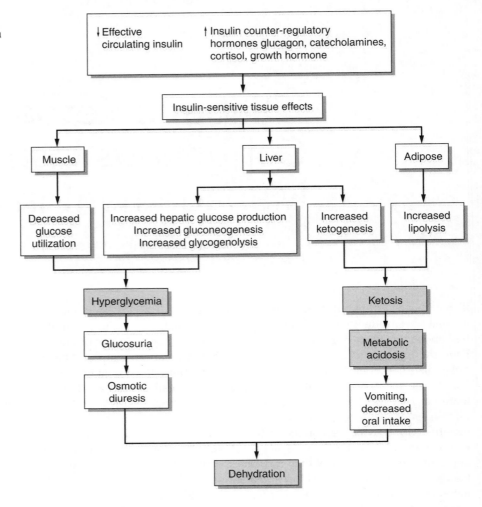

Pathophysiology of DKA

have contributed to the reduction in DKA. However, when DKA does occur, it represents a medical emergency for mother and fetus.

Patients with DKA classically present with a triad of concurrent abnormalities: dehydration, ketosis, and metabolic acidosis.[10] It occurs when there is either an absolute or relative deficiency in circulating insulin levels in the context of an excess of insulin counter-regulatory hormones.[10] The latter include catecholamines, glucagon, cortisol, and growth hormone, all of which are increased in DKA when compared to baseline.[10,11] Additional consequences associated with insulin deficiency include accelerated lipolysis, hepatic glucose and ketone production, hyperglycemia, ketonemia, depletion of water and electrolytes, increased anion gap (greater than 12), and metabolic acidemia (pH less than 7.3; bicarbonate less than 15 mEq/L). Typical symptoms of ketoacidosis include nausea and vomiting (most common during pregnancy), fruity breath, dry mouth, thirst, abdominal pain, polyuria, weakness, alteration in mental status, and labored breathing.[10]

The underlying pathophysiologic disturbances in DKA need to be assessed carefully throughout the course of treatment. Careful trending of clinical and laboratory data allows for optimal and timely treatment of underlying acidemia and hyperglycemia and prevents potentially lethal complications, such as severe hyponatremia and hypokalemia.

Pathophysiologic changes associated with DKA are depicted in Figure 10-1.[10] Overall, a shift from the normal carbohydrate metabolism of the fed state to one of primarily fat metabolism typical of the fasting state initiates the process. When carbohydrates are not available, caused either by a lack of insulin or insulin utilization at the cellular level, the body is unable to transport glucose into cells, a process that is necessary for the maintenance of normal, aerobic metabolism. With an obligatory alternate shift to fat oxidation, free fatty acids (FFAs) are produced in adipocytes and transported to the liver bound to albumin. There they are broken down into acetate, and then turned into ketoacids (e.g., acetic acid, β-hydroxybutyrate, and acetone).[12] In the absence of insulin, the liver maximally initiates this ketogenic pathway such that the supply of these moderately strong acids exceeds peripheral utilization and maternal buffering capacity in the circulation. The presence of excessive ketone bodies, combined with increased lactic acid caused by decreased peripheral uptake of glucose, results in metabolic acidosis.[13]

As glucagon levels rise, the combination of excess glucagon and insufficient insulin inhibits glycolysis and stimulates gluconeogenesis, which worsens hyperglycemia. As the degree of hyperglycemia and ketonemia increases, there is a rise in serum osmolarity. As a result, hyperglycemia and ketones serve as an osmotic reservoir, leading to diuresis, profound hypovolemia, and hypotension. Hypovolemia then stimulates other counter-regulatory stress hormones (e.g., catecholamines, growth hormone, and cortisol), which further enhance the release of glucagon. This sequence of events contributes to the continued cycle of dehydration, increased serum osmolarity, and increased release of insulin counter-regulatory stress hormones, therefore worsening acidemia that subsequently leads to acidosis.

As a result of osmotic diuresis, the loss of free water can be significant and may approach 100 to 150 mL/kg body weight. For example, a woman who weighs 165 lb (75 kg) may lose over 11 liters of free water from osmotic diuresis. The increased production of urine is accompanied by depletion of electrolytes, especially sodium, potassium, and phosphorus.

Significant dehydration secondary to DKA leads to a significantly depleted potassium level (as much as 5 mEq/kg of body weight). Consequently, low serum potassium levels may be a sign of severe hypokalemia, since potassium is lost not only at the intracellular level but also from within the circulation. Further, sodium levels may be normal, high, or low, and are proportionate to the degree of hydration and hyperglycemia. For example, for each 100 mg/dL of glucose above 100 mg/dL, serum sodium is decreased by approximately 1.6 mEq. Conversely, when glucose falls, serum sodium levels rise by a corresponding amount.

How Pregnancy Affects DKA

Select physiologic changes of pregnancy contribute to an increased predisposition for the development of DKA during pregnancy. An increase in pulmonary minute ventilation is a result of an increased tidal volume. This relative hyperventilation causes a state of respiratory alkalemia which results in a compensatory renal excretion of bicarbonate. The net effect is decreased total buffering capacity, which makes the pregnant diabetic more susceptible to development of metabolic acidemia and

TABLE 10-1

Predisposing Factors and Precipitating Events for DKA in Pregnancy

Predisposing Factors	• Decreased buffering capacity • Vomiting and dehydration (hyperemesis, gastrointestinal disorder) • "Accelerated starvation" of pregnancy • Increased insulin antagonists (HPL, prolactin, cortisol) • Stress
Precipitating Events	• Poor compliance • Infection (viral or bacterial) • Obstetrical use of steroids and beta-mimetics • Omissions of insulin doses or pump failure not recognized and treated • Diabetic gastroparesis • Newly diagnosed diabetes

DKA = diabetic ketoacidosis, HPL = human placental lactogen. Adapted from Parker, J. A., & Conway, D. L. (2007). Diabetic ketoacidosis in pregnancy. *Obstetrics and Gynecology Clinics of North America, 34,* 533–543; Montoro, M. N., Myers, V. P., Mestman, J. H., Xu, Y., Anderson, B. G., & Golde, S. H. (1993). Outcome of pregnancy in diabetic ketoacidosis. *American Journal of Perinatology, 10,* 17–20.

subsequently DKA.[13] In addition, emesis, commonly present during the first trimester, may result in dehydration significant enough to predispose to the development of DKA. Predisposing factors and events associated with the development of DKA are listed in Table 10-1.[13]

Norbert Freinkel described pregnancy as a state of "accelerated starvation." He noted that, when pregnant women skipped breakfast and had a prolonged period of fasting, lipolysis was enhanced. Measured plasma glucose concentrations in pregnant women after fasting longer than 14 hours demonstrated that final FFA and β-hydroxybutyrate levels were strongly correlated and inversely related to final plasma glucose levels. These results show why the common practice of meal skipping by personal preference or for medical testing should be avoided in pregnant women.[14]

Insulin sensitivity has been shown to decrease as gestation advances, particularly in the third trimester with decreased hepatic sensitivity to insulin, postprandial hyperglycemia, and an increased risk for ketoacidosis.[9] Increased insulin antagonists from the placenta such as human placental lactogen (HPL), prolactin, cortisol, and tumor necrosis factor (TNF) alpha act on insulin-sensitive tissues to produce alternate substrate for energy use during DKA. A concomitant rise in levels of stress hormones (e.g., glucagon, corticosteroids, catecholamines and growth hormone) further enhances hepatic gluconeogenesis, glycogenolysis, and lipolysis and contributes to the diabetogenic state.[13]

In addition to predisposing factors to DKA, there are also recognized precipitating events to DKA in pregnancy (see Table 10-1) including poor compliance with insulin regimens or meal plans, viral or bacterial infection, obstetrical use of steroids and/or administration of beta-mimetics, insulin administration failures, poor management, diabetic gastroparesis, and newly diagnosed diabetes.[13]

It is important to emphasize that pregnant women with diabetes are susceptible to the development of DKA at lower glycemic levels than non-pregnant individuals with diabetes. A study reported by Cullen showed that in pregnancies complicated by diabetes, 2 percent of patients demonstrated classic symptoms of DKA during the 10-year study period.[4] Ten of 11 patients presenting with DKA (90 percent) demonstrated nausea, vomiting, and decreased caloric intake. Plasma glucose levels of less than 200 mg/dL were present in 4 of the 11 patients (36 percent). Despite contemporary methods of diabetes care, near-normal plasma glucose levels do not preclude DKA. Nausea, vomiting, and decreased caloric intake in an otherwise normal pregnant woman with diabetes requires evaluation to exclude ketosis.[4] This has been demonstrated in women with type 1 diabetes who have had insulin withheld due to seemingly normal BG values. Therefore, insulin should not be withheld for more than a few hours in a patient with type 1 diabetes, even with a normal BG value.[7]

How DKA Affects Pregnancy

DKA in pregnancy occurs more often in women with type 1 diabetes rather than type 2 diabetes, and it is rare in GDM. Some ethnic groups have ketosis-prone type 2 diabetes, such as African Americans and Hispanics, and development is usually associated with the cessation of medication, infection, pancreatitis, or obesity.[15] Overall, the prevalence of DKA during pregnancy has declined from 16.7 percent before 1960, to 7.8 percent from 1965 to 1985, and to 1.2 to 4.1 percent from the 1990s to 2003.[16]

DKA profoundly affects both the mother and the fetus. Literature from the last decade supports a fetal loss rate of approximately 9 percent in pregnancies in which DKA occurred.[4] Maternal volume depletion and acidosis leading to decreased uterine blood flow may cause a relative fetal hypoxemia.[17] Glucose and ketones readily cross the placenta, at maternal levels.[13] Furthermore, fetal hyperglycemia by itself may contribute to osmotic diuresis, fetal intravascular volume depletion, and decreased perfusion to the placenta. A significant

decrease in maternal pH may likewise result in a corresponding decrease in the fetal pH.[13]

In the presence of maternal DKA, fetal heart rate changes such as absence of variability and the presence of late decelerations may be evident on the electronic fetal monitor tracing. There may also be a non-reassuring biophysical profile. In addition, maternal hypokalemia may cause fetal cardiac arrhythmias. These abnormalities are generally reversible with appropriately aggressive maternal treatment.[18–20]

Absent a maternal or fetal indication for prompt delivery, correction of the underlying DKA will, in the majority of cases, improve maternal condition, facilitate fetal stabilization, and allow prolongation of the pregnancy.[13]

Diagnosis of DKA

The patient with DKA typically presents with clinical symptoms such as nausea, vomiting, abdominal pain, malaise, weakness/lethargy, polyuria, polydypsia, tachypnea, hyperventilation, altered mental state, and signs of dehydration (e.g., dry mucous membranes, decreased skin turgor, hypotension and/or tachycardia, and a classic fruity odor of the breath). The patient may also be febrile, suggesting infection as a possible precipitating event.

Laboratory evaluation includes the following: complete blood count (CBC) with differential, urinalysis, serum electrolytes, BG, bicarbonate (HCO_3^-), blood urea nitrogen (BUN), creatinine, arterial blood gases, and plasma osmolality. Serum ketone β-hydroxybutyrate must be evaluated often to differentiate between mild gastrointestinal issues and DKA. Ketonuria is less sensitive than ketonemia as urine ketones are delayed by several hours from serum ketones. When elevated beyond 3.5 mmol/L, serum ketone β-hydroxybutyrate correlates better with the diagnosis of DKA than the presence of +++ urine ketones on qualitative analysis.[12,21] In addition to exploring the usual causes (insulin administration failures), additional testing may include blood and urine cultures, serum lipase, electrocardiogram, and chest X-ray.

Treatment of DKA

In order to optimize maternal and fetal outcome, the diagnosis of DKA needs to be prompt and followed by immediate initiation of treatment.[9,18] Effective therapeutic goals include the following:

- initiation of insulin to reverse metabolic abnormalities
- aggressive fluid replacement to correct volume deficit and improve tissue perfusion
- replacement of electrolytes

- management of acid–base disturbances
- detection and correction of the underlying cause of DKA, including insertion of a transurethral catheter for urine volume evaluation as well as culture and sensitivity.

A sample management protocol for the management of DKA in pregnancy is shown in Table 10-2. In addition, comprehensive guidelines regarding collaborative clinical management of the patient with DKA may also be found in the Clinical Guidelines section of this text.

Initial intravenous solution replacement consists of isotonic saline 0.9 percent infused at 1000 mL/hr over the first hour and 500 to 1000 mL/hr over the second hour. Subsequent infusions over the next 4 to 6 hours are adjusted according to electrolyte values and generally include 250 to 500 mL/hr of 0.45 to 0.9 percent NaCl. Although the IV treatment of significant dehydration is imperative, the infusion of hypotonic solutions too soon and too rapidly may create a sudden decrease in serum osmolarity, potentially resulting in cellular swelling and, rarely, cerebral edema.[22] Once serum glucose values approximate 200 mg/dL, a 5 percent dextrose/0.45 percent NaCl solution infused at 150 to 250 mL/hr is appropriate. Approximately 75 percent of the estimated fluid deficit, assumed to be approximately 100 mL/kg actual body weight on the average, is replaced over the first 24 hours of therapy with the balance over the next 24 to 48 hours.

Simultaneaous insulin administration is the cornerstone of treatment to correct metabolic alterations precipitated by DKA. The goal of initial therapy is a gradual reduction of glucose by approximately 60 to 75 mg/dL/hr. This is accomplished by an initial bolus of intravenous insulin, 0.1 unit/kg of regular insulin, followed by a continuous infusion at a rate of approximately 0.1 unit/kg/hr.

Should serum glucose fail to decrease by 50 to 70 mg/dL in the first hour, the bolus insulin infusion rate can be doubled until serum glucose reaches 200 mg/dL.[11] Thereafter, continuous infusion of regular insulin should be maintained at 0.05 to 0.1 units/kg/hr intravenous (IV) with the goal of serum glucose values between 100 and 150 mg/dL or until DKA has resolved.

Subcutaneous (SQ) insulin administration should be avoided because of the potential for inadequate absorption during crisis. However, SQ administration may resume once metabolic abnormalities have been corrected and the patient is feeling well enough to resume her prescribed meal plan.[11]

DKA is associated with significant electrolyte imbalance, especially a total body loss of potassium. The therapeutic goal is to maintain K^+ values between 4 and 5 mEq/L with adequate renal function (urine output of approximately 50 mL/hr). Caution should be exercised with the administration of potassium in initial fluids,

since the combination of contracted volume and insulin deficiency could result in a rapid rise in serum potassium and the subsequent development of cardiac arrhythmias. Initial serum potassium values guide replacement recommendations. For example, serum potassium in the range of 3 to 5 mEq/L usually prompts intravenous supplementation of 20 mEq/L of potassium chloride initially and with each subsequent liter of fluid in order to achieve serum values between 4 and 5 mEq/L. A serum potassium level less than 3 mEq/L generally requires additional supplementation; and, if the value exceeds 5 mEq/L, supplementation is withheld.[11]

Serum sodium and chloride levels are monitored during therapy and corrected through adjustment of intravenous fluid concentrations. Phosphate replacement is not normally required; however, if serum phosphate levels are less than 1.0 mg/dL, or in the presence of cardiac dysfunction, replacement therapy may include potassium phosphate.

Acute Non-DKA Insulin Infusion Management

When a pregnant woman with diabetes is hospitalized for antepartum care, labor induction, spontaneous labor, or elective Cesarean delivery, the goal of maintenance of euglycemia may necessitate insulin administration tailored to the specific needs of the patient and the specific clinical situation.

While specific detrimental outcomes of temporary hyperglycemia are not fully known, it has been established that the fetal pancreas is stimulated to overproduce insulin in accordance with elevated maternal BG levels.[23] Fetal hyperinsulinemia interferes with surfactant production in the lung, increases fetal abdominal fat deposition, and alters carbohydrate metabolism in the offspring.[24]

Evidence-based literature suggests that normal non-pregnant individuals exposed to transient glucose elevations show rapid reduction in all lymphocyte subsets.[25] In patients with diabetes, hyperglycemia is similarly associated with reduced T-cell populations for both CD-4 and CD-8 subsets, thus affecting immunity. These abnormalities are reversed when BG is lowered.[25] For maternal and fetal well-being, it is optimal to adequately address hyperglycemia associated with maternal conditions including infection and beta-mimetic and betamethasone administration. During these periods of physiologic stress, all insulin doses generally need to be doubled.

For example, maternal hyperglycemia usually ensues within 4 hours after the first injection of betamethasone. As a result, both basal and bolus insulin require modification for the following 3 to 5 days. An algorithm for increasing insulin doses during betamethasone therapy

TABLE 10-2

Sample Management Protocol for DKA in Pregnancy

Admission	Admit to unit with obstetric acute/critical care capability.
Vital signs	Daily weight, continuous pulse oximetry, strict hourly intake and output, continuous blood pressure and pulse via arterial line
	Continuous respiratory rate
Initial labs	Arterial blood gas, serum glucose, serum betahydroxybutyrate, serum electrolytes, anion gap, urinalysis, urine culture, urine ketones
Continuous fetal monitoring	• If <24 weeks gestation, check FHR every 4 hr. • If >24 weeks gestation, obtain continuous fetal monitoring.
Fluids	• Estimate fluid deficit of 100 mL/kg. Correct 75% of estimated fluid deficit over first 24 hr. Use isotonic saline (0.9% NS). • First hour, give 1 L NS (1,000 mL/hr). • Second hour, give 0.5–1 L NS (500–1000 mL/hr). • Third hour, give 0.5 L NS (500 mL/hr). • Give 0.25 L/hr of 0.45% NS (250 mL/hr); when serum glucose = 200 mg/dL, change to 5% dextrose/0.45% NS (150–250 mL/hr) • Continue 0.25 L/hr of 0.45% NS for 24–48 hr, until anion gap and acidosis have corrected and volume deficit is replaced.

Electrolytes	• Monitor electrolytes every 2–4 hr.
	• KCl is most often given for replacement—i.e., 40 mEq/L = ~5–10 mEq/hr replacement
	  • Maintain serum K^+ level at 4–5 mEq/L.
	  • If normal kidney function (normal serum creatinine in pregnancy is less than 1.0 mg/dL) all women in DKA should have replacement
	  • With replacement, maintain adequate urine output (0.5 mL/kg/hr).
	  • Suggested protocol using serum K^+:
	    • *>5 mEq/L*: No treatment
	    • *4–5 mEq/L*: Add 20 mEq/L KCl in 1,000 mL 0.9% NS as replacement to infuse at 150 mL/hr.
	    • *3–4 mEq/L*: 30–40 mEq/L KCl in 1,000 mL 0.9% NS as replacement to infuse at 150 mL/hr.
	    • *<3 mEq/L*: 40–60 mEq/L KCl in 1,000 mL 0.9% NS as replacement to infuse at 150 mL/hr.
	• Phosphate replacement not normally required. If serum phosphate is less than 1.0 mg/dL or if evidence of cardiac dysfunction, replace using potassium phosphate.
	• Calculate corrected Na^+ during fluid administration. Monitor serum Na^+ and Cl^-; adjust type of IV fluids if hypernatremia or hyperchloremia.
	• Bicarbonate replacement usually not necessary if pH >7.0
	• Assess for the presence of serum ketones every 2 hr.

Glucose monitoring	• Monitor serum glucose at least every hour. • If serum glucose is not decreased by 20% within first 2 hr, double insulin infusion rate. • Aim for a decrease in serum glucose of 60–75 mg/dL/hr.

Insulin therapy	• Give 0.1 units/kg bolus regular insulin IV.
	• Mix 500 units regular insulin in 500 mL 0.9% NS (1 mL = 1 unit).
	• Flush IV tubing with 20–50 mL of insulin solution prior to infusing it, as insulin binding to tubing occurs.
	• Administer 0.1 units/kg/hr IV continuous infusion.
	• When BG falls below 150 mg/dL, begin the following:
	  • Continue 0.45% NS at 150 mL/hr.
	  • Add a separate IV line of D_5 0.45% NS at 100 mL/hr on an IV controlled pump.
	  • Adjust insulin infusion according to the algorithm below:

Capillary Blood Glucose	*Insulin Units/hr*
<70	0
71–90	0.5
91–110	1
111–130	2
131–150	3
151–170	4

• Continue insulin therapy until bicarbonate and anion gap normalize.
• After full resolution of ketosis, maintain insulin drip until after the first subcutaneous dose of insulin is administered.

BG = blood glucose, Cl = chloride, DKA = diabetic ketoacidosis, FHR = fetal heart rate, K = potassium, KCl = potassium chloride, Na = sodium, NS = normal saline solution.

TABLE 10-3

Recommendations for Increased Insulin Needs with Betamethasone Administration

Day 1	Day 2	Day 3	Day 4
Double both basal and bolus insulin doses.	Continue with increased doses; modify as needed based on BG level.	Divide the previous day's increased dose by 50% and add that amount to the original dose	Revert to pre-betamethasone insulin doses and regime

Data from algorithm developed by Drs Larry Gavin and Jack Kitzmiller; available to providers as a laminated set of pocket-sized sheets, *Sweet Success Pocket Guide*.

can be found in Table 10-3. Similarly, BG monitoring should be increased to include fasting, before and 1 hour after the start of each meal, 2 hours following a meal, at bedtime, and at 3 a.m. until BG is within the target range and the insulin dose has returned to pre-betamethasone levels.

During hospitalization, intensive CIII or CSII pump can effectively normalize BG without unnecessary exposure to persistent hyperglycemia. CIII can replace basal insulin (NPH) using an hourly IV correction algorithm similar to that used in labor (Table 10-4). If the patient is not NPO, the premeal or bolus insulin (rapid-acting analogue) may be administered subcutaneously while using the CIII as basal insulin. This method can avoid hyperglycemia altogether but may increase the risk for hypoglycemia. Hourly self-monitoring of blood glucose (SMBG) is mandatory when using CIII or more often when symptoms of hypoglycemia are evident.

INTRAPARTUM INSULIN MANAGEMENT

The goal of intrapartum insulin management is to maintain maternal euglycemia (BG, 70 to 110 mg/dL), in order to optimize fetal tolerance of labor and prevent neonatal hypoglycemia. In the largest published experience with 233 insulin-treated pregnant women with diabetes, the lowest risk of neonatal hypoglycemia occurred when intrapartum maternal BG was maintained below 100 mg/dL. Intrapartum hyperglycemia had more effect on neonatal hypoglycemia than did antepartum BG levels.[26]

Women with GDM may not require insulin during labor because of increased insulin sensitivity and reduced insulin needs in labor in association with restriction of carbohydrate intake and uterine muscle activity. Consequently, the usual dose of intermediate-acting insulin is given at bedtime the night before induction or scheduled Cesarean delivery; however, the morning dose is withheld.[16]

To determine if insulin is needed during labor with GDMA$_2$, the BG should be assessed at least hourly and insulin initiated if 110 mg/dL or greater (see Table 10-4). In contrast, women with preexisting diabetes will likely require administration of insulin during labor to maintain BG values within the desired range. Women with type 1 diabetes need exogenous insulin to utilize glucose and therefore require insulin initiation when their BG is as low as 70 mg/dL. In contrast, a woman with type 2 diabetes who is still producing insulin and not consuming carbohydrates may have greater ability during labor to maintain a normal BG level; therefore, insulin can be initiated at a BG value of 90 to 110 mg/dL (see Table 10-4).

Intrapartum insulin is optimally delivered via IV infusion (CIII) or continuous subcutaneous insulin infusion pump (CSII), as described below.

TABLE 10-4

Intrapartum Intravenous Insulin Algorithm

Capillary Blood Glucose	Units of Insulin	mL/hr*
<70 mg/dL	0.0	0
70–90 mg/dL[†]	0.5	0.5
91–110 mg/dL	1	1
111–130 mg/dL[‡]	2	2
131–150 mg/dL	3	3
151–170 mg/dL	4	4
171–190 mg/dL	5	5
>190 mg/dL	Assess for urine ketones	Call physician or primary care provider for insulin dose

*Concentration 1 mL = 1 unit insulin.
[†]Start here for type 1 diabetes mellitus.
[‡]Start here for type 2 diabetes mellitus, gestational diabetes mellitus: GDM A$_2$.
Palmer, D., & Inturrisi, M. (1992). Insulin infusion therapy in the intrapartum period. *Journal of Perinatal and Neonatal Nursing, 16*(1), B14–25.

Box 10-1. CLINCAL ACTIONS TO MAINTAIN MATERNAL EUGLYCEMIA

- Obtain baseline capillary BG to confirm level above 70 mg/dL and below 130 mg/dL
- Start main IV with 1,000 mL plain LR at TKO rate.
- If capillary BG level is below 130 mg/dL, begin glucose infusion with 1,000 mL D_5LR (or D_5NS) at 100 mL/hr using an infusion pump. If level is above 130 mg/dL, begin insulin infusion, and start glucose infusion when capillary BG level is less than 130 mg/dL.
- Initiate insulin infusion when BG exceeds 70 mg/dL (type 1 diabetes) or 110 mg/dL (type 2 diabetes or GDMA$_2$).
- Monitor BG level every 30 minutes × 2, then every 1 hour.
- Adjust IV insulin dose according to algorithm depicted in Table 10-4 to maintain BG levels between 70 mg/dL

and 110 mg/dL. Insulin requirements decrease in the first stage of labor but may increase in the second stage.[27]
- Observe for any signs or symptoms of hypoglycemia and, if present, check BG levels immediately
- Obtain urine sample and send to lab every 8 hours (or more frequent when indicated) for ketones and protein, and consult for values +1 as necessary.
- Continue IV insulin infusion while the woman is in labor. Following delivery, BG should be reevaluated and subsequent care adjusted accordingly. Usually insulin needs are cut in half with the delivery of the placenta. The IV algorithm is halved postpartum.

D_5LR = 5 percent dextrose in lactated Ringer's solution, D_5NS = 5 percent dextrose in 0.9 percent normal saline solution, LR = Lactated Ringer's or Ringer's lactate solution, TKO = to keep open.
Data from Palmer, D, & Inturrisi, M. (1992). Insulin infusion therapy in the intrapartum period. *Journal of Perinatal and Neonatal Nursing, 6*(1), B14–25.

Intrapartum CIII

All pregnant women with diabetes who require an intravenous (IV) infusion of insulin should have a mainline infusion of fluid that does not contain glucose. This may be utilized for intrapartum administration of fluid boluses when needed for maternal or fetal cardiovascular support. All medications (e.g., magnesium sulfate, Pitocin, antibiotics) should be mixed in a solution that does not contain glucose and then administered IV piggyback through the IV hub nearest to insertion of the mainline IV. In some instances, this may require two IV insertion sites. If required, glucose should be administered by a controlled IV infusion device.[27] Consultation with the pharmacy may be necessary to determine the compatibility of IV medications.

A common method of preparing insulin for infusion involves the addition of 100 units of regular insulin to a 100-mL bag of solution (normal saline) without glucose. This mixture delivers 1 unit of regular insulin for every 1 mL of fluid. Insulin should be administered by a controlled IV infusion device. Only regular insulin or rapid acting analogues can be administered intravenously. There is no advantage to using analogs, as their action is the same as regular insulin when given IV and regular insulin is less expensive. Insulin may be absorbed by the fluid administration container and the plastic tubing and filters. The amount of insulin absorbed depends on the concentration of insulin, the surface area of the container and tubing, and the duration of contact. To improve precision of insulin titration, the IV administration set (tubing, filter) is flushed with at least 20 mL of the solution prior to infusion, which allows maximum insulin binding to plastics within the lumen. During

insulin administration, women in active labor should be NPO. If allowed in early labor, non-caloric, clear liquids should be offered, such as water, broth, or tea.

The goal of continuous intravenous insulin administration during the intrapartum period is maintenance of maternal euglycemia. Clinical actions used to accomplish this goal are presented in Box 10-1. In the event the patient develops hypoglycemia, with a BG of less than 70 mg/dL, specific clinical interventions for hypoglycemia presented in Table 10-5 are indicated.[27]

TABLE 10-5

Treatment of Hypoglycemia

Current capillary BG less than 50 mg/dL	- Stop insulin infusion. - Infuse D_5 solution at 200 mL/hr. - Give 10 mL D_{50} IV push. - Check BG every 15 minutes and repeat treatment until it exceeds 70 mg/dL. - When BG is 70 mg/dL or above, restart insulin infusion at a lower algorithm.
Current capillary BG is 50 to 70 mg/dL	- Stop insulin infusion. - Infuse D_5 solution at 200 mL/hr. - Check capillary BG every 15–20 min until it exceeds 70 mg/dL twice. - When it reaches 70 mg/dL or above, restart insulin infusion per modified algorithm.

MEMORANDUM OF AGREEMENT FOR INSULIN PUMP USE DURING HOSPITALIZATION DO NOT SIGN WITHOUT READING AND UNDERSTANDING CONTENTS

Continuous Subcutaneous Insulin Infusion Pump Therapy Patient Agreement

For your safety and optimal medical care during this hospitalization, we request that you agree to the following recommendations. If you feel you cannot agree to these recommendations, we would like to treat your diabetes with insulin injections or intravenous insulin and request that you discontinue the use of your insulin pump.

During my hospital stay:

____ I and/or my support person understand the benefits of pump therapy which includes improved blood glucose control and flexibility of diabetes management.

____ I and/or my support person understand the risks of pump therapy which includes diabetic ketoacidosis, infusion site infection, hypoglycemia and mechanical malfunction.

____ I and/or my support person have been trained in insulin pump therapy.

My support person trained:_____

Pump make and model:_____

____ I and/or my support person will provide all necessary supplies including syringe reservoir, tubing, tape, and batteries. Supplies include enough for two tubing changes.

____ During my hospital stay the nurse will have access to all bolus doses, supplements, changes in basal rates and total daily dose that I and/or my support person have performed via the pump record flow sheet that I will maintain at all times.

____ The infusion set is changed every 48–72 hours or as needed for:
    a. Skin problems, or
    b. Two blood glucose readings failing to respond to supplement insulin greater than 200 mg/dL in a row.

____ I and/or my support person will report signs of low blood sugar to the nurse.

____ I and/or my support person will report signs of any pump problems to the nurse.

____ I and/or my support person will ask questions that I may have about the use of the pump or doctor's orders.

____ If I cannot manage the pump myself, I may have my support person assist me and the medical staff with the operation of the insulin pump on condition that he or she remains in the hospital during my entire hospital stay. If my support person cannot remain in the hospital, the insulin pump will need to be disconnected.

____ If I am not physically and/or mentally capable of maintaining insulin pump operations and functions, I understand that pump therapy will be discontinued. Alternative methods to manage diabetes such as insulin injections or insulin drip will be ordered by the physicians.

____ I also understand that my pump may be discontinued and a different insulin delivery given for any of the following:
    a. Doctor's order
    b. Changes in my judgment
    c. Changes in level of awareness or consciousness
    d. Any x-ray procedure may include pump removal by tubing disconnect and/or removal of pump and tubing per physician order
    e. Other reasons deemed necessary by medical staff

Patient's Name: _____ Date of birth ___ /___ /___

Patient Signature: _____ Date _____

Family Member Signature: _____ Date _____

Witness Signature: _____ Date _____

FIGURE 10-2   Example of a collaborative patient agreement. (Courtesy of M. Inturrisi.)

Continuous Subcutaneous Insulin Infusion (CSII)

CSII pump therapy allows the woman increased flexibility as compared with multiple daily injections (MDIs). The CSII pump is programmed to deliver basal rates of short-acting analogs to control BG during specific time intervals continuously for 24 hours. Multiple basal rates can be programmed to cover changing insulin needs throughout the day. Boluses are given for meals and snacks based on pre-prandial BG values and the number of carbohydrates to be consumed. The CSII pump then calculates the premeal insulin bolus based on insulin on board from other boluses, as well as the programmed insulin to carbohydrate ratio (ICR) and the programmed insulin sensitivity factor ("Correction" or ISF). More than 20 percent of people with type 1 diabetes mellitus use CSII, and those with type 2 diabetes mellitus are also increasing their use of CSII.

Perinatal clinicians will come in contact with many women who have chosen to use the CSII pump over MDIs. Most CSII pump users do not favor removal of their pumps when they are hospitalized. They experience anxiety, loss of control, and often experience a loss of glucose control as they are switched to MDIs or IV insulin. Efforts are being made across the nation to allow pump users to maintain use of their CSII pumps while hospitalized.[28]

Intrapartum CSII

Administration of insulin via CSII pump during the intrapartum period may be considered for select patients. A highly motivated pregnant woman with diabetes who has extensive successful experience in diabetes self-management and subcutaneous insulin infusion pump therapy may, if physically and mentally able, perform all skills necessary to utilize the pump during labor. In some clinical practice venues, these patients are required to sign a document that describes specific responsibilities inherent in this collaborative agreement.

An example of an agreement is presented in Figure 10-2. This particular example includes an agreement to have the patient designate a person who agrees to be available to adjust the pump if necessary. This is someone who has demonstrated competency in skills related to the continuous subcutaneous insulin infusion pump and who has subsequently been certified by the patient's health care providers.

Criteria that should be addressed when insulin pump management is planned for a patient requiring hospitalization include:

- the presence of a written order to leave the CSII pump in place
- the type of insulin to be administered (e.g., HumaLog, NovoLog, Apridra)
- the frequency of SMBG (e.g., at least hourly during labor)
- the desired BG range (e.g., 70 to 110 mg/dL)
- the insulin dosage (e.g., current basal rate, bolus amounts, supplemental basal rates, and supplemental bolus amounts)
- intravenous fluid management recommendations based on capillary BG values (Table 10-6)
- directions for an alternate source of rapid-acting/intermediate-acting insulin should use of the pump be discontinued for more than 1 hour.

TABLE 10-6

Intravenous Fluid Algorithm for Continuous Subcutaneous Insulin Infusion Pump Use in Labor

Blood Glucose Level* (mg/dL)	IV Dextrose	LR or NS	Capillary Blood Glucose Checks
<50	Disconnect insulin pump 200 mL/hr D_5 ½NS Or 10 mL D_{50} IV push	50 mL/hr	Every 15 min until above 70 mg/dL twice then Reconnect at a lower basal rate when stable
50–69	150 mL/hr D_5 ½NS	50 mL/hr	
70–89	100 mL/hr D_5 ½NS	50 mL/hr	Every 30 min until above 90 mg/dL twice
90–110	0-50 mL/hr D_5 ½NS	0–50 mL/hr	Every hour
>110	0/hr	125 mL/hr	Every 30 min until below 110 mg/dL
≥200 Check urine ketones and notify physician or primary care provider.	Patient will correct using insulin pump bolus at ⅓ to ½ her usual dose to a capillary BG target of 100 mg/dL. If BG above target after two corrections, notify physician or primary care provider.	125 mL/hr	Every 30 min until below 110 mg/dL

D_5 = 5 percent dextrose, D_{50} = 50 percent dextrose, LR = lactated Ringer's or Ringer's lactate solution, NS = normal saline solution (0.9 percent), min = minutes.

*Change IV fluid when BG reaches these levels.

When the patient is in early labor, all CSII pump settings (ICR, ISF, basal rates) may be reduced by 20 to 30 percent, with further reduction in all settings by 50 percent (from the last pre-labor settings). The pump should not be discontinued without provision for another source of rapid-acting insulin, since the woman with type 1 diabetes may quickly become insulin depleted, which may lead to development of DKA. In addition, other variables (e.g., stress, infection, or administration of betamethasone, terbutaline, or ephedrine) may cause insulin requirements to increase temporarily. Therefore, subsequent alterations in pump basal/bolus settings may be necessary. Further, when troubleshooting unexplained high BG values and the presence of ketonuria, clinicians should consider the possibility of poor absorption caused by an inadequate or overused infusion site, ineffective insulin, or an occluded or damaged infusion catheter. Absent a desired response following administration of an initial and repeat insulin bolus, the infusion set and insertion site should be changed. Elevations of BG are corrected by SQ injection of insulin until effective CSII infusion pump function is restored.[28]

If Cesarean birth is required, the CSII pump can be continued through the surgery. It may be discontinued briefly for no more than 1 hour if providers desire. Maintenance of euglycemia enhances recovery from surgery, wound healing, and decreased infection rate.[29]

After a vaginal birth, CSII settings may be reduced again by 10 to 20 percent from those used in labor. However, immediately following Cesarean birth, insulin requirements may remain elevated due to the stress of surgery. Monitoring 30- to 60-minute BG levels in the recovery period will assist in proper adjustment. Postpartum BG targets for women with type 1 or type 2 diabetes are below 100 mg/dL fasting/premeal and below 150 mg/dL 1 to 2 hours after the start of meals.

SUMMARY

The risk for adverse pregnancy outcomes in women with diabetes has declined considerably over the last few decades. However, the incidence of complications in this subset of women remains higher than in the general obstetric population. DKA is a relatively rare but severe complication of diabetes in pregnancy and is associated with a significant risk of perinatal morbidity and mortality. Prompt diagnosis and aggressive clinical management of DKA are essential to improve perinatal outcomes. Finally, satisfactory antepartum and intrapartum insulin management in patients with diabetes will minimize the fetal and neonatal complications associated with diabetes and the increased risk for ketoacidosis.

REFERENCES

1. Centers for Disease Control and Prevention. (2005). *Diabetes fact sheet.* Atlanta, GA: Author. Retrieved from http://www.cdc.gov/nchs
2. Gabbe, S. G., Mestman, H. J., & Hibbard, L. T. (1976). Maternal mortality in diabetes mellitus: An 18-year survey. *Obstetrics and Gynecology, 48,* 549–551.
3. Kamalakannan, D., Baskar, V., Barton, D., & Abdu, T. (2003). Diabetic ketoacidosis in pregnancy. *Postgraduate Medical Journal, 79*(934), 454–457.
4. Kilvert, J. A., Nicholson, H. O., & Wright, A. D. (1993). Ketoacidosis in diabetic pregnancy. *Diabetic Medicine, 10,* 278–281.
5. Cullen, M. T., Reece, E. A., Homko, C. J., & Sivan, E. (1996). The changing presentations of diabetic ketoacidosis during pregnancy. *American Journal of Perinatology, 13,* 449–451.
6. Maislos, M., Harman-Bohem, I., & Weitzman, S. (1992). Diabetic ketoacidosis: A rare complication of gestational diabetes. *Diabetes Care, 16,* 661–662.
7. Bernstein, I. M., & Catalano, P. M. (1990). Ketoacidosis in pregnancy associated with parenteral administration of terbutaline and betamethasone: A case report. *The Journal of Reproductive Medicine, 35,* 818–820.
8. Carroll, M. A., & Yeomans, E. R. (2005). Diabetic ketoacidosis in pregnancy. *Critical Care Medicine, 33,* 347–353.
9. Kitabchi, A. E., Umpierrez, G. E., Murphy, M. B., Barrett, E. J., Kreisberg, R. A., Malone, J. I., et al. (2001). Management of hyperglycemic crises in patients with diabetes. *Diabetes Care, 24,* 131–153.
10. Parker, J. A., & Conway, D. L. (2007). Diabetic ketoacidosis in pregnancy. *Obstetrics and Gynecology Clinics of North America, 34,* 533–543.
11. Metzger, B. E., Ravnikar, V., Vileisis, R. A., Ravnikar, V., & Freinkel, N. (1982). "Accelerated starvation" and the skipped breakfast in late normal pregnancy. *Lancet, 1*(8272), 588–592.
12. Catalano, P. M., Tyzbir, E. D., Roman, N. M., Amini, S. B., & Sims, E. A. (1991). Longitudinal changes in insulin release and insulin resistance in nonobese pregnant women. *American Journal of Obstetrics and Gynecology, 165,* 1667–1672.
13. Laffel, L. (1999). Ketone bodies: A review of physiology, pathophysiology and application of monitoring to diabetes. *Diabetes/Metabolism Research Review, 15,* 412–426.
14. Montoro, M. N., Myers, V. P., Mestman, J. H., Xu, Y., Anderson, B. G., & Golde, S. H. (1993). Outcome of pregnancy in diabetic ketoacidosis. *American Journal of Perinatology, 10,* 17–20.
15. Kitabchi, A. E. (2003). Ketosis-prone diabetes: A new subgroup of patients with atypical type 1 and type 2 diabetes. *The Journal of Clinical Endocrinology & Metabolism, 88,* 5087–5089.
16. Moore, T. R. (2004). Diabetes in pregnancy. In R. K. Creasy, R. Resnik, & J. D. Iams (Eds.), *Maternal-fetal medicine: Principles and practice* (5th ed.). Philadelphia: Saunders.
17. Chauhan, S. P., & Perry, K. G., Jr. (1995). Management of diabetic ketoacidosis in the obstetric patient. *Obstetrics & Gynecology Clinics of North America, 22,* 143–155.
18. Miodovnik, M., Lavin, J. P., Harrington, D. J., Leung, L. S., Seeds, A. E., & Clark, K. E. (1982). Effect of maternal ketoacidemia on the pregnant ewe and fetus. *American Journal of Obstetrics and Gynecology, 144,* 585–593.

19. Hughes, A. B. (1987). Fetal heart rate changes during diabetic ketoacidosis. *Acta Obstetricia ET Gynecologica Scandinavica, 66,* 71–73.

20. Takahashi, Y., Kawabata, I., Shinohara, A., & Tamaya, T. (2000). Transient fetal blood flow redistribution induced by maternal diabetic ketoacidosis diagnosed by Doppler ultrasonography. *Prenatal Diagnosis, 20*(6), 524–525.

21. Sefedini, E., Prašek, M., Metelko, Ž., Novak, B., & Pinter, Z. (2008). Use of capillary β-hydroxybutyrate for the diagnosis of diabetic ketoacidosis at emergency room: Our one-year experience. *Diabetologia Croatica, 37*(3), 73–78.

22. van der Meulen, J. A., Klip, A., & Grinstein, S. (1987). Possible mechanisms for cerebral oedema in diabetic ketoacidosis. *Lancet, 330*(8554), 306–308.

23. Enis, E. D., & Kreisberg, R. A. (2000). Ketoacidosis and hyperosmolarity. In D. LeRoith, S. I. Taylor, & H. M. Olefsky (Eds.), *Diabetes mellitus: A fundamental and clinical text* (2nd ed.). Philadelphia: Lippincott Williams & Wilkins.

24. Mathiesen, E. R., Christensen, A. B., Hellmuth, E., Hornnes, P., Stage, E., & Damm, P. (2002). Insulin dose during glucocorticoid treatment for fetal lung maturation in diabetic pregnancy: Test of an algorithm. *Acta Obstetricia ET Gynecologica Scandinavica, 81*(9), 835–839.

25. Curet, L. B., Izquierdo, L. A., Gilson, G. J., Schneider, J. M., Perelman, R., & Converse, J. (1997). Relative effects of antepartum and intrapartum maternal blood glucose levels on incidence of neonatal hypoglycemia. *Journal of Perinatology, 17*(2), 113–115.

26. Kitzmiller, J. L., Block, J. M., Brown, F. M., Catalano, P. M., Conway, D. L., Coustan, D. R., ... Kirkman, M. S. (2008). Managing preexisting diabetes for pregnancy: Summary of evidence and consensus recommendations for care. *Diabetes Care, 31*(5), 1060–1079.

27. Jovanovic, L. (2004). Glucose and insulin requirements during labor and delivery: The case for normoglycemia in pregnancies complicated by diabetes. *Endocrine Practice, 10*(Suppl. 2), 40–45.

28. Journsay, D. L. (1998). Continuous subcutaneous insulin therapy during pregnancy. *Diabetes Spectrum, 11,* 26–32.

29. Inturrisi, M. (Unpublished). Guidelines for the intrapartum management of women using continuous subcutaneous insulin infusion (CSII) pump therapy. Educator, CPMC Physician Foundation Sweet Success Program. maribeth.inturrisi@kcsf.edu.

CHAPTER 11

Anesthesia Emergencies in the Obstetric Setting

Patricia M. Witcher and Keith McLendon

Anesthesia complications are responsible for 1.6 to 2.3 percent of pregnancy-related deaths in the United States.[1,2] Although the overall rate of anesthesia-related mortality has declined over the last three decades, it remains the seventh leading cause of maternal mortality.[1,3] The overall decline in maternal mortality is more likely attributed to the increased use of regional anesthesia for vaginal and Cesarean deliveries. During this same period of time, maternal mortality associated with general anesthesia has remained unchanged.[2,3] Although regional anesthesia (spinal or epidural blockade) has contributed to reducing the overall mortality risk with anesthesia in the obstetric population, regional anesthesia still carries a clinically significant risk for death or permanent impairment. Profound physiologic adaptations during pregnancy, a higher incidence of co-morbid conditions, particularly obesity, and the absolute necessity of administering general anesthesia for emergency Cesarean deliveries are all major contributing factors to higher anesthesia-related mortality and morbidity rates that are observed in the overall obstetric population.[3]

GENERAL ANESTHESIA

General anesthesia carries a mortality rate that is 16 times higher in the obstetric population compared to the mortality rate that is attributed to complications from regional anesthesia in the non-obstetric population (32 deaths per 1,000,000 live births with general anesthesia compared to 1.9 deaths per 1,000,000 live births with regional anesthesia). The majority of anesthesia-related maternal deaths occur during Cesarean delivery. Fifty percent of anesthesia-related maternal deaths involve general anesthesia despite the fact that general anesthesia accounts for only 16 percent of anesthesia for Cesarean delivery.[4] Deaths typically occur during induction of anesthesia or during the immediate recovery period.[2] Airway complications continue to

account for more than 50 percent of those deaths.[1,5] The fixed mortality rate associated with general anesthesia and the high rate of airway complications in pregnant women can most likely be attributed to the fact that general anesthesia is the only appropriate choice the anesthesia provider can select when administering anesthesia to pregnant women who require an emergent procedure, particularly women who are at highest risk for complications. The most frequent airway problems encountered with general anesthesia are aspiration pneumonitis, failed endotracheal intubation, and inadequate ventilation.[2] As a result, general anesthesia in the obstetric setting is typically reserved for those situations that necessitate surgery without delay or when regional anesthesia is contraindicated or technically unfeasible.[6]

When the decision has been made to place the obstetric patient under general anesthesia for an emergent procedure, induction of general anesthesia is typically accomplished with the administration of a rapid-acting intravenous induction agent (e.g., thiopental or propofol) and a rapid-acting muscle relaxant (e.g., succinylcholine) in order to anesthetize the patient and provide adequate muscle relaxation for intubation. Resultant respiratory depression will quickly lead to severe hypoxemia if an adequate airway cannot be established and the loss of protective airway or gag reflex, from the administration of a general anesthetic, predisposes the pregnant woman to aspiration of stomach contents. Although uncommon, failed endotracheal intubation and gastric aspiration remain the leading causes of maternal mortality related to anesthesia.[7]

Difficult or Failed Intubation

Predisposing Factors and Pathophysiologic Consequences

Many congenital and acquired physical attributes can make ventilation and intubation difficult in any individual

Box 11-1. PREDISPOSING FACTORS FOR DIFFICULT AIRWAY OR FAILED INTUBATION

- Congenital or surgically induced facial or upper airway abnormalities
- Short neck
- Limited neck mobility
- Missing or protruding teeth
- Prominent incisors
- Receding chin
- Facial edema
- Swollen tongue
- Obesity
- Emergency

undergoing general anesthesia. These include congenital or surgically induced facial or upper airway abnormalities, a short neck, an overbite, and obesity. A more comprehensive list of predisposing factors for difficult airway management appears in Box 11-1.[8] Specific factors that lead to intubation and ventilation difficulties in pregnant women include pharyngeal edema, weight gain, increased breast size, full dentition, and rapid onset of hypoxemia during induction of general anesthesia.[9]

Obese individuals can be especially problematic to intubate and maintain an airway for, because of increased adipose deposition and hemodynamic and pulmonary physiologic alterations as well as to compensate for increased body mass.[10] Obesity is discussed more completely in Chapter 22 of this text. Increased fat deposition intra-abdominally, under the diaphragm or around the chest, reduces chest wall compliance. As a result of decreased lung expansion, both expiratory reserve volume (ERV, the additional amount of air that can be exhaled after a normal expiration) and functional residual capacity (FRC, the amount of air that remains in the lungs for gas exchange after normal tidal volume exhalation) decrease. Cardiac workload increases in order to meet the metabolic demands of a body with higher body mass. Increased oxygen consumption and increased production of carbon dioxide (CO_2) promote metabolic acidosis unless there is commensurate cardiovascular compensation, or an increase in cardiac output to sustain the metabolic demand. These changes result in less pH buffering capacity and a decreased reserve supply of oxygen which make these individuals more susceptible to develop hemodynamic instability or impaired oxygenation during the induction and administration of general anesthesia. Any condition that further reduces lung compliance, such as upward displacement of the diaphragm during supine positioning or hypoventilation, leads to more rapid arterial hemoglobin oxygen desaturation and acidosis.[11]

Although failed endotracheal intubation is recognized as the most common complication of general anesthesia, Mhyre and colleagues were unable to preoperatively identify a single case of failed intubation during elective or emergency induction of general anesthesia in their study of more than 850 maternal deaths in Michigan.[2] This emphasizes that preoperative airway assessment and classification, by an experienced anesthesia care provider, is a critically important aspect of the anesthetic process used to recognize certain features or characteristics that are likely to impair ventilation and intubation. Identification of a potentially difficult airway prompts the anesthesia provider to select an alternate method of anesthesia, such as regional anesthesia. If, however, general anesthesia must be performed, a plan of action can be organized and contemplated prior to actually encountering a difficult airway. The majority of deaths in Mhyre and colleagues' study involved airway difficulty stemming from hypoventilation or airway obstruction.[2] Many of the predisposing factors encountered in their study and in general are not readily identifiable in the pre-anesthesia assessment either because they are subtle or because there is insufficient time to perform a complete airway assessment, such as in an emergency. It is important to once again emphasize that the truly emergent Cesarean delivery remains a "fixed" risk factor for morbidity and mortality in the obstetric population because it's a level of risk that cannot be changed.

Predisposing Factors Specific to Pregnancy

The incidence of failed intubation in obstetrics is 8 to 10 times higher than in the general population.[6,8] Certain physiologic changes during pregnancy, in addition to the emergent nature of many obstetric procedures, carry a greater predisposition to discover a difficult airway and/or a difficult intubation. Pregnancy-specific predisposing factors for a difficult airway are summarized in Box 11-2.[8,12] Increases in circulating blood volume and peripheral arterial vasodilation contribute to nasal mucosal vascular engorgement, which leads to edema of the oral and nasal pharynx, larynx,

Box 11-2. FAILED OR DIFFICULT INTUBATION: PREGNANCY-SPECIFIC RISK FACTORS

- Laryngeal edema
- Vascular engorgement of nasal mucosa
- Breast engorgement
- Decreased expiratory reserve volume and functional residual capacity
- Increased oxygen consumption
- Vena cava compression in supine position

and trachea.[13] These changes may obscure laryngoscopic visualization of the larynx, promote nasal obstruction in the supine position, or hinder mask ventilation.[8] Preeclampsia, in particular, is associated with even further increases in laryngeal edema because of endothelial injury and increased capillary permeability.[12] Laryngeal edema may be further compounded by prolonged strenuous expulsive effort during the second stage of labor or a concurrent respiratory tract infection. Elevated estrogen levels also contribute to hypervascularity in the upper airways, potentially increasing the likelihood that the pregnant woman will bleed during laryngoscopy, impairing visualization of anatomic landmarks that guide endotracheal intubation.[12,13] Hormonal changes during pregnancy promote changes that result in breast engorgement, which may complicate insertion of the laryngoscope if the enlarged breasts fall back against the woman's neck.[8]

Difficult or failed intubation may result in hypoventilation and/or apnea for a sufficient period to result in hypoxemia. Pregnant women are particularly vulnerable to hypoxemia because they have a significantly diminished reserve supply of oxygen arising from numerous physiologic changes in the respiratory system during pregnancy. Upward displacement of the diaphragm by the gravid uterus decreases both the residual volume (the amount of air remaining in the lungs after forceful exhalation [ERV]) and functional residual capacity (FRC). These physiologic decreases in lung volumes promote closure of the small airways and atelectasis.[13] Coupled with the state of increased oxygen consumption during normal pregnancy, these changes lead to rapid arterial oxygen desaturation in the setting of apnea or hypoventilation. Further decreases in FRC and the resultant potential for impaired oxygenation are perpetuated when oxygen consumption increases further, such as during active labor or with supine positioning because of further upward displacement of the diaphragm.[14] Inferior vena cava compression in the supine position decreases cardiac output, potentiating hemodynamic instability; this necessitates lateral displacement of the gravid uterus by placing at least a 15-degree wedge under the pregnant woman's right hip during general anesthesia. Hemodynamic instability further contributes to maternal and fetal deterioration during periods of hypoventilation. Since pregnancy evokes hyperventilation and decreased partial pressure of carbon dioxide ($PaCO_2$), metabolic compensation for respiratory alkalemia during pregnancy results in decreased pH buffering capacity, which more readily leads to metabolic acidosis in the setting of decreased oxygenation or hypoperfusion.[8,15] The physiologic changes accompanying pregnancy may also impact endotracheal intubation and ventilation.[16]

Management of Recognized or Anticipated Difficult Airway

Most airway emergencies occur when a difficult airway is not assessed and/or not recognized before the induction of general anesthesia. It is estimated that most cases of difficult intubation should be recognized and anticipated prior to induction. Many methods are used to evaluate and therefore identify a potentially difficult intubation. These include five basic methods that most, if not all anesthesia providers, use to evaluate the airway. The first is mouth opening. The woman is instructed to open her mouth; adequate opening requires at least three fingerbreadths. The second is neck extension. She should be able to lean her head far back enough to look directly at the ceiling. Third, an oropharyngeal exam is conducted by the anesthesia provider in order to visualize airway structures and classify her airway, in order to determine her risk for difficult intubation (Mallampati classification). The anesthesia provider attempts to visualize the patient's tonsillar pillars, uvula, and soft palate. Maximum identification of these structures yields a lower numerical Mallampati score (I); the score progressively increases numerically with less visualization of these structures (up to IV). A Mallampati classification of III or IV typically identifies a patient who will be difficult to intubate. The fourth method is the measured distance from the tip of the mandible to the top of the thyroid cartilage, or the thyromental distance. Thyromental distance of at least three fingerbreadths is desirable; a smaller distance indicates that the larynx will be displaced anteriorly, thereby making intubation difficult. Finally, the anesthesia provider assesses the compliance of the tissue located between the mandible and the superior aspect of the thyroid cartilage. If this tissue is supple, then displacement of the tongue with the laryngoscope during intubation should be easy. If, however, the tissue is taut, tongue displacement by the laryngoscope is anticipated to be difficult, which impairs the ability to visualize the vocal cords during intubation.[8]

Regional anesthesia is the anesthetic mode of choice in order to minimize the exposure of the patient to the risk of general anesthesia complications. Early epidural catheter placement during labor is advocated by anesthesia providers because it not only provides excellent pain relief for the laboring woman, but it can also rapidly be dosed and converted to a "Cesarean delivery–worthy" epidural should an unscheduled or emergency Cesarean delivery become necessary. The need to initiate general anesthesia remains a potential, thereby requiring maintenance of skills in airway management and ventilation with anticipation of unexpected airway problems. Restrictions or contraindications (Box 11-3) for regional anesthesia necessitate contemplation of non-routine methods of providing general anesthesia if a difficult airway is recognized before induction of anesthesia if time permits.[12]

Box 11-3. CONTRAINDICATIONS TO REGIONAL ANESTHESIA

- Severe hypovolemia
- Acute hemorrhage
- Coagulopathy
- Sepsis
- Infection over the lumbar spine
- Spinal pathology or history of extensive spinal surgery
- Emergency

Awake intubation followed by general anesthesia allows for maintenance of normal airway reflexes and allows the pregnant patient to continue to spontaneously ventilate while she is intubated. This method is time consuming and requires extensive patient preparation and cooperation. Awake intubation is typically performed using a flexible fiberoptic bronchoscopy. A flexible bronchoscope allows for the direct visualization of the vocal cords and provides a conduit for insertion of the endotracheal tube. Other adjuncts that facilitate successful intubation may be utilized by the anesthesia provider when a difficult intubation or difficult airway management is anticipated, especially when there are significant time constraints or when the difficult intubation or airway management is unexpected.

The laryngeal mask airway (LMA) is heralded by anesthesia providers as one of the best recent inventions for ventilatory support. The LMA is a tube with an inflatable cuff that is connected to a soft tube that is blindly inserted into the pharynx. The inflated cuff sits over the laryngeal inlet and does not need to be inserted into the trachea in order to support ventilation. The LMA can often provide a patent airway when all other methods have failed and the trachea cannot be intubated. The LMA can be used as a conduit for tracheal intubation, typically aided with a fiberoptic bronchoscope.[8]

An intubating LMA (ILMA) is a specific type of LMA that can be used to secure an airway when the individual cannot be intubated using direct vision laryngoscopy. The ILMA has unique features that provide better conditions for intubation than the standard LMA.[10] Another type of LMA is the ProSeal LMA. This LMA has a modified cuff and a drainage tube designed to isolate the airway from the digestive tract—a feature particularly useful in obstetric anesthesia because of the increased risk for gastric aspiration among pregnant women.

Other adjuncts or procedures for intubation include the Glidescope, Lightwand, and cricothyrotomy. Cricothyrotomy is typically reserved for intubating and establishing an airway when all other methods to intubate the patient have failed. Ultimately, cricothryotomy is the only remaining choice when an adequate airway cannot be established. Death is likely to ensue if the decision to proceed with a cricothryotomy is made too late.

Management of the Unexpected Difficult Airway

An unexpected difficult airway and/or intubation can rapidly deteriorate into an emergency situation when the anesthesia provider receives the pregnant patient in the operating room for an elective, urgent, or emergent Cesarean delivery. One of the most common scenarios preceding the unexpected airway in the obstetric population is the requirement to abandon epidural anesthesia and convert emergently to general anesthesia because of an inadequate epidural that was originally dosed for a Cesarean delivery. Unexpected, difficult intubation can present an emergency that requires rapid mobilization of supplies and resources to assist the anesthesia provider. Ideally, obstetric care providers are familiar with the location of difficult airway equipment and can assist the anesthesia provider if an anesthesiologist or another anesthetist is not immediately available. Obstetric nursing staff may be requested to assist the anesthesiologist or anesthetist with mask ventilation or be asked to apply cricoid pressure during intubation and/or ventilation during an emergency situation.

Inability to intubate the pregnant woman's trachea on the first attempt is typically accompanied by maternal hypoxemia. This requires immediate attention and usually is quickly reversed with effective positive-pressure mask ventilation with 100 percent inspired oxygen and properly applied cricoid pressure before intubation is attempted again. Cricoid pressure is accomplished by locating the cricothyroid membrane (which is the depression just inferior to the thyroid cartilage, or Adam's apple). Then, the thumb and index finger are placed on the lateral aspects of the cricoid cartilage, applying firm backward pressure on the cricoid cartilage (the only true cartilaginous rings in the larynx) to compress the underlying esophagus against the cervical vertebrae.[16] The assistant uses his or her other hand to support the patient's neck posteriorly in order to achieve appropriate cricoid pressure. Cricoid pressure is initiated upon the anesthesiologist's or anesthetist's request (usually upon the patient's loss of consciousness) and maintained throughout the entire induction period until the endotracheal tube (ETT) cuff is inflated and the anesthesia provider has confirmed appropriate ETT placement and informs the assistant that cricoid pressure is no longer required. If ETT placement is unsuccessful, cricoid pressure is maintained during mask ventilation by the anesthesiologist or anesthetist.[8] Cricoid pressure prevents passive regurgitation of gastric contents. However, cricoid pressure should be released if the patient is actively vomiting, since application of cricoid pressure during vomiting can lead to esophageal rupture if it is maintained under these circumstances. The importance of maintaining cricoid pressure on the anesthetized obstetric patient until an airway can be secured cannot be over-emphasized, because the airway remains unprotected until the trachea has been successfully intubated and the ETT cuff has been appropriately inflated. Although cricoid pressure can be beneficial and help the anesthetist or anesthesiologist intubate the anesthetized patient, it also can serve as an insurmountable hindrance if it is not appropriately applied.[17]

Repeated laryngoscopy attempts carry the potential for increased laryngeal edema and/or bleeding, which further complicate repeated attempts at intubation. If the patient cannot be intubated and she and her fetus are stable, one option is to continue mask ventilation with oxygen and awaken the patient. If, however, the woman and/or fetus are not stable, other alternatives include proceeding with general anesthesia with (1) continued mask ventilation and cricoid pressure, (2) ventilation through an LMA or a ProSeal LMA with cricoid pressure (it is difficult to properly seat a standard LMA with cricoid pressure), or (3) cricoid pressure and intubation with a Lightwand, Glidescope, or through an ILMA. Cricothyrotomy (tracheostomy), followed by securing an airway and ventilation by traditional means or by jet ventilation, is performed as a last resort if the obstetric patient's airway cannot be maintained through other methods indicated above.[8] The most significant complication associated with cricothyrotomy is not technical, but rather irreversible anoxic brain injury because the decision to proceed with cricothyrotomy is often made after several other attempts to maintain an airway have been tried and failed, with resultant worsening of hypoxia.

Perioperative Pulmonary Aspiration

Predisposing Factors and Pathophysiology

Curtis Mendelson, an obstetrician in California, reported the incidence of aspiration in a group of obstetric patients, primarily those who had been placed under general anesthesia, in a landmark publication in the 1940s.[18] The condition he described now bears his name, *Mendelson's syndrome*. Mendelson correctly postulated that the morbidity and mortality of gastric aspiration primarily depends on three variables:

- the chemical nature of the aspirate
- the physical nature of the aspirate
- the volume of the aspirate.

Increased acidity of aspirate (pH less than 2.5), particulate matter in the aspirate, and higher volume of aspirate are individually and collectively associated with increased incidence of adverse outcome.

Aspiration of acidic gastric contents induces cellular damage at the alveolar level and perpetuates an ongoing inflammatory response extending beyond the acute phase. Interstitial edema and cellular debris (e.g., fibrin, neutrophils) arise from alveolar-capillary damage and disrupt surfactant activity, which reduces lung compliance and increases intrapulmonary shunting, which leads to hypoxemia. The cellular debris within the alveoli may partially occlude the airway, which further perpetuates hypoxemia. A secondary pulmonary inflammatory response ensues immediately after cellular death, which creates even more pulmonary damage through the release of oxygen free radicals and proteases. Eventual deterioration into adult respiratory distress syndrome (ARDS) becomes more likely with increased volume and/or increased acidity of the aspirate. Aspiration of particulate matter compounds the severity of pulmonary damage (especially if the aspirate is acidic), commencing with frank bronchial obstruction and progressive inflammatory-mediated damage which leads to hypoxemia and hypercapnia. While the pathophysiologic consequences are less pronounced with aspiration of neutral, nonparticulate matter, the transient bronchospasm and impaired surfactant activity decrease oxygenation and also can potentially lead to further hypoxemia.[19] This subject is also discussed in Chapter 9 of this text.

Pregnant women are at a three-fold increased risk for perioperative aspiration because of several physiologic alterations in the gastrointestinal system.[19] Uterine enlargement alters the normal anatomic position of the distal esophagus in relation to the diaphragm and impairs lower esophageal sphincter (LES) competence, thereby predisposing the pregnant woman to regurgitation of stomach contents.[12] Increased progesterone levels during pregnancy decrease LES tone.[9] The LES is a muscular valve located at the bottom of the esophagus where it joins the top of the stomach. When the LES is closed, it prevents regurgitation of food and liquid back into the esophagus and eliminates the possibility of aspiration of gastric contents into the trachea. A rise in intra-abdominal pressure may also impair LES competence and predispose the pregnant woman to regurgitation of gastric contents. Weight gain during pregnancy and, to a greater degree, obesity promote increased intra-abdominal pressure. Labor pain and/or the concurrent administration of opioids for labor analgesia delay gastric emptying, which are also contributing factors to the elevation of intra-abdominal pressure and increased gastric volume in the obstetric population. Finally, the placenta produces gastrin, which stimulates the stomach to secrete hydrochloric acid, further increasing the acidity of gastric contents during pregnancy.[12,19] Any of these predisposing factors, combined with an obtunded gag reflex during general anesthesia, increase the risk of

TABLE 11-1

Risk Factors for Perioperative Aspiration

Predisposing Risk Factors	• Difficult airway • Previous esophageal surgery (e.g., tracheostomy) • Esophageal pathology • Concurrent administration of opioids • Recent oral intake prior to surgery • Obesity • Diabetes • Depressed level of consciousness • Operative procedure • Gastroesophageal reflux disease
Predisposing Risk Factors Specific to Pregnancy	• Upward displacement of stomach by gravid uterus • Placental production of gastrin leads to increased gastric acid secretion • Labor pain leads to delayed gastric emptying

perioperative aspiration in the pregnant woman, even if she has no symptoms of gastroesophageal reflux during pregnancy.[19,20] Predisposing risk factors for aspiration are summarized in Table 11-1.[12,19–21]

Aspiration Prophylaxis

Historically, anesthesiologists have considered a particulate gastric fluid with a pH of less than 2.5 and a gastric volume greater than 25 mL (0.4 mL/kg) to be primary risk factors for aspiration pneumonitis. Four primary principles that Mendelson advocated over 65 years ago continue to provide the foundation of anesthesia practice today:

- withholding food during labor
- administration of non-particulate antacids
- preferential use of regional anesthesia over general anesthesia for surgery
- competent administration of general anesthesia.[18]

While it is disputed whether or not pregnancy is associated with delayed gastric emptying without other risk factors, the American Society of Anesthesiologists (ASA) Task Force on Obstetric Anesthesia outlines specific recommendations for aspiration prophylaxis in the pregnant patient population, in order to minimize the risk of perioperative aspiration.[12,19,21] The ASA obstetric practice guidelines focus on anesthetic management during labor and vaginal and Cesarean deliveries, as well

as postpartum analgesia. Although the ASA Task Force on Obstetric Anesthesia concludes that clear liquid intake during labor does not increase the risk of maternal anesthesia complications, the necessity and/or timing of Cesarean delivery cannot always be predicted, which generates consensus regarding specific oral intake restrictions during labor and delivery. Ingestion of solid food is discouraged during labor and within 6 to 8 hours of scheduled Cesarean delivery or postpartum tubal ligation. Most anesthesiologists will restrict solid food intake for 8 hours prior to elective surgery in the pregnant patient, including Cesarean section and postpartum tubal ligation, because of the higher incidence of esophageal reflux in pregnant women, which is further compounded by physiological changes that have been discussed earlier. Clear liquids during labor in modest amounts are acceptable but are typically withheld 4 hours before induction of general anesthesia when possible (i.e., scheduled Cesarean delivery or postpartum tubal ligation). The presence of additional risk factors for aspiration (as described in Table 11-1) may result in further restrictions in oral intake.

Pharmacologic agents directed at reducing gastric acidity may also be routinely or selectively incorporated (based upon the presence of additional risk factors) into the preoperative preparation of the pregnant patient. These include administration of a non-particulate antacid (i.e., sodium citrate or sodium bicarbonate) or H_2 receptor antagonists (i.e., cimetidine, ranitidine, and famotidine).[21] A total of 30 mL of sodium citrate neutralizes 255 mL of gastric contents at a pH of 1.0 with an immediate onset of action and duration of 30 to 60 minutes; this duration is increased with the concomitant administration of opioids. The rapid onset of action and short duration of activity necessitate administration of non-particulate antacids just before taking the patient to the operating suite for a Cesarean delivery. Histamine receptor antagonists increase gastric pH to greater than 2.5 in about 60 percent of patients after 60 minutes and in 90 percent of patients after 90 minutes.[9] The ASA Task Force on Preoperative Fasting concluded that antacids are efficacious in raising gastric pH but they do not reduce gastric volume.[22] Therefore, metoclopramide may also be considered because it not only accelerates gastric emptying and promotes gastric motility, it also increases LES tone. However, prior administration of an opioid significantly antagonizes the effect of metoclopromide, thereby limiting its selection by anesthesia providers.[23]

Initial Clinical Presentation and Management

Perioperative aspiration usually occurs during induction of anesthesia and is typically seen in a patient with a difficult airway and/or in a patient who is difficult to intubate. Therefore, the anesthesia provider is usually actively managing the pregnant woman's airway when gastric contents are regurgitated into the hypopharynx. Despite the best preventive effort of a qualified anesthetist and/or anesthesiologist, the regurgitated contents of the stomach are often directly aspirated from the hypopharynx into the trachea, and down into the patient's lungs. Bronchospasm is the first clinical sign that is appreciated by the anesthesia provider, occurring immediately after the patient has aspirated the regurgitant material into her lungs. Typically, significant hypoxemia quickly ensues. Aspiration of particulate matter may necessitate removal of the large particles with rigid bronchoscopy to alleviate airway obstruction. Hypoxia, specifically inability of the patient to maintain hemoglobin arterial oxygen saturation (SaO_2) at 90 percent or greater, is typically accompanied by tachycardia. The first step in supportive intervention is directed at restoring oxygenation. If the aspiration is large and full of particulate matter, it may be impossible to maintain adequate oxygenation and can lead to hemodynamic instability. Restoring oxygenation is the primary supportive intervention followed by achieving a normotensive state (i.e., intravenous fluids and vasopressors).[19]

Most of these patients will require mechanical ventilation postoperatively. Vasopressors may be initiated in the operating room for hemodynamic support, after preload has been optimized with administration of crystalloids, and may be required after admission to an intensive care unit. Ventilatory and hemodynamic support may be required for a brief or extended period of time postoperatively in an intensive care unit. Morbidity and mortality following gastric aspiration during Cesarean delivery are directly related to:

- pH of gastric aspirate
- content of gastric aspirate
- whether or not the gastric aspirate was particulate
- degree of hypoxia encountered in the operating room
- length of time the patient was hypoxic
- whether or not the patient develops acute respiratory distress syndrome (ARDS).[19]

REGIONAL ANESTHESIA AND ANALGESIA

Regional anesthesia is the preferred anesthetic in obstetric patients undergoing a surgical procedure, because it significantly reduces maternal morbidity and mortality from airway complications associated with general anesthesia. Neuraxial blockade (epidural or spinal) can provide varying degrees of sensory and motor blockade by changing the specific local anesthetic used, changing the concentration of the local anesthetic, or by adding different agents to the local anesthetic such as an opioid or epinephrine. The sensory level of an epidural can be increased by administering larger volumes of local anesthetic through the epidural needle or epidural catheter. Regional *analgesia* alleviates pain during labor and vaginal delivery and typically extends to the T10 dermatome, which corresponds to the level of the umbilicus. Regional *anesthesia* for Cesarean delivery requires a denser level of sensory blockade and is accomplished by the administration of a more concentrated local anesthetic and must be extended to the T4 dermatome, which corresponds to the nipple line.[6]

Spinal anesthesia involves a single injection of local anesthetics, with or without an opioid, into the subarachnoid space, or the space that is adherent to the inside of the dura that contains the spinal cord and cerebral spinal fluid (CSF). This is illustrated in Figure 11-1. The injection of local anesthetic into the CSF quickly and easily penetrates unsheathed nerve fibers, thereby providing rapid onset of an exceptionally dense neural blockade. The speed of onset and relatively short duration of anesthesia needed are well suited for providing regional anesthesia for Cesarean delivery or postpartum tubal ligation. It may also be favored by anesthesia providers for Cesarean delivery because it involves less technical skills than the performance of an epidural blockade.

Epidural blockade involves the administration of local anesthetics, with or without opioids and/or epinephrine, through a catheter that is placed into the epidural space, which is the space between the supporting ligaments of the vertebrae and dura matter (see Fig. 11-1). Epidural blockade offers an advantage for continuous or more prolonged pain relief during labor and has a slower onset of action, which may reduce the incidence and severity of hypotension from sympathetic blockade when compared to a spinal anesthetic.[12] However, compared to spinal anesthesia, a larger volume of local anesthetic is required in order to penetrate the protective

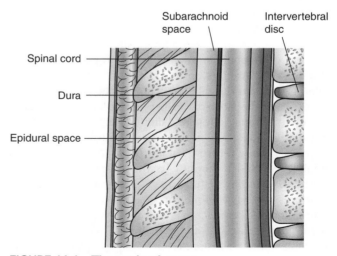

FIGURE 11-1 The epidural space.

FIGURE 11-2 Schematic of hypotension.

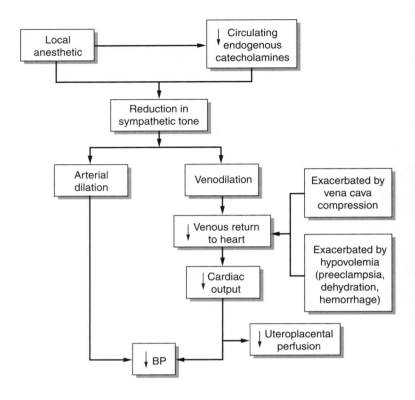

sheathing of the nerves before sensory analgesia is achieved. If the local anesthetic is inadvertently injected into the systemic circulation or subarachnoid space, significant side effects and potentially life-threatening complications can ensue.[24] Combined spinal–epidural (CSE) anesthesia blends the benefits of rapid onset spinal anesthesia and/or analgesia by dosing local anesthetic through the epidural catheter that is threaded into the epidural space following subarachnoid injection of a local anesthetic and/or an opioid.[12]

Epidural Mediated Hypotension

Sympathectomy accompanies sensory blockade at or around the dermatome level of anesthesia for a spinal or an epidural and provokes hypotension in about 10 to 30 percent of pregnant women receiving regional analgesia during labor.[7] Reduction in sympathetic tone mediates venous and arterial dilation. The effects of venodilation predominate because of the increased blood-filling capacity of the venous system and limited ability of the venous system to maintain autonomous tone.[23] Venodilation reduces venous return of blood (from increased venous pooling of blood volume) to the heart and therefore decreases cardiac output, manifesting as hypotension. Compression of the inferior vena cava by the gravid uterus further obstructs venous return. The decrease in maternal cardiac output contributes to a decrease in uteroplacental perfusion, often manifested as fetal heart rate decelerations or bradycardia. (See Figure 11-2 for

further elaboration on the physiologic consequences of sympathetic blockade.)[7] Decreased circulating volume is further exacerbated in the setting of pathophysiologic processes that promote increased capillary permeability (i.e., preeclampsia, sepsis) or depleted intravascular blood volume (i.e., diabetic ketoacidosis, hemorrhage).

The hemodynamic effects from sympathetic blockade after the placement of an epidural in the pregnant woman are predictable, and pre-hydration with at least 500 to 1000 mL of crystalloid solution is routinely employed to help decrease the incidence and severity of hypotension. Other prophylactic measures include lateral maternal positioning to alleviate vena cava compression or lateral uterine displacement with a wedge under the right hip during Cesarean delivery, along with frequent monitoring of maternal blood pressure and observation of fetal heart rate responses. Treatment of hypotension involves further intravenous volume expansion (if initial infusion was inadequate), and/or the administration of vasopressors, such as phenylephrine (intravenous doses of 50 to 100 mcg) or ephedrine (intravenous doses of 5 to 10 mg).[7] Both agents are acceptable for treating neuraxial-mediated hypotension. Ephedrine stimulates alpha and beta receptors. As a result, the increase in blood pressure from vasoconstriction may be accompanied by tachycardia. Phenylephrine mediates vasoconstriction without the beta effects on the heart. Therefore, phenylephrine may be more beneficial in the setting of reflex maternal

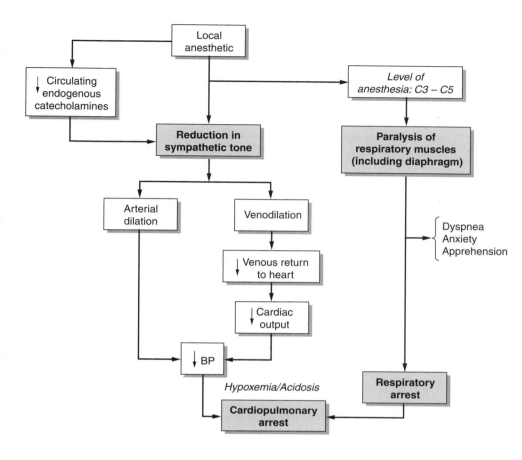

FIGURE 11-3   High spinal block.

tachycardia that accompanies hypotension, because it mediates vasoconstriction without beta stimulation, thereby decreasing or having no effect on heart rate as maternal blood pressure returns to normal.[7]

High Spinal Block

A high spinal block occurs from an "overdosage" of local anesthetic into the epidural or subarachnoid space.[25] The most common cause of a high spinal is the unintentional and unrecognized entrance through the dura into the subarachnoid (spinal) space either during the insertion of the epidural needle or when the epidural catheter is inserted through the epidural needle during the administration of an epidural. In both cases, the bolus injection of local anesthetic directly through the misplaced epidural needle or through the inadvertent placement of an epidural catheter into the subarachnoid space has the potential to result in a high spinal.[26] Epidural anesthesia requires a larger dosage of local anesthetic (5 to 10 times greater) than what would be administered for a spinal block to obtain an adequate anesthetic level for Cesarean delivery. The risk for high spinal block increases if the anesthesia provider who is administering epidural anesthesia does not recognize inadvertent insertion of the epidural needle or catheter into the subarachnoid space and

proceeds with injection of the higher dosage of local anesthetic. A test dose of 3 mL of 1.5 percent lidocaine is typically administered by the anesthesia provider through the newly inserted epidural catheter to make certain the catheter was not inadvertently placed into the subarachnoid space or blood vessel before proceeding further.

Epidural and spinal blocks rise in a segmental fashion. The potential consequence of a high spinal is paralysis of the respiratory muscles, including the diaphragm, which is innervated by the phrenic nerves (C3 to C5). Paralysis of the accessory muscles of respiration typically occurs first, often promoting apprehension, anxiety, and dyspnea. As the level of anesthesia climbs above C5 up to C3, the patient completely loses her ability to breathe and can no longer protect her airway, hence the term *total spinal*. The result of bilateral diaphragmatic paralysis is respiratory arrest. Respiratory depression or failure may be accompanied by circulatory collapse. The extremely high level of sympathetic blockade, which can actually progress to a complete sympathectomy, can lead to profound hypotension through extensive arterial and venodilation throughout the pregnant woman's body with a subsequent decrease in cardiac output.[7] If untreated, profound hypotension quickly progresses to cardiopulmonary arrest. See Figure 11-3 for the physiologic description of a high spinal block.

FIGURE 11-4 Initial management of high spinal block.

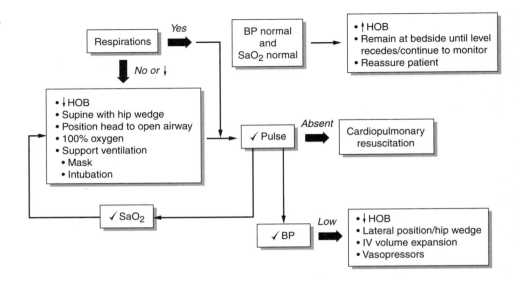

The pregnant patient's complaint of dyspnea immediately after administration of regional anesthesia requires an urgent evaluation to exclude a high spinal as the cause. The assessment begins with an evaluation of the patient's oxygenation and hemodynamic status as well as the level of anesthesia. Numbness and weakness of the fingers and hands indicates that the level of anesthesia has risen to the cervical level (C6 to C8), close to the level of innervation of the diaphragm.[7] Maternal vital signs should be evaluated, most importantly the SaO_2 and blood pressure, if she is conscious and breathing. If she is normotensive with a normal SaO_2 of greater than 95 percent, reassurance and elevation of the head of the bed to a high Fowler's position are appropriate. The head of the bed should be lowered if she is hemodynamically unstable (i.e., hypotension, tachycardia, bradycardia or pulselessness). A modified Trendelenberg position (feet elevated, head of bed lowered) increases venous return to the heart which subsequently increases cardiac output. Additionally, lowering the head of the bed is necessary to properly establish a patent airway and emergently provide mask ventilation. If the patient has lost consciousness or can no longer protect her airway she will need to be intubated and require mechanical ventilation. If she progresses to cardiopulmonary arrest, chest compressions with a rigid back support and manual lateral uterine displacement should be performed immediately. Emergent Cesarean delivery should follow in order to provide adequate cardiopulmonary resuscitation. CPR during pregnancy is presented in detail in Chapter 14 of this text. The initial management of a high spinal block is illustrated in Figure 11-4.

Although a high spinal is an event with low occurrence, the ASA's review of closed anesthesia malpractice claims revealed that cardiac arrest during neuraxial blockade is the most common damaging event with regional anesthesia.[27] The majority of claims resulted in death or permanent brain damage. Seventy percent of severe bradycardic events and/or cardiac arrests occurred with high spinal blockade. The majority of these events (82 percent) occurred outside of the operating room and recognition was delayed in more than half of these cases (55 percent), leading to a delay in resuscitation in the majority of cases. It is therefore imperative that health care professionals providing care to pregnant women receiving regional analgesia and anesthesia maintain skills in assessing the level of anesthesia, identifying and treating hemodynamic instability, and establishing adequate ventilation. Equipment and pharmacologic agents commonly required to accomplish these procedures should be immediately available and functioning properly.

Systemic Local Anesthetic Toxicity

Most often, systemic toxicity during the administration of a regional anesthetic occurs when the local anesthetic is inadvertently injected into a blood vessel instead of the epidural space.[28] Systemic local anesthetic toxicity affects both the central nervous system (CNS) and the cardiovascular system. Usually, CNS manifestations precede cardiovascular consequences and/or symptoms. These physiologic reactions are summarized in Figure 11-5. CNS toxicity ordinarily progresses in a dose-dependent manner. The patient typically will initially complain of ringing in her ears, then slurred speech, followed by excitation, disorientation with bizarre behavior, and finally tonic–clonic seizures. Sometimes the initial vascular bolus of local anesthetic is large enough to produce immediate convulsion as the first neurotoxic

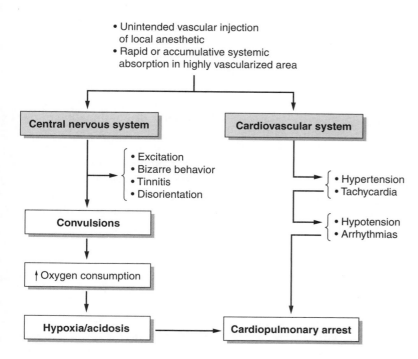

- Unintended vascular injection of local anesthetic
- Rapid or accumulative systemic absorption in highly vascularized area

Central nervous system

- Excitation
- Bizarre behavior
- Tinnitis
- Disorientation

Convulsions

↑Oxygen consumption

Hypoxia/acidosis

Cardiovascular system

- Hypertension
- Tachycardia

- Hypotension
- Arrhythmias

Cardiopulmonary arrest

FIGURE 11-5 Systemic local anesthetic toxicity.

clinical symptom after injection of the local anesthetic. Administration of a local anesthetic that contains epinephrine may result initially in cardiovascular toxicity that manifests as hypertension and tachycardia, which are followed by hypotension and dysrhythmias. Administration of a local anesthetic without epinephrine may also yield dysrhythmias or cardiac arrest as the first signs of cardiovascular toxicity. Either CNS or cardiovascular involvement may rapidly deteriorate into cardiopulmonary arrest.[7]

CNS involvement is more common than cardiovascular system involvement. However, bupivacaine is more cardiotoxic than other local anesthetics and may quickly lead to cardiopulmonary arrest secondary to arrhythmias.[29] Treatment of anesthetic toxicity is based on symptoms. The pregnant patient's report of the sensation of ringing in her ears or behavioral changes warrants immediate cessation of injection of the local anesthetic. Convulsions are treated initially with supportive interventions, such as maintaining a patent airway and implementing supplemental oxygen, followed by administration of intravenous thiopental (25 to 50 mg) or benzodiazepine (2 to 5 mg midazolam or diazepam). Respiratory depression and/or arrest should be anticipated since seizure activity causes a precipitant rise in $PaCO_2$ levels leading to hypercapnia and subsequent hypoxia, thereby necessitating immediate preparation for mask ventilation and endotracheal intubation. Succinylcholine administration may be necessary to provide paralysis for intubation and alleviate increased muscular activity if the seizure is not abated with initial interventions. Although muscle relaxants, such as

succinylcholine, block the peripheral musculoskeletal manifestations of a seizure, they do not stop the CNS seizure activity. Hemodynamic and cardiovascular support includes intravenous volume expansion, vasopressors and, in the event of complete cardiovascular collapse, chest compressions. The fetal heart rate should be evaluated only after the pregnant patient has been stabilized. Consideration should be given to delivery of the fetus within 5 minutes after the pregnant patient has suffered cardiopulmonary arrest.[7]

Intravenous lipid emulsion therapy is considered in a patient who has a toxic blood level of a local anesthetic and is presently in cardiopulmonary arrest unresponsive to standard resuscitative measures. Infusion of Intralipid is an emerging treatment for systemic local anesthetic toxicity with successful outcomes in many case reports.[29–32] Currently, guidelines and understanding of this innovative treatment are somewhat limited because of the infrequency of local anesthetic toxicity. Therefore, there is limited exposure and experience with this therapy among anesthesia providers. It is hypothesized that the intravenous lipid emulsion reverses the local anesthetic-induced myocardial depression by either binding to the local anesthetic directly, thereby reducing free plasma levels of local anesthetic, or by directly supplying the increased myocardial energy needs.[33] The timing of initiation and dosage have not achieved full consensus; however, Intralipid infusions are now often an early consideration during the resuscitation of a patient suffering from local anesthetic toxicity in order to achieve the best possible outcome. Intralipid is intravenously infused using the following guideline: bolus of 20 percent Intralipid at a rate of 1.2 to 2 mL/kg followed by a continuous infusion rate of 0.25 to 0.5 mL/kg/min.[34,35]

Epidural Hematoma

Neurologic damage, including paralysis, from regional anesthesia following vaginal or Cesarean delivery is rare, and it is often exceedingly difficult to conclude whether the etiology of the neurologic damage is anesthesia- or obstetrical-related (i.e., compression nerve injuries from positioning and/or traction).[7,24,36] Most neurologic deficits are transient and mild.[7,28] Although very infrequent, neurologic injury from spinal cord compression by an epidural hematoma of the spine that develops after administration of an epidural or spinal anesthesia is the most common cause of permanent neurologic injury associated with regional anesthesia.[7,27] An epidural hematoma most likely occurs from accidental puncture of an epidural vessel.[7] The gravid uterus leads to engorgement of the epidural venous plexus during pregnancy and may further promote inadvertent puncture of an epidural vessel.[12] The majority of epidural hematomas that develop during regional anesthesia are attributed to coagulation abnormalities, either from an intrinsic pathologic condition or from the administration of an antiplatelet or anticoagulant agent.[27]

Epidural hematomas can develop and/or extend during epidural catheter insertion or removal.[37] As a result, several precautions are typically implemented in order to avoid this complication. Although data are limited as to whether a platelet count can help predict this complication, determination of a platelet count may be helpful in patients at risk for developing a coagulopathy, including those with hypertensive disorders of pregnancy. Research has not been able to absolutely support a specific threshold platelet count that prohibits regional anesthesia. The decision to proceed with regional anesthesia is determined by the anesthesia provider who bases his or her assessment on the patient's history, physical examination, and clinical findings that predispose the pregnant woman to abnormalities in coagulation.[21]

Routine questioning about the patient's self-administered or medically prescribed antiplatelet agents, such as aspirin or ibuprofen and anticoagulant administration is ascertained on admission in order to determine if further laboratory evaluation of the patient's coagulation status is warranted and if the woman is a candidate for regional analgesia/anesthesia. While no specific recommendations exist for timing of antiplatelet drugs and regional anesthesia, the American Society of Regional Anesthesia recommends that regional anesthesia be delayed for at least 24 hours after the last

dose of low-molecular-weight heparin (LMWH) if higher-dose therapy was employed during the antepartum period. Regional needle insertion is delayed for at least 12 hours after the last dose of LMWH when lower doses or prophylactic doses have been administered.[38,39] Postoperative initiation of anticoagulation should be delayed for at least 2 hours after discontinuation of the epidural catheter. If, however, anticoagulation has been initiated after surgery, before removal of the epidural catheter, the anesthesiologist should be consulted prior to removal of the catheter. Typically, the epidural catheter remains in place until about 10 to 12 hours after the last dose of LMWH.[22] Similar precautions may be observed for unfractionated heparin.[39]

Recognition and Initial Management

Spinal cord compression by an epidural hematoma can interfere with both sensory and motor nerve impulses. Clinical signs that are consistent with spinal cord compression from an epidural hematoma include decreased muscle strength, loss of sensation in the lower extremities, or voiding difficulties.[12,40,41] Unfortunately, these clinical signs and symptoms are also consistent with the effects of a properly performed regional anesthetic without the formation of an epidural hematoma. Duration of the sensory or motor blockade from regional anesthesia is variable and is based on numerous factors, such as individual characteristics of the patient, the local anesthetic agent used, and whether or not other agents are added to the local anesthetic, such as epinephrine or opioids. The diagnosis of an epidural hematoma after a regional anesthetic is often delayed because the duration of a regional anesthetic can be so variable and the clinical presentation of an adequate regional block and an epidural hematoma with spinal cord compression often indistinguishable. Therefore, the best recommendation is to further investigate a prolonged sensory or motor blockade that is out of proportion for a particular local anesthetic administered, which typically is based upon the institution's and anesthesia providers' common routines and practices.[7,27]

Sensory and/or motor deficit is expected as a normal finding following surgery performed under regional anesthesia. Assessment for regression of the level of anesthesia and gradual resolution of sensory or motor blockade is required prior to discharging the patient from the recovery room to the postpartum area. If the regional block has not completely resolved by the time of discharge from the recovery room, the postpartum obstetric nurse should continue to evaluate for regression of the sensory and/or motor deficit. Failure of the level of anesthesia to demonstrate continued regression, persistent motor or sensory block that outlasts the anticipated duration of anesthesia, or new onset of motor or sensory deficits after such regression has occurred, requires prompt notification of the anesthesia provider to facilitate early diagnosis of an epidural hematoma, which hopefully may prevent permanent neurologic impairment.[7,27,40] If an epidural hematoma is suspected, a thorough neurologic exam by the anesthesia provider is typically followed by either magnetic resonance imaging (MRI) or a computed tomography (CT) scan. Confirmation of spinal compression by an epidural hematoma should generate an immediate request for a neurosurgical consult. Although conservative management of an epidural hematoma with corticosteroids and physical therapy in the nonobstetric population has been described in the medical literature, emergency laminectomy and surgical evacuation of the hematoma is often required.[7,27,37]

SUMMARY

The preferred selection of regional anesthesia over general anesthesia for obstetric surgery significantly reduces the overall anesthesia-related maternal mortality rate. Despite the decreased mortality risk, regional analgesia and anesthesia are still associated with a low but clinically significant rate of adverse outcomes. True obstetric emergencies reduce or eliminate the time needed for an appropriate preoperative assessment and evaluation by the anesthesia provider. Not surprisingly, many of these patients are more likely to have an unsuspected difficult airway and/or to be difficult to intubate. Additionally, pregnancy results in many physiologic changes that increase the potential for anesthesia-related complications, thereby necessitating a certain level of anticipation and preparation among obstetric as well as anesthesia health care providers. Understanding the potential impact of the physiologic alterations of pregnancy upon anesthesia as well as comprehending the fundamentals of hemodynamic stabilization, airway management and ventilation, and oxygenation in the obstetric population is essential for all professionals who provide care to pregnant women undergoing obstetric anesthesia. This preparation and understanding promote collaborative efforts between the anesthesia and obstetric care team members directed at achieving the best possible outcome for the woman and her unborn child.

REFERENCES

1. Berg, C. J., Chang, J., Callaghan, W. M., & Whitehead, S. J. (2003). Pregnancy-related mortality in the United States, 1991–1997. *Obstetrics and Gynecology, 101*(2), 289–296.
2. Mhyre, J. M., Riesner, M. N., Polley, L. S., & Naughton, N. N. (2007). A series of anesthesia-related maternal deaths in Michigan, 1985–2003. *Anesthesiology, 106*(6), 1096–1104.
3. D'Angelo, R. (2007). Anesthesia-related maternal mortality: A pat on the back or a call to arms? *Anesthesiology, 106*(6), 1082–1083.
4. Hughes, S. C., Levinson, G., & Rosen, M. A. (2002). *Schnider and Levinson's anesthesia for obstetrics* (4th ed.). Philadelphia: Lippincott Williams & Wilkins.
5. Berg, C. J., Atrash, H. K., Koonin, L. M., & Tucker, M. (1996). Pregnancy-related morality in the United States, 1987-1990. *Obstetrics and Gynecology, 88*(2), 161–167.
6. American College of Obstetrics and Gynecology. (2002). Obstetric analgesia and anesthesia. *Obstetrics and Gynecology, 100*, 177–191.
7. Hawkins, J. L., Goetzyl, L., & Chestnut, D. H. (2007). Obstetric anesthesia. In S. G. Gabbe, J. R. Niebyl, & J. L. Simpson (Eds.), *Obstetrics: Normal and problem pregnancies* (5th ed., pp. 396–427). Philadelphia: Churchill Livingstone Elsevier.
8. Thomas, J. A., & Hagberg, C. A. (2009). The difficult airway: Risks, prophylaxis, and management. In D. H. Chestnut, L. S. Polley, L. C. Tsen, & C. A. Wong (Eds.), *Obstetric anesthesia: Principles and practice* (4th ed., pp. 651–676). St. Louis, MO: Mosby.
9. Gaiser, R. (2009). Physiologic changes of pregnancy. In D. H. Chestnut, L. S. Polley, L. C. Tsen, & C. A. Wong (Eds.), *Obstetric anesthesia: Principles and practice* (4th ed., pp. 15–36). St. Louis, MO: Mosby.
10. Frappier, J., Guenoun, T., Journois, D., Philippe, H., Aka, E., Cadi, P., et al. (2003). Airway management using the intubating laryngeal mask airway for the morbidly obese patient. *Anesthesia and Analgesia, 96*(5), 1510–1515.
11. Lamvu, G., Zolnoun, D., Boggess, J., & Steege, J. F. (2004). Obesity: Physiologic changes and challenges during laparoscopy. *American Journal of Obstetrics and Gynecology, 191*(2), 669–674.
12. Wickwire, J. C., & Gross, J. B. (2004). From preop to postop: Cesarean delivery from the anesthesiologist's point of view. *Clinical Obstetrics and Gynecology, 47*(2), 299–316.
13. Norwitz, E. R., Robinson, J. N. (2010). Pregnancy-induced physiologic alterations. In M. A. Belfort, G. Saade, M. R. Foley, J. P. Phelan, & G. A. Didley III (Eds.), *Critical care obstetrics* (5th ed.). Malden, MA: Blackwell Science.
14. Pacheco, L. D., Ghulmiyyah, L. (2010). Ventilator management in critical illness. In M. A. Belfort, G. Saade, M. R. Foley, J. P. Phelan, & G. A. Didley III (Eds.), *Critical care obstetrics* (5th ed.). Malden, MA: Blackwell Science.
15. Hull, S. B., & Bennett, S. (2007). The pregnant trauma patient: Assessment and anesthetic management. *International Anesthesiology Clinics, 45*(3), 1–18.
16. Stoelting, R. K., Dierdorf, S. F., & McCammon, R. L. (2002). *Anesthesia and co-existing disease.* Philadelphia: Lippincott Williams & Wilkins.
17. McCaul, C. L., Harney, D., Ryan, M., Moran, C., Kavanagh, B. P., Boylan, J. F. (2005). Airway management in the lateral position: A randomized controlled trial. *Anesthesia & Analgesia, 101*(4), 1221–1225.
18. Mendelson, C. I. (1946). The aspiration of stomach contents into lungs during obstetric anesthesia. *American Journal of Obstetrics and Gynecology, 52,* 191–205.
19. O'Sullivan, G., & Hari, M. S. (2009). Aspiration: Risk, prophylaxis, and treatment. In D. H. Chestnut, L. S. Polley, L. C. Tsen, & C. A. Wong (Eds.), *Obstetric anesthesia: Principles and practice* (4th ed., pp. 633–650). St. Louis, MO: Mosby.
20. Sakai, T., Planinsic, R. M., Quinlan, J. J., Handley, L. J., Kim, T. Y., & Hilmi, I. A. (2006). The incidence and outcome of perioperative pulmonary aspiration in a university hospital: A 4-year retrospective analysis. *Anesthesia & Analgesia, 103*(4), 941–947.

21. American Society of Anesthesiologists Task Force on Obstetric Anesthesia. (2007). Practice guidelines for obstetric anesthesia: An updated report by the American Society of Anesthesiologists Task Force on Obstetric Anesthesia. *Anesthesiology, 106*(4), 843–863.

22. Practice guidelines for preoperative fasting and the use of pharmacologic agents to reduce the risk of pulmonary aspiration: Application to healthy patients undergoing elective procedures: A report by the American Society of Anesthesiologist Task Force on Preoperative Fasting. (1999). *Anesthesiology, 90*(3), 896–905.

23. Hey, V. M., Ostock, D. G., Mazumder, J. K., & Lord, W. D. (1981). Pethidine, metoclopramide and gastro-osophageal sphincter. A study in healthy volunteers. *Anaesthesia, 36*(2), 173–176.

24. Brown, D. L. (2010). Spinal, epidural, and caudal anesthesia. In R. D. Miller, L. I. Eriksson, L. A. Fleisher, J. P. Wiener-Kronish, & W. L. Young (Eds.), *Miller's anesthesia* (7th ed., pp. 1611–1638). Philadelphia: Churchill Livingstone.

25. Cunningham, F. G., Leveno, K. J., Bloom, S. L., Hauth, J. C., Rouse, D., & Spong, C. Y. (2010). *Williams obstetrics* (23nd ed., pp. 444–463). New York: McGraw-Hill.

26. Guay, J. (2006). The epidural test dose: A review. *Anesthesia and Analgesia, 102*(3), 921–929.

27. Lee, L. A., Posner, K. L., Domino, K. B., Caplan, R. A., & Cheney, F. W. (2004). Injuries associated with regional anesthesia in the 1980s and 1990s: A closed claim analysis. *Anesthesiology, 101*(1), 143–152.

28. Reynolds, F. (2009). Neurologic complications of labor, delivery, and regional anesthesia. In D. H. Chestnut, L. S. Polley, L. C. Tsen, & C. A. Wong (Eds.), *Obstetric anesthesia: Principles and practice* (4th ed., pp. 701–726). St. Louis, MO: Mosby.

29. Foxall, G., McCahon, R., Lamp, J., Hardman, J. G., & Bedforth, N. M. (2007). Levobupivacaine-induced seizures and cardiovascular collapse treated with Intralipid (R). *Anaesthesia, 62*(5), 516–518.

30. Litz, R. J., Popp, M., Stehr, S. N., & Koch, T. (2006). Successful resuscitation of a patient with ropivacaine-induced asystole after axillary plexus block using lipid emulsion. *Anaesthesia, 61*(8), 800–801.

31. Rosenblatt, M. A., Abel, M., Fischer, G. W., Itzkovich, C. J., & Eisenkraft, J. B. (2006). Successful use of 20% lipid emulsion to resuscitate a patient after presumed bupivacaine-related cardiac arrest. *Anesthesiology, 105*(1), 217–218.

32. Weinberg, G., Paisanthasan, C., Feinstein, D., & Hoffman, W. (2004). The effect of bupivacaine on myocardial tissue hypoxia and acidosis during ventricular fibrillation. *Anesthesia & Analgesia, 98*(3), 790–795.

33. Stehr, S. N., Ziegeler, J. C., Pexa, A., Oertel, R., Deussen, A., Koch, T., et al. (2007). The effects of lipid infusion on myocardial function and bioenergetics in 1-bupivacaine toxicity in the isolated rat heart. *Anesthesia and Analgesia, 104*(1), 186–192.

34. Rowlingson, J. C. (2007). Resuscitation of local anesthetic toxicity with Intralipid. American Society of Anesthesiologists. *ASA Newsletter, 71*(10). Retrieved from http://www.asahq.org/Knowledge-Base/Subspecialty-Interests/ASA/Resuscitation-of-Local-Anesthetic-Toxicity-with-Intralipid.aspx

35. Corman, S. L., & Skledar, S. J. (2007). Use of lipid emulsion to reverse local anesthetic-induced toxicity. *The Annals of Pharmacotherapy, 41*(11), 1873–1877.

36. Borg-Stein, J., Dugan, S., & Gruber, J. (2005). Musculoskeletal aspects of pregnancy. *American Journal of Physical Medicine & Rehabilitation, 84*(3), 180–192.

37. Herbstreit, F., Kienbaum, P., Peter, M., & Peters, J. (2002). Conservative treatment of paraplegia after removal of an epidural catheter during low-molecular-weight heparin treatment. *Anesthesiology, 97*(3), 733–734.

38. Ginsberg, J. S., & Bates, S. M. (2003). Management of venous thromboembolism during pregnancy. *Journal of Thrombosis and Haemostasis, 1*(7), 1435–1442.

39. American College of Obstetricians and Gynecologists. (2000). Thromboembolism in pregnancy. *ACOG Practice Bulletin, 19*, 1–16.

40. Litz, R. J., Hubler, M., Koch, T., & Albrect, M. (2001). Spinal-epidural hematoma following epidural anesthesia in the presence of antiplatelet and heparin therapy. *Anesthesiology, 95*(4), 1031–1033.

41. Inoue, K., Yokoyama, M., Nakatsuka, H., & Goto, K. (2002). Spontaneous resolution of epidural hematoma after continuous epidural analgesia in a patient without bleeding tendency. *Anesthesiology, 97*(3), 735–737.

CHAPTER 12

Induction of Labor

Washington C. Hill and Carol J. Harvey

Induction of labor has become one of the most common obstetric interventions in the United States. Moreover, the rate of labor induction has more than doubled from 9.5 percent in 1990 to 22.3 percent in 2005, and currently accounts for approximately 24 percent of infants born between 37 and 41 weeks gestation in the U.S.[1] The rate of induction of labor has also increased for preterm gestations. The increased incidence of induction of labor has been attributed to a number of factors, including the availability and widespread use of cervical ripening agents, logistical issues, and an increase in medical and obstetric indications for delivery. Such variables may be particularly applicable for women who have complications or critical illness during pregnancy.

A number of methods to ripen the cervix and to initiate or augment the labor process have been studied. Nonpharmacologic approaches to cervical ripening and labor induction have included herbal compounds, homeopathy, castor oil, hot baths, enemas, sexual intercourse, breast stimulation, acupuncture, and transcutaneous nerve stimulation. Mechanical methods have included cervical dilators (e.g., laminaria, synthetic hygroscopic agents such as Lamicel or Dilapan, single balloon catheters [e.g., Foley], dual balloon catheters [e.g., Atad Ripener Device], and surgical modalities (e.g., membrane stripping and amniotomy). Of these, only mechanical methods have demonstrated efficacy for timely cervical ripening or induction of labor. Surgical methods possess some efficacy in cervical ripening; however, membrane stripping and amniotomy work to efface the cervix over longer periods of time (i.e., days and weeks for membrane stripping), or only in select population groups (i.e., amniotomy in multiparous women). Pharmacologic methods, specifically prostaglandins, are used more often than other methods for cervical ripening and induction of labor due to their high rate of efficacy and ease of use.[2] Multiple randomized studies and meta-analyses have evaluated the benefits, risks, complications, and fetal outcomes of the synthetic prostaglandins (PGE_1 and PGE_2) with or without concomitant oxytocin infusions, providing clinicians more information on their use in clinical practice.[2–5] Although actual or potential risks may be associated with any method of cervical ripening or labor induction, they should be weighed against the potential benefit to the mother and/or the fetus in a specific clinical situation.

A detailed discussion of each modality available for cervical ripening or induction of labor is beyond the scope of this chapter; however, a list of cervical ripening modalities and recommendations on use or avoidance, based on current Cochrane Database Reviews on labor induction and cervical ripening methods, is presented in Table 12-1. A more detailed summary of specific methods of induction of labor can be found in Table 12-2.

Attention is also directed to recent professional organization practice guidelines for evidence-based information regarding cervical ripening or labor induction methods, including the associated risks, benefits, and safety considerations. The Association of Women's Health, Obstetric and Neonatal Nurses (AWHONN) has published a comprehensive state of the science third edition monograph on cervical ripening and induction and augmentation of labor, and the American College of Obstetricians and Gynecologists (ACOG) has published an updated Practice Bulletin on induction of labor.[2,6]

Although there are current publications to advance evidence-based practice in induction and augmentation of labor, similar recommendations for its application to high-risk and critically ill patients are absent. Labor induction in such women must be individualized based on the patient's specific clinical condition, her capacity to respond to physiologic stress, the gestational age of the pregnancy, and the degree of risk discussed with the patient during the informed consent process. To

(text continued on page 194)

TABLE 12-1

Effectiveness of Methods for Cervical Ripening

Effective methods	Mechanical cervical dilators	• *Osmotic dilators*
		  • Laminaria
		  • Lamicel
		• *Balloon devices*
		  • Foley catheter with 30- to 80-mL balloon volume
		  • Double balloon device (Atad Ripener Device)
		• *Extra-amniotic saline infusion*

	Administration of synthetic prostaglandins	PGE$_2$, dinoprostone (Cervidil, Prepidil)
	Administration of synthetic PGE$_1$ analog	Misoprostol (Cytotec)
Methods that may be effective*	Acupuncture	
	Herbal supplements	Limited data; need prospective trials
	Relaxin	• Four studies, 267 women • Role of relaxin is unclear; more studies needed • No difference in Cesarean section rates compared to placebo, but more likely to change cervix to "favorable"
	Sexual intercourse	• Only one study of 28 women • Impact remains uncertain
Ineffective methods†	Amniotomy alone	
	Corticosteroids	
	Castor oil, bath and/or enema	• Only one trial on castor oil, poor methodology • More studies are needed
	Homeopathy	• Only two trials, study quality low • Insufficient evidence, more studies needed

*Some data exist to support use of the method, more data are needed from larger studies with appropriate methodology, or data are conflicting.

†No data exist, conflicting data exist, or data exist that refute its purported effect.

Adair, C. D. (2000). Nonpharmacologic approaches to cervical priming and labor induction. *Clinical Obstetrics And Gynecology, 43,* 447–454.

Alfirevic, Z., & Weeks, A. (2006), Oral misoprostol for induction of labour. *Cochrane Database of Systematic Reviews*, Issue 2. Art. No.: CD001338. doi: 10.1002/14651858.CD001338.pub2.

Boulvain, M., Kelly, A. J., & Irion, O. (2008). Intracervical prostaglandins for induction of labour. *Cochrane Database of Systematic Reviews*, Issue 1. Art. No.: CD006971. doi: 10.1002/14651858.CD006971.

Boulvain, M., Kelly, A. J., Lohse, C., Stan, C. M., & Irion, O. (2001). Mechanical methods for induction of labour. *Cochrane Database of Systematic Reviews*, Issue 4. Art. No.: CD001233. doi: 10.1002/14651858.CD001233.

Bricker, L., & Luckas, M. (2000). Amniotomy alone for induction of labour. *Cochrane Database of Systematic Reviews*, Issue 4. Art. No.: CD002862. doi: 10.1002/14651858.CD002862.

French, L. (2001). Oral prostaglandin E2 for induction of labour. *Cochrane Database of Systematic Reviews*, Issue 2. Art. No.: CD003098. doi: 10.1002/14651858.CD003098.

Hofmeyr, G. J., & Gulmezoglu, A. M. (2010). Vaginal misoprostol for cervical ripening and induction of labour. *Cochrane Database of Systematic Reviews*, Issue 10. Art. No.: CD000941. doi: 10.1002/14651858.CD000941.pub2.

Kavanagh, J., Kelly, A. J., & Thomas, J. (2001). Sexual intercourse for cervical ripening and induction of labour. *Cochrane Database of Systematic Reviews*, Issue 2. Art. No.: CD003093. doi: 10.1002/14651858.CD003093.

Kavanagh, J., Kelly, A. J., & Thomas, J. (2006). Corticosteroids for cervical ripening and induction of labour. *Cochrane Database of Systematic Reviews*, Issue 2. Art. No.: CD003100. doi: 10.1002/14651858.CD003100.pub2.

Kelly, A. J., Kavanagh, J., & Thomas, J. (2001). Castor oil, bath and/or enema for cervical priming and induction of labour. *Cochrane Database of Systematic Reviews*, Issue 2. Art. No.: CD003099. doi: 10.1002/14651858.CD003099.

Kelly, A. J., Kavanagh, J., & Thomas, J. (2001). Relaxin for cervical ripening and induction of labour. *Cochrane Database of Systematic Reviews,* Issue 2. Art. No.: CD003103. doi: 10.1002/14651858.CD003103.

Luckas, M., & Bricker, L. (2000). Intravenous prostaglandin for induction of labour. *Cochrane Database of Systematic Reviews*, Issue 4. Art. No.: CD002864. doi: 10.1002/14651858.CD002864.

Smith, C. A. (2003). Homoeopathy for induction of labour. *Cochrane Database of Systematic Reviews*, Issue 4. Art. No.: CD003399. doi: 10.1002/14651858.CD003399.

Smith, C. A., & Crowther, C. A. (2004). Acupuncture for induction of labour. *Cochrane Database of Systematic Reviews*, Issue 1. Art. No.: CD002962. doi: 10.1002/14651858.CD002962.pub2.

TABLE 12-2

Cochrane Database Reviews on Selective Labor Induction and Cervical Ripening Methods

Method	Study/Outcomes	Reviewer Comments
Buccal or sublingual misoprostol (*Off-label use*)	Muzonzini, G., & Hofmeyr, G.J. (2004). Buccal or sublingual misoprostol for cervical ripening and induction of labour. *Cochrane Database of Systematic Reviews,* Issue 4. Art. No.: CD004221. DOI: 10.1002/14651858.CD004221.pub2 ***Total trials:*** Three trials (n = 502) *Buccal or sublingual misoprostol (off-label; route not FDA-approved) compared with vaginal misoprostol (two different doses) and oral misoprostol (two doses)* Buccal misoprostol group had slightly fewer Cesarean sections compared with vaginal misoprostol group. No other differences in outcomes. Sublingual compared to oral administration of the same dose: Women in the sublingual misoprostol group were more likely to have a vaginal delivery in 24 hours compared to the vaginal misoprostol group. However, when a smaller dose of misoprostol was studied there were no differences between the two groups.	There are limited data (only three trials) to make conclusions; however, the studies support sublingual misoprostol as being at least as effective as an identical oral dose. More studies are needed to evaluate the side effects, rates of complications and safety of sublingual or buccal misoprostol before it is used clinically. ***Summary point:*** Neither sublingual nor buccal misoprostol should be used in clinical practice (outside of a registered and approved study) until more data are made available on its overall safety.
Intracervical prostaglandins	Boulvain, M., Kelly, A.J., & Irion, O. (2008). Intracervical prostaglandins for induction of labour. *Cochrane Database of Systematic Reviews*, Issue 1. Art. No.: CD006971. DOI: 10.1002/14651858. CD006971 ***Total trials:*** 56 trials (n = 7,738) *Intracervical PGE_2 compared with placebo: 28 trials (n = 3,764)* Women who received intracervical PGE_2 were more likely to have a vaginal delivery in 24 hours compared with women in the placebo group. In a subgroup of women with intact membranes and unfavorable cervices, fewer Cesarean sections were required with PGE_2 Although the risk for tachysystole was increased in the intracervical PGE_2 group, there was no increased risk for tachysystole with FHR changes in the group. *Intracervical PGE_2 compared with intravaginal PGE_2: 29 trials (n = 3,881)* More women in the intravaginal PGE_2 group had a vaginal delivery within 24 hours compared to women in the intracervical PGE_2 group. There was no difference between the two groups in Cesarean sections or tachysystole with or without FHR changes.	Intracervical PGE_2 is more effective compared with a placebo. However, intravaginal PGE_2 is superior to intracervical PGE_2. ***Summary point:*** A better alternative than intracervical prostaglandins is intravaginal prostaglandins.

(continued)

TABLE 12-2 (Continued)

Cochrane Database Reviews on Selective Labor Induction and Cervical Ripening Methods

Method	Study/Outcomes	Reviewer Comments
Mifepristone (anti-progestins) *(Off-label use)*	Hapangama, D., & Neilson, J.P. (2009). Mifepristone for induction of labour. *Cochrane Database of Systematic Reviews,* Issue 3. Art. No.: CD002865. DOI: 10.1002/14651858.CD002865.pub2. ***Total trials:*** 10 trials (n = 1,108) *Mifepristone compared with placebo* Women who received mifepristone were more likely to ripen their cervix and be in labor at 48 hr compared to those who received a placebo. The effect continued to 96 hr. The mifepristone group was less likely to need augmentation with oxytocin or require a Cesarean section. Women in the mifepristone group were more likely to have an operative vaginal delivery compared to the placebo group, but were less likely to have a Cesarean section as a result of induction failure. There were no differences in neonatal outcomes between groups, but there were more abnormal FHR patterns in the mifepristone group. There is insufficient evidence to support a specific dose. However, 200 mg mifepristone administered as a single dose may be the lowest effective dose for cervical ripening.	Similar to other agents studied for induction of labor, there is insufficient information on the occurrence of uterine rupture or dehiscence in the reviewed studies. The study findings are of interest due to the evidence that suggests mifepristone is more effective than placebo to prevent induction failure. There are insufficient data available from clinical trials to support the use of mifepristone to induce labor. ***Summary point:*** There are not enough data to recommend the use of mifepristone at this time. More studies are needed that compare mifepristone with current meds, and that report the effect on the fetus and neonate.
Oral misoprostol *(Off-label use)*	Alfirevic, Z., Weeks A. (2006). Oral misoprostol for induction of labour. *Cochrane Database of Systematic Reviews,* Issue 2. Art. No.: CD001338. DOI: 10.1002/14651858.CD001338.pub2. ***Total trials:*** 51 *Oral misoprostol compared to placebo: 7 trials (n = 669)* Women administered oral misoprostol were more likely to have vaginal delivery within 24 hr compared to placebo; and had a lower rate of Cesarean section. *Oral misoprostol compared with vaginal dinoprostone: 10 trials (n = 3,368)* Oral misoprostol group less likely to need Cesarean section. Oral misoprostol may take longer for delivery compared to vaginal dinoprostone, but no other significant differences. *Oral misoprostol compared with intravenous oxytocin: 8 trials (n = 1,026)* No difference between the two groups except for an increase in meconium-stained fluid in the oral misoprostol group in women with ruptured membranes. *Oral misoprostol compared to vaginal PGE$_2$: 26 trials (n = 5,096)* Women who took oral misoprostol compared to IV oxytocin had no differences in maternal and neonatal outcomes or rates of vaginal deliveries. There were fewer neonates with low Apgar scores in the oral misoprostol group compared with vaginal misoprostol. May be due to less uterine tachysystole with and without FHR changes in the oral misoprostol group, but data are difficult to interpret.	Oral misoprostol is an effective induction agent. It is as effective as vaginal misoprostol and results in fewer Cesarean sections than vaginal dinoprostone. If risk for infection is high, oral misoprostol is preferred over vaginal misoprostol. Misoprostol remains off-label for induction of labor. Providers may choose to select dinoprostone due to its licensed status. ***Summary point:*** Unlike other drugs for induction and augmentation of labor, oral misoprostol is inexpensive and stable at room temperature. It can be administered orally or vaginally, and the oral route may be safer than giving it vaginally. Oral misoprostol is an effective drug for induction of labor, but the lack of large randomized trials leaves many questions regarding its safety.

TABLE 12-2 (Continued)

Cochrane Database Reviews on Selective Labor Induction and Cervical Ripening Methods

Method	Study/Outcomes	Reviewer Comments
Oral prostaglandin E2 *(Experimental)*	French, L. (2001). Oral prostaglandin E2 for induction of labour. *Cochrane Database of Systematic Reviews,* Issue 2. Art. No.: CD003098. DOI: 10.1002/14651858. CD003098 ***Total studies:*** 19 (15 compared oral or IV oxytocin with or without amniotomy) Quality of studies was poor. Only seven studies had allocation concealment. Only two studies stated the providers or subjects were blinded to treatment group. In the composite comparison of oral PGE_2 versus all oxytocin treatments (with and without amniotomy), oral PGE_2 was slightly more successful for having a vaginal delivery in 24 hr. There were no clear benefits of oral prostaglandin compared to the other methods for induction. Oral prostaglandin resulted in more GI complications, including vomiting.	Oral PGE_2 resulted in more GI effects (especially vomiting) compared with placebo or oxytocin. No clear benefit of oral PGE_2 compared to other methods of labor induction. ***Summary point:*** Overall, there is little to recommend the use of PGE_2 for the induction of labor. Other methods have been shown to be beneficial and effective in induction and augmentation, and most do not produce the significant side effects of nausea, vomiting and diarrhea associated with this drug.
Oxytocin alone	Alfirevic, Z., Kelly, A.J., & Dowswell, T. (2009). Intravenous oxytocin alone for cervical ripening and induction of labour. *Cochrane Database of Systematic Reviews,* Issue 4. Art. No.: CD003246. DOI: 10.1002/14651858.CD003246.pub ***Total trials:*** 61 trials (n = 12,819) Compared to expectant management, oxytocin increased the likelihood of vaginal birth in 24 hr. Significant increase in number of women requiring epidural anesthesia. More women were satisfied with oxytocin as an induction method. *Oxytocin compared with prostaglandins* Compared to prostaglandins, oxytocin decreased the likelihood of vaginal birth in 24 hr (prostaglandins superior to oxytocin alone). *Compared with intracervical prostaglandins* Oxytocin alone likely increased the induction failure rate and the rate of Cesarean sections. Overall, use of prostaglandins compared to oxytocin alone increases the rate of vaginal birth in 24 hr.	Most studies included women with rupture of membranes; some evidence that vaginal prostaglandins increased infection in mothers and babies; and increased use of antibiotics. The role of prostaglandins in infection needs further study. ***Summary point:*** Compared to no intervention, oxytocin is an effective agent for induction of labor. However, when oxytocin is compared to some of the prostaglandins, vaginal and intracervical prostaglandins were more effective for labor induction. Additionally, when women who had their labor induced with oxytocin were compared to those that received prostaglandins, the oxytocin group had a higher rate of epidurals.
Relaxin	Kelly, A.J., Kavanagh, J. & Thomas, J. (2001) Relaxin for cervical ripening and induction of labour. *Cochrane Database of Systematic Reviews,* Issue 2. Art. No.: CD003103. DOI: 10.1002/14651858.CD003103. ***Total studies:*** 4 studies (n = 267) *Cervical ripening and induction:* Relaxin is protein hormone. Role in parturition is unclear. Has been debated since 1950s. Most studies used relaxin derived from porcine and/or bovine sources; recombinant human relaxin is now available for study. Thought to promote cervical ripening, but inhibit uterine activity. This may produce less tachysystole. No reported cases of tachysystole in studies. No difference in Cesarean section rates compared to placebo. Cervix more likely to change to favorable.	Role of relaxin in induction and cervical ripening is unclear. ***Summary point:*** More studies are needed.

(continued)

TABLE 12-2 (Continued)

Cochrane Database Reviews on Selective Labor Induction and Cervical Ripening Methods

Method	Study/Outcomes	Reviewer Comments
Vaginal misoprostol (prostaglandin E1 analogue) *(Off-label use)*	Hofmeyr, G.J., Gulmezoglu, A.M., Pileggi, C. (2010) Vaginal misoprostol for cervical ripening and induction of labour. *Cochrane Database of Systematic Reviews,* Issue 10. Art. No.: CD000941. DOI: 10.1002/14651858.CD000941.pub2 ***Total trials:*** 70 trials *Cervical ripening or induction:* Misoprostol more likely to produce vaginal delivery in 24 hr compared to placebo. Increased uterine tachysystole without FHR changes compared to placebo. *Compared with vaginal prostaglandin E2:* Intracervical prostaglandin E2, and oxytocin, vaginal misoprostol associated with increased likelihood of vaginal delivery, less epidural use, and more tachysystole. *Compared with vaginal E2 or intracervical E2:* Oxytocin augmentation less common with misoprostol; meconium stained amniotic fluid increased with misoprostol. Higher does of misoprostol associated with more tachysystole (with and without FHR changes), and less need for oxytocin augmentation.	Vaginal misoprostol doses greater than 25 mcg every 4 hr are more effective than lower doses, but more uterine tachysystole. Studies reviewed are too small to rule out serious but rare events. Further research needed to identify the ideal dose, route of administration, and to determine if isolated case reports on uterine rupture are related to the drug. ***Summary point:*** The authors conclude that no further studies of vaginal misoprostol are required at this time due to a recent Cochrane review that demonstrated superior performance of oral misoprostol. Further information on the number of significant adverse outcomes such as uterine rupture is needed.
Vaginal prostaglandin (PGE$_2$ and PGF$_{2a}$)	Kelly, A.J., Malik, S., Smith, L., et al. (2009) Vaginal prostaglandin (PGE$_2$ and PGF$_{2a}$) for induction of labour at term. *Cochrane Database of Systematic Reviews,* Issue 4. Art. No.: CD003101. DOI: 10.1002/14651858.CD003101.pub2 ***Total trials:*** 63 trials (n = 10,441) *Induction (term): 2 trials (n = 384)* Vaginal PGE$_2$ when compared to placebo, increased likelihood of vaginal delivery in 24 hr *Cervical ripening: 5 trials (n = 467)* Increased success in cervical ripening in vaginal PGE$_2$ group. *Augmentation: 2 trials (n = 1,321)* Need for oxytocin augmentation reduced in vaginal PGE$_2$ group *Cesarean sections, tachysystole: 14 trials (n = 1,259)* No difference in Cesarean section rates between vaginal PGE$_2$ group and placebo, although rate of tachysystole with FHR changes was increased with vaginal PGE$_2$.	Sustained release vaginal PGE$_2$ superior to vaginal PGE$_2$ gel in some outcomes. ***Summary point:*** When compared to PGE$_2$ gel, sustained release PGE$_2$ has better outcomes in some studies. Methods and costs of drug delivery systems should be evaluated.

FHR = fetal heart rate.

effectively care for such complex patients, collaboration among clinicians is essential. Care providers require an understanding of normal pregnancy, uterine physiology, the effect of labor on maternal oxygen transport variables, the effect of the patient's complication and condition on labor, and the potential adverse events of the selected induction mode (e.g., mechanical, surgical, and/or medical).

This chapter addresses the indications, methods, and potential challenges of labor induction, the effect of significant complications or critical illness on the mechanisms of labor, and the effect of labor on the compromised patient. Recommended National Institutes of Child Health and Human Development (NICHD) terminology for uterine activity and fetal surveillance is incorporated throughout the chapter. Finally, strategies for clinicians to safely care for these challenging patients are presented.

UTERINE PERFUSION AND LABOR PHYSIOLOGY

Oxygen delivery (DO_2)—the amount of oxygen that is pumped from the left ventricle throughout the body via the arterial system—increases during pregnancy to meet increased demands. Specifically, DO_2 increases secondary to increased maternal cardiac output that occurs during normal pregnancy, labor, and delivery. Oxygen consumption (VO_2)—the amount of oxygen that is consumed by the body—is also increased during pregnancy to meet generalized demands, including those associated with growing fetal, placental, and maternal needs. Normal DO_2 and VO_2 prior to pregnancy, approximately 1,000 mL/minute and 250 mL/minute respectively, increase 20 to 40 percent during pregnancy. The increase in DO_2 over non-pregnant values supplies the growing fetus and placenta, which individually consume approximately 6.6 mL/kg/minute and 3.0 mL/kg/minute of O_2, respectively.[4] A more thorough discussion of hemodynamic and oxygen transport concepts may be found in Chapter 4 of this text.

To accommodate the increase in maternal cardiac output in pregnancy, maternal uterine vascular beds dilate to maximum expansion, increasing perfusion and therefore gas exchange with the placenta. In fact, the internal lumen of the uterine artery doubles in size without thickening of the vessel wall.[7] The expansion provides a dilated vasculature that accommodates larger volumes of blood and oxygen to the uterus and further to the placental membrane barrier. To fill the expanded vasculature, uteroplacental blood flow increases during pregnancy from a baseline volume of less than 50 mL/minute to 750 to 1000 mL/minute at term.[7] It is important to note, however, that despite the increase in volume of blood flow, the uterine arteries lose auto-regulation capability during pregnancy, which may limit the maintenance of maternal blood pressure during periods of diminished flow. Since uterine blood flow is dependent upon uterine perfusion, the *quantity* of uterine blood flow dictates the quantity of oxygen delivered to the fetus.[8] Normal maternal cardiac output and blood pressure are therefore vital for the maintenance of uterine perfusion, placental blood flow and fetal oxygenation. To maintain constant oxygen delivery during periods of decreased uterine perfusion pressures (e.g., post

epidural anesthesia with vasodilation of maternal vasculature), the fetus is able to increase the oxygen extraction. However, the ability for a fetus to accomplish this feat assumes the fetus is at term, healthy, and that the uterine perfusion (maternal cardiac output) is at maximum volume prior to the decrease.[8] When these conditions cannot be met in pregnancies of women with reduced cardiac output or decreased DO_2, the fetus is less likely to tolerate episodes of reduced blood flow and is at a greater risk for deterioration and compromise.

LABOR

Once labor begins, maternal, fetal and placental demands for oxygen dramatically increase, not only from the physical "work" of labor but also from catecholamine release related to maternal pain, anxiety and other psychosocial factors. Maternal VO_2 increases approximately 86 percent (between 35 and 140 percent) during the course of labor compared to pre-labor values.[4] In patients without anesthesia or analgesia, second-stage VO_2 may elevate 200 to 300 percent over third trimester values. Therefore, for patients with marginal oxygen delivery, the use of effective analgesia and anesthesia during labor and delivery is essential.

Labor is defined as progressive maternal cervical effacement and dilation associated with intermittent regular uterine contractions. The establishment of progressive cervical dilation from repetitive uterine contractions relies in part on the effectiveness of intermittent pressure transferred to the fetal presenting part that is applied to the maternal cervix. The uterine myometrium produces this pressure by coordinated shortening and relaxing of muscle fibers to thin the lower uterine segment and dilate the cervix. This synchronized "work" of the uterus is dependent upon multiple maternal and fetal physiologic factors, some of which are yet to be realized. Effective myometrial activity is dependent upon adequate calcium stores, functioning calcium channels, normal uterine perfusion pressures, normal pH balance, absence of metabolic acidosis, absence of over-stretched muscle fibers, adequate glycogen stores, the availability of oxygen to maintain aerobic metabolism, and similar physiologic steady states.[9,10] Additionally, the movement of calcium through channels may be further dependent on maternal lipid concentrations. An elevated concentration of serum lipids may be a factor in the increased incidence of dysfunctional labor reported in obese women.[9]

Each uterine contraction during labor expresses 300 to 500 mL of blood from the uterine vessels into the maternal systemic circulation.[11] This transient increase in blood volume slightly decreases the maternal heart rate; increases mean arterial pressure, central venous pressure, pulmonary artery pressures, and left ventricular filling pressures; and increases cardiac output by approximately 20 to 30 percent.[12,13] These changes may significantly alter maternal cardiovascular profiles during contractions; thus, assessment and measurement of non-invasive and, if utilized, invasive hemodynamic and pulmonary parameters should be performed between contractions when the uterus is at rest.

THE EFFECT OF MATERNAL COMPROMISE ON LABOR

Oxygen transport and maternal pH status have been shown to affect uterine activity associated with both spontaneous and induced labor. Acute hypoxemia and/or disruption of maternal oxygen transport below a critical threshold can lead to uterine contractions, progressive cervical dilation, and delivery of the fetus at any gestational age.[11] In contrast, chronic hypoxemia in some situations may work in an opposite manner to down-regulate precursors responsible for uterine contractions.[9] This may help explain why a number of critically ill pregnant women continue their pregnancies for several days and/or weeks prior to the onset of labor, whereas other women exhibit uterine contractions around the time they become physiologically unstable. It is important to note that there are critical levels of maternal hypoxemia beyond which a pregnancy cannot be successfully maintained. The end result may include fetal death, spontaneous uterine expulsion of the pregnancy, or both.

Quenby and colleagues studied the effect of myometrial pH and lactate levels both *in vitro* and *in vivo* to determine their effects on uterine contractions.[10] The researchers hypothesized that during a contraction the myometrium may become locally hypoxic from the loss of oxygenated vascular blood that is "squeezed" from the uterine vessels. Consequently, if the time between contractions does not permit re-establishment of vascular flow, the smooth muscle is unable to maintain aerobic metabolism; subsequently, pH values decrease and lactate levels increase. The group further found that when myometrial tissue had a low pH it was more likely to be associated with ineffective contractions compared to myometrium with a normal pH.[10] From these observations, Quenby and colleagues speculated that dysfunctional labor in both critically ill and normal women may be the result of either inadequate uterine rest or tachysystole.[10] It is also important to note from the same study that myometrial pH had an almost identical effect on spontaneous labor contractions versus induced labor contractions. Conditions common in patients with significant complications or critical illness that are known to negatively affect uterine activity are listed in Table 12-3.

TABLE 12-3

Maternal Conditions that Negatively Affect Myometrial Function

- Decreased pH
  - From maternal systemic acidosis
  - From decreased perfusion (causes localized acidosis due to inadequate "wash out" of hydrogen ions [H^+] between contractions)
- Arterial carbon dioxide (CO_2) less than 20 mmHg (due to hyperventilation)
- Decreased cardiac output
- Decreased mixed venous oxygen saturation (SvO_2)
- Hypotension (decreased mean arterial pressure)
- Hypothermia
- Metabolic acidosis
- Hypocalcemia (rare, extremely low ionized calcium [Ca^+])
- Maternal medications
  - *Examples*: Calcium channel blockers, epinephrine, halothane (and other general anesthesia agents)

Arakawa, T. K., Mlynarczyk, M., Kaushal, K. M., Zhang, L., & Ducsay, C. A. (2004). Long-term hypoxia alters calcium regulation in near-term ovine myometrium. *Biology of Reproduction, 71*(1), 156–162.

Bursztyn, L., Eytan, O., Jaffa, A. J., & Elad, D. (2007). Mathematical model of excitation-contraction in a uterine smooth muscle cell. *American Journal of Cell Physiology, 292*, C1816–C1829; Bursztyn, L., Eytan, O., Jaffa, A. J., & Elad, D. (2007). Modeling myometrial smooth muscle contraction. *Annals of the New York Academy of Sciences, 1101*, 110–138.

Monir-Bishty, E., Pierce, S. J., Kupittayanant, S., Shmygol, A., & Wray, S. (2003). The effects of metabolic inhibition on intracellular calcium and contractility of human myometrium. *BJOG, 110*(12), 1050–1056.

Quenby, S., Pierce, S. J., Brigham, S., & Wray, S. (2004). Dysfunctional labor and myometrial lactic acidosis. *Obstetrics and Gynecology, 103*(4), 718–723.

Wray, S. (2007). Insights into the uterus. *Experimental Physiology, 92*, 621–631.

THE EFFECT OF LABOR ON COMPROMISED PATIENTS

Once a woman has been identified as a candidate for induction of labor, further analysis of her ability to tolerate labor should be considered and specific plans made for labor management, delivery, and postpartum care. The same extensive cardiopulmonary alterations of pregnancy, labor, and birth that normal pregnant women experience and generally tolerate without problems, may have deleterious effects on patients who have complications prior to the process. Patients who are at risk for oxygen transport deterioration will be maximally challenged during the second stage of labor and immediately postpartum—two instances that produce the most dramatic changes in fluid shifts, intra-cardiac pressures, cardiac output, oxygen demand, and pulmonary capillary permeability. These normal changes of pregnancy make the critically ill parturient and her fetus more vulnerable to decreases in maternal cardiac output and oxygen delivery.[14]

Induction of labor to achieve a vaginal delivery is a goal for many pregnant women with significant complications or critical illness. Vaginal delivery requires less oxygen and metabolic demand when compared to Cesarean delivery and carries a lower risk for pulmonary embolism and surgical site infection. Additionally, more blood may be lost during Cesarean versus vaginal delivery, thereby decreasing the patient's oxygen carrying capacity and increasing her risk for inadequate DO_2. Patients with left outflow obstructive cardiac lesions and/or patients with severe pulmonary hypertension may not tolerate the sudden reduction of maternal abdominal pressure when the abdominal muscles and peritoneum are opened during surgery. Such patients are dependent upon elevated ventricular filling pressures to maintain forward blood flow through the heart in order to adapt to the demand by increasing intra-thoracic pressure. If intra-thoracic pressure is reduced to near zero, rapid deterioration, reversal of blood flow, and cardiac arrest may follow. Cesarean birth is associated with increased rates of fluid overload, electrolyte imbalance, hypotension from regional anesthesia, and other surgical complications. Further, morbidly obese patients are at increased risk for difficult intubation, wound breakdown, longer operating times, and the need for additional surgical procedures at the time of Cesarean delivery.[15] Table 12-4 lists additional benefits and risks of Cesarean and vaginal deliveries for all women.

To optimize the probability of a vaginal delivery, care must be taken to stabilize the parturient with significant complications or compromise prior to induction. Also, if adverse changes develop in maternal or fetal status during labor, clinicians should consider factors that may have developed that negatively impact oxygen transport. When these precipitating or contributing issues are identified, care should be directed to ameliorate the condition or significantly reduce its effect. Fetal surveillance during maternal instability via continuous electronic fetal monitoring (EFM) may assist clinicians to rule out real-time episodes of inadequate maternal DO_2 and the resultant oxygen transport deficits. EFM in such patients may demonstrate abnormal fetal heart rate (FHR) characteristics and may assist clinicians in timely assessment and intervention to improve maternal DO_2.

UTERINE ACTIVITY AND FHR TERMINOLOGY IN INDUCTION OF LABOR

To improve communication among physicians and nurses responsible for the interpretation of EFM data, updated terminology and a new category system of assessment have been introduced.[16]

The Eunice Kennedy Shriver National Institute of Child Health and Human Development (NICHD) convened workshops in the mid-1990s to develop standardized definitions for use in the interpretation of FHR tracings generated from continuous EFM. The recommendations for FHR terminology published in 1997 (NICHD I) have since been endorsed by ACOG, AWHONN, and the Academy of Certified Nurse Midwives (ACNM).[17,18] Approximately one decade later, a new NICHD workgroup (NICHD II) reviewed and refined EFM terminology and presented new definitions for the characteristics of uterine activity (NICHD II).[16] The revised terms for uterine activity are presented in Table 12-5.

The NICHD II committee recommended that the terms *hyperstimulation* and *hypercontractility* should not be used because both are inconsistent in meaning. Rather, the term *tachysystole* is recommended to describe uterine activity (contractions) that exceeds normal intervals (more than five contractions in a 10-minute window, evaluated over three consecutive 10-minute windows). Additionally, when tachysystole is identified, a change or lack of change in the FHR should be noted. In the same publication, the NICHD II committee further refined the definitions for FHR decelerations (Table 12-6). The committee recommended that providers use these terms when communicating the findings of specific FHR responses in antepartum and intrapartum settings.[16]

A new parameter for EFM interpretation was added in the 2008 NICHD publication: A three-tiered system to categorize integration and synthesis of individual features of the FHR during a 10-minute or greater segment of time.[16] The categories are numbered I, II, and III and generally describe tracings that range from "normal" and thought to rule out fetal metabolic acidosis (Category I), to the opposite end of the spectrum with tracings that may be associated with fetal hypoxia and metabolic acidosis (Category III). Category II tracings consist of characteristics that meet neither Category I nor Category III criteria.[16] A detailed description of the three categories is presented in Table 12-7. The recommended responses to tracings in each category are described in Table 12-8.

FETAL CONSIDERATIONS

To maintain adequate fetal oxygenation levels, oxygen must leave the maternal circulation, pass through the

TABLE 12-4

Benefits and Risks of Vaginal Delivery Versus Scheduled Cesarean Section

	Vaginal Delivery	Scheduled Cesarean Section
Benefits	Smaller amount of blood loss (~500 mL)	Scheduled, planned
	Reduced total VO_2/oxygen demand compared to Cesarean section	Surgery can be scheduled when maximum amount of resources are available for mother and baby
	Avoids rapid drop in intra-abdominal pressure (when peritoneum is opened), preventing sudden decrease in right heart filling pressures	Selection of a specific operating room can be accomplished (large room, C-arm equipped, etc.); experienced personnel can be scheduled to be present, etc.
	Increased hemodynamic stability	Analgesia/anesthesia easier to manage in a scheduled as opposed to an emergency Cesarean section
	Faster recovery postpartum	Avoids repetitive increases in VO_2, VE, CVP, PAP, PCOP, CO, MAP during labor from contractions
	Less postpartum complications such as pain, infection, wound breakdown, pulmonary edema, abdominal compartment syndrome, DVT, PE, et al.	Invasive hemodynamic catheters, central line access introducers and non-invasive monitors can be placed under sterile conditions without urgency.
Risks	Timing of delivery less predictable (off-shifts, weekends or holidays)	Increased blood loss (~1000 mL)
	Length of labor may be prolonged	Increased need for deeper anesthesia during surgery
	Drugs used for induction of labor may increase VO_2	Increased catecholamines (increased pain, anxiety, stress) postpartum
	Increased catecholamines from contractions, pushing and delivery (pain, anxiety, stress)	Sudden drop in intra-abdominal pressures when peritoneum is opened, dramatic decrease in preload
	Fetal condition during labor may be difficult to determine if maternal medications cross placenta, influence EFM interpretation	Increased risks of postoperative complications (bleeding, infection, thrombosis, etc.)
	If emergency Cesarean section needed for obstetric needs, complications increased compared to scheduled Cesarean section	Increased total VO_2
		If emergency Cesarean section, may not be adequate time to place invasive monitors, acquire special equipment (rapid volume infusers, difficult airway cart, blood products, etc.) and summon experienced staff.

CO = cardiac output, CVP = central venous pressure, DVT = deep venous thrombosis, EFM = electronic fetal monitoring, MAP = mean arterial pressure, PAP = pulmonary artery pressure, PCOP = pulmonary capillary occlusion pressure, PE = pulmonary embolus, VE = minute ventilation, VO_2 = oxygen consumption.

Carvalho, B., & Jackson, E. (2008). Structural heart disease in pregnant women. In D. R. Gambling, M. J. Douglas, & R. S. McKay (Eds.), *Obstetric anesthesia and uncommon disorders* (2nd ed., pp. 1–27). New York: Cambridge University Press.

Witcher, P. M., & Harvey, C. J. (2006). Modifying labor routines for the woman with cardiac disease. *Journal of Perinatal and Neonatal Nursing, 20,* 303–310.

intervillous space of the placenta, and bind with fetal hemoglobin. Oxygen movement across the placenta from the mother to the fetus is accomplished by diffusion, the passive movement of particles from an area of higher concentration to an area of lower concentration. In normal pregnancy, the maternal partial pressure of oxygen in both the arterial and venous systems (PaO_2, PvO_2) increases. Likewise, the partial pressure of carbon dioxide ($PaCO_2$, $PvCO_2$) decreases. This enhances the diffusion gradient between the maternal and fetal systems and encourages the movement of O_2 from the mother to the fetus and the dispersal of CO_2 from the fetus to the mother. Despite an increase of maternal O_2 levels above pre-pregnancy values, the fetus lives in a comparatively low-oxygen environment (maximum fetal PaO_2 is approximately 35 mmHg). To compensate, the fetus has a higher cardiac

TABLE 12-5

NICHD Electronic Fetal Monitoring Terminology for Uterine Activity

Term	Description
Normal Tachysystole	• Five or less contractions in 10 minutes, averaged over a 30-minute window • More than five contractions in 10 minutes, averaged over a 30-minute window • Should be quantified for presence or absence of associated FHR decelerations • Term applies to spontaneous or stimulated labor • Clinical response may differ depending on whether contractions are spontaneous or stimulated
Hyperstimulation and Hypercontractility	• Terms not defined and should be abandoned

FHR = fetal heart rate, NICHD = National Institute of Child Health and Human Development.

Macones, G. A., Hankins, G. D., Spong, C. Y., Hauth, J., & Moore, T. (2008). The 2008 National Institute of Child Health and Human Development workshop report on electronic fetal monitoring: update on definitions, interpretation, and research guidelines. *Journal of Obstetric, Gynecologic, and Neonatal Nursing, 37,* 510–515 and *Obstetrics and Gynecology, 112*(3), 661–666.

TABLE 12-6

NICHD II Characteristics of Fetal Heart Rate Decelerations

Late Deceleration	• Visually apparent usually symmetrical *gradual* decrease and return of FHR associated with a uterine contraction. • A *gradual* FHR decrease is defined as from the onset to FHR nadir of 30 seconds or longer. • The decrease in FHR is calculated from the onset to the nadir of the deceleration. • The deceleration is delayed in timing, with the nadir of the deceleration occurring after the peak of the contraction. • In most cases, the onset, nadir, and recovery of the deceleration occur after the beginning, peak, and ending of the contraction, respectively.
Early Deceleration	• Visually apparent, usually symmetrical, *gradual* decrease and return of FHR associated with a uterine contraction • A *gradual* FHR decrease as one from the onset to FHR nadir of 30 seconds or longer. • The decrease in FHR is defined as from the onset to the nadir of the deceleration. • The nadir of the deceleration occurs at the same time as the peak of the contraction. • In most cases, the onset, nadir, and recovery of the deceleration are coincident with the beginning, peak, and ending of the contraction, respectively.
Variable Deceleration	• Visually apparent *abrupt* decrease in FHR. • An *abrupt* FHR decrease is defined from the onset of the deceleration to the *beginning* of the nadir of less than 30 seconds. • The decrease in FHR is calculated from the onset to the nadir of the deceleration. • The decrease in FHR is 15 beats or more per minute, lasting 15 seconds or more, and less than 2 minutes in duration. • When variable decelerations are associated with uterine contractions, their onset, depth, and duration commonly vary with successive uterine contractions.
Prolonged Deceleration	• Visually apparent decrease in FHR from the baseline that is greater than or equal to 15 beats per minute, lasting more than 2 minutes but less than 10 minutes. • A deceleration that lasts more than 10 minutes is a *baseline change*.

FHR = fetal heart rate.

Macones, G. A., Hankins, G. D., Spong, C. Y., Hauth, J., & Moore, T. (2008). The 2008 National Institute of Child Health and Human Development workshop report on electronic fetal monitoring: Update on definitions, interpretation, and research guidelines. *Journal of Obstetric, Gynecologic, and Neonatal Nursing, 37,* 510–515 and *Obstetrics and Gynecology, 112*(3), 661–666.

TABLE 12-7

NICHD 3-Tier Fetal Heart Rate Category System

Category I Includes **all** of those listed:	• Baseline rate: 110–160 beats per minute • Baseline FHR variability: Moderate • Late or variable decelerations: Absent • Early decelerations: Present or absent • Accelerations: Present or absent
Category II Includes tracings **not categorized** as Category I or III. May represent an appreciable fraction of those encountered in clinical care. Examples of Category II tracings include any of those listed:	Baseline rate • Bradycardia not accompanied by absent baseline variability • Tachycardia Baseline FHR variability • Minimal • Absent (not accompanied by recurrent decelerations) • Marked variability Accelerations • Absent after fetal stimulation Periodic or episodic decelerations • Recurrent variable decelerations with minimal or moderate variability • Prolonged deceleration 2 min or more and less than 10 min • Recurrent late decelerations with moderate variability • Variable decelerations with other characteristics (slow return to baseline, "overshoots," or "shoulders")
Category III Includes **either** of those listed:	Absent baseline FHR variability and any of the following: • Recurrent late decelerations • Recurrent variable decelerations • Bradycardia Sinusoidal pattern

FHR = fetal heart rate.
Macones, G. A., Hankins, G. D., Spong, C. Y., Hauth, J., & Moore, T. (2008). The 2008 National Institute of Child Health and Human Development workshop report on electronic fetal monitoring: update on definitions, interpretation, and research guidelines. *Journal of Obstetric, Gynecologic, and Neonatal Nursing, 37,* 510–515 and *Obstetrics and Gynecology, 112*(3), 661–666.

output by weight compared to the adult and remains in aerobic metabolism by shifting the oxyhemoglobin curve to the left, resulting in greater binding of oxygen to fetal hemoglobin (Fig. 12-1).[11,13,19] This allows for greater hemoglobin saturation with oxygen at much lower partial pressures of oxygen when compared to an adult.

It is important to note that fetal pO_2 values will never be greater than maternal values; likewise, the concentration of fetal CO_2 will never be less than maternal CO_2. Therefore, conditions that interfere with or affect the concentration of dissolved gases in the maternal arterial and venous systems will directly impact the fetus. If all other variables of fetal DO_2 are normal and the fetus has hemoglobin saturations greater than 30 to 35 percent, aerobic metabolism will be maintained.[19]

FETAL SURVEILLANCE AS AN INDIRECT INDICATOR OF MATERNAL CONDITION

Because the fetus may demonstrate alterations in FHR patterns prior to a measurable change in the mother's vital signs, it is possible to use fetal surveillance observations as an element of maternal assessment. This observation is based on the method by which

TABLE 12-8

Recommendations for Practice with the NICHD 3-Tier Category System of EFM Interpretation

Interpretation	Category I **Normal**	Category II **Indeterminate**	Category III **Abnormal**
Baseline rate	Normal: 110–160 bpm	Abnormal: <110 or >160 bpm	Sinusoidal pattern
• Tachycardia	No	YES	—
• Bradycardia	No	YES without decelerations (but with variability)	YES with absent variability
Variability	Moderate	ALL *Examples*: • Absent – without recurrent decelerations • Minimal – with bradycardia or tachycardia • Minimal – with variable decelerations • Moderate – with recurrent late decelerations • Moderate – with variable decelerations • MARKED	ABSENT – • with bradycardia • with recurrent late decelerations • with recurrent variable decelerations
Accelerations	Yes or No	NO	NO
Decelerations			
• Early	Yes or No		
• Late	No	YES – • Recurrent late decelerations with moderate variability	YES – • Recurrent late decelerations with absent variability
• Variable	No	YES – • Recurrent variable decelerations with minimal or moderate variability • variable decelerations with other features: slow return to baseline, overshoots, or shoulders	YES – • Recurrent variables with absent variability
Prolonged Deceleration	No	YES – independent of other features	—
Recommended Actions	None	• Evaluation • Continued surveillance • Reevaluation • Take in entire clinical circumstances	PROMPT EVALUATION Depending on the clinical situation, efforts to expeditiously resolve the *abnormal* FHR pattern may include, but are not limited to: • Maternal O_2 • Position change • Discontinue oxytocin/stimulants • Treat maternal hypotension
Follow-up	Routine	If no improvement with intervention, move to Category III; consider delivery	Resolve abnormal FHR pattern; prepare for delivery

Characteristics of some variable decelerations; clinical significance unknown and requires further investigation.
O_2 = oxygen, FHR = fetal heart rate.
Macones, G. A., Hankins, G. D., Spong, C. Y., Hauth, J., & Moore, T. (2008). The 2008 National Institute of Child Health and Human Development workshop report on electronic fetal monitoring: Update on definitions, interpretation, and research guidelines. *Journal of Obstetric, Gynecologic, and Neonatal Nursing, 37*, 510–515 and *Obstetrics and Gynecology, 112*(3), 661–666.

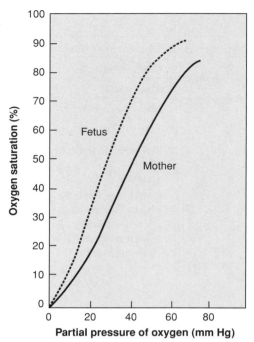

FIGURE 12-1 Maternal and fetal oxyhemoglobin dissociation curves. The fetal oxyhemoglobin dissociation curve demonstrates a left shift. The maternal oxyhemoglobin dissociation curve demonstrates a right shift. These changes enhance oxygen binding to fetal hemoglobin. This allows the fetus higher levels of hemoglobin saturation at lower amounts of dissolved oxygen when compared to the adult.

the fetus receives oxygen and the influence maternal hemodynamic compensatory actions have on uterine blood flow. As presented above, the fetus is dependent upon the volume and pressure of uterine blood flow for fetal oxygen content. Uterine blood flow, which originates from the maternal aorta, does not have the ability to preferentially shunt blood to higher functioning areas of the placenta/intervillous space because uterine vessels lose the ability to constrict and/or compensate during pregnancy. The other vessels of the arterial system, however, maintain this function and will react to decreased oxygen delivery by shunting maternal blood to the body's most vital organs for survival—the heart, brain, and adrenals. Inversely, periods of maternal physiologic stress that reduce oxygen delivery stimulate the shunting of blood away from non-vital systems, of which the uterus is considered to be one.

The reduced volume of blood flow that reaches the uterine arteries decreases perfusion pressures of the blood that will ultimately enter the placental vascular beds. Low pressures disrupt the diffusion gradients of dissolved gases and may reduce oxygen levels in the fetus. Additionally, if the oxygen content in the reduced

blood flow is low, the fetus can have abrupt changes in oxygen delivery that may stimulate reflexive and/or autonomic changes in heart rate. As an example, when a patient receives epidural anesthesia that dilates her vasculature, the arterial system is not maximally filled and "relaxes" compared to total blood volume. The reduction in arterial pressures decreases the amount of venous blood that returns to the heart, thereby decreasing preload. The reduced preload lowers ventricular contractility and cardiac output which, in turn, increases afterload and shunts blood away from lesser organ systems. As a consequence, the uterine arteries receive a smaller than normal amount of blood, which further reduces uterine blood flow. The normal fetus at term typically reacts to a reduction in oxygen delivery by increasing the baseline FHR to compensate for less oxygen content.

If the reduction in oxygen delivery is preceded by an increase in placental vascular resistance, FHR may decrease abruptly (i.e., prolonged FHR deceleration, bradycardia, etc.). Further, if uterine contractions are present, the fetus may demonstrate a pattern of late decelerations or a prolonged deceleration in association with them. Again, interpretation of the continuous EFM tracing may provide clinicians with an indirect assessment of maternal oxygen transport. Specifically, such alterations in FHR, especially in a patient with no external signs of a condition change, may alert clinicians to further assess the mother for hemodynamic and oxygen transport deterioration, which may ultimately result in the shift to anaerobic metabolism.

FHR surveillance is particularly important in the management of complicated and critically ill patients for the confirmation of fetal well-being. If the fetus has a normal EFM tracing with accelerations or moderate variability, it is reasonable to conclude that the mother has adequate cardiac output and oxygen content at the time the tracing was observed.

EFM is recommended as a method of fetal surveillance in labor.[6,20,21] Patients who require induction of labor and/or those who require uterine stimulants are considered patients with risk factors that should have continuous EFM during active phase labor and delivery.[6] The intervals for FHR and uterine activity assessment in such pregnancies under those conditions are every 15 minutes in the active phase of labor and every 5 minutes during the second stage of labor (pushing).[6] When the EFM tracing is saved as a part of the patient's permanent medical record, frequent fetal assessments (i.e., every 5 minutes) can be documented periodically as a summary chart entry at longer time intervals. This allows the nurse to care for the patient and neonate, and employ a more efficient method of documentation when compared to historical practice.[6]

TABLE 12-9

Maternal and Fetal Indications for Induction

Maternal	• Abruptio placentae
	• Chorioamnionitis
	• Preeclampsia, eclampsia
	• Chronic hypertension
	• Premature rupture of membranes
	• Post-term pregnancy
	• Diabetes mellitus
	• Renal disease
	• Pulmonary disease
	• Cardiac disease
	• Antiphospholipid syndrome
	• Hepatic disease, failure
	• Malignancy
	• Recurrent fetal death
Fetal	• Oligohydramnios
	• Isoimmunization
	• Severe fetal growth restriction
	• Fetal demise
	• Prolonged gestation
	• Major anomalies
	• Non-reassuring antepartum fetal testing
Other	• Chronic fetal stress/intolerance
	• Evidenced by biochemical or biophysical indicators
	• Logistic, psychosocial

American College of Obstetricians & Gynecologists. (2009). ACOG Practice Bulletin No. 107: Induction of labor. *Obstetrics and Gynecology, 114,* 386–397.

National Collaborating Centre for Women's and Children's Health. (2008). *Clinical guideline: Induction of labour.* London: ROGC Press, p. 124. Retrieved from http://www.nice.org.uk/nicemedia/live/12012/41255/41255.pdf

TABLE 12-10

Maternal and Fetal Contraindications to Labor Induction

Maternal Contraindications*	• Complete placenta previa
	• Vasa previa
	• Classical uterine incision scar
	• Extensive myomectomy (entering endometrial cavity)
	• Pelvic structural deformities
	• Active or culture-proved genital herpes infection
	• Invasive cervical carcinoma
	• Maternal exhaustion
Relative Maternal Contraindications	• Grand multiparity
	• Uterine over-distention
	• Polyhydramnios
	• Multiple gestation
	• Breech presentation
	• Previous Cesarean section(s) (*avoid prostaglandin use*)
Fetal Contraindications	• Umbilical cord prolapse
	• Abnormal presentation
	• Transverse lie
	• Funic (cord) presentation
	• Presenting part above pelvic inlet
	• Presence of abnormal fetal heart rate patterns – Category III, prior to fetal status testing

*Contraindications are generally the same as those for spontaneous labor and vaginal delivery. They include but are not limited to the maternal and fetal conditions.

American College of Obstetricians & Gynecologists. (2009). ACOG Practice Bulletin No. 107: Induction of labor. *Obstetrics and Gynecology, 114,* 386–397.

Battista, L., Chung, J. H., Lagrew, D. C., & Wing, D. A. (2007). Complications of labor induction among multiparous women in a community-based hospital system. *American Journal of Obstetrics and Gynecology, 197*(3), 241.e1–7; discussion 322–323.

Wing, D. A., & Gaffaney, C. A. (2006). Vaginal misoprostol administration for cervical ripening and labor induction. *Clinical Obstetrics and Gynecology, 49,* 627–641.

Individualization of care is paramount in critically ill patients to achieve a safe induction of labor without maternal and/or fetal compromise.

INDICATIONS FOR INDUCTION OF LABOR

Candidates for induction of labor generally have maternal or fetal conditions for which delivery offers greater benefit than the risk of continuation of the pregnancy (Table 12-9). These general indications for induction, however, are not inclusive of all maternal and fetal conditions that may prompt providers to consider induction of labor and/or Cesarean delivery in a given clinical situation. Equally important to note are women who are not candidates for induction (Table 12-10). Patients in this category have contraindications to labor in general and are at increased risk for adverse outcome from labor and/or vaginal delivery.

Bishop Score

The probability that an induction of labor will result in progressive dilation and vaginal delivery for an individual patient may be estimated based on the patient's cervical status prior to the start of the procedure. The Bishop Score (Table 12-11) is one of the most commonly used methods to determine if a patient's cervix is likely to progress in labor during an induction.

TABLE 12-11

Bishop's Pelvic Scoring

	0	1	2	3
Dilation (cm)	0	1–2	3–4	5–6
Effacement (%)	0–30	40–50	60–70	80
Station	–3	–2	–1 to 0	+1 to +2
Consistency	Firm	Medium	Soft	
Position	Posterior	Midposition	Anterior	

Bishop, E. H. (1964). Pelvic scoring for elective induction. *Obstetrics and Gynecology, 24,* 266–268.

Lyndrup, J., Legarth, J., Weber, T., Nickelsen, C., & Guldbaek, E. (1992). Predictive value of pelvic scores for induction of labor by local PGE2. *European Journal of Obstetrics, Gynecology, and Reproductive Biology, 47*(1), 17–23.

It is a numeric score assigned based on assessment of the cervix to evaluate position, effacement, dilation, and consistency. The scores determined for each of these elements are added to obtain the total Bishop Score. An *unfavorable cervix,* describing the cervix that is less likely to demonstrate progressive cervical dilation and effacement when exposed to oxytocin, is generally defined as one with a Bishop Score of 6 or less. A score above 8 is highly predictive of vaginal delivery in most randomized trials.[2]

For patients with significant complications or who are critically ill and require cervical ripening prior to induction of labor, providers should consider the ripening method (mechanical or medical) in light of the parturient's oxygen transport status. Critically ill patients with unstable hemodynamic or pulmonary status due to maximized and/or inadequate DO_2 and VO_2 may benefit from mechanical methods such as balloon catheters (e.g., Foley, Atad Ripener Device, etc.), that may ripen the cervix at a lower total oxygen and energy expenditure when compared to prostaglandins.[2]

PHARMACOLOGIC METHODS FOR INDUCTION OF LABOR

Common drugs prescribed for induction of labor in healthy women are oxytocin (e.g., Syntocinon, Syntocin, Pitocin), dinosprostone (Cervidil, Prepidil, Prostin E2), and misoprostol (Cytotec). These medications are utilized in the care of patients with pregnancy complications unless there are specific contraindications for use in association with the patient's condition or disease. Clinicians who care for patients undergoing labor induction should be familiar with common side effects and/or adverse effects of the medications to identify drug hypersensitivity or intolerance. For more detailed information on the side effects of common drugs used in induction, see Table 12-12.

Oxytocin

"Oxytocin" comes from the Greek words that mean "quick birth" and was so named after its discovery in 1906.[22] Oxytocin is a nonapeptide found in the pituitary extracts of mammals.[23] It is the most common drug prescribed in obstetrics and is used to abate uterine bleeding after delivery and to initiate or augment labor when delivery is desired and spontaneous labor has not begun or uterine contractions have begun but are not effective in creating progressive cervical change.[24,25] It stimulates the uterus to contract by binding with the myometrial oxytocin receptors. The degree of uterine muscle sensitivity to oxytocin is dependent in part on the number of myometrial oxytocin receptors. Oxytocin receptors are present in the uterus as early as 13 weeks and increase over 300 percent compared with the nonpregnant state.[26] As pregnancy progresses, the concentration of receptors increases and undergoes an accelerated rise around 30 weeks and then plateaus until term.[25] As the receptor concentration increases during pregnancy, myometrial sensitivity to oxytocin increases as well. Compared to earlier in the gestation, the term uterus requires much lower doses of oxytocin to contract. Thus, a patient's response to oxytocin is in part dependent upon the gestational age of the fetus, a finding that supports the use of lower doses of the drug the closer the fetus is to term.[26]

Synthetic analogues of oxytocin (e.g., Pitocin) are available and are approved by the U.S. Food and Drug Administration (FDA) and the Health Products and Food Branch of Health Canada for intravenous (IV) or intramuscular (IM) routes. For antepartum and intrapartum patients, the FDA only approves the IV route for administration of oxytocin.

TABLE 12-12

Adverse Affects of Common Drugs Used for Labor Induction

	Oxytocin	Dinoprostone	Misoprostol
Trade Name Key points	Syntocinon, Pitocin, etc. • Maternal death from water intoxication (e.g., severe hyponatremia) continues to occur. Administer in isotonic solution (e.g., 0.9% NaCl, LR, etc.) to avoid electrolyte imbalance. Use isotonic solutions for all IVs.	Cervidil, Prepidil, Prostin E2 • CAUTION: Avoid in patients with asthma (may cause bronchospasm, coughing, dyspnea, wheezing, respiratory distress), glaucoma, increased ocular pressure, hypo- or hypertension. • Use with caution in pts with cardiac, renal, or hepatic disease; anemia, jaundice, diabetes, epilepsy, and GU infections.	Cytotec • AVOID: aluminum hydroxide and magnesium carbonate antacids (may reduce the bioavailability of misoprostol acid). • AVOID: magnesium-containing antacids (exacerbates diarrhea). • Eliminated through kidneys; use with caution in pts with renal failure.
Cardiac	• Hypertension, hypotension, PVCs, sinus tachycardia, other arrhythmias • Neonatal: bradycardia, PVCs, other arrhythmias.	• Transient decrease in BP, syncope, cardiac arrhythmias	
CNS	• Mania-like affect, seizures (from water intox.), coma	• Headache, anxiety, tension, paresthesia, weakness	• Headache (2%)
Metabolic	• Water intoxication	• Flushing, fever, chills	• Chills
Hyper-sensitivity	• Anaphylaxis	• Anaphylaxis, bronchospasm, cardiac arrhythmias, seizure	• Anaphylaxis
GU	• Pelvic hematoma, spasm, uterine tachysystole, prolonged contractions, uterine rupture	• Uterine contractions with or without FHR changes, tachysystole, uterine rupture, amnionitis	• Urinary incontinence
Hematologic	• Fatal afibrinogemia, postpartum hemorrhage	• Increased risk PP-DIC (<1 in 1,000)	• Thrombocytopenia, purpura, abnormal WBC differential
Hepatic	• Neonatal jaundice		
GI	• N&V	• N&V, diarrhea, abd pain (<1%), anorexia	• Diarrhea, abd pain, nausea, gas, vomiting
Respiratory	• Pulmonary edema	• Bronchospasm, coughing, dyspnea, wheezing	• Dyspnea (in overdose)
Renal	• Decreased GFR, RPF		
Ocular	• Neonatal retinal hemorrhages	• Blurred vision, eye pain	
Other	• Low Apgar scores at 5 min, fetal death • Neonatal seizures, CNS injury	• FHR abnormalities, fetal bradycardia, decelerations, sepsis, 1 min Apgar <7, acidosis	• Higher rate of C/S (in one study) for attempted VBAC; • Many complications associated with doses >25 mcg

abd = abdominal, BP = blood pressure, C/S = Cesarean section, CNS = central nervous system, FHR = fetal heart rate, GFR = glomerular filtration rate, GU = genitourinary, intox = intoxication, NaCl = sodium chloride, PP-DIC = postpartum disseminated intravascular coagulation, pts = patients, PVCs = premature ventricular contractions, N&V = nausea and vomiting, resp = respiratory, RPF = renal plasma flow, min = minute(s), VBAC = vaginal birth after Cesarean section, WBC = white blood cells.

AHFS Consumer Medication Information. (2011). *Misoprostol.* Retrieved from http://www.nlm.nih.gov/medlineplus/druginfo/meds/a689009.html

Drugs.com. (2009). *Oxytocin.* Retrieved from http://www.drugs.com/ppa/oxytocin.html

RxList–The Internet Drug Index. (2011). *Pitocin drug description.* Retrieved from http://www.rxlist.com/pitocin-drug.htm

The most common complication of oxytocin administration is tachysystole, which can initially be treated by reducing or discontinuing the oxytocin infusion. Oxytocin has an approximate onset of action between 3 and 5 minutes from the start of the IV infusion, and reaches steady state concentration in 40 minutes.[2] The medication is diluted in intravenous fluid and administered via an electronic infusion pump. Because most of the medication errors in which oxytocin infusion plays a key role are dosing errors, it is recommended that the drug be mixed in a standardized concentration.[27,24] To further reduce calculation errors, the solution of oxytocin should yield a concentration such that 1 mL of fluid contains 1 mU of oxytocin.[27] This is possible by having the pharmacy mix 30 units of oxytocin in 500 mL of normal saline or lactated Ringer's solution.

There are numerous protocols and guidelines for initial and incremental increases in oxytocin. In general, oxytocin protocols are either low-dose (e.g., begin with a low dose and increase by 1 to 2 milliunits per minute [mU/min] at intervals of 15 to 40 minutes), or high dose (i.e., begin at a higher initial dose of 6 mU/min and increase by 3 to 6 mU/min every 15 to 40 minutes).[2] Table 12-13 shows examples of low-dose and high-dose oxytocin protocols.

Fetal surveillance is intensified when an oxytocin infusion is in progress due to the potential for tachysystole and/or fetal intolerance of labor. Figure 12-2 is an FHR tracing that illustrates tachysystole during an induction of labor. Tachysystole, the presence of more than five contractions in 10 minutes averaged over 30 minutes, is considered present with or without changes in FHR. The identification of tachysystole during induction or augmentation of labor is typically treated by turning the oxytocin drip down or temporarily stopping the infusion. There are no prospective data to guide the clinician responsible for the oxytocin infusion on the strength or rate of further increases after the drug has been discontinued secondary to tachysystole. Thus, current guidelines on the subject are based in part on expert opinion and the known pharmacodynamics of the drug.

FETAL DEPENDENCE ON MATERNAL HEMODYNAMIC STATUS

Induction of labor is employed when maternal or fetal compromise necessitates clinical interventions to increase the probability of maternal and/or fetal survival. Specifically, it is utilized to:

- evacuate a specific source of physiologic stress (e.g., infection, coagulopathy, pulmonary/diaphragm obstruction, etc.)
- reduce the oxygen delivery and consumption demands of the pregnancy
- improve the cardiovascular stability of the mother
- allow treatment of the mother or fetus that is not possible during pregnancy
- hasten the mother's return to the non-pregnant state.

Negative maternal oxygen transport balance that produces hypoxia and/or acid–base derangements may initiate the process of spontaneous labor. The contractions that accompany the labor may be ineffective due to acidosis and may require augmentation with oxytocin to prevent prolonged labor.[14,28,29]

Smooth muscle cells in the myometrial layer of the uterus are responsible for uterine contractions and are functionally dependent upon the cycle of calcium ions moving in and out of the cell via the calcium channels. The movement and work of the uterus requires increased amounts of oxygen and nutrients to dilate the cervix and progressively advance the fetus through the maternal pelvis. Adequate maternal DO_2 may be threatened by uterine contractions and the resultant demand for increased amounts of oxygen. Therefore, the goals of induction and/or augmentation of labor are to produce forceful uterine contractions to shorten the duration of labor and to prevent maternal oxygen deficits from the increased demand of contractions, labor, and birth.[30]

Clinicians formulate an individual plan of care for induction or augmentation based on the premise that fetal health and survival are dependent on maternal health and survival. Consequently, interventions to optimize maternal cardiovascular stability and prevent a negative oxygen delivery/consumption balance are used rather than a default list of interventions widely used for parturients without complications. As an

TABLE 12-13

Sample High-Dose and Low-Dose Oxytocin Protocols

Regimen	Starting Dose (mU/min)	Increase (mU/min)	Time Interval for Increases (minutes)
Low-dose	0.5–2	1–2	15–60
High-dose	4–6	3–6	15–40

mU/min = milliunit per minute.
American College of Obstetricians & Gynecologists. (2009). ACOG practice bulletin no. 107: Induction of labor. *Obstetrics and Gynecology, 114*, 386–397.
Smith, J. G., & Merrill, D. C. (2006). Oxytocin for induction of labor. *Clinical Obstetrics and Gynecology, 49*, 594–608.

Tachysystole: Six or more contractions in 10 minutes, for three
consecutive 10-minute periods, total of 30 minutes.

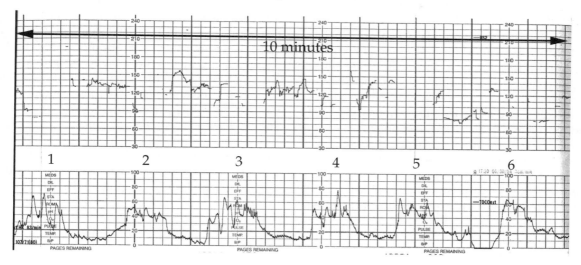

*Six contractions in 10 minutes. If the preceding 20 minutes
or the following 20 minutes also have 6 contractions in both 10-
minute segments, tachysystole exists.*

FIGURE 12-2   Fetal heart rate tracing demonstrating uterine tachysystole during induction
of labor.

example, an antepartum patient who is diagnosed with septic shock may require mechanical ventilation, vasopressor drugs, inotropic therapy, antimicrobial therapy, and heavy sedation or, rarely, paralysis. The presence of the fetus does not prevent aggressive management of the parturient's condition as the fetus will most likely benefit from prompt recognition of the disease, maternal stabilization measures, and ventilation support.

The plan of care for critically ill obstetric patients is based on the knowledge that maternal stabilization and survival are the goals of clinical care, and interventions for the fetus that may negatively impact the mother's oxygen transport are avoided. As an illustrative example, if fetal surveillance modalities demonstrate FHR decelerations, an abnormal FHR baseline, and/or other features that meet the criteria for a Category II or III tracing, conventional interventions for improvement in fetal condition may not be performed if there is a risk of worsening the maternal condition. As a result, actions such as positioning the patient laterally, administering a fluid bolus, delivering supplemental oxygen greater than maternal needs, administering beta-adrenergic agents for tocolysis, and/or performing an emergency Cesarean delivery may not be carried out if the intervention conflicts with maternal stability and/or survival. For the parturient with cardiac disease and pulmonary edema from volume overload, further fluid boluses may not be administered in the event the fetus

demonstrates late decelerations, tachycardia, prolonged decelerations, and/or a Category II or III tracing. The reason for holding and questioning the actions is due to the interventions' risk of exacerbating the maternal pulmonary edema. This may further reduce oxygen content in the mother and fetus and ultimately worsen the condition of both. Rather, such a patient may require placement of an arterial line and pulmonary artery catheter to determine the specific type of pulmonary edema present, selection of treatment options based on the patient's hemodynamic profile (e.g., medications, patient positioning, fluid management, reduction of VO_2, etc.), and positioning the patient to optimize maternal hemodynamic status and improve gas exchange in the mid to lower lungs.

BALANCING MATERNAL AND FETAL OXYGEN TRANSPORT DEMANDS

Independent of the causative factor, maternal hypoxemia and acidemia can result in fetal acidemia. When the mother becomes hemodynamically unstable, the uterine vasculature will not receive an increase in perfusion to assist fetal survival. When maternal hypoxemia and acidemia result in decreased oxygen delivery to the placenta, the processes responsible for the initiation of labor may be activated.[14] This can further compromise both maternal and fetal conditions by increasing oxygen demand from uterine activity and decreasing fetal oxygen transfer during contractions.[14] Stable patients with underlying disease or conditions frequently demonstrate cardiopulmonary compromise when labor begins. A patient with a cardiac defect that obstructs left ventricular outflow (e.g., severe aortic stenosis, mitral valve stenosis, etc.) may first show signs of cardiac failure when labor begins and contractions increase in frequency, duration, and intensity. Eliasson measured VO_2 using indirect calorimetry in a group of pregnant women by tracking the concentration of oxygen of inhaled and exhaled air, and reported that healthy low-risk patients in the third trimester increase oxygen consumption (VO_2) approximately 86 percent in active-phase labor.[31] This is likely due to not only an increase in maternal cardiac output (CO) but also a significant increase in minute ventilation (VE) of greater than 160 percent.[31] For patients who are not able to increase both CO and VE to increase their DO_2, maternal compromise may rapidly ensue and result in both maternal and fetal acidemia. Table 12-14 indicates interventions for antepartum and intrapartum patients that may assist providers to balance maternal and fetal demands for oxygen delivery.

Oxygen consumption is a dynamic minute-to-minute variable in oxygen transport physiology. It increases and decreases based on the maternal condition and the types of procedures, interventions, stress, pain, etc., that the patient experiences. When the maternal DO_2 no longer meets the body's demand, actions to reduce the body's demand may temporize the development of acidosis.

TABLE 12-14

Actions to Promote Maternal Stability and Reduce VO_2 During Induction of Labor

	Goal	Collaborative Interventions	Considerations
Antepartum/Early Labor/Latent Phase			
Anxiety	Reduce anxiety to decrease VO_2 before and during labor induction	• Increase patient knowledge regarding disease/condition, plan of care, anticipated procedures, options for pain control, possibility of surgical interventions, newborn stabilization, potential for adult ICU and/or NICU admission (if anticipated). • Allow and encourage partner and/or family members to remain with patient at all times.	• Consider early sedation of patient if tachycardic or other signs or anxiety • *Avoid* FDA Category-X benzodiazepines; may use a pain-reducing agent such as morphine (to reduce VO_2)
Limit ambulation in latent phase	Estimate current and predicted DO_2 and VO_2 requirements for labor and delivery.	• Allow limited ambulation (if no contraindications) if patient desires. Or, encourage pt to find position in which she is most comfortable in bed. • Instruct patient and family re: reducing VO_2.	• Ambulation has not been shown to decrease the time for the cervix to dilate or efface. Encourage conservation of energy in latent phase.
Nutrients/Food	Provide kilocalories intake for energy expenditure during labor and delivery.	• If NPO, clear liquids and/or ice chips only, begin intravenous (IV) fluids with isotonic fluid and dextrose (e.g., D_5RL; $D_5$0.9%NaCl). Do not fluid bolus with this solution. Run as continuous infusion IV piggyback as ordered. • Fluid bolus with non-dextrose solution.	• If surgical delivery likely, clear fluids and ice chips only if anesthesia agrees. • Consult IV nutrition services if pt NPO >24 hr.

(text continued on page 211)

TABLE 12-14 (Continued)

Actions to Promote Maternal Stability and Reduce VO_2 During Induction of Labor

Intrapartum Phase

	Goal	Collaborative Interventions	Considerations
Optimize DO$_2$: *Cardiac*	Optimize CO, SaO$_2$ Avoid maternal hypotension from hypovolemia	• Lateral positioning if tolerated by patient • Maintain maternal MAP >60–65 mmHg • Optimize PCWP for patient condition. Target higher normal values while avoiding pulmonary edema. • If epidural, discuss opioid v. anesthetic	• Associated with high CO in pregnancy • Assure optimum preload for best ventricular performance • Do not increase PCWP greater than COP, *if possible*
	Maintain CO in normal ranges for stage of labor	• Optimize preload – PCWP (see above) • Assess afterload, ventricular work loads, contractility. Correct as indicated. • Correct severe abnormalities in SVR • Start positive inotropes *(if pt condition allows)* for low CO unresponsive to increased preload, low contractility (per specific pt condition).	• After adequate fluid volume is obtained, and patient remains hypotensive, assess calculated hemodynamic parameters. • If contractility low, CO low, PCWP elevated – consider maternal echocardiogram for possible undiagnosed cardiac lesion, CHF.
	Maintain "normal" oxyhemoglobin curve	• Keep patient warm (if indicated, use active warming devices; warming blankets, etc.) • Maintain maternal core temperature approximately approximately 99° F/37.5° C	• Oxyheme curve shifts further to left if pt cold, O$_2$ less likely to be delivered to cells. • Hypothermia accompanied by acidosis increases mortality rates.
Optimize DO$_2$: *Pulmonary*	Optimize SaO$_2$ Maintain SaO$_2$ >95%	• Use humidified supplemental oxygen as needed. • Obtain consult for intubation and mechanical ventilation when indicated (e.g., SaO$_2$ <90%–92%. If antepartum and fetus viable, consult with perinatology/intensivist to determine range of desired maternal SaO$_2$ to support fetus (~92%–94%).	Limited data on minimal SaO$_2$/PaO$_2$ levels for fetal survival.
	Maintain Hgb >7g/dL	• Evaluate need for Hgb transfusion if severely anemic prior to induction.	• Transfusion of packed red blood cells in critically ill patients (*NOT* experiencing hemorrhage) increases morbidity/mortality in some groups. • Transfusion is considered when the patient's hgb is <7. • If patient scheduled for Cesarean section, consider Cell Saver use in operating room (collection and re-infusion of patient's blood)

(continued)

TABLE 12-14 (Continued)

Actions to Promote Maternal Stability and Reduce VO$_2$ During Induction of Labor

Intrapartum Phase

	Goal	Collaborative Interventions	Considerations
Reduce VO$_2$	Maintain adequate ventilation (VE)	• Position patient with HOB elevated >30–45 degrees • Use hemodynamic profile, locate pt position that optimizes SaO$_2$ and CO.	• May improve lung expansion; reduces ventilator acquired pneumonia • Maintain hip roll • Turning/position changes may help non-functioning alveoli to open at lower hydrostatic pressures (i.e. change positions of lung zones) • Fluid administration guided by PAC values
	Reduce intrapulmonary shunt (Qs/Qt)	• Recruit non-functioning alveoli to reduce shunt • Frequently turn patient to place various lobes of lungs in independent positions. • Measure increase in PCWP during contractions; may need to decrease PCWP to prevent pulmonary edema secondary to autotransfusion • Consider specialized pulmonary ICU patient bed for continuous pulmonary treatments	
	Prevent ventilator-acquired pneumonia (intubated patients)	*See Chapter 4 on mechanical ventilation during pregnancy.*	
	Decrease VO$_2$: identify and treat/prevent known expenditures of O$_2$	• Liberal use of sedation, aggressively treat pain • Consult OB anesthesia, perinatology for acceptable methods of analgesia/anesthesia based on pt disease or condition • Limit patient's physical exertion • Avoid ambulation in early labor • Offer bedpan rather than ambulating to bathroom • Limit activities known to increase VO$_2$ • If limiting activity, DVT prophylaxis (screen prior to induction)	• Pain is one of the largest contributors to increased oxygen demand during labor • Common interventions during labor and delivery may accelerate the loss of adequate oxygen reserves • Reduce position changes, vaginal exams, ambulation, pushing, etc. Space out interventions to allow recovery for O$_2$/energy expenditures.
	Prevent infections: chorioamnionitis, UTI, central line, etc.	• Limit vaginal exams once membranes ruptured, (when possible) • Use bedpan rather than Foley catheter, (prevent catheter associated UTI) • Avoid/delay artificial rupture of membranes, (when possible); AROM does not significantly reduce the time to delivery. • Adhere to CDC's recommended guidelines for central line catheter insertion and maintenance procedures • Evaluate for prophylactic antibiotics	• Closely monitor temperature. Treat temp elevations early. • Avoid maternal tachycardia • Ruptured membranes >12 hours increases infection risk • Infection increases VO$_2$ • Fever increases VO$_2$ • To prevent central line infection

T A B L E   1 2 - 1 4 (Continued)

Actions to Promote Maternal Stability and Reduce VO₂ During Induction of Labor

Intrapartum Phase

Goal	Collaborative Interventions	Considerations
Avoid excessive VO₂ demands in second stage	• Use "laboring down," (delayed pushing until Ferguson's reflex felt by mother). • Open glottis pushing, avoid breath-holding • Non-coached pushing • May need to shorten second stage with forceps, vacuum • Avoid excessive uterine activity from oxytocin	• Uterine contractions increase VO₂ • Tachysystole increases VO₂

AROM = artificial rupture of membranes, CDC = Centers for Disease Control and Prevention, CHF = congestive heart failure, CO = cardiac output, COP = colloid oncotic pressure, DO₂ = oxygen delivery, DVT = deep venous thrombosis, FDA = Food and Drug Administration, Hgb = hemoglobin, HOB = head of bed, ICU = intensive care unit, MAP = mean arterial pressure, NaCl = sodium chloride, NICU = neonatal intensive care unit, NPO = nothing by mouth, PAC = pulmonary artery catheter, PaO₂ = partial pressure of oxygen in arterial blood, PAOP = pulmonary artery occlusion pressure, PCWP = pulmonary capillary wedge pressure, SaO₂ = oxygen saturation, SVR = systemic vascular resistance, UTI = urinary tract infection, VO₂ = oxygen consumption.

American College of Obstetricians & Gynecologists. (2009). ACOG practice bulletin no. 107: Induction of labor. *Obstetrics and Gynecology, 114,* 386–397.

Bobrowski, R. A. (2004). Maternal-fetal blood gas physiology. In G. A. Dildy, M. A. Belfort, G. R. Saade, Phelan, J. P., Hankins, G. D. V., and Clark, S. L. (Eds.), *Critical care obstetrics* (4th ed., pp. 43–59). Malden, MA: Blackwell Science.

Eliasson, A. H., Phillips, Y. Y., Stajduhar, K. C., Carome, M. A., & Cowsar, J. D. (1992). Oxygen consumption and ventilation during normal labor. *Chest, 102*(2), 467–471.

Garite, T. J. (2004). Fetal considerations in the critical care patient. In M. R. Foley, T. H. Strong, & T. J. Garite (Eds.), *Obstetric intensive care manual* (2nd ed., pp. 282–297). New York: McGraw-Hill.

Hankins, G. D., Harvey, C. J., Clark, S. L., Uckan, E. M., & Hook, J. W. (1996). The effects of maternal position and cardiac output on intrapulmonary shunt in normal third-trimester pregnancy. *Obstetrics and Gynecology, 88*(3), 327–330.

Witcher, P. M. (2006). Promoting fetal stabilization during maternal hemodynamic instability or respiratory insufficiency. *Critical Care Nursing Quarterly, 29,* 70–76.

SUMMARY

Induction or augmentation of labor in critically ill patients requires balancing the oxygen transport needs of both mother and fetus with the desire to induce effective uterine contractions to bring about delivery. The increased oxygen demand of the mother as labor progresses may deprive the myometrial muscle cells from the oxygen needed to produce effective uterine contractions. Conversely, the uterine contractions and resulting increase in oxygen demand may result in inadequate DO₂ to other maternal systems, increasing the risk for maternal anaerobic metabolism. Thus, effective clinical management of induction and augmentation relies on the skilled delivery of select medications to bring about cervical ripening and uterine contractions in a manner that does not exhaust current maternal oxygen stores. In addition, assessment of fetal status using EFM with its inherent challenges of interpretation and communication is vital during the induction process and may be improved by using a common language for EFM management. Finally, inherent to the role of clinical providers in planning and guiding uterine activity to bring about a vaginal delivery in critically ill patients is to actively assess both mother and fetus for indicators of oxygen transport adequacy, to respond to factors that may alter oxygen transport and to actively work to balance the VO₂ requirements of both.

REFERENCES

1. Martin, J. A., Hamilton, B. E., Sutton, P. D., Ventura, S. J., Menacker, F., Kirmeyer, S., et al. Centers for Disease Control and Prevention National Center for Health Statistics National Vital Statistics System. (2007). Births: Final data for 2005. *National Vital Statistics Reports, 56*(6), 1–103.
2. American College of Obstetricians & Gynecologists. (2009). ACOG practice bulletin no. 107: Induction of labor. *Obstetrics and Gynecology, 114,* 386–397.
3. Boulvain, M., Kelly, A. J., & Irion, O. (2008). Intracervical prostaglandins for induction of labour. *Cochrane Database of Systematic Reviews,* Issue 1. Art. No.: CD006971. doi: 10.1002/14651858.CD006971

4. French, L. (2001). Oral prostaglandin E2 for induction of labour. *Cochrane Database of Systematic Reviews,* Issue 2. Art. No.: CD003098. doi: 10.1002/14651858.CD003098

5. Hofmeyr, G. J., & Gulmezoglu, A. M. (2010). Vaginal misoprostol for cervical ripening and induction of labour. *Cochrane Database of Systematic Reviews,* Issue 10. Art. No.: CD000941. doi: 10.1002/14651858.CD000941.pub2

6. Simpson, K. R. (2008). *AWHONN Practice Monograph: Cervical ripening and induction and augmentation of labor* (3rd ed., pp. 1–46). Washington, DC: Association of Women's Health, Obstetric and Neonatal Nurses.

7. Osol, G., & Mandala, M. (2009). Maternal uterine vascular remodeling during pregnancy. *Physiology (Bethesda), 24,* 58–71.

8. Greiss, F. (2008). Uterine and placental blood flow. *Global Library of Women's Medicine.* Retrieved from http://www.glowm.com/?p=glowm.cml/section_view&articleid=197#sectionView

9. Wray, S. (2007). Insights into the uterus. *Experimental Physiology, 92,* 621–631.

10. Quenby, S., Pierce, S. J., Brigham, S., & Wray, S. (2004). Dysfunctional labor and myometrial lactic acidosis. *Obstetrics and Gynecology, 103*(4), 718–723.

11. Witcher, P. M. (2006). Promoting fetal stabilization during maternal hemodynamic instability or respiratory insufficiency. *Critical Care Nursing Quarterly, 29,* 70–76.

12. Hendricks, C. H. (1958). The hemodynamics of a uterine contraction. *American Journal of Obstetrics and Gynecology, 76,* 969–982.

13. Bobrowski, R. A. (2004). Maternal-fetal blood gas physiology. In G. A. Dildy, M. A. Belfort, G. R. Saade, Phelan, J. P., Hankins, G. D. V., and Clark, S. L. (Eds.), *Critical care obstetrics* (4th ed., pp. 43–59). Malden, MA: Blackwell Science.

14. Witcher, P. M., & Harvey, C. J. (2006). Modifying labor routines for the woman with cardiac disease. *Journal of Perinatal and Neonatal Nursing, 20,* 303–310.

15. Alanis, M. C., Villers, M. S., Law, T. L., Steadman, E. M., & Robinson, C. J. (2010). Complications of cesarean delivery in the massively obese parturient. *American Journal of Obstetrics and Gynecology, 203*(3), 271.e1–7.

16. Macones, G. A., Hankins, G. D., Spong, C. Y., Hauth, J., & Moore, T. (2008). The 2008 National Institute of Child Health and Human Development Planning Workshop report on electronic fetal monitoring: Update on definitions, interpretation, and research guidelines. *Journal of Obstetric, Gynecologic, and Neonatal Nursing, 37,* 510–515 and *Obstetrics and Gynecology, 112*(3), 661–666.

17. Electronic fetal heart rate monitoring: Research guidelines for interpretation. The National Institute of Child Health and Human Development Research Planning Workshop. (1997). *American Journal of Obstetrics and Gynecology, 177*(6), 1385–1390.

18. Electronic fetal heart rate monitoring: Research guidelines for interpretation. The National Institute of Child Health and Human Development Research Planning Workshop. (1997). *Journal of Obstetric, Gynecologic, and Neonatal Nursing, 26,* 635–640.

19. Garite, T. J. (2004). Fetal considerations in the critical care patient. In M. R. Foley, T. H. Strong, & T. J. Garite (Eds.), *Obstetric intensive care manual* (2nd ed., pp. 282–297). New York: McGraw-Hill.

20. American Academy of Pediatrics & American College of Obstetricians and Gynecologists. (2007). *Guidelines for perinatal care* (6th ed., pp. 139–201). Elk Grove, IL: Authors.

21. Liston, R., Sawchuck, D., & Young, D. (2007). Fetal health surveillance: Antepartum and intrapartum consensus guideline. *JOGC, 29,* 1–56.

22. Lee, H. J., Macbeth, A. H., Pagani, J. H., & Young, W. S. 3rd. (2009). Oxytocin: The great facilitator of life. *Progress in Neurobiology, 88,* 127–151.

23. RxList–The Internet Drug Index. (2011). *Pitocin drug description.* Retrieved from http://www.rxlist.com/pitocin-drug.htm

24. Clark, S. L., Simpson, K. R., Knox, G. E., & Garite, T. J. (2009). Oxytocin: New perspectives on an old drug. *American Journal of Obstetrics and Gynecology, 200*(1), 35.e1–6.

25. Moleti, C. A. (2009). Trends and controversies in labor induction. *MCN: American Journal of Maternal Child Nursing, 34,* 40–47; quiz 48–49.

26. Smith, J. G., & Merrill, D. C. (2006). Oxytocin for induction of labor. *Clinical Obstetrics and Gynecology, 49,* 594–608.

27. Simpson, K. R., & Knox, G. E. (2009). Oxytocin as a high-alert medication: Implications for perinatal patient safety. *MCN: American Journal of Maternal Child Nursing, 34,* 8–15; quiz 16–17.

28. George, R., Berkenbosch, J. W., Fraser, R. F. II, & Tobias, J. D. (2001). Mechanical ventilation during pregnancy using a helium-oxygen mixture in a patient with respiratory failure due to status asthmaticus. *Journal of Perinatology, 21*(6), 395–398.

29. Graves, C. R. (2002). Acute pulmonary complications during pregnancy. *Clinical Obstetrics and Gynecology, 45,* 369–376.

30. Arakawa, T. K., Mlynarczyk, M., Kaushal, K. M., Zhang, L., & Ducsay, C. A. (2004). Long-term hypoxia alters calcium regulation in near-term ovine myometrium. *Biology of Reproduction, 71*(1), 156–162.

31. Eliasson, A. H., Phillips, Y. Y., Stajduhar, K. C., Carome, M. A., & Cowsar, J. D. (1992). Oxygen consumption and ventilation during normal labor. *Chest, 102*(2), 467–471.

CHAPTER 13

Acute Renal Failure

Betsy B. Kennedy, Carol J. Harvey, and George R. Saade

Acute renal failure (ARF), also referred to as acute kidney injury (AKI), broadly refers to a condition characterized by a relatively sudden and sustained decline in renal function. Criteria for ARF, described by the Second International Consensus Conference of the Acute Dialysis Quality Initiative (ADQI) Group, include an abrupt reduction in kidney function, defined as an absolute increase in serum creatinine of more than 0.3 mg/dL or more than 25 micromoles/L, a 50 percent increase in serum creatinine, or oliguria, defined as less than 0.5 mL/kg/hr for more than 6 hours.[1]

The consequences of this dysfunction include failure of the kidneys to adequately excrete nitrogenous waste products, resulting in increased serum levels of protein metabolism derivatives (i.e., azotemia), an inability to maintain fluid and electrolyte balance, and increased risk of significant sequelae. The development of ARF in any patient increases the risk for death and is further increased if renal replacement therapy (e.g., dialysis) is needed.

Theoretically, rapid-onset ARF in a patient with no history of renal impairment is a reversible condition that does not always leave a patient with permanent impairment. However, the likelihood of recovery is dependent upon the type of ARF and its duration. To prevent progression of ARF requiring maintenance dialysis or a renal transplant, it is important to assess for ARF based on a high degree of suspicion, to quickly correct the underlying condition that is causing ARF, and to prevent further complications in the patient to enhance the chance for recovery.

This chapter addresses normal renal physiology, the impact of pregnancy on renal physiology, classification systems for ARF, common causes of ARF in pregnancy, and current trends in the management of ARF in pregnancy, including renal replacement therapies. Brief clinical case excerpts are presented to highlight significant differences between types of ARF.

INCIDENCE OF ARF

The exact incidence of ARF in pregnancy is difficult to determine as historically there have been no standard definitions of ARF in any population. Over the last 50 years the incidence in pregnancy has decreased in industrialized countries from 1 per 3,000 pregnancies to 1 per 15,000 to 20,000 pregnancies in women with no history of renal impairment.[2,3] The decrease has been attributed to the reduction of septic abortions (secondary to the legalization of abortion in industrialized nations) and the increase in accessible prenatal care with a resultant decrease in maternal deaths.[2,3] Prakash and colleagues in India recently reported a significant (p < 0.001) fall in the incidence of cortical necrosis related to ARF in pregnancy in a patient group from 1992 to 2002 compared to a similar group from 1982 to 1991. They concluded that the changing trends in obstetric ARF in their population were mainly related to a decrease in the number of septic abortions, puerperal sepsis, and maternal mortality.[2] Although ARF occurs infrequently in the general pregnant population, it remains a common complication in critically ill patients and independently increases the risk for maternal mortality.[4]

The exact incidence of ARF and related mortality rates is elusive not only because of the prior use of non-standardized definitions of the disease, but also the lack of consistent use of International Classification of Disease (ICD) Clinical Modifications 9 and/or 10 codes for ARF, including diagnoses, types, and mortality secondary to the disease. Thus, epidemiologic study of ARF in various population groups and its outcomes is challenging. The incidence of ARF in all patients has been reported at 1 to 5 percent of hospital admissions, and mortality rates have ranged from 25 to 90 percent.

Similarly dismal has been the suggestion that there have been no measurable improvements in morbidity and mortality rates over the past two decades.[5,6] In an attempt to counter this suggestion, two large retrospective studies based on administrative databases reported that although the overall rate of ARF had increased, morbidity and mortality rates had decreased over time.[7,8] Although the studies share the same limitations as other reports that rely upon extrapolated data from Medicare databases, state death certificates, and/or ICD-9 coding reports, a statistically significant improvement in outcome measures agrees with current clinical commentary on improved patient outcomes when evidence-based treatment plans are implemented. However, even when the improvement is accounted for, the outcomes of patients with ARF remain poor.[9]

In light of current reports, it may be reasonable to say that the rate of renal insufficiency has increased in the general population across all age groups and that approximately 4 to 5 percent of non-pregnant hospitalized patients develop ARF, which may lead to further complications and death, frequently from infection and/or cardiopulmonary collapse. Although the rate has decreased over the past 15 to 20 years, 40 to 70 percent of all patients admitted to an intensive care unit (ICU) without a history of renal impairment continue to die from ARF.[10] Morbidity and mortality rates for pregnant women who develop ARF are largely indeterminate, again related to the lack of a national database to follow the small number of pregnant patients admitted to ICUs. Additionally, the definition of ARF in pregnancy, like other specialties has only recently been developed.

Most cases of ARF in pregnancy occur in women with no previous renal disease. However, women with underlying chronic renal dysfunction (serum creatinine of 1.4 mg/dL or above) are at significantly increased risk for further loss of renal function during pregnancy.[11] Approximately 40 percent of these women will have an added loss in renal function, and many will present with abrupt onset and progression.[6] Thus the absence of ARF in pregnancy at any gestational age does not preclude the possibility that the woman may develop sudden-onset ARF and have a rapid deterioration of renal function.

ARF during pregnancy is rare, but when present, the concomitant risks pose clinical challenges for care providers. Because of associated mortality risks and potential for long-term morbidity, a multidisciplinary team of care providers that represents critical care, maternal-fetal medicine, obstetric critical care, and nephrology and neonatology specialties is recommended for clinical management.

NORMAL KIDNEY FUNCTION

Early identification and classification of ARF is commonly based on the interpretation of serum and urine laboratory tests that reflect kidney function. A brief review of renal anatomic and physiologic principles is presented, in order to better understand changes associated with ARF.

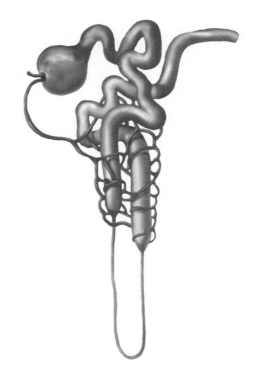

FIGURE 13-1 Functional unit of the kidney—the nephron.

Normally, the renal/urinary system is composed of two kidneys, bilateral ureters, the urinary bladder, and the urethra. The functional unit of the kidney is the nephron, illustrated in Figure 13-1, with each adult kidney containing approximately 1 to 1.5 million nephrons. The nephron consists of a vascular and tubular component. Blood flows from the abdominal aorta into the renal arteries, the smaller renal arteries and arterioles, ending in the afferent arteriole, and ultimately in the glomerulus. The highly permeable capillaries in the glomerulus reform into the efferent arteriole, which then branches into the peritubular capillaries and vasa recta. The peritubular capillaries and vasa recta communicate with the renal tubules, to facilitate movement of water and solutes (secretion and reabsorption) between the plasma (peritubular capillaries and vasa recta), and filtrate (renal tubules).

Bowman's capsule surrounds the glomerulus and is considered the starting point of the tubule that participates in secretion and reabsorption (Fig. 13-2). The tubule is a continuous structure, divided into the proximal convoluted straight tubule, the descending limb, the ascending limb (together referred to as the loop of Henle), the distal convoluted tubule, and the cortical and medullary collecting ducts. The tubule is responsible for reabsorption of water, electrolytes, and other substances back into the blood of the peritubular capillaries, and into the systemic circulation (Fig. 13-3). The tubule exits into the collecting ducts, creating urine, which is drained into the ureters and stored in the bladder.

Nephrons produce urine via three processes: tubular reabsorption, tubular secretion, and glomerular

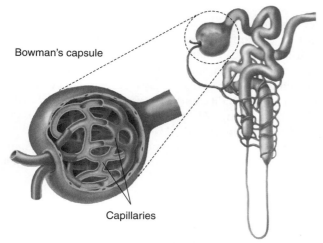

FIGURE 13-2 Bowman's capsule surrounds the glomerulus and is considered the starting point of the tubule that participates in secretion and reabsorption.

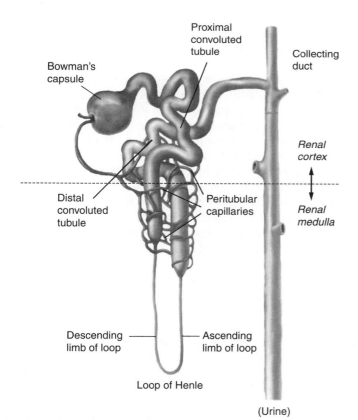

FIGURE 13-3 The tubule is a continuous structure divided into the proximal convoluted straight tubule, the descending limb, the ascending limb (together referred to as the loop of Henle), the distal convoluted tubule, and the cortical and medullary collecting ducts. The tubule is responsible for reabsorption of water, electrolytes, and other substances back into the blood of the peritubular capillaries, and into the systemic circulation.

filtration.[12] The kidneys receive up to 25 percent of cardiac output per minute, resulting in a continuous filtration of fluid from the glomerular capillary bed into Bowman's capsule. The glomerular filtration rate (GFR) affects the amount of urine produced, waste products excreted, electrolyte balance, fluid balance, and acid base balance. The kidneys are usually able to autoregulate to maintain the GFR despite variations in arterial blood pressure and renal perfusion pressure. Even wide changes in arterial blood pressure, within the normal limits of 70 mmHg to 160 mmHg, have little to no effect on GFR. The juxtaglomerular apparatus (JGA), a group of cells positioned where the distal convoluted tubule of each nephron meets the angle of the afferent and efferent arterioles, controls tubuloglomerular feedback (renal autoregulation). Changes in the tubular fluid volume and electrolytes are sensed by the macula densa and relayed to the JGA. The JGA stimulates afferent arteriole vasodilation or constriction, affecting blood flow and glomerular capillary bed hydrostatic pressure, in order to maintain GFR.

Hydration status causes the kidneys to alter the amount of urine output. Fluid volume excess causes decreased tubular reabsorption of filtrate, resulting in large amounts of dilute urine. Fluid volume deficit causes maximal reabsorption of tubular filtrate, resulting in a small amount of concentrated urine. The kidneys are responsible for excretion of metabolic waste products including, but not limited to, urea, creatinine, uric acid, bilirubin, and metabolic acid.

While the respiratory system is primarily responsible for the regulation of acid–base balance, excreting large amounts of carbon dioxide each day, the kidneys excrete fixed acids (acid anion and associated hydrogen ion), for which there is no other means of removal. The kidneys are also responsible for reabsorption of filtered bicarbonate, the most important buffer for fixed acids.

In summary, select essential functions of the kidneys are: maintenance of intravascular volume; regulation of water balance, electrolyte balance, and plasma osmolality; regulation of acid–base balance in association with the respiratory and buffer systems; excretion of the end-products of metabolism and some exogenous substances (drugs); and participation in blood pressure regulation.[13]

EFFECTS OF PREGNANCY ON KIDNEY FUNCTION

During pregnancy, GFR increases approximately 40 to 65 percent, and renal blood flow increases even more, to approximately 50 to 85 percent.[6,14] This increased perfusion leads to a 50 percent increase in the GFR and, in combination with the increase in renal plasma flow, accounts for more efficient clearance of several substances from

TABLE 13-1

Normal Alterations of Renal Function in Pregnancy

Renal Function	Alteration in Pregnancy
Anatomical	• Dilation of renal collecting system
	• Kidney enlargement
	• Some hydronephrosis normal
	• More effects on right side
Hemodynamic	• Decrease in peripheral vascular resistance
	• Decreased renal vascular resistance
	• Arteriolar underfilling – leads to systemic responses
	• Increased cardiac output
	• Increased plasma volume
	• Decreased blood pressure – mid-gestation
	• Increased renal plasma flow/ Increased GFR
Solute handling	• Some proteinuria is normal (<300 mg/24hr)
	• Some glucosuria is normal
Acid–base balance	• Increased minute ventilation
	• Respiratory alkalosis
	• Kidneys compensate by decreasing serum HCO_3.
	• Decreased HCO_3 reduces buffering capacity if needed

Data from Grammill, H. S., & Jeyabalan, A. (2005). Acute renal failure in pregnancy. *Critical Care Medicine, 33*(Suppl. 10), S372–S384.

the blood, including creatinine and urea. This leads to lower serum levels of both substances. A normal creatinine level in pregnancy is 0.46 mg/dL, whereas a normal blood urea nitrogen (BUN) is 8.24 mg/dL. There is also a physiologic decrease in plasma osmolality as early as the first trimester. Sodium and water are retained during the course of pregnancy, with approximately 950 mEq of sodium and 6 to 8 liters of water accumulated. Thus, it can be said that pregnancy is a state of "super" or augmented renal clearance, impacting the function of the renal system and diagnostic criteria for ARF.[15]

Specific physiologic and anatomic changes associated with pregnancy that affect the renal system are described in Table 13-1. Hydronephrosis and hydroureter, which normally occur in pregnancy, affect renal function as evidenced by adjustments in laboratory parameter reference ranges.

ASSESSMENT OF KIDNEY FUNCTION

Evaluation of kidney function includes serum and urine laboratory analyses and, commonly, renal imaging studies. Patient condition and assessment findings determine the level of diagnostic testing.

One of the fundamental components of assessment is urine output in milliliters per hour (mL/hr). Precise measurement is important in the diagnosis of ARF, as the volume of urine output plays a role in the prediction of patient morbidity and mortality rates. Oliguric ARF (less than 400 mL/24 hr) has a worse prognosis compared to nonoliguric ARF.[5]

A comparison of normal non-pregnant and pregnant values for select serum and urine indices is presented in Table 13-2.

DEFINITION AND CLASSIFICATIONS OF ARF

Patients at Risk

Patients at highest risk for ARF include those with co-morbidities such as diabetes mellitus, preexisting renal insufficiency, cardiac failure, or sepsis.[16] The kidneys are dependent upon adequate oxygen delivery and consumption to maintain metabolic efficiency and avoid ischemic or hypoxemic injury. Physiologic stress produces a series of orchestrated measures to best manage overall survival. Predetermined measures will eventually result in the interruption of oxygen delivery to select organ systems that are not critical for survival. Common "non-critical" systems include integumentary, gastrointestinal, reproductive, and renal. Adaptive responses shunt arterial blood from these systems to more critical organs involved in survival: the heart, brain, and adrenal glands. Hence, all patients in unstable physiologic states are at risk for developing ARF. Acute clinical conditions associated with development of renal failure in hospitalized patients are extensive. These conditions include but are not limited to sepsis, septic shock, hypotension, hemorrhage, volume depletion, cardiac/vascular surgery, organ transplantation surgery, abdominal compartment syndrome, and mechanical ventilation.[16,17]

Risk factors for ARF in pregnant patients are the same as those for the general population. Risk is also affected by the patient's age, physiologic status prior to hospital admission, specific etiology of the renal insult, and timing of identification and treatment. Risk factors often present in cases of ARF during pregnancy include hypertension, disseminated intravascular coagulation (DIC), infection, hypovolemia, and obstruction by the gravid uterus.[6] Hypertensive complications that increase risk for ARF are most commonly preeclampsia-eclampsia, principally with co-morbidities such as placental abruption, pulmonary edema, or hemorrhage. The exact rate of ARF in preeclampsia

TABLE 13-2

Normal Laboratory Values in the Pregnant and Non-Pregnant Woman

Parameter	Pregnancy Values	Non - Pregnancy Values
Blood urea nitrogen (BUN)	5–12 mg/dL	10–20 mg/dL
Serum creatinine	<1.0 mg/dL	<1.5 mg/dL
Serum uric acid	1.2–4.5 mg/dL	1.5–6.0 mg/dL
Serum osmolality	275–280 mOsm/kg	285–295 mOsm/kg
Serum sodium	130–140 mEq/L	136–145 mEq/L
Serum potassium	3.3–4.1 mEq/L	3.5–5.0 mEq/L
Urine protein	<300 mg/day	<150 mg/day
Urine sodium	37–150 mmol/24 hr	100–260 mmol/24 hrs
Urine creatinine – clearance	50–166 mL/min	91–130 mL/min
Urine creatinine – excretion	10.2–11.4 mmol/24 hr	8.8–14 mmol/24 hr

remains debatable, but current data suggest that 1.5 to 2 percent of women with preeclampsia develop ARF, and in patients with HELLP syndrome (see Chapter 7), the rate increases to greater than 7 percent.[6] Causes of ARF in pregnancy and the most common times of onset are presented in Table 13-3.

The RIFLE Criteria

Until recently, there was no agreement on an objective and measurable definition of ARF, which has hindered the investigation of the incidence and subsequent morbidity and mortality in patients with renal failure. In 2004, the

TABLE 13-3

Causes of ARF/AKI in Early Pregnancy, Late Pregnancy, and Postpartum

Causes of AKI	Common Timing of Onset		
	Early pregnancy	Late pregnancy	Postpartum
Pyelonephritis	×	×	×
Obstructive uropathy	×	×	×
Nephrolithiasis (renal stones)	×	×	×
Hyperemesis gravidarum	×		
Spontaneous abortion	×		
Hemorrhage (antepartum)	×		
Septic abortion with shock	×		
Gram-negative sepsis (especially *E. coli*)	×		
Myoglobulinuria (due to *Clostridium*-induced myonecrosis of uterus)	×		
Preeclampsia/HELLP syndrome		×	
Placental abruption		×	
Acute fatty liver of pregnancy (AFLP)		×	
Hemorrhage (intrapartum and postpartum)		×	×
Amniotic fluid embolism		×	×
Thrombotic microangiopathies: Thrombotic thrombocytopenia purpura (TTP), hemolytic uremic syndrome (HUS)		×	×
Disseminated intravascular coagulation (DIC)		×	×
Postpartum acute renal failure			×

Data from:

Krane, N. K., Agraharkar, M., Agraharkar, A., et al. (2010). Renal disease and pregnancy. Retrieved from http://emedicine.medscape.com/article/246123-overview

Agraharkar, M., Gupta, R., & Workeneh, B. T. (2007). Acute renal failure. E-medicine. Retrieved from http://www.emedicine.com/med/TOPIC1595.HTM

Krane, N. K., & Hamrahian, M. (2007). Core curriculum in nephrology. Pregnancy: Kidney diseases and hypertension. *American Journal of Kidney Diseases, 49*(2), 336–345.

TABLE 13-4

RIFLE Criteria to Determine Risk for ARF

	Serum Creatinine/GFR	Urine Ouput
Risk	Serum Cr increased 1.5× or GFR decreased more than 25%	Less than 0.5 mL/kg/hr for 6 hr
Injury	Serum Cr increased 2.0× or GFR decreased more than 50%	Less than 0.5 mL/kg/hr for 12 hr
Failure (hours)	Serum Cr increased 3.0× or GFR decreased more than 75% or Serum Cr greater than 4 mg/dL or Serum Cr acute rise greater than 0.5 mg/dL	Less than 0.3 mL/kg/hr for 24 hr *or* anuria for 12 hr
Loss	Persistent AKI; complete loss of kidney function for more than 4 weeks	
ESKD	End stage kidney disease for longer than 3 months	

Note:
Because ARF can occur superimposed on chronic disease, these laboratory values may differ.
AKI = acute kidney injury, GFR = glomerular filtration rate, Cr = creatinine, ESKD = end-stage kidney disease.

Acute Dialysis Quality Initiative (ADQI) group convened an International Consensus Conference of experts in the field and agreed upon a definition of ARF. Furthermore, the group created the "RIFLE" classification system based on changes from the patient's baseline either in serum creatinine level or GFR, urine output, or both.[18] The purpose of RIFLE, which is the acronym for Risk, Injury, Failure, Loss, and End-stage kidney disease (ESKD), is to classify patients at separate risk for development of ARF.[19] The criteria are described in Table 13-4. A component of the RIFLE system is the use of urine output as a predictor of renal failure. The categorization of anuric, oliguric, nonoliguric, or polyuric urine output levels are defined in Table 13-5.

Classification

ARF can be classified as one of three general etiologic types: prerenal (hypoperfusion), intrinsic (intrarenal), or postrenal (obstructive) failure, depending upon the anatomic location of the problem.

Prerenal failure is the result of disruption of oxygen and nutrient transport to the kidney. In pregnancy, the cause of decreased transport is frequently decreased cardiac output secondary to hemorrhage, hypovolemia,

TABLE 13-5

Definitions and Categories of Urine Output

Anuria	<100 mL in 24 hr
Oliguria	<400 mL in 24 hr
Nonoliguria	>400 mL in 24 hr
Polyuria	>6 L in 24 hr

or hypotension. The primary etiology may be postpartum hemorrhage, septic shock, placental abruption, ruptured ectopic pregnancy, or DIC. If the kidneys are not perfused and oxygen and nutrient delivery restored, nephrons will become ischemic, which results in alteration of renal function based on the number of nephrons damaged. This type of renal failure is classified as intrinsic failure. Acute tubular necrosis (ATN) is one type of intrinsic failure. Postrenal failure, also termed obstructive renal failure, is caused by the obstruction of urine flow at any location. Frequently associated with hydronephrosis related to engorgement of the kidneys with urine, postrenal failure may cause nephron damage if left undiagnosed and/or untreated.

Each of the three types of renal failure has associated etiologies, history and physical assessment findings, and laboratory determinants. It is paramount for care providers to quickly identify the insult, correct the problem, reperfuse the kidneys, and provide supportive measures for the patient until recovery occurs.

Prerenal Failure

Prerenal azotemia is the most common form of ARF and results from an insult that occurs before blood reaches the kidneys. The kidneys receive approximately 20 to 25 percent of cardiac output per minute. When cardiac output is adequate, a mean arterial pressure (MAP) greater than 70 mmHg should maintain adequate renal perfusion. During periods of hypovolemia or decreased cardiac output from other causes, there is evidence that patients with a MAP less than 65 mmHg have an increased risk for ARF.[20] Any condition that decreases cardiac output or limits systemic perfusion pressure, such as decreased intravascular volume and decreased vascular tone, may lead to hypoperfusion of the kidneys. Initially, the normal kidneys adapt by afferent arteriole dilation and efferent arteriole constriction to maintain normal GFR (autoregulation), and by renin release. Renin activates a cascade of events that results in peripheral vasoconstriction, increased water reabsorption, and increased serum BUN concentration. Although the structure of the kidneys is normal, the glomeruli eventually become unable to filter blood secondary to reduction in blood flow. Glucose and oxygen delivery to the tubular cells is decreased, and there is retention of metabolic wastes. The outcome is decreased adenosine triphosphate (ATP) synthesis in renal tubular cells. Many tubular processes are ATP-dependent, so numerous dysfunctions occur as a result of inadequate oxygen, glucose, and ATP. Elevated serum concentration of the nitrogenous waste products eventually occurs, and the kidneys progress to failure if the source is not identified and treated.

The adaptive response of functioning kidneys with intact nephrons to decreased oxygen and nutrient delivery includes release and activation of angiotensin II, aldosterone, and antidiuretic hormone (ADH). These produce increased reabsorption of sodium (Na^+) and urea in nephrons. The increased level of serum Na^+ results in increased intravascular volume and causes decreased urine output and, commonly, oliguria. This results in an increased concentration of urine (increased urine osmolality) and a decrease in urine Na^+.

With timely identification and rectification of the underlying cause to reestablish systemic and therefore renal perfusion, the condition can be reversible. Treatment needs to be based on the etiology of the prerenal problem. Fluid administration with intravenous normal saline solution (0.9% NaCl), and/or blood transfusion in cases of hemorrhage or anemia, is most often a cornerstone of initial treatment of prerenal failure. If hypoperfusion persists and is not recognized or ineffectively managed, the protective mechanisms of the kidneys become depleted. The resulting ischemic damage may be permanent and lead to intrinsic failure (e.g., ATN). The amount of damage is dependent on the duration of the insult and the baseline health of the kidneys at the time of insult. Etiologies of prerenal failure can be found in Table 13-6.

TABLE 13-6

Etiologies of Prerenal Failure

Cardiac disorders which limit/reduce cardiac output	• Congestive heart failure • Myocardial infarction • Arrhythmias • Pulmonary embolus • Mechanical ventilation (PEEP)
Hypovolemia	• Hemorrhage – abruption, postpartum hemorrhage, uterine rupture, surgical blood loss • Dehydration – hyperemesis • Burns • Shock
Altered peripheral vascular resistance	• Severe preeclampsia/hypertension • Hypotension • Sepsis/shock • Antihypertensive medications • DIC/AFE
Renal artery disorders	• Emboli/thrombi • Stenosis • Aneurysm • Occlusion • Trauma
Oxygen and nutrient transport disorders	• Reduced cardiac output (see above) • Reduced oxygen delivery capacity (decreased Hgb) • Reduced Hgb saturation (decreased SaO_2) • Reduced O_2 affinity

DIC/AFE = disseminated intravascular coagulation/amniotic fluid embolism syndrome, Hgb = hemoglobin, O_2 = oxygen, PEEP = positive end-expiratory pressure, SaO_2 = saturation of arterial hemoglobin with oxygen.

Adapted from:

Agraharkar, M., Gupta, R., & Workeneh, B. T. (2007). Acute renal failure. *E-medicine.* Retrieved from http://www.emedicine.com/med/TOPIC1595.HTM

Prerenal azotemia is the most common type of renal failure in pregnancy. Volume depletion significant enough to cause renal ischemia is often caused by obstetric hemorrhage, severe hyperemesis gravidarum, or volume shifts.[6] Management is directed at the cause, with a goal of volume and blood product replacement to re-establish renal perfusion before progression to intrinsic failure. Obstetric hemorrhage is particularly concerning due to the added risk of associated coagulopathies such as DIC, which can cause direct tubular damage and failure.[6]

Case Excerpt: Prerenal Failure. The patient, a 27-year-old gravida 2 para 2 0 0 2, had a history of an uncomplicated pregnancy and vaginal delivery followed by severe postpartum hemorrhage secondary to uterine atony. The estimated blood loss at the time of delivery was noted to be 3,000 mL. Treatment included administration of 2 liters of D_5LR and 6 liters of 0.9% NaCl. Assessment findings—including vital signs, serum and urine renal indices—approximately 16 hours following the diagnosis of postpartum hemorrhage, are presented in Table 13-7.

Intrinsic Failure

Intrinsic (parenchymal) renal failure is the result of direct damage to the kidney parenchyma. It is precipitated by an ischemic event, exposure to nephrotoxins, immunologic/inflammatory mechanisms, or a combination of two or more. Structural damage to the kidneys is the main feature of intrinsic ARF. Intrinsic renal failure can be grouped as tubular injury necrosis, vasculitis, acute glomerulonephritis, and/or acute interstitial nephritis.[6] The most common form is ATN that is either ischemic or cytotoxic.[5] Ischemic ARF is secondary to a severe, prolonged decrease in renal blood flow and hypoperfusion. A sustained MAP of less than 60 to 70 mmHg initiates several pathways that result in the loss of autoregulation by afferent and efferent arterioles, loss of sympathetic nervous system regulatory response, and decreased GFR. The ischemic event results in the death of susceptible tubular cells (ATN) and damage to the basement membrane, which is a supportive layer on the outside of the tubular cells. The degree of damage to the renal cells is proportional to the duration of ischemia.

Additional damage secondary to free (superoxide) radicals may also ensue. Free radicals are extremely active oxygen derivatives with a single electron in their outer shell. All cells that have oxidative metabolism can produce free radicals as by-products, and under certain circumstances these free radicals can degrade membranes, proteins, and DNA, and thereby destroy the cell. With reoxygenation after ischemia, increased damage by free radicals may occur. Thus, after ischemic anoxia, an increase in the production of free radicals and a decrease in the cellular defense mechanisms allow these agents to cause increasing cell damage. Consequently, a para-

dox develops following ischemic anoxia. The cells need oxygen to survive, but oxygen also produces increased free radicals which can destroy the cell.

Acute renal failure from exposure to cytotoxic substances (nephrotoxins) is caused by direct damage of the tubular cells and subsequent necrosis. Nephrotoxins may be responsible for as much as 50 percent of all cases of acute or chronic renal failure in non-pregnant patients. The tubules are highly susceptible to toxic damage due to repeated exposure to circulating toxins during filtration of the blood. In addition, there are frequently high renal intracellular concentrations of these injurious substances as they await excretion. If there is existing renal dysfunction, dehydration, or diabetes mellitus, exposure to multiple nephrotoxins exacerbates the potential for ARF. If injuries from nephrotoxins affect the renal tubular cells, but not necessarily the basement membrane, the resulting ATN may be reversible. However, recovery is dependent upon the repair and regeneration of new non-necrotic renal cells. A list of nephrotoxic substances is displayed in Table 13-8.

ATN often, but not always, follows a four-phase clinical course: onset, oliguric/anuric phase, diuretic phase, and recovery phase. These phases are described in Table 13-9.

Differentiating the diagnosis of ATN from prerenal failure presents a common clinical challenge. Prerenal azotemia corresponds with the onset of ATN; however, prerenal azotemia may be reversible, while injury from ATN may be permanent. Evaluation of serum and urine laboratory values provide important clues. Typical laboratory values for prerenal failure, ATN, and postrenal failure are presented together in Table 13-10. A key marker for prerenal failure is a low fractional excretion of sodium ($FeNa^+$)—the portion of sodium, after being filtered at the glomerulus, that remains in the urine and is excreted.[6] When blood and oxygen transport to the kidneys is reduced, normally functioning nephrons increase the uptake of sodium from the urine to bring it back into the bloodstream. The sodium attracts water in an attempt to maintain intravascular volume status to promote a positive fluid balance. Thus, increasing serum levels of sodium and simultaneously decreasing urine levels of sodium are indicative of prerenal failure. $FeNa^+$, the fractional excretion of sodium, is a calculated value using this formula:

$$FeNa^+ = \frac{UNa \times PCr}{PNa \times UCr} \times 100$$

in which PCr = plasma creatinine, PNa = plasma sodium, UCr = urine creatinine, and UNa = urine sodium.

In patients with normal kidney function, $FeNa^+$ is less than 1 percent; that is, the percentage of Na^+ not reabsorbed by the kidneys and allowed to pass into the urine is a small percentage of the total Na^+ that was filtered from the blood. If the kidneys are working, the

TABLE 13-7

Case Excerpt: Prerenal Failure

Vital Signs		Comments
Heart Rate	128 bpm	
Blood Pressure (mean arterial pressure)	88/50 mmHg (63)	
Respirations	24 per minute	
Temperature	98.0° F (36.7°C)	
Labs – CBC		
RBC	3.13 million/mm^3	
Hgb	9.5 g/dl	
Hct	28.4%	
Platelets	101,000/mm^3	
Labs – Chemistry		
BUN	51 mg/dL (H)	
Creatinine	2.2 mg/dL (H)	
Sodium	140 mg/dL	
Potassium	3.7 mEq/L	
Chloride	105 mEq/L	
Labs – Urine		
Specific gravity	1.045	
pH	7.0	
Protein	Trace	
Glucose, Ketone, Bile, Blood, Nitrite, Leucocyte estimate	Negative	
WBC, RBC, Epithelial, Bacteria	Negative	
Comments	Normal sediment	
Prerenal vs. Intrarenal AKI		
BUN:Creatinine ratio	23:1	c/w prerenal
Urine volume	Oliguria	
Urinary sediment	Normal	c/w prerenal
Specific gravity	1.041	Concentrated – prerenal
Osmolality (mOsm/Kg H$_2$O)	High (>500)	Concentrated – prerenal
Ratio: Osm Urine to Osm plasma	>1.5	
Urine Na (mEq/L)	14.3	low
Urine urea (g/24 hr)	13	low
Hemoglobinuria	none	
Leukocyturia	none	
Proteinuria	Trace to none*	c/w prerenal
Fractional excretion of Na$^+$ $$FENa = \frac{(U_{Na}/P_{Na})}{(U_{Cr}/P_{Cr})} \times 100$$	≤1%	c/w prerenal
Fractional excretion of urea $$FEUrea = \frac{(U_{urea}/P_{urea})}{(U_{Cr}/P_{Cr})} \times 100$$	<35%	

bpm = beats per minute, BUN = blood urea nitrogen, c/w = consistent with, Hct = hematocrit, Hgb = hemoglobin, MAP = mean arterial pressure, Na = sodium, Osm = osmolality, PCr = plasma creatinine, PNa = plasma sodium, Purea = plasma urea, RBC = red blood cell, UCr = urine creatinine, UNa = urine sodium, Uurea = urine urea, WBC = white blood cell.

Discussion

The values listed are most consistent with renal compensation for decreased intravascular blood flow. BUN and Na+ are selectively reabsorbed to promote the movement of water into the intravascular space. The urine is concentrated with no abnormal cells, and the patient's tachycardia and blood pressure also suggest hypovolemia and/or low oxygen delivery from the blood loss. Treatment will most commonly be aimed at correcting intravascular volume, evaluating the need for blood transfusions to increase oxygen content and supporting hemodynamic status until renal oxygen delivery can be optimized.

TABLE 13-8

Select Examples of Nephrotoxic Agents

Categories	Types	Examples
Drugs	Anesthetics	halothane
		methoxyflurane
	Antibiotics	aminoglycosides (gentamicin, tobramycin, amikacin, netilmicin)
		amphotericin B
		cephalosporins
		ciprofloxacin
		demeclocycline
		penicillins
		pentamidine
		polymixins
		rifampin
		sulfonamides
		tetracycline
		vancomycin
	Antivirals	acyclovir
		cidovir
		foscarnet
		valacyclovir
	Anti-inflammatories	NSAIDs (ibuprofen, indomethacin, naproxen, toradol)
	Chemotherapeutic agents	adriamycin
		cisplatin
		methotrexate
		mitomycin C
		nitrosoureas
	Immunosupressants	cyclosporin A
		tacrolimus
	Vasoactives	captopril
		enalopril
		lisinopril
		losartan
	Others	acetaminophen
		cimetidine
		hydralazine
		lindane
		lithium
		lovastatin
		mannitol
		procainamide
		thiazides
Contrast media	Ionic	diatrizoate
		lomustine
	Nonionic	metrizamide
Biologic substances	Blood pigments	hemoglobin
	Tumor produced toxins	myoglobin
	Others	calcium
		cystine
		oxalate
		uric acid

TABLE 13-8 (Continued)

Select Examples of Nephrotoxic Agents

Categories	Types	Examples
Heavy metals		arsenic
		bismuth
		cadmium
		gold
		lead
		mercury
		uranium
Plant and animal substances		mushrooms
		snake venom
Environmental substances	Pesticides	
	Fungicides	
	Organic solvents	carbon tetrachloride
		diesel fuel
		ethylene glycol
		phenol
		unleaded gasoline

FeNa$^+$ should remain very low. Conversely, if the woman proceeds to develop ATN, renal cells become damaged and can no longer reabsorb the Na$^+$ filtered from the blood. This produces an increase in the FeNa$^+$, frequently to greater than 3 percent. It is important to note that the calculated values for FeNa$^+$ are not diagnostic if diuretics or volume replacement are administered to the patient. When loop and other types of diuretics are used as treatment of ARF, alternative renal indices must be used to differentiate between prerenal failure and

ATN. One recommendation is the measurement of the fractional excretion of urea, which is calculated by the formula:

$$Fe_{urea} = \left[\frac{U_{urea} \times P_{Cr}}{U_{Cr} \times P_{urea}} \right] \times 100$$

The recommendation is based on the principle that urea is not affected by diuretics.[5] However, other laboratory indices should be evaluated to differentiate between prerenal and intrinsic renal AKI.

TABLE 13-9

Phases of Acute Tubular Necrosis

Phase	Duration	Characteristics	Treatment Goals
Onset/initiating phase	Hours to days (Time from ischemic or nephrotoxic insult to cell injury)	↓ GFR ↓ urine output	Identification and treatment of cause
Oliguric/anuric phase (maintenance phase)	5–8 days in nonoliguric patient 10–16 days in oliguric patient	Severely ↓ GFR 50% of patients will be oliguric/anuric 50% of patients will be nonoliguric	Prevention of life-threatening complications from infection, fluid and electrolyte imbalances, and metabolic acidosis
Diuretic phase	7–14 days	Renal tubular patency restored ↑ GFR Polyuria (as high as 2–4L/day)* Inability to concentrate urine Able to clear volume, but not solute	Observation for and prevention of volume depletion, hypokalemia, and infection
Recovery/convalescent phase	Months to 1 or 2 years, depending on degree of parenchymal damage	Renal function slowly returns to normal or near normal ↑ urine output	Patient education on follow-up care and prevention

*Polyuria may not be evident in patients receiving hemodialysis.

TABLE 13-10

Characteristic Laboratory Findings in Prerenal Failure, ATN, and Postrenal Failure

	Prerenal	ATN	Postrenal
BUN:Creatinine ratio	20:1–40:1	10:1–15:1 (normal)	Normal to slightly increased
Urine volume	Oliguria	Oliguria or nonoliguria	Variable: oliguria, polyuria, or abrupt anuria
Urinary sediment	Normal hyaline casts	Debris Granular or cellular casts: WBCs RBCs	No casts, WBCs, RBCs
Specific gravity	High	Low	Variable
Urine Osmolality	High (>500 mOsm/Kg H_2O)	Low (<300 mOsm/Kg H_2O) (isosthenuria)	Variable Increased or similar to plasma (isosthenuria)
Ratio (Osm Urine to Osm plasma)	>1.5	<1.2	
Urine Na⁺	Low (<20 mEq/L)	Increased over prerenal (>40 mEq/L)	Variable: decreased
Urine urea	Low (15 g/24 hr)	Low (5 g/24 hr)	Low
Hemoglobinuria	None	Variable	Variable
Leukocyturia	None	Variable	Variable
Proteinuria	Trace to none*	Mild to moderate*	Trace to none*
Fractional excretion of Na⁺ (FENa)†	≤1%	>1%	
Fractional excretion of urea‡	<35%	Not established	Not established

*In patients without preeclampsia, eclampsia, or proteinuric hypertension.
†FENa is not accurate when done within 8 to 12 hours of administration of loop diuretics or volume replacement.
‡If diuretics have been administered within 8 to 12 hours, FEUrea may be obtained because urea transport is not affected by diuretics.

Agraharkar, M., Gupta, R., & Workeneh, B. T. (2007). Acute renal failure. *E-medicine*. Retrieved Mar 3, 2011. Available Online at: http://www.emedicine.com/med/TOPIC1595.HTM, Last updated Jan 11, 2011.

Case Excerpt: Intrinsic Renal Failure. The patient, a 26-year-old gravida 1, para 0 at 29 4/7 weeks gestation, was diagnosed with severe preeclampsia and admitted to the hospital for stabilization. Placental abruption ensued and an emergency Cesarean section was performed secondary to nonreassuring fetal heart rate findings. The patient experienced acute and significant blood loss, hypotension, severe anemia, and DIC, and required multiple transfusions of blood products.

On postoperative day 2, the patient was diagnosed with pulmonary edema, had a temperature of 104.8°F/40.4°C, and experienced two episodes of hypotension requiring volume resuscitation and intermittent administration of a vasopressor. Urine output was 20 to 60 mL/hr for 6 hours, and the urine was dark brown with visual sediment. Renal laboratory indices were evaluated and are presented in Table 13-11.

Postrenal Failure

Postrenal failure is caused by the obstruction or disruption of the flow of urine from the collecting ducts of the kidneys, through the ureters, into the bladder and out of the body. Obstruction of urine causes decreased GFR and eventual ARF via an increase in tubular hydrostatic pressure and vasoconstriction. Postrenal failure accounts for 10 percent or less of all cases of ARF in non-pregnant patients but may have a higher incidence during pregnancy due to the increasing size of the gravid uterus. The obstruction can be mechanical or functional and can occur anywhere from the calyces to the urethral meatus. Etiologies of postrenal failure are listed in Box 13-1.

Intratubular obstruction may be caused by crystal formation from uric acid, calcium oxalate, calcium phosphate, or acyclovir. For renal failure to occur, the obstruction must be bilateral (or affect a single functioning kidney). Unilateral obstruction is not usually sufficient to cause ARF but it can cause loss of the one kidney that is obstructed.

In pregnancy, obstruction can have a variety of origins. The gravid uterus is capable of causing compression of the entire urinary system, particularly in the third trimester. Uterine distention from polyhydramnios, multiple gestation, or uterine fibroids increases the potential for compression. The incidence of nephrolithiasis (kidney stones) in pregnancy is the same as

TABLE 13-11

Case Excerpt: Intrinsic Renal Failure

Labs – Chemistry		Comments
BUN	42 mg/dL	
Serum creatinine	3.7 mg/dL	
Prerenal vs. Intrarenal AKI		
BUN:Creatinine ratio	11:1	c/w intrinsic
Urine volume	non-oliguria	c/w intrinsic
Urinary sediment	epithelial cells, RBC casts	c/w intrinsic
Specific gravity	1.006	c/w/ intrinsic
Urine Na⁺	54 mEq/L	c/w intrinsic
Proteinuria	moderate	c/w intrinsic
Fractional excretion of Na⁺ (FENa)	2.3%	c/w intrinsic

BUN = blood urea nitrogen, c/w = consistent with, Na^+ = sodium.

Discussion

Intrinsic renal failure is represented by the above lab values that demonstrate failure of the damaged nephrons to adequately filter protein from the urine, selectively reabsorb Na and urea, and failure to concentrate the urine. Additionally, dead renal epithelial cells that have sloughed off the tubule walls are present in the abnormal urine sediment. In total, the labs reflect dying or dead nephrons.

that of non-pregnant women and should be considered as a potential cause of obstruction.

When a temporary obstruction is relieved in a timely fashion, postrenal azotemia is reversible. If obstruction is prolonged, compression of the parenchymal tissue may lead to permanent injury. Complete recovery, therefore, is dependent upon early discovery of the obstruction followed by timely and effective interventions.

Although postrenal failure accounts for a small percentage of cases of ARF, it is considered first in the pursuit of the diagnosis in all ARF cases, especially if there is a sudden onset of anuria, persistent oliguria, or if, based on history and assessment findings, the possibility of obstruction is raised. Signs and symptoms of postrenal failure include severe flank pain, hematuria, nausea and vomiting, and/or changes in urine flow. When obstruction is suspected, evaluation begins with urinary catheterization. If a urinary catheter is already present, it is checked for position, flushed with sterile normal saline, and replaced if necessary. Renal ultrasonography performed at the bedside has become the mainstay as the first method to rule out obstruction. Specialized imaging studies such as diagnostic imaging of the kidneys, ureters, and bladder (KUB), intravenous pyelogram, cystoscopy, or computed tomography (CT) scan, may also be utilized in evaluation of postrenal failure. When imaging studies are employed to ascertain the presence or absence of an obstruction, consideration should be given to avoiding nephrotoxic contrast media or using a contrast medium that has lower toxicity (compared to traditional agents) to potentially avoid further damage to the kidneys.

Relief from the obstruction and return of urine flow are the goals of treatment. Retrograde ureteral stent placement or percutaneous nephrostomy, and/or delivery of the fetus (depending on gestational age) may be required to relieve the obstruction.

Box 13-1. ETIOLOGY OF POSTRENAL FAILURE

Obstruction of flow can result from any of the following:
- Foley catheter obstruction
- Renal calculi/Nephrolithiasis
- Ureter twisting
- Blood clots
- Urethral strictures
- Edema
- Abdominal and pelvic neoplasms, retroperitoneal malignancies
- Compression from gravid uterus, lymphocele, hematoma
- Spinal cord disease (neurogenic bladder)
- Diabetic neuropathy
- Bladder rupture
- Congenital abnormalities

Source:
Agraharkar, M., Gupta, R., & Workeneh, B. T. (2007). Acute renal failure. *E-medicine*. Retrieved Mar 3, 2011. Available Online at: http://www.emedicine.com/med/TOPIC1595.HTM, Last updated Jan 11, 2011.

Case Excerpt: Postrenal (Obstructive) Failure. The patient, a 27-year-old gravida 3, para 0, blood type A negative, was admitted to the hospital at 22 weeks gestation. Her history was significant for Rh sensitization after her first pregnancy that ended with a spontaneous abortion at 17 weeks. Rh immune globulin (Rhogam) was ordered but not administered during her hospitalization. Her second pregnancy resulted in an intrauterine fetal demise (IUFD) at 23 weeks. Her current prenatal course was complicated by severe fetal ascites, which was managed by intermittent fetal transfusions. The maternal abdomen was noted to be significantly distended secondary to increasing polyhydramnios.

The patient presented with symptoms that included malaise, nausea, and vomiting occurring four times per day. She was admitted to the Labor and Delivery unit, and was unable to provide a urine sample. Urinary catheterization produced a return of 18 mL of dark brown urine. Her vital signs at the time of admission included a blood pressure of 110/70 mmHg, heart rate of 118 beats per minute, respirations of 20 per minute, and temperature of 99.2°F (37.3°C). Laboratory data are presented in Table 13-12.

TABLE 13-12

Case Excerpt: Serum and Urine Lab Values

Lab Test	Results
BUN	40 mg/dL
Serum creatinine	1.5 mg/dL
BUN:Creatinine ratio	27:1
Urine volume (per hour)	18 mL; 22 mL; 10 mL
Urinalysis	
Specific gravity	1.011
pH	7.4
Protein	trace
Glucose	Negative
Ketone	Negative
Blood	Positive (see below)
Leuc. EST	Occ
WBC	Occ
RBC	Numerous
Epith	Negative
Bacteria	Occ
Comments: sediment	Numerous RBCs, WBCs, occ casts
Urine Osmolality	300 mOsm/Kg H_2O
Urine Na^+	32 mEq/L
$FeNa^+$	.87%

Discussion

Renal ultrasound showed severe bilateral hydronephrosis, dilated ureters, and a relatively empty bladder. Diagnosis was obstructive postrenal failure from distended uterus secondary to polyhydramnios. Treatment was carried out to decompress the uterus and 1400 mL of amniotic fluid was slowly removed. With repositioning of patient, urine output increased to 400 mL the first hour and 620 mL the second hour. An additional 700 mL of amniotic fluid was removed from the uterus on the second day of hospitalization. The woman's renal labs returned to normal pregnancy values within 72 hours of treatment.

ARF in Special Populations

The causes of ARF in patients with preeclampsia are multifactorial. Severe preeclampsia may cause prerenal failure by the mechanisms of intravascular volume depletion, renal vasospasm, or vasoconstriction, which all limit renal perfusion. Frustratingly, when patients with preeclampsia and oliguria have laboratory tests that suggest early hypoperfusion (prerenal ARF) of the kidneys (elevated urine osmolarity, low urine Na^+, $FeNa^+$ <1 percent, etc.), interventions aimed at increasing preload via hydration may not be prudent in all patients. The rationale is that preeclampsia can produce renal cell ischemia related to arteriole vasoconstriction, activated inflammatory pathways, and decreased oxygen delivery and consumption from alterations in oxyhemoglobin dissociation. In this instance, treatment of ARF is focused on alleviating the underlying disorder (preeclampsia) with maternal stabilization and delivery of the fetus when indicated.

Sepsis, septic shock, and systemic inflammatory response syndrome (SIRS) create hemodynamic instability and volume depletion or third-spacing of fluid through damaged endothelium, which ultimately results in decreased renal perfusion. Susceptibility to infection is increased during pregnancy related to physiologic, immunologic, and anatomic changes. In addition, pregnant women demonstrate an increased sensitivity to endotoxins. Pyelonephritis is the most frequently occurring infectious process in pregnancy, caused by ascending untreated bacterial infection. Other common causes of sepsis in pregnancy include chorioamnionitis and pneumonia. Hemodynamic support, including volume replacement and administration of vasoactive agents, is the goal of treatment, along with administration of antimicrobials. For a more detailed discussion on sepsis, septic shock, and SIRS in pregnancy, refer to Chapter 18 of this text.

Glomerulonephritis, an infrequent occurrence in pregnancy, can complicate pregnancy and cause intrinsic renal failure. Acute glomerulonephritis, or inflammation and injury of the glomerulus, occurs when antigen/antibody complexes are trapped in the basement membrane. Symptoms of acute glomerulonephritis are very similar to those of preeclampsia, making differentiation difficult. Further discussion on the differential diagnosis of preeclampsia from glomerulonephritis may be found in Chapter 7 of this text.

Bilateral cortical renal necrosis (BCRN) is also an uncommon cause of ARF in pregnancy and is caused by necrosis of the renal cortex. BCRN occurs in the presence of decreased arterial perfusion secondary to vascular spasm, microvascular injury, and/or DIC.[20] The pathogenesis remains unclear, but the most likely initiating factor is vasospasm of the small vessels.

BCRN is associated with septic abortion as there appears to be endotoxin-mediated vascular damage that results in thrombosis.[21] It is confirmed by angiogram or biopsy. In pregnancy, BCRN has also occurred with placental abruption, potentially from the hypercoaguable state of pregnancy, endothelial injury, and intravascular thrombosis.[21] Although BCRN accounts for only 2 percent of ARF in non-pregnant adults, it may account for up to 20 percent of ARF with third trimester onset.

Diagnostic Principles

Diagnosis of ARF is based on the patient's history, physical examination, and an assessment and interpretation of indices of renal function. One obstacle to diagnosis is that there is no sensitive marker for early detection of ARF.[22] The diagnosis can be made when a quick decline (hours to days) in GFR is manifested in a rapidly increased BUN and serum creatinine. Urine output may or may not be decreased. The method for diagnosis of ARF begins with the patient's history and physical examination and includes the elements of serum and urine sample collection and analyses.

History and Physical Examination

Undiagnosed chronic renal failure (CRF) is more common in the general population than originally thought. Therefore, it is important to first distinguish ARF from an unknown underlying CRF by searching the patient's history for physical changes or complaints over time such as anorexia, persistent nausea, weight loss, fatigue, and itching. The presence of one or more of these conditions is more likely associated with CRF when compared to ARF. Most patients who develop ARF in the hospital have no history of CRF or are not aware of any underlying reduced renal function. In obstetric patients, ARF is commonly associated with a history of hemorrhage, hypertension (new onset or chronic), and blood transfusions.

Patients with ARF from prerenal failure may have a recent history of diarrhea, vomiting, heat exhaustion, excessive fluid loss, concurrent illness that produced decreased appetite and fluid intake, hypotension, hemorrhage, liver disease, new-onset heart failure, diabetes insipidus, and/or recent use and/or adjustment of antihypertensive medications. In patients with intrinsic failure the history may include any of the above problems with the added complication of prolonged duration of the problem without successful correction. Additionally, a history of edema, congestive heart failure, shock, sepsis/SIRS/septic shock, hemorrhage, type 1 diabetes mellitus, hypertension, systemic lupus erythematosus (SLE), hepatitis B or C, syphilis, multiple myeloma and/or AIDS are associated with intrinsic ARF.

Obtaining the patient's medication history may result in the identification of a nephrotoxic agent such as recent or current antibiotic therapy, nonsteroidal anti-inflammatory drugs (NSAIDs), angiotensin converting enzyme (ACE) inhibitors, diuretics, herbal remedies, dietary supplements, chemical exposure, and/or intravenous drug abuse. Nephrotoxic causes of ARF generally produce intrinsic failure.

When a patient presents with ATN or glomerular nephritis and there is no known coexisting medical complication, a travel history, food exposure history, and recall of recent contact with foreign travelers may reveal uncommon causes of renal failure from infectious disease, an emerging challenge for all health care providers. Immunologic changes in pregnancy alter the woman's susceptibility to the severity of infectious diseases. Pregnancy increases a patient's susceptibility to listeriosis and toxoplasmosis and is thought to increase the severity of influenza and varicella.[23] Recent causes of ARF from infectious disease in all populations include listeriosis (*Listeria monocytogenes*), tuberculosis, *E. coli* (*Escherichia coli* O157:H7), and hemorrhagic fever with renal syndrome (HFRS), which is a group of similar illnesses caused by hantaviruses.[24]

Patients in postrenal failure may have a history of renal colic, dysuria, frequency, hesitation, urgency, incontinence, single ureter, pelvic malignancy, or history of pelvic irradiation. These patients may also have nausea and vomiting, lethargy, and other signs and symptoms of uremia.

The patient's history, physical, and laboratory indices together offer the core information to formulate a working diagnosis. Isolation of the woman's type of ARF involves excluding other potential etiologies and disease states.

Kidney Biopsy

The goals of renal biopsy in pregnancy are no different than in non-pregnant patients. Biopsy is typically performed when noninvasive methods to diagnose the etiology of ARF do not point to a specific insulting origin or when targeted therapy is not effective. In non-pregnant patients it has been demonstrated that biopsy changes the management plan of 70 percent of patients and is associated with less than a 1 percent complication rate.[6] During pregnancy, however, conflicting complication rates have been reported with results as high as 4.4 percent of pregnant patients having severe sequelae, including one maternal death.[6,25,26] More recent investigations of renal biopsy during pregnancy have demonstrated much lower complication rates, a finding that is more probably related to improved techniques of tissue acquisition under ultrasound guidance rather than any significant change in the population. The most common serious complication of biopsy in the pregnant patient is bleeding under the capsule into the kidney, hematoma formation, and subsequent compression. Currently, biopsy is considered in select pregnancies when ARF occurs prior to 32 weeks gestation without an apparent etiology.[6,26] Benefits are weighed against potential complications, and patient consent is obtained prior to the procedure.

Clinical Management

The lack of dramatic improvement in morbidity and mortality among hospitalized patients with ARF in the past decade has resulted in scientific questioning of the effectiveness of traditional management strategies, and is reflected in current recommendations that concentrate more on the avoidance of further damage to the kidney. There are data to suggest that patients who receive consultation from a nephrologist have improved survival rates when compared to those who do not have consultation.[27] Also, those patients who had a nephrology consult at lower BUN values (less than 80 mg/dL) had higher survival rates compared to patients who had consults at higher BUN values (greater than 100 mg/dL).

The immediate treatment of ARF centers on correction of hypovolemia, early diagnosis, treatment of the underlying cause(s), prevention of further damage, and the provision of physiologic support while recovery occurs.[6] Hydration with intravenous 0.9% NaCl (normal saline) is more beneficial when compared to oral hydration for the prevention or reduction of contrast nephropathy.[28] Normal saline is also more beneficial compared to intravenous 0.45% NaCl for the same indications.[28] There are no data that currently demonstrate significant benefit from colloid solutions in the prevention or treatment of ARF. Thus, albumin-based solutions are not recommended in the immediate management of hypovolemia or oliguria.[28] There is no evidence of benefit in using glucose-containing solutions (e.g., $D_5$0.9%NaCl, D_5RL, etc.) in the treatment of hypovolemia in patients with ARF, and further use of glucose-containing solutions for energy requirements requires the same glucose control protocols using intravenous insulin drips commonly prescribed for non-pregnant critically ill patients.

Pharmacotherapeutics

Historically, pharmacologic strategies to prevent or treat ARF were intended to increase renal perfusion or decrease renal oxygen consumption to theoretically reduce injury to the kidneys.[28] Common prior interventions included the use of loop diuretics [e.g., furosemide (Lasix)], low-dose dopamine, and/or mannitol, to name a few. These pharmacotherapeutics, when evaluated using prospective randomized trials and/or meta-analyses, did not produce a significant improvement in

the outcomes of patients with ARF, and they may have been harmful. The dearth of effective treatment for ARF has been one of the rationales for the overall modest improvement in outcomes of patients over the past decade.

Renal Replacement Therapy

Because there are limited, if any, effective pharmacological interventions for ARF, external filtration of blood is frequently required. When caring for obstetric patients with ARF prior to recovery of renal function, it may be necessary to institute renal replacement therapy (RRT) to aggressively treat fluid overload, azotemia, electrolyte imbalance, acid–base imbalance, excessive drug levels, and to reduce circulating inflammatory mediators.[29]

The rationale for RRT in critically ill patients has changed from one of "replacing" renal function to one of "supporting" renal function. The change is based on the premise that critically ill patients may need and benefit from a different type RRT than traditional hemodialysis (HD) or peritoneal dialysis used in patients with long-term, end-stage renal disease (ESRD). Providers are encouraged to approach ARF as a multisystem disease rather than the isolated failure of one organ and to consider therapy that is not only beneficial for the kidneys but supportive to other organ systems and in concert with the treatment plan. Therefore, it is hypothesized that the use of RRT early in the progression of a disease may offer improved morbidity and mortality rates. In support of this paradigm shift of early initiation of RRT, data from the Program to Improve Care in Acute Renal Disease (PICARD)—a large multicenter study of ARF—showed that RRT initiated in patients at higher BUN levels was associated with greater mortality rates compared to those who had lower values at initiation.[10] Although the study data and conclusions have variables that may have had a significant impact on the results, the idea of earlier treatment remains appealing.

RRT is indicated for management of ARF when supportive measures are not effective. Specific indications are listed in Table 13-13. The two general categories of RRT are dialysis and filtration. Dialysis works on the basic principles of diffusion and osmosis of solutes in fluid, and works by moving electrolytes, urea, creatine, and free water across a semipermeable membrane. In hemodialysis, the patient's blood is pumped and filtered through a dialyzer, which is a plastic-encased group of semipermeable filters/fibers surrounded by a solution called the dialysate. The dialysate fluid contains prescribed concentrations of electrolytes and solutes, such as Na^+, K^+, Cl^+, Ca^{++}, bicarbonate, magnesium, glucose, and others. For example, if the patient's K^+ level is elevated to a critical level, a dialysate with either a low concentration of K^+ or zero K^+ will be used to promote the diffusion of K^+ out of the patient's blood, across the

TABLE 13-13

Indications for Renal Replacement Therapy

Life-threatening	• Fluid overload • Pulmonary edema/hypoxia • Metabolic acidosis • Azotemia (increased BUN and/or creatinine) • Cardiac failure (decreased cardiac output, LVSWI, and/or ventricular ejection fraction) • Platelet dysfunction • Hyperkalemia • ECG abnormalities (peaked T-waves, ST-segment depression, bundle branch blocks, widening QRS, increases in PR interval, decreased amplitude of P wave, ventricular tachycardia • Seizures • Cerebral edema • Hepatic failure • Neurological signs: confusion, change in mental status, agitation, paresthesias, paralysis
Recently reported	• Sepsis or systemic inflammatory response syndrome (SIRS) • Multisystem organ failure (MSOF) • Adult respiratory distress syndrome (ARDS) • Tumor lysis syndrome • Chronic heart failure • Rhabdomyolysis (myoglobin released during muscle injury) • Cancer chemotherapy

Data from:

Dirkes, S., & Hodge, K. (2007). Continuous renal replacement therapy in the adult intensive care unit: history and current trends. *Critical Care Nurse, 27*(2), 61–80.

Kes, P., Ljutić, D., Basić-Jukić, N., & Brunetta, B. (2003). Indications for continuous renal function replacement therapy. *Acta Medica Croatica, 57*(1), 71–75.

Mehta, R. L. (2001). Indications for dialysis in the ICU: Renal replacement vs. renal support. *Blood Purification, 19,* 227–232.

semipermeable filter, and into the dialysate solution, thereby lowering the patient's serum K^+. If the patient also has a metabolic acidemia, the nephrologist will prescribe a dialysate with a higher concentration of bicarbonate than the blood to move more of the buffer into the patient's system to neutralize the acidemia. By altering the composition of the dialysate to achieve the desired changes in the patient's chemistry and water balance, successful dialysis can correct metabolic acidosis, normalize electrolytes, and remove excessive fluid.

Similar to hemodialysis, another type of dialysis is peritoneal dialysis (PD), where the patient's peritoneum is used as a filtering membrane. Rather than accessing the woman's vascular system and pumping the blood through a dialyzer, the dialysate solution is placed into her peritoneal cavity through a dialysis catheter. Solutes are removed from the blood and into the peritoneal cavity via vascular areas that surround the intestines.

Hemodialysis is the mainstay treatment for outpatients with ESRD. Ambulatory patients who are not pregnant undergo dialysis every 2 to 3 days to remove waste products from metabolism and control fluid balance. When pregnant, patients undergoing hemodialysis will typically increase their days for dialysis to every other day, with some eventually requiring daily dialysis.

Stable inpatients with ESRD have hemodialysis in an attempt to replace renal function to allow the patient to recover from surgery or illness and to be discharged. The process of hemodialysis, however, is associated with hypotension and potentially adds further ischemic injury to the kidneys. Therefore, its use in critically ill patients is somewhat limited and has been replaced with methods of continuous filtration that produce less hypotensive and/or cardiovascular compromise. They are frequently performed on a continuous basis and called continuous renal replacement therapy (CRRT).

CRRT is the acronym for newer types of RRT initially based on filtration and ultrafiltration, but currently may include integrated modes of dialysis by adding a dialyzer into the system. CRRT may be further stratified by the specific method(s) of blood filtering. A list of common types of CRRT and acronyms are presented in Table 13-14.[32]

RRT has undergone advancements that include improved patient selection, evidenced-based methodology, new technology, prescriptive use of dialysates, starting and stopping protocols, and others. Nonetheless, there are limited data to guide the type of modality used on a specific population group, starting parameters, timing of the procedures, use of specific membranes or solutions, and/or dose of therapy.[33] Trends include the use of CRRT with additional therapeutic technologies, the use of combination methods as patients recover renal function, and earlier initiation of RRT.[34]

Complications of RRT are frequently serious, may add further ischemic insult to the kidneys, and may be life-threatening. At the Acute Dialysis Quality Initiative's (ADQI) 4th International Consensus Conference, Baldwin and colleagues reported on complications of RRT and categorized the complications into broad groups:

• Complications related to vascular or peritoneal access
• Complications from the extracorporeal circuit
• Complications from hemodynamic instability and compromise
• Complications of electrolyte and metabolism
• Complications related to human error.[35,1]

TABLE 13-14

Types of Continuous Renal Replacement Therapy

Type	Acronym	Comments
Slow continuous ultrafiltration	SCUF	• Goal is fluid removal. • Patients who may benefit include those with fluid overload; and/or congestive heart failure
Continuous venovenous hemofiltration	CVVH	• Goal is fluid volume management with moderate solute removal. • Patients who may benefit include those who have moderate electrolyte imbalances, are oliguric and need parenteral nutrition or blood products, those in septic shock, and those who are resistant to diuretics. • CVVH uses ultrafiltration and convection to remove fluids and solutes.
Continuous venovenous hemodialysis	CVVHD	• The goal of CVVHD is fluid volume management with a greater level of solute removal than CVVH. • Patients who may benefit include those who are hemodynamically unstable and volume overloaded, azotemic or uremic, have electrolyte disturbances and acidosis, and those who require parenteral nutrition despite fluid overload. • CVVHD uses the process of diffusion to enhance solute clearance.
Continuous venovenous hemodiafiltration	CVVHDF	• The treatment goal of CVVHDF is maximal fluid and solute removal. • Patients who may benefit from this mode include those with severe azotemia and fluid overload, extreme electrolyte imbalances, and hemodynamic instability. • CVVHDF uses convection and diffusion, combining the principles of CVVH and CVVHD to provide maximal solute clearance.

Data from:
Paton, M. E. (2007). CRRT: Help for acute renal failure. *Nursing Made Incredibly Easy,* Sept/Oct, 28–38.

A more comprehensive list of complications is presented in Table 13-15.

When RRT is considered for an individual patient, the benefits of the procedure are weighed against the risks involved. To maximize patient benefit and reduce complications or human error, RRT is ideally performed in hospitals and units with extensive experience in the method of RRT prescribed for the patient. For critically ill obstetric patients, the need for RRT may necessitate transport to a medical center that has a critical care obstetrics unit with concomitant nephrology services experienced in RRT during pregnancy.

FETAL CONSIDERATIONS

The spectrum of ARF, together with the causative conditions and resulting end-organ system pathology, is extremely diverse, making prediction of fetal outcome difficult in most pregnancies. Dissimilar from prognostic variables in chronic renal disease, there is disagreement with respect to the effects that proteinuria, hypertension, and serum creatinine levels play in the prediction of pregnancy outcome. There is some agreement that preeclampsia-eclampsia and/or HELLP syndrome are associated with an increased incidence of preterm delivery, low birth weight, stillbirth, and overall neonatal morbidity and death. Additionally, the need

for RRT for any indication during pregnancy increases the risk of miscarriage, stillbirth, preterm delivery, and neonatal morbidity and death.

Not surprisingly, there are no randomized prospective trials on methods of fetal surveillance during ARF in pregnancy. Recommendations on antepartum methods and/or recommended protocols to monitor fetal health are based on expert opinion and/or extrapolated from other series of fetal outcome data.

When patients and families are counseled on the subject of elective early delivery of a preterm pregnancy, the inclusion of the team's neonatology care providers is important. Information communicated to the patient may include survival statistics relative to the institution's experience and outcomes for the estimated gestational age. The patient is informed about risks and benefits of the proposed medical plan of care, probabilities of maternal and fetal outcomes if the plan is accepted or rejected, and alternative care if feasible, with the intent to allow the woman to make an informed choice and/or have input regarding pregnancy management.

PREVENTION

Because the etiologies and risk factors for ARF remain elusive, identification of preventive measures has been

TABLE 13-15

Complications of Renal Replacement Therapy (RRT)

Access Related Complications

Infection
- Local (exit site, subcutaneous tunnel)
- Systemic (bacteremia, sepsis)
- Peritonitis (in peritoneal dialysis)

Hemorrhage

Catheter-associated vascular thrombosis

Vascular or visceral organ injury

Access malfunction

Extracorporeal Circuit Associated Complications

Bio-incompatibility

Mechanical dysfunction
- Hemolysis
- Air embolism
- Fluid balance errors

Microbiological contamination

Chemical contamination

Anticoagulation
- Inadequate anticoagulation/thrombosis
- Excessive anticoagulation/hemorrhage
- Heparin-associated thrombocytopenia

Hemodynamic Compromise/Hypotension

Volume depletion

Vasodilation

Electrolyte and Metabolic Complications

Prescriptive errors

Errors in compounding fluids

Acid–base disturbances

Vitamin and micronutrient depletion

Hormone depletion

Amino acid depletion

Thermal balance

Human Factors

Physician error

Nursing error

Pharmacist error

Biomedical technician error

Adapted from:
Palevsky, P. M., Baldwin, I., Davenport, A., Goldstein, S., & Paganini, E. (2005). Renal replacement therapy and the kidney: Minimizing the impact of renal replacement therapy on recovery of acute renal failure. *Curr Opin Crit Care, 11*, 584–554.

based mostly on expert opinion rather than prospective randomized clinical trials. However, the ADQI, in its 2004 Consensus Conference, presented evidence-based recommendations for ARF prevention, and/or early identification and treatment. Corresponding grades and/or levels of supportive data can be found in the Consensus Conference Proceedings.[36]

In general, the following clinical questions may be addressed from current recommendations in care.

1. *Which obstetric patients are most likely to develop azotemia and, potentially, ARF?*

Patients with a history of or a current diagnosis of renal insufficiency, renal disease, chronic ESRD, ongoing dialysis, and/or renal transplant are at significant risk for developing progressive renal failure during pregnancy. The next highest risk group are women with diabetes mellitus with vascular involvement, active lupus, and/or sepsis/septic shock/SIRS. Factors unique to pregnancy that increase the risk of azotemia and ARF include preeclampsia-eclampsia, HELLP syndrome, amniotic fluid embolism, and acute fatty liver of pregnancy. Finally, any disease that disrupts adequate perfusion and ventilation increases the woman's risk for developing ARF. Common diagnoses that meet criteria in critically ill pregnant patients include heart failure, pulmonary edema, respiratory failure, severe anemia from hemorrhage or hemolysis, DIC, hemolytic uremic syndrome, trauma, uncorrected hypovolemia, hypotension, and shock.

When providing care to these patients, it may be beneficial to assess renal function laboratory indices earlier during hospitalization compared to historical practice. For example, guidelines may be created to expedite diagnosis by recommending renal function studies for women who have an obstetric hemorrhage that decreased hemoglobin or hematocrit to less than 9.0 g/dL or 27 percent, respectively; or, for patients who require a vasoactive drug (e.g., epinephrine) to maintain blood pressure.

2. *Which renal function tests can be used for "screening" patients for ARF?*

Screening for ARF should be done in patients at risk, because there are no early signs and symptoms of renal failure. GFR has to decrease by over 50 percent before serum levels of creatinine start to increase. There are no perfect renal function tests that measure GFR, but experts agree that serum and urine creatinine and BUN, when measured at the same time, show evidence of renal insufficiency. Therefore, renal function screening tests include serum creatinine, BUN, sodium, potassium, and osmolality; urine tests consist of creatinine, urea, sodium, osmolality, and specific gravity. From these laboratory values, the BUN: creatinine ratio (serum) and $FeNa^+$ are calculated. Screening is performed on patients at risk for ARF and when the patient condition(s) meets criteria. A reasonable frequency of screening critically ill patients is approximately every 8 to 12 hours, or after an episode of hemodynamic instability, or decreased oxygen delivery, or increased oxygen extraction ratio. Once azotemia is identified, additional testing is warranted to further discern the cause.

3. *Where and who should care for and manage pregnant women in ARF?*

Studies show a benefit in outcomes for patients managed in an adult ICU with early consultation with a nephrologist. An obstetric ICU with immediate access to a nephrology service and experience with RRT in pregnant women may be the ideal setting for such patients.

4. *What type of intravenous fluids should be prescribed for patients at risk for ARF?*

First, all colloid-containing solutions are avoided. Normal saline without dextrose (0.9% NaCl) has been shown to prevent further injury to the kidneys in patients at risk for or with ARF compared to 0.45% NaCl without dextrose solutions. If dextrose solutions are administered, it should be with extreme caution, in amounts that are physiologic and appropriate for calorie expenditure, and with ongoing tight glucose measurements and glycemic control. Specific values for serum glucose levels that improve outcome in patients with ARF have not been established, but most experts recommend using the tight glucose controls suggested for other critically ill and/or cardiac surgical patients.

Therefore, the administration of dextrose-containing solutions and/or intravenous or gastric feedings is accompanied by frequent testing of serum glucose levels, utilization of a continuous insulin infusion/pump, and meticulous attention to the institution's insulin administration guidelines to achieve glucose control.

5. *When patients become oliguric and do not respond to a fluid challenge or other fluid therapy, is there any benefit in administering diuretics or low-dose dopamine to improve urine output?*

No. Administration of diuretics, particularly the loop diuretics (furosemide [Lasix], etc.) to increase urine output has not reduced the rate of ARF, and in some patients (cardiac surgery) the use of these agents has increased the rate of kidney injury. Low-dose dopamine shares the same analysis: when used in oliguric patients to increase urine output, dopamine did not reduce the risk of ARF and did not effectively treat ARF when present. The opposite desired effect occurred with dopamine; use of the agent increased the incidence of ARF in patients who received the medication. Additionally, in patients with identified azotemia and ARF, the use of dopamine amplified kidney damage.

6. *What is one of the most common overlooked opportunities that clinicians have to decrease the risk for ARF?*

When patients are at risk for ARF and begin to have reduced GFR or azotemia, radiographic studies are frequently needed to rule out obstruction, and/or determine the etiology of injury. Such patients benefit from isotonic intravenous fluid therapy to dilute the nephrotoxic contrast agents used in the procedures. To further reduce the incidence of ARF, the use of low-osmolality contrast media or possibly iso-osmolar media in imaging studies may be discussed with consulting radiology team members.

The prevention of ARF has received recent attention and new ideas to reduce ESRD in the general population, their dependency on dialysis, and the incidence of premature organ system failure and death are under investigation. Avoidance of known nephrotoxic agents, abandonment of traditional therapies that offer no benefit and may cause harm, and earlier recognition and treatment of ARF are the tenets for reducing the rates of ARF in all populations.

SUMMARY

Until the recent past, patients with oliguric azotemia and/or ARF were frequently treated with continuous low-dose dopamine infusions and intermittent boluses of loop diuretics to promote increases in urine output. Injudicious volume expansion with colloids or dextrose-containing crystalloids was also carried out without the use of invasive hemodynamic monitoring or control of serum hyperglycemia. Now, there is evidence that the prior model of care did not offer protection from further kidney injury, but rather may have contributed to further damage.

Current tenets of managing patients with ARF include the early support of functioning nephrons with adequate renal arterial perfusion pressures and oxygen availability to the renal cells, avoidance of nephrotoxic medications and treatments, and use of alternative iso-osmolar contrast agents when imaging studies are required. The use of invasive hemodynamic monitoring to monitor hemodynamic and oxygen transport status in patients with azotemia may also promote improved patient outcomes.

Prevention and early diagnosis of ARF have emerged as the cornerstones of current clinical management and will remain until successful and specific markers for the disease and effective treatments are found. Promising research includes the study of specific biomarkers that would identify pregnant patients in early ARF, allowing earlier intervention that may assist in reducing the progression of ARF to permanent injury and/or chronic disease.

REFERENCES

1. Bellomo, R., Ronco, C., Kellum, J. A., Mehta, R. L., & Palevsky, P. (2004). Acute renal failure – definition, outcome measures, animal models, fluid therapy and information technology needs: Second International Consensus

Conference of the Acute Dialysis Quality Initiative (ADQI) Group. *Critical Care, 8,* R204–R212.

2. Prakash, J., Kumar, H., Kar, B., et al. (2003). Acute renal failure in pregnancy: Twenty years journey. *Nephrology, Dialysis, Transplantation, 18*(Suppl. 4), 665.

3. Zeier, M. Z. (2002). Post-partum 'acute renal failure.' *Nephrology, Dialysis, Transplantation, 17,* 1703–1705.

4. Krane, N. K., & Hamrahian, M. (2007). Core curriculum in nephrology. Pregnancy: Kidney diseases and hypertension. *American Journal of Kidney Diseases, 49*(2), 336–345.

5. Agraharkar, M., Gupta, R., Agraharkar, A., & Workeneh, B. T. (2007). Acute renal failure. *E-medicine.* Retrieved from http://www.emedicine.com/med/TOPIC1595.HTM

6. Grammill, H. S., & Jeyabalan, A. (2005). Acute renal failure in pregnancy. *Critical Care Medicine, 33*(Suppl. 10), S372–S384.

7. Xue, J. L., Daniels, F., Star, R. A., Kimmel, P. L., Eggers, P. W., Molitoris, B. A., et al. (2006). Incidence and mortality of acute renal failure in Medicare beneficiaries, 1992 to 2001. *Journal of the American Society of Nephrology, 17,* 1135–1142.

8. Waikar, S. S., Curhan, G. C., Wald, R., McCarthy, E. P., & Chertow, G. M. (2006). Declining mortality in patients with acute renal failure, 1988 to 2002. *Journal of the American Society of Nephrology, 17,* 1143–1150.

9. Lameire, N., Van Biesen, W., & Vanholder, R. (2006). The rise of prevalence and the fall of mortality of patients with acute renal failure: What the analysis of two databases does and does not tell us. *Journal of the American Society of Nephrology, 17,* 923–925.

10. Liu, K. D., Himmelfarb, J., Paganini, E., Ikizler, T. A., Soroko, S. H., Mehta, R. L., et al. (2006). Timing of initiation of dialysis in critically ill patients with acute kidney injury. *Clinical Journal of the American Society of Nephrology, 1,* 915–919.

11. Jones, D. C., & Hayslett, J. P. (1996). Outcome of pregnancy in women with moderate or severe renal insufficiency. *The New England Journal of Medicine, 335,* 226–232.

12. Ward, K. (2005). Kidneys, don't fail me now. *Nursing Made Incredibly Easy!* March/April, 18–26.

13. Campbell, D. (2003). How acute renal failure puts the brakes on kidney function. *Nursing, 33*(1), 59–63.

14. Davison, J. D. (2001). Renal disorders in pregnancy. *Current Opinion in Obstetrics and Gynecology, 13,* 109–114.

15. Barraclough, K., Leone, E., & Chiu, A. (2007). Renal replacement therapy for acute kidney injury in pregnancy. *Nephrology, Dialysis, Transplantation, 22,* 2395–2397.

16. Leblanc, M., Kellum, J. A., Gibney, R. N., Lieberthal, W., Tumlin, J., & Mehta, R. (2005). Risk factors for acute renal failure: Inherent and modifiable risks. *Current Opinion in Critical Care, 11*(6), 533–536.

17. Krane, N. K., Agraharkar, M., Agraharkar, A., et al. (2010). *Renal disease and pregnancy.* Retrieved from http://emedicine.medscape.com/article/246123-overview

18. Peacock, P. R., & Sinert, R. (2010). *Renal failure, acute.* Retrieved from http://emedicine.medscape.com/article/777845-overview

19. Bellomo, R. (2005). Defining, quantifying, and classifying acute renal failure. *Critical Care Clinics, 21,* 223–237.

20. Bellomo, R., Bonventre, J., Macias, W., & Pinsky, M. (2005). Management of early acute renal failure: Focus on post-injury prevention. *Current Opinion in Critical Care, 11,* 542–547.

21. Erkan, E., & Devarajan, P. (2010). *Renal cortical necrosis.* Retrieved from http://emedicine.medscape.com/article/983599-overview

22. Spevetz, A. (2007). Management and prevention of acute renal failure: Notes from the ICC conference. *Critical Connections, 6*(4), 13.

23. Jamieson, D. J., Theiler, R. N., & Rasmussen, S. A. (2006). Emerging infections and pregnancy. *Emerging Infectious Disease, 12*(11), 1638–1643.

24. Chang, H. H., Tserenpuntsag, B., Kacica, M., Smith, P. F., & Morse, D. L. (2004). Hemolytic uremic syndrome incidence in New York. *Emerging Infectious Diseases, 10*(5), 928–931.

25. Schewitz, L., Friedman, I., & Pollack, V. (1965). Bleeding after renal biopsy in pregnancy. *Obstetrics and Gynecology, 26,* 295–304.

26. Lindheimer, M. D., & Davison, J. M. (1987). Renal biopsy during pregnancy: "to b... or not to b...?" *British Journal of Obstetrics and Gynaecology, 94,* 932–934.

27. Mehta, R. L., Farkas, A., Fowler, W., & Pascual, M. (1955). *Effect of delayed consultation on outcome from acute renal failure in the ICU* (abstract). 28th Annual Meeting of the American Society of Nephrology, Nov 1995.

28. Kellum, J., Leblanc, M., & VenKataraman, R. (2007). Acute renal failure. *BMJ.* Clinical Evidence, Web publication date: 01 Jan 2007, pp. 1–4.

29. Mehta, R. L. (2001). Indications for dialysis in the ICU: Renal replacement vs. renal support. *Blood Purification, 19,* 227–232.

30. Dirkes, S., & Hodge, K. (2007). Continuous renal replacement therapy in the adult intensive care unit: History and current trends. *Critical Care Nurse, 27*(2), 61–80.

31. Kes, P., Ljuti, D., Basi-Juki, N., & Brunetta, B. (2003). Indications for continuous renal function replacement therapy. *Acta Medica Croatica, 57*(1), 71–75.

32. Paton, M. E. (2007). CRRT: Help for acute renal failure. *Nursing Made Incredibly Easy! 5*(5), 28–38.

33. Weisbord, S. D., & Palevsky, P. M. (2006). Acute renal failure in the intensive care unit. *Seminars in Respiratory and Critical Care Medicine, 27*(3), 262–273.

34. Hegarty, J., Middleton, R. J., Krebs, M., Hussain, H., Cheung, C., Ledson, T., et al. (2005). Severe acute renal failure in adults: Place of care, incidence and outcomes. *QJM, 98*(9), 661–666. [Epub 2005 Jul 29.]

35. Palevsky, P. M., Baldwin, I., Davenport, A., Goldstein, S., & Paganini, E. (2005). Renal replacement therapy and the kidney: Minimizing the impact of renal replacement therapy on recovery of acute renal failure. *Current Opinion in Critical Care, 11,* 584–554.

36. Kellum, J. A., Leblanc, M., Gibney, N., Tumlin, J., Lieberthal, W., & Ronco, C. (2005). Primary prevention of acute renal failure in the critically ill. *Current Opinion in Critical Care, 11,* 537–541.

CHAPTER 14

Cardiopulmonary Resuscitation in Pregnancy

Deborah Anne Cruz, Patricia Marie Constanty, and Shailen S. Shah

Cardiopulmonary arrest is the abrupt cessation of spontaneous and effective ventilation and systemic perfusion. Sudden cardiac arrest (SCA) is a leading cause of death in the United States (U.S.) and Canada.[1–3] Data from the Centers for Disease Control and Prevention (CDC) estimate that in the U.S. approximately 300,000 people die annually in out-of-hospital and emergency department settings from coronary heart disease.[1,2,4,5] Approximately 250,000 of these deaths occur in an out-of-hospital setting.[1,6] The annual incidence of SCA in North America is approximately 0.55 per 1,000 population.[3,4] With respect to the obstetric patient population, cardiopulmonary arrest occurs in approximately 1 in 30,000 pregnancies.[7,8]

The goal of cardiopulmonary resuscitation (CPR) is prompt initiation of basic life support (BLS) to provide artificial ventilation and perfusion until advanced cardiac life support (ACLS) can be initiated. The desired outcome of resuscitation efforts is restoration of spontaneous and effective cardiopulmonary function. When cardiopulmonary arrest occurs during pregnancy, normal physiologic alterations of pregnancy should be integrated into resuscitation protocols recommended for the nonpregnant population, in order to facilitate optimal outcomes for both the pregnant woman and the fetus.

Since publication of the second edition of this text, several important changes in managing CPR and emergency cardiac care (ECC) have been recommended.[9] As with all versions of the ECC guidelines published since 1974, the 2010 American Heart Association Guidelines for CPR and ECC contain recommendations designed to improve survival from SCA and acute life-threatening cardiopulmonary problems.

This chapter addresses the causes of cardiopulmonary arrest and presents updated recommendations for basic and advanced resuscitation techniques. The effects of pregnancy on CPR are described including modifications to resuscitation techniques that should be considered during pregnancy. The role of perimortem

Cesarean delivery and infant survival data are presented. Potential complications associated with resuscitation efforts are identified. Finally, the vital need for collaboration among members of the health care team and advance preparation to facilitate optimal response to this relatively rare emergency event in pregnancy are reinforced.

CAUSES OF CARDIOPULMONARY ARREST

Outside the hospital and in a coronary care unit setting, the most frequent cause of circulatory arrest is tachyarrhythmia, which occurs most often in patients with underlying heart disease. The most frequent initial rhythm in witnessed SCA is ventricular fibrillation (VF), the treatment for which centers around electrical defibrillation. The probability of successful defibrillation diminishes rapidly over time, and VF tends to deteriorate to asystole within a few minutes. For every minute that passes between collapse and defibrillation, survival rates from witnessed VF SCA decrease 7 to 10 percent if no CPR is provided.[10] When bystander CPR is provided, the decrease in survival rates is more gradual and averages 3 to 4 percent per minute from collapse to defibrillation.[10–12] If bystanders provide immediate CPR, many adults in VF can survive with intact neurologic function, especially if defibrillation is performed within approximately 5 minutes following SCA.[13] This fact underscores the utility of the installation of automated external defibrillators (AEDs) in public places.

In contrast, primary respiratory events are much more common in hospitalized patients. Such events may be caused by acute respiratory failure, excessive sedation, pulmonary embolism, or airway obstruction. These principles should be kept in mind upon initiation of and throughout resuscitation efforts. For example, because an arrhythmia is likely to be the cause of sudden death in the coronary care unit, a patient in cardiopulmonary arrest is almost always treated immediately with unsynchronized direct current (DC) cardioversion. In contrast, arrest situations on a general hospital unit are much more likely to be managed successfully if initial attention is devoted to airway management and oxygenation followed by a search for the cause of the crisis.

Primary Pulmonary Events

The term *respiratory arrest* refers to a situation in which a patient becomes unresponsive and without respirations, but an effective pulse is present. Failure to rapidly achieve effective ventilation and oxygenation results in progressive hypoxemia and acidemia that culminate in cardiovascular dysfunction, hypotension, and eventual circulatory collapse. The cause of many respiratory arrests relates to either respiratory center depression (e.g., excessive sedation) or to failure of respiratory muscles (e.g., excessive workload, impaired mechanical efficiency, excessive sedation, mucus plugging, or muscle weakness). The first compensatory response to respiratory compromise is usually tachypnea. However, as the increased workload of breathing continues, the respiratory effort and rhythm become slow, dysfunctional, and eventually cease.

Soon after ventilation ceases, the partial pressure of arterial oxygen (PaO_2) dramatically decreases. Available stores of oxygen are limited and are consumed quickly. In contrast, carbon dioxide has a large storage reserve and an effective buffering system. If effective circulation is maintained, the partial pressure of arterial carbon dioxide ($PaCO_2$) builds rather slowly, at a rate of 6 to 9 mmHg in the first apneic minute and 3 to 6 mmHg per minute thereafter.[14] If the patient remains apneic and develops metabolic acidemia, H^+ combines with HCO_3 to generate carbon dioxide and water, dramatically increasing the rate of carbon dioxide production. Thus, life-threatening hypoxemia occurs long before significant respiratory acidemia.

Profound hypoxemia depresses neural function and produces bradycardia that is refractory to sympathetic and parasympatholytic influences. Cardiac output, the product of heart rate and stroke volume, thus decreases, which further impairs oxygen transport. The result of this process is a *pulmocardiac arrest*. Nearly half of hospitalized patients who suffer cardiac arrest exhibit an initial bradycardic rhythm, strongly suggesting a primary respiratory etiology.[14]

Primary Cardiovascular Events

The heart may become unable to maintain an adequate cardiac output because of a new arrhythmia or adverse alterations in preload, afterload, contractility, or heart rate. Intrinsic compensatory mechanisms, regulated via neurohormonal release of catecholamines, are subsequently activated in an attempt to improve cardiac output and oxygen transport. If appropriate interventions to correct the underlying problem are not initiated in a timely fashion, or if such interventions are not successful, profound hypoxemia ensues.

Neural tissue is disproportionately susceptible to hypoxemia and acidemia caused by decreased cardiac output. Circulatory arrest always produces loss of consciousness within seconds, and respiratory rhythm ceases very rapidly thereafter.[14] The result of this process is a *cardiopulmonary arrest*. Thus, ongoing respiratory efforts indicate very recent cardiovascular collapse.

Although it is useful to consider cardiopulmonary arrest situations as primarily cardiac or pulmonary in origin, the context within which the event occurs should also be considered. Probable causes of cardiopulmonary arrest in common clinical settings and appropriate initial considerations are presented in Table 14-1.[14]

Causes of Cardiopulmonary Arrest in Pregnancy

Although it occurs infrequently during pregnancy, cardiopulmonary arrest is a complication for which the outcome is critically dependent on the underlying cause of the arrest and prompt initiation of resuscitation efforts. The causes of cardiopulmonary arrest during pregnancy have generally been divided into three categories: preexisting medical conditions, obstetric complications, and random, catastrophic events. In addition, iatrogenic factors also contribute to the incidence of cardiopulmonary arrest in pregnancy. The major causes of cardiac arrest during pregnancy that have been reported in the literature are listed in Box 14-1.[15]

GUIDELINES FOR CARDIOPULMONARY RESUSCITATION

CPR is not a single skill but rather refers to a series of assessments and interventions. In addition, cardiopulmonary arrest is not a single problem. As a consequence, the steps of CPR may vary depending on the type or etiology of the arrest. Because survival declines dramatically with time after arrest, most successfully resuscitated patients are revived within 5 to 10 minutes. The primary activities of resuscitation include:

- airway management and ventilation
- cardioversion/defibrillation
- circulatory support
- establishment of intravenous access
- administration of drugs
- performance of specialized procedures.

TABLE 14-1

Common Clinical Scenarios of Cardiopulmonary Arrest

Setting	Likely Etiology	Interventions
Early during mechanical ventilation	Misplaced ET tube	Confirm proper location by visualization, auscultation, CO_2 detector
	Tension pneumothorax	Physical examination, chest tube placement
	Hypovolemia	Volume resuscitation
	Auto-PEEP	Reduce V_E, increase expiratory time, bronchodilator, suction airway
	Profound hypoxemia	Check ET tube placement, check SaO_2, administer 100% O_2 ($FiO_2 = 1.0$)
During chronic mechanical ventilation	ET tube displacement	Confirm proper placement of ET tube by auscultation and chest radiograph
	Hypoxemia	Confirm oxygenation by oximeter or ABG, increase FiO_2
	Tension pneumothorax	Physical examination, chest tube placement
	Auto-PEEP	Reduce V_E, increase expiratory time, bronchodilator
	Mucus plugging	Suction airway
After central line placement/ attempt	Tension pneumothorax	Physical examination, chest tube placement
	Tachyarrhythmia	Withdraw intracardiac catheter or wires, try cardioversion/antiarrhythmic
	Bradycardia/heart block	Withdraw intracardiac catheter or wires, try chronotropic drugs, temporary pacing
During dialysis or plasmapheresis	Hypovolemia	Fluid therapy
	Transfusion reaction	Stop transfusion, treat anaphylaxis
	IgA deficiency: allergic reaction	Stop transfusion, treat anaphylaxis
	Hyperkalemia	Check K^+, treat empirically if ECG suggests hyperkalemia
After first dose of a new medicine (e.g., antibiotics)	Anaphylaxis	Stop drug; administer fluid, epinephrine

ABG = arterial blood gas, ECG = electrocardiogram, ET = endotracheal tube, FiO_2 = fraction of inspired oxygen, K^+ = potassium, PEEP = positive end-expiratory pressure, SaO_2 = oxygen saturation in arterial blood, VE = minute volume.

Box 14-1. CAUSES OF CARDIOPULMONARY ARREST IN PREGNANCY

Venous thromboembolism
Preeclampsia/eclampsia
Sepsis
Amniotic fluid embolism (anaphylactoid syndrome of pregnancy)
Hemorrhage
    Placental abruption
    Placenta previa
    Uterine atony
    Disseminated intravascular coagulation
Trauma
Iatrogenic
    Medication errors or allergy
    Anesthetic complications
    Hypermagnesemia
Preexisting heart disease
    Congenital
    Acquired

Basic Life Support

The steps of Basic Life Support (BLS) for adult patients consist of a series of sequential assessments and actions. These steps are depicted in the Simplified Adult BLS Healthcare Provider Algorithm presented in Figure 14-1. This algorithm incorporates evidence-based changes recommended by the AHA to promote more effective CPR.[9] Key issues and major changes were included in the 2010 American Heart Association (AHA) Guidelines for CPR and ECC. These changes are designed to simplify lay rescuer training and to continue to emphasize the need to provide early chest compressions for the victim of a sudden cardiac arrest. A summary of changes in the 2010 AHA guidelines is presented in Table 14-2.

Recent studies have shown that half of all chest compressions administered by professional rescuers during CPR were too shallow and were interrupted too often.[9] It is important to note that chest compressions administered by a rescuer generate only a small amount of blood flow compared to that generated by normal cardiac

TABLE 14-2

Summary of Key 2010 BLS Components for Adults

Component	Recommendations for Adults
Recognition	• Unresponsive • Not breathing, not breathing normally (e.g., gasping) • No pulse palpated within 10 seconds (HCP only)
CPR sequence	• CAB
Compression rate	• At least 100/minute
Compression depth	• At least 2 inches (5 cm)
Chest wall recoil	• Allow complete recoil between compressions. • HCPs rotate compressors every 2 minutes.
Interruptions	• Attempt to limit interruptions to less than 10 seconds.
Airway	• Head tilt-chin lift (HCP trauma: jaw thrust)
Compression to ventilation ratio (until advanced airway placed)	• 30:2 • (1 or 2 rescuers)
Ventilations: when rescuer untrained or trained and not proficient	• Compressions only
Ventilations with advanced airway (HCP)	• 1 breath every 6–8 seconds (8–10 breaths/minute). • Asynchronous with chest compressions. • About 1 second per breath. • Visible chest rise
Defibrillation	• Attach and use AED as soon as available. Minimize interruptions in chest compression before and after shock, resume CPR beginning with compressions immediately after each shock.

BLS = basic life support, HCP = health care provider, CPR = cardiopulmonary resuscitation, CAB = circulation-airway-breathing, cm = centimeters, AED = automated external defibrillator.

function. For this reason, the more effective the compressions, the more blood flow generated to perfuse vital organ systems. Furthermore, blood flow stops every time compressions are interrupted. When compressions are resumed, the first few are not as effective as later compressions. For these reasons, the current AHA guidelines emphasize effective chest compressions with limited interruptions. The guidelines indicate to "push hard and push fast" for a compression rate of at least 100 per minute for all victims of arrest (except newborns).

FIGURE 14-1   Simplified adult basic life support algorithm.

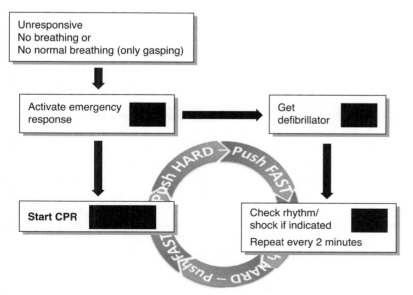

The current AHA guidelines suggest that for most victims, ventilation is not as important as chest compressions during the first few minutes of CPR following cardiac arrest. However, in cases of hypoxic arrest (e.g., drug overdose), ventilation is paramount. For this reason, chest compression–only CPR is not recommended. Chest compression–only CPR is easier for untrained rescuers to perform and can be more readily guided by dispatchers over the telephone. However, because the health care provider should be trained, the recommendation remains for the health care provider to perform both compressions and ventilations. In such situations, a compression-to-ventilation ratio of 30:2 is recommended.

During the first few minutes of CPR, arterial oxygen content (CaO_2) remains adequate. As cardiac output decreases, oxygen delivery to vital organs decreases, including perfusion of the lungs. It is estimated that blood flow to the lungs during CPR is approximately 25 to 33 percent of normal flow.[9] For this reason, rescuers can use shorter ventilation efforts than previously recommended. Current AHA guidelines include the recommendation to deliver 1-second breaths during CPR efforts.

Advanced Cardiac Life Support (ACLS)

Four rhythms produce pulseless cardiac arrest: ventricular fibrillation (VF), rapid ventricular tachycardia (VT), pulseless electrical activity (PEA), and asystole. Survival from these arrest rhythms requires both BLS and ACLS. The conventional ACLS Cardiac Arrest Algorithm, presented in Figure 14-2, has been simplified and streamlined to emphasize the importance of high-quality CPR and the fact that ACLS actions should be organized around uninterrupted periods of CPR. A detailed discussion of drugs included in these algorithms may be found in Chapter 6 of this text.

The foundation of ACLS is performance of good BLS, beginning with prompt high-quality CPR and, for VF/pulseless VT, attempted defibrillation within minutes of arrest. Following these interventions, venous access should be established. Medications recommended in resuscitation algorithms may be administered via large-bore peripheral venous catheter or central venous catheter. Drugs typically require 1 to 2 minutes to reach the central circulation when given via peripheral vein but require less time when given via central venous access.[16] For this reason, if a drug is administered via peripheral vein, it should be administered by bolus injection and followed by a small fluid bolus. In addition, the extremity used for injection should also be elevated to facilitate venous return.[16] Intraosseous cannulation provides access to a noncollapsible venous plexus, enabling drug delivery similar to that achieved by central venous access. If IV and intraosseous access cannot be established, some resuscitation drugs may be administered via endotracheal tube. Drugs that may be administered by this route include lidocaine, epinephrine, atropine, naloxone, and vasopressin. However, it should be noted that drugs administered via endotracheal tube achieve lower blood concentrations than the same doses given intravascularly. Furthermore, recent studies suggest that the lower epinephrine concentrations achieved when the drug is given by endotracheal tube may produce transient beta-adrenergic effects.[17,18] These effects may be detrimental, causing hypotension, decreased coronary artery perfusion pressure and flow, and reduced potential for return of spontaneous circulation. Thus, although endotracheal administration of some resuscitation drugs is possible, IV or intraosseous drug administration is preferred, because it will provide more predictable drug delivery and pharmacologic effect.

EFFECTS OF PREGNANCY ON CPR

Physiologic adaptations that accompany normal pregnancy may limit the effectiveness of CPR efforts. The impact of selected physiologic alterations is evident when one reviews specific issues related to CPR. The current algorithm for cardiopulmonary resuscitation during pregnancy is presented in Figure 14-3.

Airway and Breathing

The incidence of failed intubation in an obstetric population during a surgical procedure is seven times greater than in the general population.[19] This increased risk is related to airway alterations of pregnancy. The larynx is located more anteriorly, and capillary engorgement of the mucosa throughout the respiratory tract causes edema of the pharynx, larynx, and trachea.[8]

Displacement of the gastrointestinal tract occurs during normal pregnancy. The gravid uterus causes cephalad displacement of the stomach, and hormonal influences allow relaxation of the gastric sphincter. Gastric contents have a decreased pH, which subsequently increases the risk of morbidity and mortality if aspiration occurs.

Minute ventilation, alveolar ventilation, and tidal volume are increased by 40 to 70 percent. Maternal oxygen consumption increases by at least 20 percent. A minimal increase in the respiratory rate and a significant increase in tidal volume assist in meeting both maternal and fetal oxygen demands. Hyperventilation increases expiration of carbon dioxide, which stimulates excretion of serum bicarbonate. Maternal arterial blood gases reflect the end result of these changes. Pregnancy is a state of compensated respiratory alkalemia. This facilitates maternal/fetal gas exchange across the placenta.

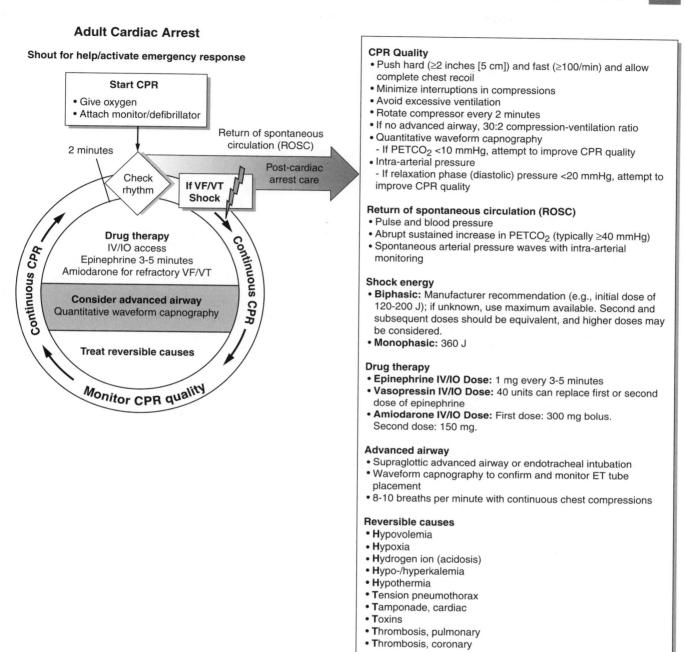

FIGURE 14-2   ACLS adult cardiac arrest circular algorithm.

Pregnancy significantly decreases respiratory reserves, which can impede the effectiveness of resuscitation measures. The gravid uterus displaces the diaphragm by 4 to 7 cm, which decreases functional residual capacity (FRC) and chest wall compliance. Although the overall lung capacity is not changed, the FRC is decreased by at least 20 percent. The pulmonary changes associated with pregnancy allow for more efficient gas exchange, but the decrease in FRC decreases oxygen reserve and increases the potential for hypoxia in the presence of apnea. Decreased serum bicarbonate makes it more difficult to correct acidemia associated with hypoxemia. Therefore, it is important that hypoventilation and hypoxemia are corrected as soon as possible when resuscitating a pregnant woman.

The problems associated with the increased risk of aspiration are compounded by the decreased functional residual lung capacity and oxygen consumption associated with normal pregnancy. Early endotracheal

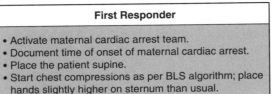

First Responder

- Activate maternal cardiac arrest team.
- Document time of onset of maternal cardiac arrest.
- Place the patient supine.
- Start chest compressions as per BLS algorithm; place hands slightly higher on sternum than usual.

Subsequent Responders

Maternal interventions

Treat per BLS and ACLS algorithms

- Do not delay defibrillation.
- Give typical ACLS drugs and doses.
- Ventilate with 100% oxygen.
- Monitor waveform capnography and CPR quality.
- Provide post-cardiac arrest care as appropriate.

Maternal modifications

- Start IV access above the diaphragm.
- Assess for hypovolemia and give fluid bolus when required.
- Anticipate difficult airway; experienced provider preferred for advanced airway placement.
- If patient receiving IV/IO magnesium prearrest, stop magnesium and give IV/IO calcium gluconate 30 mL in 10% solution.
- Continue all maternal resuscitation interventions (CPR, positioning, defibrillation, drugs, and fluids) during and after cesarean section.

Obstetric interventions for patient with an obviously gravid uterus*

- Perform manual left uterine displacement (LUD) – displace uterus to the patient's left to relieve aortocaval compression.
- Remove both internal and external fetal monitors if present.

Obstetric and neonatal teams should immediately prepare for possible emergency cesarean section

- If no ROSC by 4 minutes of resuscitative efforts, consider performing immediate emergency cesarean section.
- Aim for delivery within 5 minutes of onset of maternal arrest.

*An obviously gravid uterus is a uterus that is deemed clinically to be sufficiently large to cause aortocaval compression.

Search for and treat possible contributing factors (BEAU_CHOPS)

Bleeding/DIC
Embolism: coronary/pulmonary/amniotic fluid embolism
Anesthetic complications
Uterine atony
Cardiac disease (MI/ischemia/aortic dissection/cardiomyopathy)
Hypertension preeclampsia/eclampsia
Other: differential diagnosis of standard ACLS guidelines
Placenta abruptio/previa
Sepsis

FIGURE 14-3 Maternal cardiac arrest algorithm.

intubation should be considered because of the increased risk of aspiration. Edema of the respiratory tract further increases the potential difficulty of intubation, and decreased respiratory reserve necessitates that the procedure be performed in as timely a manner as possible.

Circulation

The cardiovascular changes associated with normal pregnancy promote a high-flow, low-resistant state with a high cardiac output and low systemic vascular resistance (SVR). The uterus, with minimal resistance, receives up to 30 percent of the cardiac output, compared with 2 to 3 percent in the non-pregnant patient. These adaptations are necessary to meet both maternal and fetal demands during pregnancy.

Effective CPR may be impeded by structural and physiologic changes that occur during pregnancy. The gravid uterus poses a potential threat to venous return and cardiac output if a pregnant woman is placed in the supine position. This risk is compounded by decreased vascular resistance of the iliac arteries, inferior vena cava, and abdominal aorta. Compression of these vessels occurs when the pregnant woman is in the supine position, especially when the estimated gestational age is 20 weeks or longer. As a consequence, uteroplacental perfusion and fetal oxygenation may be significantly diminished. Furthermore, the gravid uterus poses an obstruction to forward blood flow, particularly when arterial pressure and volume are decreased, as occurs in cardiac arrest. For these reasons it is important that the uterus is displaced laterally during CPR of the pregnant woman.

Drugs

Changes in the pregnant woman's response to drugs may also hinder resuscitation efforts. Vasopressors recommended in ACLS, especially alpha-adrenergic or combined alpha and beta agents, may produce uteroplacental vasoconstriction. This may further reduce fetal oxygenation and impair the elimination of carbon dioxide.

Clinical experience with the pharmacologic agents used in ACLS is limited in pregnancy. Data concerning the fetal effects of these drugs are mostly generated from studies that involve chronic use rather than limited dosing in the acute arrest setting. In addition, the volume of distribution and drug metabolism may vary from non-pregnant norms. Multiple factors contribute to the alterations in therapeutic blood levels of drugs in pregnancy. These include increased intravascular volume, reduced drug protein binding, increased clearance of renally excreted drugs, progesterone-activated increased hepatic metabolism, and altered gastrointestinal absorption related to changes in gastric secretion and gut motility.[20]

As noted above, the effectiveness of medications may be altered during normal pregnancy. However, there are no data to support modifications in the recommended ACLS algorithms with respect to administration of pharmacologic agents during pregnancy.

FETAL PHYSIOLOGY

Oxygenation of the fetus depends on maternal cardiac output and arterial oxygen content (CaO_2). In turn, CaO_2 depends on the amount of oxygen chemically bound to maternal hemoglobin and the amount of oxygen dissolved under pressure in the maternal plasma (PaO_2). These concepts are discussed at length in Chapter 4 of this text. Because of the high-flow, low-resistance state of the vasculature during pregnancy, the uterine vessels are normally maximally dilated. Maternal conditions that lead to hypotension and hypoxia subsequently decrease uteroplacental perfusion. Impairment of fetal oxygenation may lead to fetal acidosis.

The fetus is dependent on a pattern of placental circulation that does not permit the PO_2 of the umbilical vein to exceed the PO_2 of the maternal uterine vein. Because of this, blood in the umbilical vein that delivers oxygen to the fetus has a low oxygen tension.[21] Adequate oxygen content is maintained in part because of a normal left shift of the fetal oxyhemoglobin dissociation curve and an increased level of hemoglobin in the fetus. Therefore, fetal hemoglobin has a higher affinity for oxygen. However, because of this left shift in the fetal oxyhemoglobin dissociation curve, a small decrease in the fetal PO_2 may cause a significant change in the fetal oxygen saturation.

Current understanding of the acid–base pathophysiology during cardiopulmonary arrest indicates that carbon dioxide generated in maternal tissues is not well cleared when there is low blood flow.[22] Adequate ventilation and restoration of perfusion are therefore the mainstays of control of maternal and fetal acid–base balance during cardiac arrest. It should be noted that administration of bicarbonate to correct acidemia that occurs secondary to maternal cardiac arrest does not benefit the mother or fetus.[23]

PERIMORTEM CESAREAN DELIVERY

It has been suggested that perimortem Cesarean delivery may not only be of benefit to the infant, but may also facilitate maternal resuscitation.[24] In the non-pregnant patient, external chest compressions produce a cardiac output approximately 30 percent of normal. The gravid uterus obstructs venous return, especially if the patient is in the supine position. Lateral tilt can mitigate this, but the rotation of the patient's torso compromises compression force during CPR. Also, the low-resistance, high-volume uteroplacental unit sequesters blood, further hindering effective CPR. Consequently, chest compression in pregnancy can be expected to produce a cardiac output less than 30 percent of normal.[25] The pregnant woman becomes acidotic more quickly than her nonpregnant counterpart. Without adequate cerebral perfusion, irreversible brain damage may occur within 4 to 6 minutes.[26] This is especially true when the pregnant woman is pulseless and anoxic.[27,28]

The timing of delivery is also critical with respect to infant survival and subsequent morbidity. Neonatal survival and intact neurologic status is likely when delivery is accomplished within 15 minutes of maternal cardiac arrest. However, the highest incidence of intact neurologic survival has been reported when delivery occurs within 5 minutes of maternal arrest.[29,30] Perimortem Cesarean delivery and surviving infant outcomes from the time of arrest until delivery are summarized in Table 14-3.

TABLE 14-3

Outcome of Surviving Infants: Time of Arrest Until Perimortem Cesarean Delivery

Time Between Arrest and Delivery (Minutes)	Sample	Intact Neurologic Status (%)
0–5	n = 45 infants	98
6–15	n = 18 infants	83
16–25	n = 9 infants	33
26–35	n = 4 infants	25
36+	n = 1 infant	0

Delivery of the fetus decreases compression or obstruction of the maternal great vessels, improves the effectiveness of external chest compressions, and may increase cardiac output by approximately 25 percent. Therefore, it is generally recommended that Cesarean delivery be considered 4 minutes after a parturient has experienced cardiopulmonary arrest, if resuscitation efforts have been unsuccessful. Delivery within this time frame may assist CPR efforts, decrease fetal exposure to medications, and improve survival and neurologic outcomes for both the pregnant woman and her infant. For this reason, *delivery* is considered a component of CPR during pregnancy. It should be emphasized, however, that no data exist to support *actual* maternal benefit of perimortem Cesarean section. Therefore, this recommendation is based upon theoretical extrapolation of physiologic information and case reports. While desirable, these time-limited goals may be difficult to achieve in actual clinical practice. Furthermore, sporadic reports document instances of infant survival at longer intervals following arrest. Therefore, delivery in the third trimester should be considered following maternal arrest, if signs of fetal life are present.[31] It has been suggested that perimortem Cesarean delivery should be considered in cases of unsuccessful initial CPR after 20 weeks gestation regardless of viability to improve maternal outcome.[32] However, it should be noted that maternal death remains the most likely outcome, regardless of the arrest-to-delivery interval.[33,34]

The technique of Cesarean delivery is well known to obstetric care providers. In the setting of perimortem delivery, efficiency is the paramount issue, and the following modifications of the usual techniques are useful:

1. Final closure of the uterus and abdominal cavity can be delayed until successful restoration of maternal pulse and blood pressure. The abdominal wound should be packed with wet lap packs until successful resuscitation.

2. Usual surgical preparation and draping are not performed. The goal of delivery within 5 minutes of maternal arrest precludes transfer of the mother to an operating suite. If resuscitation is successful, administer broad-spectrum antibiotics to decrease risk of infection.

COMPLICATIONS OF CPR

While CPR is essential for a pregnant woman who experiences cardiopulmonary arrest, clinicians should be aware of potential complications that may ensue. Both the mother and fetus may sustain injuries. The presence of such injuries does not imply that resuscitation efforts were performed incorrectly.

Maternal complications may include rib or sternum fractures, hemothorax, hemopericardium, rupture of the spleen or uterus, and liver laceration. Fetal complications may include medication toxicity, reduced uteroplacental perfusion, fetal hypoxemia, and acidemia. While fetal monitoring may be used to assess fetal status, successful maternal resuscitation should remain the primary goal.[30]

Prognosis

CPR was originally designed to temporarily support circulation in otherwise healthy patients who suffered sudden cardiac death. In most cases, acute myocardial infarction or primary arrhythmia was the inciting event. However, since its inception, the use of CPR has been expanded to include nearly all patients who suffer the cessation of circulatory function. Because of this wide applicability, its success rate has, understandably, declined.[14] CPR initially returns circulatory function in 40 to 50 percent of patients to whom it is applied. Significantly fewer than one half of the initial survivors will survive to hospital discharge. Further, at least one half of patients who survive to the time of hospital discharge suffer significant neurologic damage.

Survival declines dramatically with time after arrest. This concept is illustrated in Figure 14-4. As this figure illustrates, most patients who are successfully resuscitated are revived within 5 to 10 minutes.

Certain clinical disorders are associated with an extremely poor long-term prognosis. These include refractory widely-metastatic carcinoma, end-stage acquired immunodeficiency syndrome (AIDS), and multiple organ system failure. CPR is rarely successful if cardiac arrest ensues as the final manifestation of days or weeks of multiple organ failure.

In some cases, a decision may be made to forego resuscitation efforts. Each case must be considered individually with regard for the physical condition of the

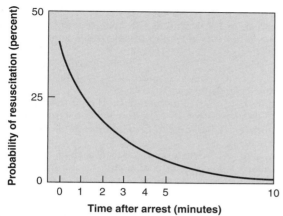

FIGURE 14-4   Probability of successful resuscitation after cardiopulmonary arrest.

patient, the expressed wishes of the patient and family, and the likelihood that CPR can succeed if performed.

During ongoing CPR, neurologic signs and arterial blood gases are unreliable predictors of outcome and should not be used in the decision-making process regarding termination of resuscitation efforts. However, resuscitation seldom is successful when more than 20 minutes are required to establish coordinated ventricular activity. With rare exceptions, failure to respond to 30 minutes of advanced life support predictably results in death. Best results occur when sudden electrical events are corrected promptly with cardioversion. Prolonged resuscitation with intact neurologic survival may occur when hypothermia or profound pharmacologic central nervous system dysfunction (e.g., barbiturates) precipitates the arrest.

ADVANCE PREPARATION

Development of staff proficiency for emergency situations remains an ongoing challenge. In the event of maternal cardiopulmonary arrest, prompt initiation of resuscitation efforts by the health care team is essential. It is important that obstetric care providers possess current knowledge of and demonstrate proficiency in BLS, including the ability to locate and properly use emergency equipment. In addition, clinicians should demonstrate proficiency in resuscitation measures and logistics specific to the pregnant woman and her fetus. Combined with the capability to rapidly access resources and personnel for ACLS, this advance preparation should markedly enhance resuscitation efforts.

Advance preparation also includes continuing professional education related to high-risk and critical care obstetric topics. Patients often show signs of impending collapse prior to cardiopulmonary arrest. An Australian retrospective study identified that patients demon-

strated evidence of deterioration an average of 6.5 hours prior to an unanticipated event, identified as cardiopulmonary arrest or admission to an ICU.[35] These data were further supported by Franklin and Schein, who reported that the majority of patients demonstrated evidence of instability within 6 to 8 hours prior to an emergency event.[36,37] In 2005, the Institute of Healthcare Improvement (IHI) initiated the "100,000 Lives Campaign" that recommended the development of a systematic approach to the management of patient deterioration in acute settings before cardiac or respiratory arrest occurs.[38]

The need for collaboration among clinicians cannot be overemphasized. In July 2004, the Joint Commission issued Sentinel Event Alert #30: Preventing Infant Death and Injury during Delivery.[39] In a review of 47 sentinel event reports that led to a rate of 6.9 deaths per 1,000 live births, the general themes of identified root causes included:

- communication issues (72 percent)
- organizational culture created a barrier to effective communication and teamwork (55 percent)
- inadequate staff competency (47 percent)
- inadequate orientation and training process (40 percent).

As a result, the Joint Commission brought forth recommendations to address these issues. Among these was the recommendation to conduct team training in perinatal clinical areas to teach staff to work together and communicate more effectively.

For select high-risk events such as maternal cardiopulmonary arrest, the Joint Commission recommended that clinical drills should be conducted to help staff prepare for such events when they actually occur. The purpose of such drills is to facilitate effective provision of maternal and neonatal resuscitation efforts including perimortem Cesarean delivery. Guidelines for emergent notification of necessary personnel should be established in each institution. Deployment of resuscitation equipment should also be considered in institutional maternal resuscitation guidelines.

SUMMARY

The likelihood of successful CPR depends on the population to whom the procedures are applied, the time elapsed before resuscitation is initiated, and the duration of resuscitation required before circulation is restored. When cardiopulmonary arrest occurs during pregnancy, initial resuscitation efforts include initiation of BLS and ACLS. Specific physiologic alterations associated with pregnancy should be incorporated into resuscitation measures. Consideration of fetal status is secondary to maternal resuscitation efforts. However, perimortem Cesarean delivery should be considered in the event the pregnant woman remains unresponsive to resuscitation efforts after 4 minutes of CPR. Fetal outcome is directly related to the condition of the mother. Delivery of the fetus may have maternal resuscitative benefit by improving venous return and cardiac output. Because cardiopulmonary arrest is relatively rare during pregnancy, development of applicable guidelines and utilization of team drills may facilitate clinical responses that optimize maternal and fetal outcomes.

REFERENCES

1. Zheng, Z. J., Croft, J. B., Giles, W. H., & Mensah, G. A. (2001). Sudden cardiac death in the United States, 1989 to 1998. *Circulation, 104,* 2158–2163.
2. Chugh, S. S., Jui, J., Gunson, K., Stecker, E. C., John, B. T., Thompson, B., et al. (2004). Current burden of sudden cardiac death: Multiple source surveillance versus retrospective death certificate-based review in a large US community. *Journal of the American College of Cardiology, 44,* 1268–1275.
3. Vaillancourt, C., & Stiell, I. G. (2004). Cardiac arrest care and emergency medical services in Canada. *Canadian Journal of Cardiology, 20,* 1081–1090.
4. Rea, T. D., Eisenberg, M. S., Sinibaldi, G., & White, R. D. (2004). Incidence of EMS-treated out-of-hospital cardiac arrest in the United States. *Resuscitation, 63,* 17–24.
5. Cobb, L. A., Fahrenbruch, C. E., Olsufka, M., & Copass, M. D. (2002). Changing incidence of out-of-hospital ventricular fibrillation, 1980-2000. *JAMA, 288,* 3008–3013.
6. Centers for Disease Control and Prevention. (2011). *Injury prevention & control: Data & statistics (WISQARS).* Atlanta, GA: Author. Retrieved from http://www.cdc.gov/injury/wisqars/index.html
7. Dildy, G. A., & Clark, S. L. (1995). Cardiac arrest during pregnancy. *Obstetrics and Gynecology Clinics of North America, 22,* 303–314.
8. Peters, C. W., Layon, A. J, and Edwards, R. K. (2005). Cardiac arrest during pregnancy. *Journal of Clinical Anesthesia, 17,* 229–234.
9. Hazinski, M. F., Nolan, J. P., Billi, J. E., Bottiger, B. W., Bossaert, L., de Caen, A. R., et al. (2010). 2010 International Consensus on Cardiopulmonary Resuscitation and Emergency Cardiovascular Care Science with Treatment. Part I: Executive Summary. *Circulation, 122,* S250–S275.
10. Larsen, M. P., Eisenberg, M. S., Cummins, R. O., & Hallstrom, A. P. (1993). Predicting survival from out-of-hospital cardiac arrest: A graphic model. *Annals of Emergency Medicine, 22,* 1652–1658.
11. Valenzuela, T. D., Roe, D. J., Cretin, S., Spaite, D. W., & Larsen, M. P. (1997). Estimating effectiveness of cardiac arrest interventions: A logistic regression survival model. *Circulation, 96,* 3308–3313.
12. Swor, R. A., Jackson, R. E., Cynar, M., Sadler, E., Basse, E., Boji, B. (1995). Bystander CPR, ventricular fibrillation, and survival in witnessed, unmonitored out-of-hospital cardiac arrest. *Annals of Emergency Medicine, 25,* 780–784.
13. Cobb, L. A., Fahrenbruch, C. E., Walsh, T. R., Copass, M. K., Olsufka, M., Breskin, M., et al. (1999). Influence of cardiopulmonary resuscitation prior to defibrillation in patients with out-of-hospital ventricular fibrillation. *JAMA, 281,* 1182–1188.
14. Marini, J. J., & Wheeler, A. P. (2010). Cardiopulmonary arrest. In J. J. Marini & A. P. Wheeler (Eds.), *Critical care medicine: the essentials* (3rd ed.). Philadelphia: Lippincott Williams & Wilkins, 361–374.
15. Mallampalli, A., & Guy, E. (2005). Cardiac arrest in pregnancy and somatic support after brain death. *Critical Care Medicine, 33*(Suppl. 10), S325–S331.
16. Emerman, C. L., Pinchak, A. C., Hancock, D., & Hagen, J. F. (1988). Effect of injection site on circulation times during cardiac arrest. *Critical Care Medicine, 16,* 1138–1141.
17. Vaknin, Z., Manisterski, Y., Ben-Abraham, R., Efrati, O., Lotan, D., Barzilay, Z., et al. (2001). Is endotracheal adrenaline deleterious because of the beta adrenergic effect? *Anesthesia and Analgesia, 92,* 1408–1412.
18. Manisterski, Y., Vaknin, Z., Ben-Abraham, R., Efrati, O., Lotan, D., Berkovitch, M., et al. (2002). Endotracheal epinephrine: A call for larger doses. *Anesthesia and Analgesia, 95,* 1037–1041.
19. Hawkins, J. (2003). Anesthesia related maternal mortality. *Clinical Obstetrics and Gynecology, 46*(3), 679–687.
20. Page, R. L. (1995). Treatment of arrhythmias during pregnancy. *American Heart Journal, 130,* 871–876.
21. Lapinsky, C. J. (2005). Cardiopulmonary complications of pregnancy. *Critical Care Medicine, 33*(7), 1616–1622.
22. Androgue, H. J., Rashad, M. N., Gorin, A. B., Yacoub, J., & Madias, N. E. (1989). Assessing acid-base status in circulatory failure: Differences between arterial and central venous blood flow. *The New England Journal of Medicine, 320,* 1312–1316.
23. Niemann, J. T. (1992). Cardiopulmonary resuscitation. *The New England Journal of Medicine, 327,* 1075–1080.
24. Cunningham, F. G., Leveno, K. J, Bloom, S. L., Hauth, J. C., Rouse, D. J., & Spong, C. Y. (Eds.). (2001). *Williams obstetrics* (23rd ed.). New York: McGraw-Hill.
25. Katz, J., Dotters, D. J., & Droegemueller, W. (1986). Perimortem cesarean delivery. *Obstetrics and Gynecology, 68,* 571–576.
26. Archer, G. W., & Marx, G. F. (1974). Arterial oxygen tension during apnoea in parturient women. *British Journal of Anaesthesia, 46,* 358–360.
27. DePace, N. L., Betesh, J. S., & Kotler, M. N. (1982). 'Postmortem' cesarean section with recovery of both mother and offspring. *JAMA, 248*(8), 971–973.
28. O'Connor, R. L., & Sevarino, F. B. (1994). Cardiopulmonary arrest in a pregnant patient: A report of successful resuscitation. *Journal of Clinical Anesthesia, 6,* 66–68.
29. Clark, S. J., Hankins, G. D. V., Dudley, D. A., Dildy, G. A., and Flint Porter, T. (1995). Amniotic fluid embolism: Analysis of the national registry. *American Journal of Obstetrics and Gynecology, 172,* 1939.
30. Hueppchen, N. A., Satin, A. J., Phelan, J.P., Hankins, G. D. V., and Clark, S. L. (2004). Cardiopulmonary resuscitation. In G. A. Dildy, M. A. Belfort, G. R. Saade, M. (Eds.), *Critical care obstetrics* (4th ed.). Malden, MA: Blackwell Science, 87–103.
31. Selden, B. S., & Burke, T. J. (1988). Complete maternal and fetal recovery after prolonged cardiac arrest. *Annals of Emergency Medicine, 17,* 346–349.
32. Johnson, M. D., Luppi, C. J. and Over, D. C. (1998). Cardiopulmonary resuscitation In: Gambling, D. R. and Douglas, M. J. (Eds). *Obstetric. anesthesia and uncommon disorders.* Philadelphia: W.B. Saunders, 51–74.
33. Karetzky, M., Zubair, M., & Parikh, J. (1995). Cardiopulmonary resuscitation in intensive care unit and non-intensive care unit patients: Immediate and long-term survival. *Archives of Internal Medicine, 155*(12), 1277–1280.

34. Diem, S. J., Lantos, J. D., & Tulsky, J. A. (1996). Cardiopulmonary resuscitation on television: Miracles and misinformation. *The New England Journal of Medicine, 334,* 1578–1582.

35. Bruist, M. D., Jarmolowski, E., Burton, P. R., Bernard, S. A., Waxman, B. P., & Anderson, J. (1999). Recognising clinical instability in hospital patients before cardiac arrest or unplanned admission to intensive care: A pilot study in a tertiary-care hospital. *The Medical Journal of Australia, 171*(1), 22–25.

36. Franklin, C., & Matthew, J. (1994). Developing strategies to prevent in-hospital cardiac arrest: Analyzing responses of physicians and nurses in the hours before the event. *Critical Care Medicine, 22*(2), 244–247.

37. Schein, R. M., Hazday, N., Pena, M., Ruben, B. H., & Sprung, C. L. (1990). Clinical antecedents to in-hospital cardiopulmonary arrest. *Chest, 98*(6), 1388–1392.

38. Institute of Healthcare Improvement. (n.d.). *Intensive care.* Cambridge, MA: Author. Retrieved from www.ihi.org/IHI/Topics/Criticalcare/IntensiveCare

39. Joint Commission. (2004). *Sentinel event alert, issue 30. Preventing infant death and injury during delivery.* Washington, DC: Author. Retrieved from http://www.jointcommission.org/assets/1/18/SEA_30.PDF

CHAPTER 15

Obstetric Hemorrhage

Carol J. Harvey and Gary A. Dildy

Obstetric hemorrhage remains one of the top three causes of maternal mortality in industrialized and developing nations.[1] The overwhelming majority of maternal deaths occur in developing nations. Data from the World Health Organization estimate that the global maternal death rate exceeds 536,000 per annum. Data also indicate that 25 percent of the total number of maternal deaths were because of severe bleeding.[2] It is important to note that obstetric hemorrhage is a potentially life-threatening condition not limited to any specific geographic boundary or patient population.

Berg and colleagues estimate that 90 percent of maternal deaths secondary to postpartum hemorrhage (PPH) are preventable.[3] Clark and colleagues, in their report of data from a series of 95 maternal deaths in a large U.S. health care organization, estimate that 73 percent of deaths due to PPH were preventable.[3,4] Prevention of adverse outcome is dependent upon recognition of risk factors, timely identification of abnormal bleeding, and prompt initiation of appropriate clinical management. Prompt management requires detection of abnormal bleeding, laboratory assessment, pharmacologic intervention, and in some cases blood component therapy and surgical intervention.

The American College of Obstetricians and Gynecologists' (ACOG) position on PPH is quite clear: "All obstetric units and practitioners must have the facilities, personnel, and equipment in place to manage this emergency properly."[5] Thus, all practitioners of obstetrics should be prepared to identify and appropriately respond to this potentially life-threatening complication of pregnancy.

The purpose of this chapter is to address the following concepts: normal physiology of pregnancy with regard to blood volume expansion and peripartum blood loss, etiologies of hemorrhage, clinical estimation of blood loss, clinical management of hemorrhage, and blood component therapy. The inherent need for col-laboration is reinforced. Clinical case excerpts are presented to reinforce application of concepts to practice.

PHYSIOLOGY OF PREGNANCY AND PERIPARTUM BLOOD LOSS

During pregnancy the maternal plasma volume expands by approximately 42 percent, while red blood cell (RBC) volume increases 24 percent, increasing overall blood volume while at the same time producing the so-called "physiologic anemia of pregnancy" phenomenon.[6] This net increase in blood volume is generally sufficient to compensate for blood loss that normally occurs during the third stage of labor when the placenta detaches. Women with hypertensive disorders of pregnancy have diminished maternal plasma volume expansion; as such, they are not only less able to tolerate hemorrhage, but are also at greater risk for hemorrhage.

Average blood losses at spontaneous vaginal delivery, Cesarean delivery, and elective Cesarean hysterectomy are approximately 500 mL, 1000 mL, and 1500 mL, respectively.[7] Expressed as a percentage of total blood volume, average blood losses at spontaneous vaginal delivery, Cesarean delivery, and elective Cesarean hysterectomy are approximately 10 percent, 25 percent, and 33 percent, respectively. However, when emergency Cesarean hysterectomy is performed, average blood loss has been estimated to be 3500 mL, which represents more than 75 percent of the total maternal blood volume at term.[8] It has been estimated that women who undergo operative vaginal delivery (forceps and/or vacuum) lose as much blood as those who undergo Cesarean delivery.[9] It has also been shown that the degree of any perineal laceration correlates positively with the degree of blood loss, such that women with third- or fourth-degree lacerations may lose as much blood as women who undergo Cesarean delivery.[9]

Postpartum hemorrhage has been traditionally defined as an estimated blood loss in excess of 500 mL. However this definition is somewhat arbitrary, and as noted above, half of all women lose at least 500 mL at spontaneous vaginal delivery. This discrepancy can be partly explained by the fact that blood loss at delivery is usually underestimated.[10] The incidence of PPH, based on a definition of a 10 percent drop in hemoglobin and/or hematocrit, or the need for a blood transfusion, is approximately 4 percent of vaginal deliveries and 6 percent of Cesarean deliveries.[11] Thus, approximately 1 in 20 women will experience PPH.

PPH is classified as *primary* when the bleeding occurs in the first 24 hours after birth and *secondary* if excessive blood loss from the vagina begins more than 24 hours postpartum and prior to 6 weeks following delivery.

There is no consensus with respect to the definition of massive transfusion in the obstetric patient. For the purpose of this chapter, massive transfusion is defined as replacement of the patient's total blood volume within 24 hours. For actively bleeding patients, massive transfusion is defined as transfusion of 10 or more units of packed red blood cells (PRBCs) within 24 hours. Massive transfusion most commonly occurs in patients with significant traumatic injuries, gastrointestinal bleeding, or PPH.[12] Frequently, patients with obstetric hemorrhage and coagulopathy will require 10 or more units of PRBCs in 2 hours or less.[12] This patient population is at significant risk for exsanguination, vascular collapse, and death.

ETIOLOGIES OF OBSTETRIC HEMORRHAGE

Obstetric hemorrhage is a clinical sign, not a diagnosis. In order to provide proper therapy, a correct diagnosis must be made. A thorough discussion of all potential etiologies for obstetric hemorrhage is beyond the scope of this chapter. Although some concepts presented in this chapter apply to any patient with obstetric hemorrhage, PPH is a focus of the text. For example, etiologies of PPH are listed in Table 15-1. The most common etiology of PPH is uterine atony, followed by retained placenta and lower genital tract lacerations. This list is not exhaustive; thus, hemorrhage should be considered even when the patient's uterus is firm and visual inspection of the lower genital tract is negative. Continued vaginal bleeding in the presence of a firmly contracted uterus should prompt the delivery provider to specifically assess for cervical and/or vaginal lacerations.

TABLE 15-1	
Etiologies of Obstetric Hemorrhage	
Antepartum	• Uterine rupture • Placental abruption • Placenta previa • Vasa previa
Intrapartum	• Uterine rupture • Placental abruption
Postpartum	• Uterine atony • Retained placenta • Lower genital tract lacerations (cervix, vagina, perineum) • Upper genital tract lacerations (uterine rupture) • Placenta accreta, increta, percreta • Uterine inversion • Inherited coagulopathy (e.g., von Willebrand's disease) • Acquired coagulopathy (abruption, amniotic fluid embolism, retained dead fetus syndrome)

Patients at Risk for Obstetric Hemorrhage

Risk factors for hemorrhage are prevalent in the general obstetric population, and some women who develop hemorrhage will have no obvious risk factors. Since obstetric hemorrhage is relatively common, clinicians should be well versed and prepared to care for patients who develop this complication. Prolonged labor, uterine over-distention (e.g., large baby, multiple gestation, polyhydramnios), and intrapartum infection are all associated with an increased risk for PPH. Additional risk factors for PPH are presented in Table 15-2. It should be appreciated that some antenatal conditions that involve abnormal placentation or maternal complications (e.g., placenta previa, placenta percreta, placental abruption) may result in obstetric hemorrhage with increased risk for maternal–fetal morbidity and mortality. In a large series of pregnancies complicated by placenta percreta, a 7 percent maternal mortality rate was reported; half of these deaths occurred in cases where percreta was suspected prenatally.[13]

There are different levels of pre-delivery preparations applied to these conditions. For the woman who has a protracted labor with a large baby and suspected intrapartum chorioamnionitis, preparation would include establishment of adequate intravenous access, type and crossmatch of PRBCs and fresh frozen plasma (FFP), and arrangement for the immediate availability of uterotonic agents. For the woman with suspected abnormal placentation (e.g., percreta), pre-delivery preparation becomes more intricate and may

TABLE 15-2
Risk Factors for Postpartum Hemorrhage

Uterine factors	• Previous Cesarean section • Prolonged labor • Precipitous labor • Exposure to exogenous oxytocin (e.g., induction, augmentation) • Fetal macrosomia • Polyhydramnios • Chorioamnionitis • Episiotomy with 3rd/4th degree laceration • Operative vaginal delivery (forceps/vacuum) • Grand multiparity • Maternal obesity • Multiple gestation
Placental factors	• Placental abruption • Placenta previa • Placenta accreta • Placenta percreta • Placenta increta • Abnormally adherent placenta • Hypertension
Coagulation Deficits: Acquired	• Hemoglobin <9.0 or hematocrit <27.0 • Thrombocytopenia • Anticoagulation therapy (e.g., patients with mechanical heart valves) • Liver disease • Prolonged activated partial thromboplastin time • Sepsis/septic shock • Severe preeclampsia • Amniotic fluid embolus
Coagulation Deficits: Congenital	• von Willebrand's disease • Antibodies to Factor VIII • Factors X, XI, XIII deficiencies

Data from Reference 67.

include establishment of central venous access with insertion of a catheter type approved for high-pressure infusions, placement of an intra-arterial catheter for continuous blood pressure assessment and obtaining samples for arterial blood gas analysis, femoral intra-arterial access for large vessel embolization, preparation of a cell salvage device, availability of a Level I or rapid-volume infuser, crossmatch for a larger number and variety of blood components, active patient warming devices, multidisciplinary consultation, and preparation for special approaches to hysterectomy.[14]

ASSESSMENT OF BLOOD LOSS

Underestimation of blood loss is common. This can lead to delay in treatment and subsequent increased risk for morbidity and mortality. The triennial reports of the Confidential Enquiries into Maternal Deaths showed that many maternal deaths secondary to hemorrhage in the United Kingdom are attributed to delayed diagnosis and delayed blood component therapy.[15] Studies assessing estimation of blood loss have shown that accuracy is not dependent upon the clinician's age or years of experience, and that improvement in a clinician's ability to accurately estimate blood loss can be achieved using simple educational methods.[10]

In everyday clinical practice, blood loss estimation can be performed by subjective visual means as well as by objective methods involving measurement of blood volume collected in containers or weighing surgical materials such as laparotomy (lap) sponges. As a general rule, 1 mL of blood weighs approximately 1 gram; thus, a 75-gram lap sponge contains approximately 75 mL of blood (minus the weight of the lap sponge). Another useful parameter to remember is that a fully saturated standard 18-inch × 18-inch lap sponge holds approximately 100 mL of whole blood. Figure 15-1 illustrates the approximate amount of blood contained on saturated surgical laps and sponges.

The accurate estimation of blood loss is critical in planning interventions for the patient who is actively bleeding and can be done by multiple providers.

Shock

Shock is defined as inadequate oxygen delivery and tissue perfusion secondary to decreased intravascular volume; it may progress to cellular hypoxia, acidosis, organ system damage, and death.[16] Shock is commonly classified by causative etiologies, which are listed in Table 15-3.

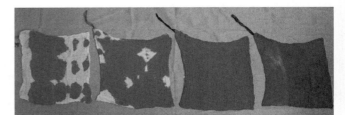

FIGURE 15-1 Estimating blood loss. Blood absorption characteristics of a dry 18-inch × 18-inch laparotomy sponge. From left to right: 25 mL of blood saturates about 50% of the surface area, 50 mL of blood saturates about 75% of the surface area, 75 mL of blood saturates the entire surface, and 100 mL of blood will saturate and drip from the sponge. If this were an actual clinical scenario, actual blood loss would be 250 mL. Photo courtesy Gary Dildy, M.D.

TABLE 15-3

Shock: Etiologies and Differential Diagnosis

Type of Shock	Etiology	Examples
Hypovolemic	Inadequate circulating volume from blood volume loss	• Burns
		• Hemorrhage
Cardiogenic	Inadequate cardiac output from decreased contractility	• Arrhythmias
		• Myocardial ischemia
Obstructive	Extra-cardiac obstruction to blood flow	• Cardiac tamponade
		• Pneumothorax
		• Pulmonary embolus
Distributive	Inadequate circulating volume from decreased vascular tone	• Acute adrenal insufficiency
		• Anaphylaxis
		• Inflammatory
		• Neurogenic
		• Sepsis

Data from Reference 70.

Because the body attempts to compensate for a decrease in intravascular volume by vasoconstriction and preferential shunting of arterial blood to the heart and brain, the onset of shock may not initially be accompanied by hypotension. Additionally, some obstetric patients may not demonstrate a compensatory increase in their heart rate during the early stages of shock, which may mislead the practitioner and complicate timely diagnosis and early treatment.

PHARMACOLOGIC THERAPY FOR UTERINE ATONY

Initial management of uterine atony involves bi-manual uterine massage performed by the delivering provider and medical therapy to enhance uterine contractility. A detailed presentation of concepts related to pharmacologic adjuncts in the care of obstetric patients with selected complications is included in Chapter 6 of this text. Achievement of normal uterine tone may be augmented by draining the urinary bladder if it is over-distended. Pharmacologic therapy is summarized in Table 15-4 and consists of administration of oxytocin, ergot alkaloids, and/or prostaglandins. Providers should be trained in the estimation of blood loss and respond collaboratively to acquire uterotonic drugs, provide safe administration of the agents, and assess the woman's hemodynamic status and response to therapy. Oxytocin is generally considered the first line of therapy, as it is commonly administered as a prophylactic measure and has few contraindications (e.g., the patient reports a known/suspected allergy). There is no consensus with respect to the order in which prostaglandins (E or F class) and ergot alkaloids should be administered. Ergot alkaloids should be avoided in hypertensive women, and the F-class prostaglandins should be avoided in women with reactive airway disease such as asthma.

Misoprostol (Cytotec) is a PGE_1 analogue, originally marketed for the prevention and treatment of peptic ulcer disease, commonly used off-label in obstetrics because of its effect on uterine contractility. A thorough discussion of this pharmacologic agent is presented in Chapter 12 of this text. This drug is advantageous because it is inexpensive, light and heat stable, and has a long shelf life. Misoprostol is probably safe in the setting of hypertension, has been studied extensively in the routine management of the third stage of labor, and is rapidly absorbed via the oral, vaginal, and rectal routes. While not demonstrated to be superior to other drugs in the prevention of PPH, a small randomized clinical trial demonstrated that misoprostol (800 mcg per rectum) is superior to oxytocin and ergot alkaloids in the primary treatment of PPH.[17] Further randomized controlled trials are required to identify the best drug combination, route, and dose for the treatment of PPH.[18] In the presence of PPH, misoprostol should be administered rectally or orally, depending on the patient's condition and potential need for surgery and general anesthesia.

GENERAL MANAGEMENT OF OBSTETRIC HEMORRHAGE

Prevention of hemorrhage-related complications includes early recognition of abnormal blood loss and early mobilization of resources. Careful assessment and interpretation of maternal vital signs are critical in patient care during active bleeding. Obstetric patients, however, may not

TABLE 15-4

Pharmacologic Management of PPH: Uterotonic Agents

Drug Name	Dose	Intervals	Contraindications	Adverse Effects	Comments

oxytocin (Pitocin, Syntocinon)
• 10-units/mL vials.
• Premix solutions of concentrations up to 40 units in 500 mL available.
	<u>IV</u>:
	• 10–40 units in 1000 mL NS or LR
	• Premix solution of 10–40 units in 500 or 1000 mL NS or LR.
	• Infuse at rates of 20–50 mL/min
	<u>IM</u>:
	• 10–20 units
		Continuous infusion	Hypersensitivity	• IV push at high doses – hypotension
				• IV push may be associated with myocardial ischemia
				• Myocardial ischemia:
				  • chest pain
				  • difficulty breathing
				  • confusion
				  • fast or irregular heartbeat
				  • severe headache
				• Water intoxication after prolonged use, especially when mixed in non-isotonic solutions
					• Avoid mixing in dextrose-containing solutions.
					• Unless an emergency, only use pre-mixed solutions.
					• Do not administer with water-containing IV solutions.
					• Maintain intake and output.

methylergo novine (Methergine) 0.2 mg/mL	<u>IM</u>: • 0.2 mg	q 2-4 hr	Hypertension Heart disease Do not co-administer with potent CYP 3A4 inhibitors including macrolide antibiotics (e.g., erythromycin), HIV protease or reverse transcriptase inhibitors, or azole antifungals. Less potent CYP 3A4 inhibitors should be administered with caution.	• Hypertension • Seizure and/or headache • Hypotension • Nausea, vomiting • Acute MI (rare) • Chest pains (rare) • Seizures • Cerebral ischemia • Cerebral vascular accident (when administered with other ergots, macrolide antibiotics, protease inhibitors)	• Avoid use, if possible, in pts with preeclampsia or preexisting hypertension. • Avoid administering IV. If IV route deemed life-saving, administer slowly over at least 60 seconds and monitor BP (increased risk of HTN crisis and CVA).

carboprost tromethamine (15 S)-15 methyl analogue of prostaglandin F2α, (15 S)-15-methyl PGF2α-THAM (Hemabate)	<u>IM</u>:
	0.25 mg
		q 15 to 90 min
		Total dose of Hemabate should not exceed 2 mg (8 doses of 0.25 mg)
			• Asthma
			• Known hypersensitivity to Hemabate solution
			• Acute pelvic inflammatory disease
			• Use with caution in patients with a history of –
			  • hypotension
			  • hypertension
			  • cardiovascular disease
			  • renal impairment
			  • hepatic disease
			  • anemia
			  • jaundice
			  • diabetes
			  • epilepsy
				• Vomiting
				• Diarrhea
				• Nausea
				• Temperature increase greater than 2° F
				• Flushing
					• Hemabate must be refrigerated at 2° to 8° C (36° to 46° F).
					• Pretreat or concurrently administer anti-emetic and antidiarrheal drugs
					Hemabate may augment the activity of other oxytocic agents.

TABLE 15-4 (Continued)

Pharmacologic Management of PPH: Uterotonic Agents

Drug Name	Dose	Intervals	Contraindications	Adverse Effects	Comments
dinoprostone (Prostin E2)	Vaginal or rectal suppository: 20 mg • Administer rectally if patient has excessive vaginal blood flow.		Use with caution in patients with a history of – • hypotension • hypertension • cardiovascular disease • renal impairment • hepatic disease • anemia • jaundice • diabetes • epilepsy	• Vomiting (67%) • Temperature elevations (50%) • Diarrhea (40%) • Nausea (33%) • Headache (10%) • Shivering and chills (10%) • Transient diastolic blood pressure decreases of greater than 20 mmHg (10%)	• Store in a freezer not above –20°C (–4°F) but bring to room temperature just prior to use. • Remove foil before use.
misoprostol (Cytotec)	Rectal suppository: 800–1000 mcg Cytotec available as: • 100-mcg tablets • 200-mcg tablets	Maximum dose not established >2 hr between first and second doses If first dose followed by pyrexia or shivering, wait at least 6 hr for second dose	History of allergy to prostaglandins	• Pyrexia • Shivering, chills • Nausea, vomiting • Diarrhea • Abdominal pain. • Hyperstimulation of the uterus, uterine tetany, uterine rupture, amniotic fluid embolism • Pelvic pain, retained placenta, genital bleeding, shock, and maternal death have been reported.	

BP = blood pressure, CVA = cerebral vascular accident, HTN = hypertension, IM = intramuscular, IV = intravenous, LR = lactated Ringer's solution, MI = myocardial infarction, NS = normal saline.
Data from References 66–68.

TABLE 15-5

Classification of Hemorrhage Based on Clinical Assessment

Parameter	Class I	Class II*	Class III	Class IV
Estimated blood loss (%)	15	15–30	30–40	>40
Pulse (beats/minute)	<100	>100	>120	>140
Pulse pressure	N	↓	↓	↓
Blood pressure	Normal or ↑	↓	↓	↓
Respiratory rate (breaths/min)	Normal	20–30	30–40	>40
Urine output (mL/hr)	>30	20–30	5–15	Negligible

*May not occur, or may occur late, in obstetric patients.

show signs and symptoms usually observed in nonpregnant patients with hemorrhage until approximately *one-third* of the woman's entire blood volume is lost.

In the setting of postpartum bleeding, vital signs usually trend such that pulse rate increases, blood pressure decreases, and pulse pressure decreases as blood loss progresses. This concept is presented in Table 15-5. Urine output also declines as hypovolemia worsens. Tachycardia may be compensatory or occur secondary to other influences such as infection and pain.

Irrespective of the cause, maternal tachycardia in the postpartum woman should alert the clinician to the possibility of hypovolemic shock, as the potential for serious blood loss may occur when the maternal pulse exceeds 100 beats per minute.

When potentially significant blood loss is suspected, the etiology should be determined and steps implemented to facilitate prompt resuscitation and stabilization as needed. A frequent clinical error is delay in laboratory assessment of hemoglobin and/or hematocrit and clotting function, thus producing a delay in availability of blood products for transfusion. Early laboratory evaluation is recommended to establish a baseline and assess for the presence of anemia and/or coagulopathy with follow-up re-evaluation as clinically indicated by the degree of ongoing blood loss and change in vital signs.

Nonsurgical and Surgical Management of Postpartum Hemorrhage

There are no data from prospective randomized studies that define the optimum sequence of nonsurgical and surgical interventions to best treat PPH. Most recommendations are based on expert opinion, retrospective case studies, or studies with small samples of heterogeneous subjects. Therefore, the following interventions may not be in sequence for effective management of all patients with obstetric hemorrhage. Providers should individualize care based on patient history, current clinical condition, available resources, and updated clinical guidelines and recommendations for obstetric management of PPH.

Uterine Packing and Intrauterine Tamponade Balloons

Uterine packing for placental site bleeding and uterine atony has fallen out of favor in recent years but is still used by some practitioners with satisfactory results.[19] Others have reported success in bleeding cessation with the use of intrauterine balloon tamponade modalities including condoms, Foley catheters, the Sengstaken-Blakemore tube (C.R. Bard, Inc., Covington, GA) and the Rusch urologic catheter. The SOS Bakri Tamponade Balloon Catheter (Cook Medical, Inc., Bloomington, IN) is a surgical obstetric silicone fluid-filled balloon (up to 500 mL capacity) approved by the U.S. Food and Drug Administration (FDA) in 2002 and designed for tamponade function.[20] FDA labeling lists contraindications to its use in several settings, including coagulopathy, arterial bleeding requiring surgical exploration or angiographic embolization, bleeding requiring immediate hysterectomy, and others. A similar product, the BT-Cath (Utah Medical Products, Midvale, UT) balloon tamponade catheter (up to 500 mL capacity) is also commercially available. The FDA has also recently approved the Belfort-Dildy Obstetric Tamponade System (Glenveigh Surgical, LLC, Suwanee, GA) that employs dual balloons and is indicated for providing temporary control or reduction of postpartum uterine bleeding. Inflation of the vaginal balloon anchors the uterine balloon and provides tamponade if vaginal bleeding is present. All three tamponade balloons share the same contraindications.

Balloon tamponade devices are particularly appealing to address placental-site bleeding including that from a low-lying placenta or placenta previa. In a systematic review of PPH management with balloon catheters for uterine tamponade, Doumouchtsis and colleagues reported an overall success rate of 84 percent (Fig. 15-2).[21] The study evaluated the performance of the Foley urinary, Sengstaken–Blakemore esophageal balloon, Rusch balloon, and other unidentified catheters, and condoms. The high rate of hemorrhage abatement with the use of balloon catheters may encourage increased utilization of such devices in the control of uterine bleeding when future fertility is desired and/or as a temporizing intervention prior to surgical intervention in the unstable coagulopathic patient. There are currently no studies that compare and/or measure the effectiveness among individual types of balloon tamponade catheters.

Interventional Radiology

Selective arterial embolization (SAE) is a procedure performed by interventional radiologists in which a catheter is guided fluoroscopically through a peripheral artery (usually femoral) to the appropriate uterine vessel, which is then injected and embolized with various materials to occlude the artery. Uterine artery embolization (UAE) via arterial catheterization under fluoroscopic guidance has been used successfully in gynecologic patients in the treatment of pain and heavy

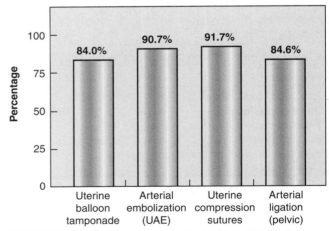

Success rates of treatment for PPH

FIGURE 15-2 Percentage of patients who had their bleeding controlled by one of four methods used in PPH management. Balloon catheters inserted into the uterus and expanded according to manufacturer instruction may offer an effective nonsurgical method to control postpartum hemorrhage.

bleeding from uterine fibroids. It has also been used in the management of PPH to decrease blood supply to the uterus and thereby decrease blood loss. UAE for PPH has a reported 90.7 percent success rate in controlling bleeding and preventing hysterectomy, and appears particularly useful in cases of expanding retroperitoneal hematomas, where open surgical exploration may be difficult and dangerous.[22] Its use, however, is limited to the availability of interventional radiologic teams and may not be feasible in the massively bleeding hemodynamically unstable intra-operative patient.

Uterine artery balloon placement is another interventional radiological procedure used in patients with extremely high probability for massive PPH, such as women with known placenta percreta. Prior to Cesarean delivery, intra-arterial sheaths (large bore catheters) are placed in both the right and left femoral arteries under fluoroscopic guidance. Balloon catheters (deflated) are then threaded through the sheaths and into the iliac arteries. The balloons are inflated after delivery of the infant to decrease blood supply to the uterus and thereby decrease blood loss. A relatively new procedure for the treatment of PPH, it has been used for temporary obstruction of blood supply in the iliac arteries. Post-procedure balloon re-inflation is performed in accordance with prescribed amounts of fluid in each balloon. Protocols and care guidelines for balloon placement, inflation volume, timed intervals of deflation and ongoing vascular assessments are defined by clinical guidelines and are beyond the scope of this chapter.

When nonsurgical management options do not stop the hemorrhage, providers should prepare for surgical intervention. Surgical procedures commonly used to treat obstetric patients with massive PPH are presented in Box 15-1.

Modalities include laceration repair, curettage, and hypogastric or uterine artery ligation or the use of a compression suture. The latter is particularly useful for women who have experienced uterine atony and who have responded well to bimanual compression. The B-Lynch compression suture is one example, first utilized successfully in 1997 as an innovative technique to man-age uterine atony. The procedure involves placement of a continuous suture to envelope and mechanically compress the uterus in an attempt to avoid hysterectomy.

Hysterectomy

The incidence of obstetric hysterectomy ranges between 0.33 and 0.70 per 1000 deliveries.[23–26] Maternal mortality associated with obstetric hysterectomy is substantial (0.6 to 4.5 percent) for a number of reasons, including the moribund condition of the patient at the onset of the operation, and the technical difficulty of the procedure, especially in the setting of ongoing hemorrhage.[24,26,27] The average estimated blood loss during emergency obstetric hysterectomy has been reported at approximately 3500 mL, so one can expect the average patient undergoing emergency obstetric hysterectomy to lose at least half of her total blood volume.[8] Concomitant coagulopathy often exists, particularly in patients requiring hysterectomy for abnormal placentation. Complications related to the procedure itself may include vascular, ureteral, bowel, and bladder injuries.

COAGULOPATHY AND OBSTETRIC HEMORRHAGE

Numerous professional organizations have published guidelines to direct contemporary blood replacement therapy (Table 15-6). Most of these guidelines strongly recommend intermittent laboratory analysis of bleeding profiles to guide transfusion therapy. Results of bleeding profiles may require a minimum of 30 to 40 minutes for analysis and thus may not reflect real-time clotting factor concentration during acute loss of blood. The expansion of point-of-care (POC) testing for hemostasis and fibrinolysis into operating rooms, intensive care units, outpatient clinics, etc., offers expedited results when compared to traditional laboratory testing. POC testing may offer obstetric providers similar benefits during obstetric hemorrhage; however, there are no randomized trials that have evaluated the impact of POC testing on patient outcomes in the setting of obstetric hemorrhage.

It is critical to note that the perfect test for hemostasis does not yet exist. Current laboratory tests do not accurately measure or reflect true *in vivo* coagulation. The prothrombin time (PT), activated partial thromboplastin time (aPTT), and International Normalized Ratio (INR) were developed to assess and adjust dosing of anticoagulant medications such as warfarin (INR) and heparin (aPTT). Laboratory tests have also been used in unsuccessful attempts to predict the risk for intraoperative and postoperative blood loss from coagulation deficiencies in patients undergoing invasive procedures. It is evident that more specific tests are needed to assess the ability of blood to remain liquid and yet

Box 15-1. SURGICAL MANAGEMENT OF POSTPARTUM HEMORRHAGE

1. Uterine curettage
2. Vaginal/cervical laceration repair
3. Uterine packing or balloon tamponade
4. Hypogastric artery ligation
5. Uterine artery ligation
6. B-Lynch stitch or other compression stitch
7. Hysterectomy
8. Pelvic packing

Data from References 66 and 69.

TABLE 15-6

National and International Guidelines in Blood Transfusion Therapy

Organization	Guideline
American Society of Anesthesiologists (ASA, 2006)[28]	*Practice Guidelines for Perioperative Blood Transfusion and Adjuvant Therapies: An Updated Report by the American Society of Anesthesiologists Task Force on Perioperative Blood Transfusion and Adjuvant Therapies*
American College of Obstetricians and Gynecologists (ACOG, 2006)[5]	*ACOG Practice Bulletin No. 76 Postpartum Hemorrhage*
Society of Obstetricians and Gynaecologists of Canada (SOGC, 2002)[29]	*SOGC Clinical Practice Guidelines No. 115: Hemorrhagic Shock*
British Committee for Standards in Haematology, National Blood Service (2006)[30]	*Guidelines on the Management of Massive Blood Loss*
National Health Service Guideline (England) (NHS, 2006)[30]	*Management of Massive Bleeding and Coagulopathy*
Australia Department of Health, New South Wales (2010)[31]	*Maternity – Prevention, Early Recognition & Management of Postpartum Haemorrhage (PPH) (Policy Directive)*
European Guideline (2007)[32] Endorsed by the European Society of Anaesthesiologists, the European Society of Intensive Care Medicine, the European Shock Society, the European Trauma Society, and the European Society for Emergency Medicine	*Management of bleeding following major trauma: A European guideline*
American College of Critical Care Medicine Taskforce of Society of Critical Care Medicine (2009)[33]	*Red blood cell transfusion in adult trauma and critical care*

produce appropriate clotting when demanded by the body. Better understanding of the role of platelets in hemostasis, including the number and characteristics of platelets necessary to prevent active bleeding in the obstetric patient, is also important.

The dynamics of coagulopathy secondary to obstetric hemorrhage has recently been compared to the diathesis of bleeding found in trauma patients with significant penetrating and non-penetrating injuries.[34] The rapid onset of coagulopathy that occurs at or around the time the uterus is emptied and the tissue factor–rich placenta detaches from the uterine wall to allow contraction of the myometrium; or that occurs when the placenta fails to detach, most likely has a multi-factorial cause. In these circumstances, bleeding in the obstetric patient appears similar in its rate of onset and subsequent volume of blood loss seen in young, previously healthy patients with traumatic injuries. Therefore, select management principles that have improved survival outcomes in trauma victims are recommended for incorporation into obstetric practice.[35]

Current trauma resuscitation protocols/guidelines are based on recent findings that a percentage of trauma patients present to emergency departments (EDs) or trauma centers with the presence of coagulopathy on admission.[36–38] These patients have a four- to five-fold increase in mortality compared to non-coagulopathic

trauma victims and are more likely to require resuscitation that includes massive transfusion of blood products.[36] A thorough discussion of trauma during pregnancy is presented in Chapter 21 of this text.

A percentage of obstetric patients who experience obstetric hemorrhage also develop disseminated intravascular coagulation (DIC), a coagulopathy that occurs after delivery of the infant, or following disruption of the placental attachment sites. Similar to that in combat and trauma victims, coagulopathy that complicates obstetric hemorrhage is not likely caused by dilutional anemia from resuscitation fluids but rather may have its origin in an undetermined endothelial "triggering" event that results in consumptive clotting and fibrinolysis. Additional research is needed to fully elucidate the etiology of this coagulopathy and to give obstetric providers an opportunity to prevent the resultant complications. A thorough discussion of DIC in the obstetric patient is presented in Chapter 16 of this text.

CRITICAL MANAGEMENT PRINCIPLES

"Bloody Vicious Cycle"

Hemorrhage is the most common cause of death for non-pregnant trauma patients in the hospital setting.[39]

As previously noted, similarities have been identified between patients with obstetric hemorrhage and previously healthy patients with selected traumatic injuries. For this reason, knowledge of critical concepts related to trauma management may be applicable to the care of patients with obstetric hemorrhage.

The highest mortality rates are observed in the subgroup of patients with hypothermia, coagulopathy, and acidosis.[39] Historically labeled the *"bloody vicious cycle"* or the *"deadly triad,"* this complication of hemorrhage and massive blood transfusions has been well documented for over two decades.[40] Hypothermia has been identified in patients with an apparent cyclic process of worsening acidosis, hypotension, and bleeding that is associated with death if not aggressively treated and hemostasis is not achieved. Hypothermia has also been linked with acute trauma and coagulopathy when hypoperfusion and acidosis trigger DIC.[40,41]

Hypothermia is defined as a body temperature lower than 35°C (95.0°F). Each 1°C drop in temperature is associated with a 10 percent decrease in the function of clotting factors. Additionally, hypothermia inhibits platelet function and results in fibrinolysis.[32] Normal coagulation requires that enzymes interact with clotting factors to produce the fibrin polymer strands that build a stable clot. In critically ill patients, both hemodilution and hypoperfusion are contributing factors to hypothermia, coagulopathy, and acidosis; but hypothermia alone can cause significant alterations in hemostasis.[39,42] Moreover, the enzymes that participate in the clotting cascade are temperature sensitive and are significantly inhibited in the presence of a low temperature. The patient's core temperature should be assessed, documented, and communicated to laboratory personnel when such blood samples are obtained and assessed. Otherwise, laboratory results may not accurately reflect the patient's coagulation status.

A key principle in current hemorrhage management is prevention of hypothermia via use of external adjuncts for patient warming. Such adjuncts include operating room table warmers, heating blankets, intravenous fluid infusion warmers, and blood warmers.

Volume Replacement Therapy

To facilitate rapid administration of intravenous fluid to patients with obstetric hemorrhage, large bore (14G or 16G) catheters-over-needles are used for intravenous access. Once hemorrhage is identified, at least two large bore IV lines are recommended for the management of volume and blood replacement therapy. Additionally, establishment of central venous access provides a route for rapid blood replacement therapy using a Level I or rapid volume infuser. Selection of the specific type and gauge of central hemodynamic catheter should be based on the internal lumens' diameters for rapid crystalloid and blood transfusion. Commercially available "trauma" infusion catheters and tubing sets have features such as single peripheral catheters that are inserted over existing IV lines to increase lumen size; dual lumen peripheral intravenous catheters with 18G and 20G lumens, respectively; and single, double, and triple lumen high volume central venous catheters that meet manufacturing specifications for blood transfusions and for rapid volume infusers' forced pressures (e.g., Arrow EID, Arrow Trauma Products, Arrow International, Inc., Reading, PA).

The choice of crystalloids versus colloids in the initial treatment of shock has long been debated, and providers responsible for volume resuscitation are able to cite studies supporting the use of either.[43] Studies have measured outcomes of patients treated primarily with colloids or crystalloids; however, most failed to prospectively classify the underlying pathology that prompted the need for volume transfusion. Additional criticisms have been directed at poor study design and/or insufficient sample size. The result has been an ongoing exchange of study results that have both supported and condemned the use of albumin for volume replacement.

A 2004 Cochrane review, updated in 2008, investigated mortality rates in patients receiving albumin and plasma protein fraction (PPF) [e.g., Plasmanate (Human) 5%] versus patients who were treated with crystalloid solutions [e.g., normal saline (0.9% NaCl)] when volume was needed for resuscitation and/or hypovolemia. From a meta-analysis based on 37 studies that involved more than 8,000 patients, the reviewers concluded that there was no evidence to support the use of albumin/PPF for the treatment of hypovolemia.[44] The relative risk of death in all patients that received albumin was 1.04 (95 percent confidence interval 0.96 to 1.13). Specifically, the relative risk of death in patients treated with albumin for hypovolemia was 1.01 (95 percent confidence interval 0.93 to 1.11); burns, 2.52 (95 percent confidence interval 1.22 to 5.22); and hypoalbuminemia, 1.20 (95 percent confidence interval 0.87 to 1.64).[44] The authors acknowledged that further studies are needed to determine if albumin is beneficial in other populations. The selection of normal saline versus lactated Ringer's solution requires more data from randomized control trials that address maternal and fetal outcomes after use of each fluid type in resuscitation protocols.

The administration of isotonic, non-dextrose crystalloid solutions (i.e., normal saline, lactated Ringer's solution) in a 3 to 1 ratio (three liters of solution for every one liter of blood loss) is currently recommended for initial volume expansion during obstetric hemorrhage. Importantly, glucose-containing solutions (e.g.,

D_5LR, D_5 0.9% NaCl) are avoided due to evidence of increased mortality in critically ill patients resuscitated with glucose solutions.

Blood Component Therapy

Hemodynamically Stable Patients Without Coagulopathy

In 2006, the American Society of Anesthesiologists (ASA) Task Force on Perioperative Blood Transfusion and Adjuvant Therapies presented recommendations for blood replacement therapy via prescriptive formulas for individual blood components based on hematologic indices and patient weight.[28] Table 15-7 is an example of a transfusion algorithm based on the current guidelines.

ASA guidelines primarily address the transfusion demands of the hemorrhage patient when medical and/or surgical interventions are successful in controlling bleeding and/or the rate of bleeding allows time to obtain results from laboratory clotting studies. Other professional organizations have published recommendations for transfusion during massive hemorrhage when bleeding is uncontrolled and coagulopathy is present or imminent; recommendations for each of these clinical situations are discussed below.

CASE EXCERPT: Blood replacement therapy in the hemodynamically stable patient
Patients who are hemodynamically stable and are no longer bleeding may be transfused based on the recommended targeted laboratory value goals presented in Table 15-7. The patient in this case excerpt, a 24-year-old gravida 1 para 1, is 3 hours postpartum. Immediately after spontaneous vaginal delivery, it was noted that the uterus was atonic with associated moderate to heavy vaginal bleeding. The sequential use of bimanual uterine massage, intravenous administration of 1000 mL of crystalloid (0.9% NaCl) with 40 units of oxytocin, and intramuscular methylergonovine maleate (Methergine) was effective in achieving hemostasis. Estimated blood loss was documented as 750 mL. One hour later, the patient remained tachycardic, tachypneic, and hypotensive. A complete blood count was ordered, and the results are listed in Table 15-8. The number of units of PRBCs administered to the patient suggests that underestimation of blood loss may have occurred.

Hemodynamically Unstable Patients With Coagulopathy

Transfusion of blood products is integral to the comprehensive management of hemorrhagic shock in the obstetric patient. Although blood transfusion in the patient with obstetric hemorrhage who is no longer actively bleeding is generally guided by laboratory parameters (e.g., hemoglobin, hematocrit, platelet count, PT, aPTT, and fibrinogen), administration of blood products in the patient with continued active bleeding should not be delayed in order to wait for laboratory evaluation of coagulation indices. In the setting of acute hemorrhage that requires massive transfusion therapy, aggressive transfusion of blood products without laboratory results is often part of resuscitation, in order to decrease the risk for hemorrhagic shock and acute cardiovascular collapse. Management decisions are guided by estimation of blood loss and patient assessment data. For example, in the setting of uterine atony with an estimated blood loss of 1000 mL, the demonstrated ability to form a clot combined with normal maternal vital signs, it would be reasonable to order laboratory tests, type and crossmatch for PRBCs, and await the results of the laboratory assessment prior to consideration and initiation of transfusion therapy. In the setting of severe bleeding (e.g., an estimated blood loss greater than 1500 mL), demonstrated inability of blood to clot, and abnormal maternal vital signs, immediate transfusion with PRBCs, FFP, platelets, and possibly cryoprecipitate may be indicated prior to the availability of laboratory results. An example of collaborative clinical guidelines to assist in the management of the hemodynamically unstable patient is presented in Table 15-9.

Blood Components

Red Blood Cells

The purpose of PRBC transfusion is to improve the oxygen-carrying capacity of the blood. A thorough discussion of hemodynamic and oxygen transport concepts applicable to obstetrics is presented in Chapter 4 of this text. The decision to begin transfusion of PRBCs in the intra-operative setting is based on estimation of blood loss within the surgical field. The decision to initiate transfusion is also based on assessment and estimation of vaginal bleeding, laboratory data consistent with anemia or inability to adequately maintain hemostasis, abnormal vital signs, and/or evidence of organ system dysfunction. Decreased systolic or mean arterial pressure (MAP), tachycardia, and/or decreased urine output suggest inadequate preload and cardiac output in the obstetric patient. An initial drop in preload may or may not be accompanied by maternal tachycardia; thus, the absence of an elevated heart rate in the presence of bleeding or a history of significant blood loss does not preclude the need for administration of PRBCs, additional blood components, or both. A decrease in oxygen delivery to organ systems, if not corrected, results in the conversion from aerobic to anaerobic metabolism. Metabolic acidosis may develop with a resultant decrease in arterial pH, reduction of bicarbonate (HCO_3), and an increase in serum lactate. Consequently, intermittent assessment of maternal acid–base status via arterial blood gas measurements for

TABLE 15-7

Transfusion of Blood Components: Recommendations Based on Serial Laboratory Values

Component	Content	Volume	Expected Change in Labs	Indication/Trigger	Goals of Transfusion
Warm fresh whole blood	• Same components in same percentages as blood loss	400–500 mL	1 unit replaces all components of blood loss in similar ratio without loss of individual component function from storage.	• Hgb <8.0 g/dL in bleeding patient. • If patient stable and not bleeding, Hgb <6.0 g/dL; or Hgb <8.0 g/dL and patient is symptomatic.	Hgb 10 g/dL, or Hct 30%
Packed red blood cells (PRBCs)	• RBCs, preservative and anticoagulant solutions may vary. • Hct 50%–65% • Hgb approximately 42.5–80 g • Iron approximately 147–278 mg	128–240 mL red blood cells; plus contains average 50 mL donor plasma (range 20–150 mL); plus anticoagulant and preservative.	1 unit PRBC increases Hgb approximately 1 g/dL or Hct by 3% (assumes pt not bleeding or hemolyzing).	• Hgb <8.0 g/dL in bleeding patient. • If patient stable and not bleeding, Hgb <6.0 g/dL; or Hgb <8.0 g/dL and patient is symptomatic.	Hgb 10 g/dL, or Hct 30%
Platelets	• Random donor platelets (RDPs) should contain ≥5.5 × 10^{10} platelets in 50 mL plasma. Four to 10 RDPs are pooled prior to transfusion. • Platelets apheresis: Single donor platelets (SDPs) should contain ≥3.0 × 10^{11} (average is 3.5–4.0 × 10^{11} per bag) in 250 mL plasma. • SDPs are ready for transfusion – no thawing needed.	Platelets (RDPs): 50 mL plasma × number of RDPs in the pool. Platelets Apheresis (SDPs): 250 mL of plasma.	For each RDP given, count increases 7,000–10,000/μL. For each SDP apheresis pack given, count increases 30,000–60,000/μL	• <50,000–70,000/μL in actively bleeding patients • <20,000/μL in unstable non-bleeding patients • <10,000/μL in stable, non-bleeding patients.	>100,000/μL in actively bleeding patients

(continued)

TABLE 15-7 (Continued)

Transfusion of Blood Components: Recommendations Based on Serial Laboratory Values

Component	Content	Volume	Expected Change in Labs	Indication/Trigger	Goals of Transfusion
Fresh frozen plasma (FFP)	• Non-cellular portion of blood that is separated from whole blood and frozen. Contains all coagulation factors. • Dosing is based on patient's current weight; or, in uncontrolled bleeding, given as close as possible to a 1:1 PRBC:FFP ratio.	Approximately 200–250 mL in one unit. Apheresis-derived units may be 400–600 mL.		PT >1.5 times the mid range of normal aPTT >1.5 times high normal range or factor assay less than 25%.	PT ≤1.5 × control, aPTT ≤1.5 × control, fibrinogen >100 mg/dL
Cryo-precipitated Antihemolytic Factor (AHF)	• Each unit of cryoprecipitate AHF (Cryo) should contain at least 80 IU Factor VIII:C, and 150 mg of fibrinogen in 5 to 20 mL of plasma. • Cryo also contains Factor VIII:vWF (von Willebrand factor), Factor XIII, and fibronectin.	5–20 mL per unit; see label for total number of units included.	Typical dose for stable hypo-fibrinogenemia is one unit per 7–10 kg of body weight; increases fibrinogen levels by 50 mg/dL in the absence of bleeding or consumption. In hemorrhage, Cryo may be given in increased doses of 1 unit/5 kg or 2 units/10 kg; and repeated as needed to maintain fibrinogen levels >100 mg/dL.	Fibrinogen <100 mg/dL	Fibrinogen >100 mg/dL

aPPT = activated partial thromboplastin time, Hgb = hemoglobin, Hct = hematocrit, IU = international units, PT = prothrombin time.
Data from References 71–76.

TABLE 15-8

Case Excerpt: Labs and Calculations for Blood Replacement Therapy

	Prior to Delivery	4 Hours Postpartum
Vital signs		
Heart rate (beats/min)	90	138
Blood pressure (mmHg)	110/76	100/42
Mean arterial pressure (mmHg)	87	61
Respirations (breaths/min)	18	22
Temperature	99.0°F (37.3°C)	97.0°F (36.1°C)
Test results		
Hgb (g/dL)	12.0	5.2
Platelets (/L)	340,000	105,000
PT (seconds)	—	—
aPTT (seconds)	—	—
FSP/FDP	—	—
D-dimer (mcg/dL)	—	—
Fibrinogen (mg/dL)	—	—

FDP = fibrin degradation products, FSP = fibrin split products, Hgb = hemoglobin, MTP – massive transfusion protocol, PT = prothrombin time, aPTT = partial thromboplastin time.

Note:

The patient's Hgb level was 5.2 g/dL, which was less than the 7.0 g/dL "trigger" to consider packed red blood cell (PRBC) replacement. Further assessment revealed the patient was symptomatic (see vital signs), and urine output since delivery was less than 100 mL.

To "correct" the Hgb level, the goal for transfusion was set at 10 g/dL. One unit of PRBCs increases Hgb by approximately 1 g/dL; thus, the number of units of PRBCs for transfusion was calculated to be 4.8 (rounded up to 5). Five units of PRBCs were transfused, and a follow-up Hgb level was assessed to determine the patient's need for further transfusion of PRBCs.

The patient's platelets were greater than 100,000/μL and indicated that a transfusion of platelets was not required at that time.

the duration of hemorrhage offers objective feedback with respect to the adequacy of erythrocyte replacement and restoration of adequate perfusion. Worsening acidemia may indicate the need for more aggressive transfusion of PRBCs and optimization of intravascular volume. Pharmacologic therapy may be indicated, including administration of agents for inotropic support, which improves ventricular contractility and cardiac output. Administration of vasopressors to increase blood pressure may be indicated; however, such medications should be initiated after preload has been optimized.

Measurements of hemoglobin (Hgb) and/or hematocrit (Hct) during the initial and/or acute phases of

hemorrhage rarely reflect the actual concentration of RBCs in the maternal circulation. Periodic (every 20 to 30 minutes) laboratory assessments of Hgb and/or Hct levels may be necessary to assess and appreciate the dynamic alterations of these values in cases of obstetric hemorrhage. Because most blood gas analyzers report the patient's Hgb with the gas results, it may be useful to order arterial blood gases every 20 to 30 minutes to have periodic estimates of the patient's RBC concentration.

In the *actively bleeding patient*, Hgb less than 8 g/dL indicates the immediate need for RBC replacement. Each unit of PRBCs increases the patient's Hgb by approximately 1 g/dL (Hct by approximately 3 percent). The goal of PRBC transfusion is to administer the amount of packed red cells required to correct the arterial concentration to a Hgb of at least 10 g/dL. Hence, if the patient has stopped bleeding, is hemodynamically stable, and has a Hgb of 5.0 g/dL, approximately 5 units of PRBCs will most likely be necessary to increase her Hgb to 10 g/dL. It should be noted that few patients with massive hemorrhage are hemodynamically stable and thus require not only rapid replacement of lost erythrocytes but also require transfusion of additional PRBCs to optimize oxygen carrying capacity via RBCs during ongoing blood loss.[28]

Another factor that may impact survival after transfusion with 6 or more units of PRBCs is the age of the donated blood at the time of infusion. Weinberg and colleagues reported results from a study of a group of patients who received 6 or more units of PRBCs of which 3 or more of the units were *less than* 14 days old. Data from this group were compared to data from a second group who received 6 or more units of PRBCs but 3 or more of the units were *greater than* 14 days old. The group that received 3 or more units of blood older than 14 days had a 7.8-fold increased risk of death compared to a lower 3.8-fold increased odds of death in those who received the "younger" PRBCs.[45] Therefore, it may be beneficial in the massively bleeding patient to request from the blood bank the freshest units of blood products.

Fresh Frozen Plasma

Blood plasma contains coagulation factors, fibrinogen, and proteins required to support the steady state oncotic/osmotic pressures of blood and normal hemostasis. FFP is used during blood replacement therapy to avoid and/or treat DIC and to facilitate hemostasis. When possible, FFP transfusions are guided by the analysis of the patient's PT, aPTT, and fibrinogen level. During massive hemorrhage the clinical assessment of the patient's clotting function is more important than laboratory results. As with Hgb evaluation, laboratory values from clotting profiles in early and/or acute hemorrhage rarely reflect current depletion of fibrinogen and clotting factors.

TABLE 15-9

Collaborative Guidelines for Massive Obstetric Hemorrhage in a Hemodynamically Unstable Patient*

Parameter	Actions	Comments
• Hemorrhage suspected	• Early diagnosis of possible hemorrhage • *Early move of patient to large OR* • Communicate emergency to HT leader • HT leader evaluates situation and declares the hemorrhage event. • HT pagers/phones activated for 'all call' of team.	• Notify anesthesia on transfer to OR. • Anesthesia monitoring per ASA standards • HT leader (e.g., L&D charge nurse, shift supervisor, etc.) takes charge; OBH "command center" based at nurses' station closest to patient (typically the OR nurses' station). HT leader assigns unit secretary to staff OBH desk. • HT leader initiates notification protocol.
• Volume resuscitation with normal saline until blood products (type O Rh[D]-negative) available	• Start IV access in large veins in both arms (avoid hands); use 14G–16G catheters over needles. • Place CVC with multi-lumens with large diameters (e.g., 16G, and 18G in triple lumen). Or, place CVC/PAC introducer "cordis" • Request type O Rh(D)-negative blood from BB—4 to 6 units PRBCs now and prepare packs of 4 to send until crossmatched blood is available. • Request type O Rh(D)-negative FFP—4 to 6 units of thawed FFP now and prepare packs of 4 to send when additional units thawed and/or available. • Request BB to start thawing all frozen products for the "OB Hemorrhage Pack" • Request 1 apheresis platelet pack O Rh(D)-negative. If Rh(D)-negative not available, screen for RhoGAM need after transfusion.	• There is no benefit of colloids over crystalloids for volume resuscitation. • Give pre-warmed fluids. • Use normal saline (0.9% NaCl) without glucose. • Do not delay initial transfusion due to lack of crossmatched blood if patient hemorrhaging (use O-negative). • Negotiate with BB to keep 4 to 6 units of FFP thawed at all times (for hospitals that normally utilize numerous units FFP/day in general surgery or other departments). Once thawed, units should be used within 24 hr of thawing. (By staging FFP thawing throughout the day, several units can be thawed and used in scheduled surgeries and/or transfusions while providing a large pool of thawed FFP at any one time for emergencies.)

• Send type and crossmatch.
• Assess Hgb/Hct and coagulation profile
• Order "OB Hemorrhage Massive Transfusion Pack"
  • 8 units PRBCs
  • 6–8 units FFP
  • 2 platelet apheresis packs
  • 2 cryoprecipitate adult doses/bags
	• Draw two to three tubes of blood for ongoing type and crossmatch
	• Draw additional blood and send for CBC, DIC profile (PT, aPTT, platelets, fibrinogen, FDP and/or D-dimer), Chemistry, (electrolytes)
		• BB requires several tubes of blood to type and cross larger volumes of blood products.
		• Create proactive plan for ordering blood (i.e., BB continues to prepare and send blood products in the same sequence as initial orders unless notified).
		• Note: BB will require additional tubes of "fresh" blood for ongoing crossmatching during transfusion.

TABLE 15-9 (Continued)

Collaborative Guidelines for Massive Obstetric Hemorrhage in a Hemodynamically Unstable Patient*

Parameter	Actions	Comments
• If patient is hemorrhaging, begin administration of O-negative blood. • Do not wait for crossmatch or Hgb/Hct values; transfuse based on clinical picture. • Transfuse PRBCs; maintain Hgb >8 g/dL • Transfuse enough PRBCs to reach goal of 10 g/dL (provides margin of safety).	• Transfuse PRBCs, FFP, and platelets simultaneously or by alternating 1 unit of PRBCs with 1 unit FFP ongoing basis. • Transfuse platelets a the same time in another IV site to avoid platelet destruction from high volume flow of PRBCs and FFP. • If blood not available, request and transfuse Group O Rh(D)-negative (begin with 4 to 6 units) • 1 unit of PRBCs increases Hgb 1 g/dL (e.g., current Hgb 5, transfuse at least 5 units PRBCs to correct for stable patient). • If patient bleeding, add more units for continuing blood loss. • 2-person check for "right patient–right blood" • Use blood warmer, blood filter from blood bank, blood tubing. • May use pressure bags with PRBCs and FFP. • Use 0.9% NaCl as mainline solution to run blood products. • Use rapid volume infuser if available (must be model that warms blood); must use correct tubing and connect to approved site. • Notify cell-saver team.	• Continue to use O-negative; then ABO group specific when blood group identified by BB. • If patient hemorrhaging, do not delay initial transfusion due to lack of crossmatched blood. • BB to auto send blood when crossmatch complete. • Number 1 reason for blood transfusion reactions is that patient receives wrong blood. Confirm patient ID with two identifiers, armband, two licensed witnesses, standardized guidelines. • Assign two additional RNs, licensed anesthesia care providers, or a combination of the two to witness blood in OR to prevent delay in transfusion • Continue to send BB tubes of blood as requested for ongoing crossmatching. • Replace blood filters every 2 units PRBCs or per BB policy. • Do not use lactated Ringer's or any solution with calcium (reacts with citrate preservative in blood and precipitates out).
• Maintain platelets >75,000 µL. • Transfuse to 100,000 as goal (provides margin of safety).	• Transfuse 1 platelet apheresis large pack. • Anticipate platelets <50,000 µL after 2× blood volume loss. • One unit platelet aphaeresis increases platelet count by 35,000 µL to 50,000 µL. • Do not use pressure bag for platelets.	• Anticipate large percentage of platelets rendered useless in transfusion. • Have second apheresis pack ready. • Do not use pressure bag on platelets. • Do not squeeze bag. • Do not shake platelets. • Use filter that BB provides for platelets.
• Maintain PT and aPTT <1.5 × control. • Maintain fibrinogen >100 mg/dL.	• Transfuse FFP in 1:1 or 1:1.5 ratio to PRBC. • Anticipate need to transfuse FFP early.	• Transfuse early to prevent and/or abate DIC. • Takes 30 minutes to thaw, order early. • OB patient may need more than non-pregnant patient due to increased blood volume.
• Fibrinogen <80 mg/dL	• Transfuse cryoprecipitate.	• Hemostasis no longer occurs if fibrinogen <75 mg/dL. • Critically low fibrinogen level likely reached when 1.5 × blood volume lost. • 4 units FFP increase fibrinogen 200–500 mg/L (volume = 1,000 mL or 1 liter). • 2 pools of cryoprecipitate increase fibrinogen 320–400 mg/L (volume = 150–200 mL); complete dose can be administered more rapidly than fibrinogen equivalent.

(continued)

TABLE 15-9 (Continued)

Collaborative Guidelines for Massive Obstetric Hemorrhage in a Hemodynamically Unstable Patient*

Parameter	Actions	Comments
• If DIC present, blood products ineffective, evaluate patient for undiagnosed von Willebrand factor deficiency. If this congenital bleeding disorder is known or suspected, administer DDAVP	• Transfuse DDAVP. • Dose 0.3 mcg/kg • Limit repeat doses to every 6 to 8 hours	• DDAVP promotes release of von Willebrand factor from vascular endothelium. • Improves hemostasis in healthy volunteers and patients with disorders related to aspirin, NSAIDs, or cirrhosis, but its effect in massive hemorrhage is unknown.
• If DIC present, blood products are ineffective for hemostasis, and patient is unstable and deteriorating, consider recombinant factor VIIa (rFVIIa)	• Give rFVIIa. • 90 mcg/kg (dose not standardized) [NovoSeven Coagulation Factor VIIa (Recombinant), Novo Nordisk Health Care AG, USA.]	• FDA off-label use has been reported in OB literature. Side effects may include thrombosis and its sequelae. • Dose supplied in powder form. Reconstitute prior to administration; dose based on patient weight. • Repeat rFVIIa dose 2 hours after first dose. May need to continue dosing every 2–4 hours first 12–24 hours (limited data available in OB pts).
• Maintain core temperature ≥37° C (≥98.6° F)		• Prevent or treat "deadly triad:" hypothermia, acidosis, hemorrhage.

aPTT = activated partial thromboplastin time, ASA = American Society of Anesthesiologists, BB = blood bank, CBC = complete blood count, CVC = central venous catheter, DDAVP = desmopressin, DIC = disseminated intravascular coagulation, FFP = fresh frozen plasma, Hct = hematocrit, Hgb = hemoglobin, HT = hemorrhage team, L&D = labor and delivery, NSAID = nonsteroidal anti-inflammatory drug, OBH = obstetric hemorrhage, OR = operating room, PAC = pulmonary artery catheter, PRBCs = packed red blood cells, PT = prothrombin time.

*This guideline does not define or imply the standard of care for post PPH patients. The purpose of the content is for education of providers only.

Data from References 69–71 and 74–77.

Agreement on evidence-based protocols does not yet exist to recommend an exact amount or timing of FFP transfusions in massive hemorrhage. Recent guidelines from the ASA recommend transfusing FFP required to achieve a minimum of 30 percent of normal coagulation factors present in plasma, an amount that is reached by transfusing 10 to 15 mL/kg FFP.[28] As an example, in an obstetric patient who weighs 165 pounds (75 kg), the estimated volume of FFP needed to correct a slightly prolonged PT/aPTT is 750 to 1125 mL, or three to four 250-mL units. For patients who weigh approximately 200 pounds (91 kg), the volume of FFP required increases to 910 to 1365 mL, or four to five units of FFP.

Historically there has been limited agreement on when and in what order blood products should be transfused; however, transfusion of FFP should be accomplished to improve patient survival. The dilemma of early administration of FFP to prevent coagulopathy versus limited plasma use to avoid transfusion-related acute lung injury (TRALI) frequently resulted in the deferral of FFP until there was clinical evidence of a coagulopathy. More recently, prospective randomized trials that studied casualties in combat zone hospitals and civilian trauma victims in the United States (U.S.) have helped to establish new recommendations and guidelines for the use of FFP during massive hemorrhage. Data show a significant improvement in mortality rates of injured soldiers who received at least 2 to 3 units of plasma for every 3 units of PRBCs (mortality rate 19 percent) compared to casualties who were given the more traditional ratio of 1 unit of plasma for every 4 units of PRBCs (mortality rate 65 percent).[46] Results from this study and others at the Army Hospital in the Green Zone in Baghdad have generated new paradigms for transfusion guidelines and have resulted in a network of U.S. trauma centers implementing a 1:1 (PRBC:FFP) transfusion ratio and more recently a 1:1:1 (PRBC:FFP:Platelets–apheresis platelet pack) transfusion ratio for replacement transfusions in patients with massive hemorrhage.[46]

Platelets

Platelets are administered when serum levels fall to 50,000 to 100,000/uL during active hemorrhage when additional blood loss is anticipated, or when values decrease to less than 50,000/uL in the stable patient. The goal of platelet transfusion in the hemorrhaging patient is to restore and maintain serum levels at approximately 100,000/ uL. Many blood banks in North America now supply platelets in large apheresis packs. Apheresis or platelet pheresis is the process by which a donor is connected to a closed system where blood is collected and centrifuged to separate components. Platelets are collected and the remaining blood components are returned to the donor. One platelet apheresis pack is standardized to contain a minimum of 35,000 platelets, and most have almost 50,000 platelets per bag. Platelets are usually stored in the blood bank at room temperature and are associated with an increased risk of infection due to the loss of protective cooling on infectious organisms. Platelets are a fragile component of whole blood and are easily damaged or destroyed during rapid transfusions. Platelets may be rendered inactive from increased velocity or turbulence from pressure bag compression, producing rapid flow through tubing, blood filters, and intravascular access catheters. For this reason, pressure bags should not to be used during platelet transfusions, and the need for platelet replacement should be considered early during the process to allow additional time for non-mechanized infusion.

Cryoprecipitate

Cryoprecipitated antihemolytic factor (commonly called Cryo) is the layer of precipitate that is formed when 1 unit of FFP is thawed at 1°C to 6°C. A concentrated volume of 10 to 15 mL is produced from each unit of whole blood and contains 200 mg to 300 mg of fibrinogen, 100 units of factor VIII (80 to 100 IU), von Willebrand factor (80 to 100 IU), factor XIII (50 to 100 IU), and 55 mg fibronectin. The resultant collection bag has a volume of approximately 15 to 20 mL and carries the identical infection risk as 1 unit of whole blood or packed cells. Cryoprecipitate is administered during massive hemorrhage when the patient is bleeding at a rate faster than FFP can be transfused, when fibrinogen levels fall below 100 mg/dL, or when the larger volume associated with FFP transfusion is contraindicated.[47] It is important to note that Cryo does not contain all clotting factors and plasma proteins needed for coagulation. Thus, the continued transfusion of FFP is typically indicated when Cryo is included in massive transfusion therapy.

Complications of Blood Transfusion

Administering human blood and its products carries risks to the intended recipient, ranging from mild allergic reactions to cardiovascular collapse and death. In Table 15-10, the categories of blood transfusion reactions and patient signs and symptoms of specific complications are presented. Despite multiple processes added over the years for screening, crossmatching, and selecting the precise blood products for an individual patient, the most common cause of transfusion reactions and complications remains *administering the wrong unit of blood to the wrong patient.*

Other Products Used in Hemorrhage

Desmopressin

Desmopressin (DDAVP), a synthetic derivative of vasopressin, is FDA approved for use in patients with von Willebrand's disease and some types of hemophilia. Von Willebrand's disease is a genetic disorder and is manifested by reduced levels of von Willebrand factor (VWF) or reduced levels of functioning VWF. Von Willebrand's disease results in a bleeding disorder whereby the body's ability to stop bleeding from common sources (tooth extractions, menstruation, cuts, trauma, surgery, etc.) is impaired. DDAVP works by stimulating the release of VWF from the endothelium and increasing levels of factor VIII. Von Willebrand's disease affects approximately 0.6 to 1.3 percent of the population when newer screening methods are employed.[48] Because of its relative frequency in the population at large, and because pregnancy may be the first time a patient experiences a large blood loss, it is recommended that providers consider administering DDAVP during unrelenting hemorrhage in the event the patient has 'yet-to-be diagnosed' von Willebrand's disease.[28,48]

The National Heart, Lung, and Blood Institute (NHLBI) published evidenced-based guidelines for the management of von Willebrand's disease in pregnancy, including intrapartum recommendations for testing and optimum ranges for laboratory tests results.[48] The complete guideline can be accessed at the NHLBI website at http://www.nhlbi.nih.gov/guidelines/vwd/vwd.pdf.

Recombinant Activated Factor VII (rFVIIa)

Recombinant activated factor VIIa [(rFVIIa), NovoSeven RT, Novo Nordisk A/S Bagsværd, Denmark] is approved by the FDA for use in patients with congenital factor VII deficiency or hemophilia A or B who have inhibitors to or deficiencies of factor VIII and factor IX. It controls hemorrhage in the setting of coagulopathy by promoting thrombin generation and clot stabilization. Since licensure of the drug in 1999, there have been numerous reports of off-label use of rFVIIa in patients without hemophilia but with uncontrolled hemorrhage in a variety of settings.[49–51] It is estimated that thousands of patients have received the drug as the result of participation in a study protocol or at the direction of a physician independent of research protocols.[52] Current reports of off-label use include diagnoses associated with massive hemorrhage such as trauma, surgical bleeding, esophageal varices, etc.; intracranial hemorrhage; as

TABLE 15-10

Transfusion Reactions and Complications

Category	Reaction	Clinical Manifestations and Comments
Immunologic— Immediate *(may occur during infusion or within minutes to hours after blood product infused)*	Hemolytic transfusion reaction	• Increased temp, HR • Chills • Dyspnea • Chest or back pain • Abnormal bleeding • Shock • Hypotension • DIC • Hemoglobinemia • Hemoglobinuria • Elevated serum bilirubin • Recipient's antibodies attach to transfused PRBCs
	Immune-mediated platelet destruction	• Markedly reduces survival time of transfused platelets
	Febrile nonhemolytic reaction	• Temperature elevation of ≥1° C or ≥2° F occurring during or shortly after transfusion • Sudden chills • Headache • Anxiety • Caused by hypersensitivity to donor WBCs, platelets, or plasma proteins
	Allergic reactions	• Uticaria • Wheezing • Angioedematous reactions • Anaphylaxis • Caused by sensitivity to plasma protein or donor antibody–reacts with antigens of recipient
	Anaphylactoid reactions	• Autonomic dysregulation • Severe dyspnea • Pulmonary and/or laryngeal edema
	TRALI	• Massive pulmonary edema within 6 hours of transfusion
Immunologic—Delayed	Delayed hemolytic reaction	• 2–14 days after transfusion • Fever • Positive direct antiglobulin test • Unexplained decrease in Hgb/Hct • Elevated LDH, bilirubin • Mild jaundice
	Alloimmunization	• Days or weeks after the immunizing event • Usually does not cause any symptoms or physiologic changes
	PTP	• Rare • Dramatic, sudden, and self-limited thrombocytopenia • 7–10 days after transfusion • Patient has history of sensitization either by pregnancy or transfusion
	GVHD	• Rare • Extremely dangerous • T-lymphocytes in transfused component engraft in recipient and react against tissue antigens in recipient • Severely immunocompromised patients at risk • Erythematous skin rash • Abnormal liver function tests • Profuse, watery diarrhea

TABLE 15-10 (Continued)

Transfusion Reactions and Complications

Category	Reaction	Clinical Manifestations and Comments
Non-immunologic	Transmission of infectious disease	• Sudden chills • High fever • Nausea, vomiting, diarrhea • Hypotension • Transfusion of blood product contaminated with bacteria, viruses • Other infectious agents • Creutzfeldt-Jakob disease agent and variant Creutzfeldt-Jakob disease agent
	Bacterial contamination	• Rare • Onset of high fever (≥2°C or ≥3.5°F rise in temperature) • Severe chills • Hypotension • Circulatory collapse
	Circulatory overload	• Pulmonary edema • Distended neck veins • Dyspnea, cough • Increased risk in elderly, patients with chronic severe anemia • Pregnant patients (increase in plasma volume with decreased colloid osmotic pressure) may be a greater risk
	Hypothermia	• Cardiac arrhythmias • Cardiac arrest
	Metabolic complications	• Citrate "toxicity" • Low ionized Ca+ level • Ventricular arrhythmias • Acidosis/alkalosis • Hypokalemia/hyperkalemia
	Iron overload (hemosiderosis)	• Deposit of iron in heart, endocrine organs, liver, spleen, skin, and other organs as a result of long-term transfusions (aplastic anemia thalassemia) • Decreased thyroid function • Arrhythmias • Cardiac failure
Fatal Transfusion Reactions	When a fatality occurs as complication of blood transfusion, FDA should be notified within 1 business day.	Consult blood bank for notification policy.

HR = heart rate, DIC = disseminated intravascular coagulation, FDA = U.S. Food and Drug Administration, GVHD = Graft-versus-host disease, Hct = hematocrit, Hgb = hemoglobin, LDH = lactic dehydrogenase, PRBCs = packed red blood cells, PTP = post-transfusion purpura, TRALI = transfusion-related acute lung injury, WBCs = white blood cells.

a preventive therapy in patients with preoperative thrombocytopenia and other blood disorders; and in obstetric hemorrhage.[50]

In 2005–2006, investigators and providers were warned of a series of serious adverse events reported to the FDA's Adverse Event Reporting System after patients were given rFVIIa.[53] At that time, 431 adverse events for rFVIIa existed in the FDA's database that covered the time period from FDA approval (March 25, 1999) to December 31, 2004. One hundred and sixty-five reports described 185 thromboembolic complications that became the focus of the report.[49] Thromboembolic events included:

• thromboembolic cerebrovascular accident (n = 39)
• myocardial infarction (n = 34)
• pulmonary embolism (n = 32)
• other arterial thromboses (n = 26)
• deep vein and other venous thromboses (n = 42)
• clot occlusion of invasive devices (n = 10).

Additionally, more adverse events were reported in patients who did not have hemophilia or other on-label indications. With regard to the thromboembolic events, 21 percent occurred within 2 hours of rFVIIa administration and 51 percent occurred within the first 24 hours of therapy. There were 50 deaths in the thromboembolic group, of which 72 percent were thought to be from the embolic event. The authors of the publication emphasized that the results did not confirm or determine a direct cause and effect relationship, perhaps due to the volunteer reporting system, the complexity of patient management, and the high baseline morbidity of the patients that received rFVIIa. The results also did not establish the frequency of adverse events. Rather, commentary from the FDA raised the question of a possible relationship.[49]

By 2008, several more clinical trials were published describing the off-label use of rFVIIa in various patient populations. From such trails, Hsia and colleagues performed a meta-analysis to question the benefits of rFVIIa and the incidence and impact of adverse outcomes.[54] Twenty-two randomized controlled trials met inclusion criteria, including 3184 total subjects; 2080 subjects received rFVIIa and 1104 received placebo. Subjects in the rFVIIa group received significantly less PRBC transfusion compared to the placebo group. Thromboembolic events and death occurred in each group. The incidence of stroke, unspecified arterial thromboembolism, venous thromboembolism, deep vein thrombosis, pulmonary embolism, and nonspecific venous thromboembolism was not significantly different between groups. All events of arterial embolization, however, were significantly higher in the rFVIIa group versus placebo, and the incidence of myocardial infarction was also higher in the rFVIIa group. The authors estimated an absolute risk increase of arterial thromboembolism to be approximately 1 percent.[54] There were no randomized controlled trials on obstetric patients with hemorrhage included in the meta-analysis.

The use of rFVIIa in obstetric patients has been reported. There is not, however, a completed prospective randomized double-blind trial on the use of the drug in obstetric patients during hemorrhage or in the prevention of hemorrhage at the time of delivery. It is unknown if the hypercoagulable state of pregnancy alters the drug's profile or if it will increase the relative risk of thromboembolic events. It is recommended that providers consider use of rFVIIa in the treatment of obstetric hemorrhage requiring massive transfusion only when standard therapy is not effective and the potential benefits outweigh the risks of not using the drug.

The therapeutic dosing of rFVIIa for pregnant patients with massive hemorrhage is unknown at this time. The standard dose for patients with hemophilia is 90 micrograms/kg (mcg/kg). However, in studies of trauma victims, some protocol doses have been as high as 100 to 200 mcg/kg. The initial dose was repeated at approximately 2-hour intervals until hemostasis was achieved and bleeding controlled.

In a recent literature review of the use of rFVIIa in obstetric patients, Franchini and colleagues report that neither the response to the drug nor adverse events were dose dependent.[55] Further, the authors recommend administration of 90 mcg/kg of rFVIIa intravenously over 3 to 5 minutes. Interestingly, the authors suggested that administering the dose prior to performing a hysterectomy may prevent the need for such surgery. Most important is to critically treat and correct patient conditions that are known to inhibit the effectiveness of rFVIIa; thus, correction of acid–base imbalance, hypothermia, hypocalcemia, and hyperkalemia in addition to transfusion of PRBC, FFP, platelets and Cryo are necessary *before* rFVIIa is administered. Franchini and colleagues also recommend a second dose of rFVIIa (90 mcg/kg) if there is no improvement after approximately 20 minutes.[55] However, the manufacturer recommends repeating the therapeutic dose 2 to 3 hours after initial administration and periodically throughout the subsequent 24-hour period. There is currently no consensus regarding this recommendation for therapy in postpartum patients.

Assessment of patients after administration of rFVIIa includes evaluation for ongoing bleeding as well as the onset of arterial and/or venous thromboembolic events.

Anti-fibrinolytics

Anti-fibrinolytics are administered to stop or prevent bleeding when fibinolysis is the suspected cause. Two of the most studied (and FDA approved) anti-fibrinolytics are aminocaproic acid (Amicar) and tranexamic acid (TXA) (Lysteda, Cyklokapron). Both are lysine acid derivatives that block fibrinolysis by preventing the formation and activation of plasmin, thereby allowing thrombi to strengthen the clot and prevent lysis.[12,56] The two drugs are similar in action, although TXA is 10 times more potent than aminocaproic acid.

Anti-fibrinolytics are used in patients with congenital (rare) or acquired hyperfibrinolysis (e.g., hepatic failure); hemophilia prior to dental procedures or other surgery; severe thrombocytopenia; and a high risk for blood loss from surgeries such as cardiac bypass, liver transplantation, and orthopedic procedures.[12] Specifically, anti-fibrinolytics are administered to reduce blood loss, thereby decreasing the number of patients that require blood transfusions.[57]

Reported adverse events from anti-fibrinolytics are commonly the result of excessive clot formation. Myocardial infarction, embolic stroke, deep venous thrombosis, and renal dysfunction have all been reported after administration of these drugs.

There are limited to no prospective randomized data with regard to the use of anti-fibrinolytics during pregnancy, excluding case studies on women with pre-existing fibrinolytic disease states. The effect of the hypercoaguable state of pregnancy on the incidence of thrombotic complications in patients treated with anti-fibrinolytics is unknown.

In 2009, investigators at the London School of Hygiene and Tropical Medicine commenced enrolling patients in the World Maternal Antifibrinolytic Trial (WOMAN). The purpose of the study is to measure the outcomes in women who are given an anti-fibrinolytic (TXA) during PPH. This ambitious study will attempt to recruit and randomize 15,000 women who experience hemorrhage after delivery to either tranexamic acid or placebo and report the outcomes of the subjects up to 42 days after delivery.[58] Completion of the study is scheduled for 2015.

Cell Saver Use During Cesarean Section

Autotransfusion (cell saver, cell salvage) devices scavenge surgical site blood by suction, which is then anticoagulated, filtered, differentially centrifuged, re-filtered, and infused back into the venous circulation (Fig. 15-3). The safety profile of the procedure has been established in several types of surgery, but there remain two major concerns about cell salvaging during Cesarean delivery or other obstetric procedures. One is rhesus immunization in the Rh-negative mother with an Rh-positive fetus and the second is amniotic fluid embolism (AFE). During collection of obstetric surgical site blood, there is frequently mixing of mater-nal and fetal red blood cells, amniotic fluid, and irriga-tion fluids into the vacuum of the cell saver. The addi-tion of an advanced leukocyte reduction filter (Leukoguard RS Filter) has been used for the majority of recently reported cases and has been shown to effectively remove or reduce fetal squamous cells, leu-kocytes, bacteria, and other surgical field contami-nants.[59] Fetal RBCs, however, are not reduced and are found in higher concentrations in cell salvage blood when compared to maternal venous blood.[59] Therefore, patients at risk for isoimmunization should receive anti-D immune globulin (RhoGAM). A qualitative test for the amount of fetal hemoglobin in maternal blood should be performed after salvaged blood transfusion to guide the amount of anti-D immune globulin needed.[59]

There has been general concern in the past regard-ing transfusion of blood collected at the time of deliv-ery, for fear of causing AFE. However, laboratory stud-ies have shown that amniotic fluid, fetal debris, and

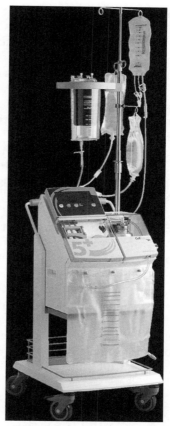

FIGURE 15-3 Commercially available cell saver device, the Cell Saver 5, Autologous Blood Transfusion System (Photo courtesy of Haemonetics Corp., Braintree, MA.)

tissue factor can be effectively separated from RBCs with the use of a leukocyte reduction filter, which should theoretically reduce the risk of AFE.[59,60] Interestingly, there have been more than 100 cases of successful cell saver use during Cesarean delivery in Great Britain prior to 2000, which is the year the cur-rent leukocyte reduction filters were made available for use.

Cell salvage use has been reported in a number of published cases, including a series of 139 women who received autotransfusion at the time of Cesarean deliv-ery.[61] None of these patients experienced DIC or AFE. ACOG recommends that cell saver technology be con-sidered in obstetric cases such as placenta accreta, where heavy blood loss is anticipated.[5]

The operation of a cell salvage device has been reportedly performed by perfusionists, anesthesia pro-viders, and specially trained nurses who typically have experience and expertise in operating cardiac bypass machines or who work in institutions that perform high-volume surgery. Thus, cell salvage teams may not be available in many hospitals, making the decision of where to deliver a patient with a high probability of PPH more challenging.

Jehovah's Witness Patients and Cell Saver Use

The maternal mortality rate for Jehovah's Witnesses is 44 times that of the general population, according to a recent study from New York.[62] Cell saver technology is acceptable to many of these women because the collected blood product is not perceived as removed from the circulation. Women who decline blood component therapy should be identified prenatally and counseled regarding their beliefs and preferences; signed informed consent can then be obtained, specifying which technologies, such as autotransfusion, would be acceptable to them in the setting of a hemorrhagic emergency.

CASE EXCERPT: Blood replacement therapy in the hemodynamically unstable patient: Use of massive transfusion protocol

Obstetric patients who become hemodynamically unstable require urgent assessment for the etiology of PPH and targeted aggressive management. The patient in this case excerpt, a 30-year-old, gravida 2 para 2, is post Cesarean delivery for failure to progress and fetal intolerance to labor augmentation. The surgical procedure was uneventful but, after delivery of the infant, an abnormally adherent placenta was discovered. Uterotonic agents were administered but were not effective. The patient's blood pressure dropped and she became severely tachycardic and unresponsive. The patient was intubated and converted to general anesthesia. The uterus did not adequately contract, and bleeding continued. Estimated blood loss at that time was 2500 mL. The hospital's OB hemorrhage protocol was initiated; surgical, nursing, and anesthesia resources were summoned. Stat blood samples were drawn (CBC, PT, aPTT, fibrinogen, FSP/SDP, D-dimer), and the results are presented in Table 15-11. Important to note is the lack of delay in the transfusion of blood products by not waiting for the lab results. Rather, the hospital's OB hemorrhage protocol prompted the order for one "Massive Transfusion Pack" (MTP). The MTP consisted of 6 units of PRBCs, 6 units of FFP, 1 apheresis platelet pack, and 1 adult dose of Cryo. To expedite the transfusion, the blood bank immediately released 6 units of type O-negative (O-neg) PRBCs and 6 units of thawed FFP (per policy, the hospital's blood bank routinely kept 4 to 6 units of O-neg FFP thawed at all times) were immediately delivered to the operating

TABLE 15-11

Case Example #2: Massive Hemorrhage

	After the PPH		After 1st MTP		After 2nd and 3rd MTPs
Vital Signs					
Heart rate (beats/min)	140		152		122
Blood Pressure (mmHg)	70/36		85/46		108/60
Mean Arterial Pressure (mmHg)	47		59		76
Respirations (breaths/min)	32	Blood transfusion (1st MTP) • 6 PRBCs • 4 FFP • 1 Platelets (apheresis) • 1 Cryo adult dose	Ventilator	Blood transfusion (2nd and 3rd MTPs) • 12 PRBCs • 8 FFP • 2 Platelets (apheresis) • 2 Cryo adult doses	Ventilator
Temperature	97.4°F (36.3°C)		97.1°F (36.2°C)		99.0°F (37.2°C) (with active warming)
Lab Tests					
Hgb (g/dL)	7.5		6.6		9.2
Platelets (mm³)	68,000		49,000		88,000
PT (seconds)	19		53		36
aPTT (seconds)	71		>120		55
Fibrinogen (mg/dL)	141		81		125
FSP/FDP	negative		negative		positive
D-dimer	WNL		positive		positive

aPTT = activated partial thromboplastin time, Cryo = cryoprecipitate, FFP = fresh frozen platelets, FDP = fibrin degradation products, FSP = fibrin split products, Hgb = hemoglobin, MTP = massive transfusion pack, PPH = postpartum hemorrhage, PRBCs = packed red blood cells, PT = Prothrombin time, WNL = within normal limits.

room. The platelets were delivered approximately 5 minutes later, and Cryo arrived approximately 20 minutes after the platelets.

Massive transfusion guidelines recommend the "simultaneous" administration of PRBCs, FFP, and platelets. To accomplish this, anesthesia personnel obtained central venous access and inserted a 7-french triple lumen CVC with two 18-gauge lumens and one 16-gauge lumen. Two units of PRBCs were infused followed by 2 units of FFP; the apheresis platelets were concurrently transfused via a separate peripheral IV line (to avoid turbulence with the CVC infusions).

Based on visual assessment of ongoing patient bleeding and consideration of the lab results, a second MTP was ordered. A vasoactive drip was started by anesthesia to increase perfusion pressures. Arterial blood gas (ABG) analysis during the hemorrhage showed a decreased arterial pH and decreased bicarbonate level. Repeat lab results revealed minimal improvement. A rapid volume infuser was brought into the operating room. The third MTP pack was ordered and transfused. During this time, the surgeons were able to control bleeding and anesthesia personnel utilized active warming devices for prevention of hypothermia. Table 15-11 also shows the follow-up lab studies and vital signs after the third MTP pack was administered.

When the patient was stabilized and no further bleeding occurred, the transfusion of blood products changed to the "hemodynamically stable" patient guidelines that focused on correcting abnormal laboratory results. The patient eventually required 4 more units of PRBCs and 3 units of FFP that were initiated in the OR and completed in the adult intensive care unit. Repeat arterial blood gases (every 30 to 40 minutes) demonstrated an improving pH.

The patient remained in the ICU for 4 days and was discharged home on postpartum day 7. She had transient renal failure that resolved without dialysis, and she demonstrated no long-term organ system dysfunction at 18 weeks post discharge.

COMPLICATIONS OF MASSIVE HEMORRHAGE

In most cases of PPH, the patient develops anemia not requiring transfusion and recovers with no long-term complications. As described above, PPH has the very real potential of leading to hypovolemic shock, cardiac arrest, and maternal death. In cases of survival after severe hemorrhage and shock, long-term sequelae such as panhypopituitarism, cerebral injury, and complications of blood transfusion therapy (viral infection, graft-versus-host disease, etc.) lead to chronic disability. These adverse outcomes are avoidable in many situations by prompt recognition of abnormal bleeding, treatment of the cause of bleeding, and preparation for resuscitation and blood transfusion.

Reperfusion Injury

After periods of ischemia (from inadequate oxygen delivery and utilization at the cellular level), when blood flow is re-established the tissue will react and create an inflammatory response producing oxidative damage of cellular membranes and DNA. It is one mechanism by which survivors of massive hemorrhage may go on to develop multisystem organ failure, cerebral injury, and death. Assessment of post-transfusion/resuscitation patients should include surveillance to monitor organ systems for damage from superoxides and hydroxyl radicals.[63,64]

Post-resuscitation assessment of organ system dysfunction includes ongoing vital sign measurements, physical assessment, and laboratory studies of key organ systems. Arterial blood gases are useful to evaluate the patient's current acid–base balance, oxygen delivery variables, and base deficit levels to assess the need for post-resuscitation supplemental bicarbonate administration or alternative therapies. Because the kidneys are highly susceptible to decreased oxygenation, urine and blood analysis of renal function may be useful in establishing baseline status to compare future analyses for evidence of renal injury. The evaluation of cardiac enzymes is usually indicated if the rate of hemorrhage produced maternal tachycardia in excess of 140 bpm and/or if electrocardiogram (ECG) changes were present and suggestive of ischemia (elevated S-T segments, inverted T-waves, ectopy, etc.); or if maternal MAP was less than 60 to 65 mmHg for more than 10 to 15 minutes. Patients that are post massive transfusion are at risk for infection, ileus, electrolyte imbalances, pulmonary edema, cerebral edema, adult respiratory distress syndrome (ARDS), and other sequelae.[63]

Rh Sensitization

Rh sensitization can occur in a Rh(D)-negative mother who received Rh(D)-positive blood products during transfusion. Additionally, if a condition existed that increased the risk of maternal exposure to fetal blood (placental abruption, abnormal placentation, etc.), the risk for Rh sensitization may be high. After PPH and transfusion of Rh(D)-negative women, testing for the presence of fetal cells in the maternal blood is performed. Maternal blood analysis with a Kleihauer-Betke test or flow cytometry is done to determine the amount of Rh Immune Globulin (Human) (RhoGAM) needed to suppress the immune system and prevent the development of the anti-Rh(D) antibodies of isoimmunization.

COLLABORATIVE MANAGEMENT OF MASSIVE POSTPARTUM HEMORRHAGE AND PATIENT SAFETY

Contemporary management of obstetric emergencies such as PPH requires the rapid mobilization of a multidisciplinary team with clear communication, strong leadership, and appropriate decision-making to ensure a positive patient outcome. This includes efforts toward establishing institutional protocol-driven, rapid response capabilities in accordance with current practice recommendations. One recommended activity in the preparation of PPH team members to effectively respond to patients with massive hemorrhage is the use of clinical simulation drills. The benefits of simulation training have long been employed in other industries, including commercial airline, nuclear power, and disaster preparedness. When used to prepare for a rare but life-threatening clinical event such as obstetric hemorrhage, it may reduce response time, improve team communication, and decrease delays in patient care. When simulation is repeated, providers continue to refine knowledge derived from past experiences and apply lessons learned toward performance improvement for the next actual event. It is recommended that units and hospitals create hemorrhage clinical guidelines, utilize simulation as an educational tool to improve clinical response and patient outcomes, and address specific unit challenges to hemorrhage resuscitation.[65]

Analysis of clinical errors and significant delays in the care of women experiencing obstetric hemorrhage identify components of care that, when not employed or performed after significant delay, lead to increased maternal morbidity and mortality. Box 15-2 is a list of the common errors identified in the management of obstetric hemorrhage.

SUMMARY

Obstetric hemorrhage remains a significant contributor to maternal morbidity and mortality across all geographical and socioeconomic spectra worldwide. Complications may be prevented by prompt recognition, timely initiation of appropriate clinical management strategies, and collaborative interventions. With proper education and preparation, the health care provider, as an individual and as part of the health care team, may significantly reduce the incidence of poor outcomes from this common complication of childbirth.

Box 15-2. COMMON ERRORS IN THE MANAGEMENT OF POSTPARTUM HEMORRHAGE

- Failure or delay to identify hemorrhage
- Failure or delay in using alternative uterotonic agents other than oxytocin
- Failure or delay in calling for help/notification of unit managers/anesthesia/second surgeon
- Failure or delay in moving patient to an operating room
- Failure or delay in recognizing maternal vital signs consistent with postpartum hemorrhage
- Failure or delay in moving a post–Cesarean section patient from the post-anesthesia care unit to an operating room
- Failure or delay in typing, crossmatching, and ordering blood products
- Failure or delay in administering blood products
- Failure or delay in administering fresh frozen plasma and/or platelets until large volumes of packed red blood cells have been transfused
- Failure of or incomplete communication between and among medicine, nursing, laboratory personnel, blood bank personnel, anesthesia, vascular surgery, others

Data from References 78–80.

REFERENCES

1. Chang, J., Elam-Evans, L. D., Berg, C. J., Herndon, J., Flowers, L., & Seed, K. A. (2003). Pregnancy-related mortality surveillance–United States, 1991–1999. *MMWR Surveillance Summaries, 52*(2), 1–8.
2. World Health Organization. (2009). *World Health Statistics 2009* (p. 149). Geneva: WHO Press.
3. Berg, C. J., Harper, M. A., Atkinson, S. M., Bell, E. A., Brown, H. L., Hage, M. L., et al. (2005). Preventability of pregnancy-related deaths: Results of a state-wide review. *Obstetrics and Gynecology, 106*(6), 1228–1234.
4. Clark, S. L., Belfort, M. A., Dildy, G. A., Herbst, M. A., Meyers, J. A., & Hankins, G. D. (2008). Maternal death in the 21st century: Causes, prevention, and relationship to cesarean delivery. *American Journal of Obstetrics and Gynecology, 199*(1), 36 e1–5; discussion 91–2 e7–11.
5. American College of Obstetricians and Gynecologists. (2006). Postpartum hemorrhage. ACOG Practice Bulletin No. 76. *Obstetrics and Gynecology, 108*, 1039–1047.
6. Chesley, L. C. (1972). Plasma and red cell volumes during pregnancy. *American Journal of Obstetrics and Gynecology, 112*(3), 440–450.
7. Pritchard, J. A. (1962). Blood volume changes in pregnancy and the puerperium II. Red blood cell loss and changes in apparent blood volume during and following vaginal delivery, cesarean section, and cesarean section plus total hysterectomy. *American Journal of Obstetrics and Gynecology, 84*, 1272–1282.
8. Clark, S. L., Yeh, S. Y., Phelan, J. P., Bruce, S., & Paul, R. H. (1984). Emergency hysterectomy for obstetric hemorrhage. *Obstetrics and Gynecology, 64*(3), 376–380.

9. Stafford, I., Dildy, G. A., Clark, S. L., & Belfort, M. A. (2008). Visually estimated and calculated blood loss in vaginal and cesarean delivery. *American Journal of Obstetrics and Gynecology, 199*(5), 519 e1–7.

10. Dildy, G. A., Paine, A. R., George, N. C., & Velasco, C. (2004). Estimating blood loss: Can teaching significantly improve visual estimation? *Obstetrics and Gynecology, 104*(3), 601–606.

11. Combs, C. A., Murphy, E. L., & Laros, R. K., Jr. (1991). Factors associated with hemorrhage in cesarean deliveries. *Obstetrics and Gynecology, 77*(1), 77–82.

12. Deloughery, T. G. (2007). Update in hematology. *Annals of Internal Medicine, 147*(10), 717–724.

13. O'Brien, P., El-Refaey, H., Gordon, A., Geary, M., & Rodeck, C. H. (1998). Rectally administered misoprostol for the treatment of postpartum hemorrhage unresponsive to oxytocin and ergometrine: A descriptive study. *Obstetrics and Gynecology, 92*, 212–214.

14. Pelosi, M. A., 3rd, & Pelosi, M. A. (1999). Modified cesarean hysterectomy for placenta previa percreta with bladder invasion: Retrovesical lower uterine segment bypass. *Obstetrics and Gynecology, 93*(5 Pt 2), 830–833.

15. Lewis, G. (2004). *Why mothers die 2000–2002: The sixth report of confidential enquiries into maternal death in the United Kingdom* (p. 338). London: RCOG Press.

16. Gutierrez, G., Reines, H. D., & Wulf-Gutierrez, M. E. (2004). Clinical review: Hemorrhagic shock. *Critical Care (London, England), 8*(5), 373–381.

17. Lokugamage, A., Sullivan, K., Niculescu, I., Tigere, P., Onyangunga, F., El Refaey, H., et al. (2001). A randomized study comparing rectally administered misoprostol versus Syntometrine combined with an oxytocin infusion for the cessation of primary post partum hemorrhage. *Acta Obstetricia Et Gynecologica Scandinavica, 80*(9), 835–839.

18. Mousa, H. A., & Alfirevic, Z. (2003). Treatment for primary postpartum haemorrhage.[update in Cochrane Database Syst Rev. 2007;(1):CD003249; PMID: 17253486]. *The Cochrane Database of Systematic Reviews.* (1):CD003249.

19. Maier, R. C. (1993). Control of postpartum hemorrhage with uterine packing. *American Journal of Obstetrics and Gynecology, 169*(2 Pt 1), 317–321; discussion 21–3.

20. Bakri, Y. N., Amri, A., & Abdul Jabbar, F. (2001). Tamponade-balloon for obstetrical bleeding. *International Journal Gynaecologica and Obstetrica, 74*(2), 139–142.

21. Doumouchtsis, S. K., Papageorghiou, A. T., & Arulkumaran, S. (2007). Systematic review of conservative management of postpartum hemorrhage: What to do when medical treatment fails. *Obstetrical and Gynecological Survey, 62*(8), 540–547.

22. Doumouchtsis, S. K., Papageorghiou, A. T., & Arulkumaran, S. (2009). The surgical management of intractable postpartum hemorrhage.[comment]. *Acta Obstetricia Et Gynecologica Scandinavica, 88*(4), 489–490; author reply 90–92.

23. Baskett, T. F. (2003). Emergency obstetric hysterectomy. *Journal of Obstetrics and Gynaecology, 23*(4), 353–355.

24. Eniola, O. A., Bewley, S., Waterstone, M., Hooper, R., & Wolfe, C. D. (2006). Obstetric hysterectomy in a population of South East England. *Journal of Obstetrics and Gynaecology, 26*(2), 104–109.

25. Lau, W. C., Fung, H. Y., & Rogers, M. S. (1997). Ten years experience of caesarean and postpartum hysterectomy in a teaching hospital in Hong Kong. *European Journal of Obstetrics, Gynecology, and Reproductive Biology, 74*(2), 133–137.

26. Kwee, A., Bots, M. L., Visser, G. H., & Bruinse, H. W. (2006). Emergency peripartum hysterectomy: A prospective study in The Netherlands. *European Journal of Obstetrics, Gynecology, and Reproductive Biology, 124,* 187–192.

27. Knight, M., & Ukoss, O. B. O. (2007). Peripartum hysterectomy in the UK: Management and outcomes of the associated haemorrhage. *BJOG, 114*(11), 1380–1387.

28. American Society of Anesthesiologists. (2006). Practice guidelines for perioperative blood transfusion and adjuvant therapies an updated report by the American Society of Anesthesiologists Task Force on Perioperative Blood Transfusion and Adjuvant Therapies. *Anesthesiology, 105,* 198–208.

29. Martel, M. -J. (2002). SOGC clinical practice guidelines no. 115: Hemorrhagic shock. *Journal of Obstetrics and Gynaecology Canada, 24*(6), 504–511.

30. British Committee for Standards in Haematology. (2006). Guidelines on the management of massive blood loss. *British Journal of Haematology, 135*(5), 634–641.

31. Primary Health and Community Partnerships. (2010). Maternity – prevention, early recognition & management of postpartum haemorrhage (PPH). Policy Director, NSW Department of Health. Retrieved from http://www.health.nsw.gov.au/policies/pd/2010/pdf/PD2010_064.pdf

32. Spahn, D. R., Cerny, V., Coats, T. J., Duranteau, J., Fernández-Mondéjar, E., Gordini, G., et al. Task Force for Advanced Bleeding Care in Trauma (2007). Management of bleeding following major trauma: A European guideline. *Critical Care, 11*(1), R17.

33. Napolitano, L. M., Kurek, S., Luchette, F. A., Corwin, H. L., Barie, P. S., Tisherman, S. A., et al. Eastern Association for the Surgery of Trauma Practice Management Workgroup. (2009). Clinical practice guideline: Red blood cell transfusion in adult trauma and critical care. *Critical Care Medicine, 37*(12), 3124–3157.

34. Padmanabhan, A., Schwartz, J., & Spitalnik, S. L. (2009) Transfusion therapy in postpartum hemorrhage. *Seminars in Perinatology, 33*(2), 124–127.

35. Barbieri, R. L. (2009). Planning reduces the risk of maternal death: This tool helps. *OBG Management, 21*(8), 8, 10a, 10b.

36. Macleod, J. B., Lynn, M., Mckenney, M. G., Cohn, S. M., & Murtha, M. (2003). Early coagulopathy predicts mortality in trauma. *The Journal of Trauma, 55*(1), 39–44.

37. Gonzalez, E. A., Moore, F. A., Holcomb, J. B., Miller, C. C., Kozar, R. A., Todd, S. R., et al. (2007). Fresh frozen plasma should be given earlier to patients requiring massive transfusion. *The Journal of Trauma, 62*(1), 112–119.

38. Holcomb, J. B., Wade, C. E., Michalek, J. E., Chisholm, G. B., Zarzabal, L. A., Schreiber, M. A., et al. (2008). Increased plasma and platelet to red blood cell ratios improves outcome in 466 massively transfused civilian trauma patients. *Annals of Surgery, 248*(3), 447–458.

39. Dirkmann, D., Hanke, A. A., Gorlinger, K., & Peters, J. (2008). Hypothermia and acidosis synergistically impair coagulation in human whole blood. *Anesthesia and Analgesia, 106*(6), 1627–1632.

40. Mikhail, J. (1999). The trauma triad of death: Hypothermia, acidosis, and coagulopathy. *AACN Clinical Issues, 10,* 85–94.

41. Brohi, K., Cohen, M. J., Ganter, M. T., Matthay, M. A., Mackersie, R. C., & Pittet, J. F. (2007). Acute traumatic coagulopathy: Initiated by hypoperfusion modulated through the protein C pathway? *Annals of Surgery, 245*(5), 812–818.

42. Fukudome, E. Y., & Alam, H. B. (2009). Hypothermia in multisystem trauma. *Critical Care Medicine, 37*(Suppl. 7), S265–S272.

43. Liolios, A. (2004). *Volume resuscitation: The crystalloid vs colloid debate revisited.* Retrieved from http://www.med-scape.com/viewarticle/480288

44. The Albumin Reviewers (Alderson P, Bunn, F., Li Wan Po, A., Li, L., Pearson, M., Roberts, I., & Schierhout G). (2004). Human albumin solution for resuscitation and volume expansion in critically ill patients. *The Cochrane Database of Systematic Reviews, 4,* CD001208. DOI: 10.1002/14651858. CD001208.pub2

45. Weinberg, J. A., Mcgwin, G., Jr., Griffin, R. L., Huynh, V. Q., Cherry, S. A. 3rd., Marques, M. B., ... Rue, L. W. 3rd. (2008). Age of transfused blood: An independent predictor of mortality despite universal leukoreduction. *The Journal of Trauma, 65*(2), 279–282; discussion 82–84.

46. Hess, J. R., Dutton, R. B., Holcomb, J. B., & Scalea, T. M. (2008). Giving plasma at a 1:1 ratio with red cells in resuscitation: Who might benefit? *Transfusion, 48,* 1763–1765.

47. Santoso, J. T., Saunders, B. A., & Grosshart, K. (2005), Massive blood loss and transfusion in obstetrics and gynecology. *Obstetrical and Gynecological Survey, 60*(12), 827–837.

48. National Institutes of Health National Heart, Lung, and Blood Institute. (2007). *The diagnosis, evaluation, and management of von Willebrand disease.* Retrieved from http://www.nhlbi.nih.gov/guidelines/vwd/vwd.pdf

49. O'Connell, K. A., Wood, J. J., Wise, R. P., Lozier, J. N., & Braun, M. M. (2006). Thromboembolic adverse events after use of recombinant human coagulation Factor VIIa. *JAMA, 295*(3), 293–298.

50. Rose, L. (2007). Recombinant factor VIIa: Review of current "off license" indications and implications for practice. *AACN Advanced Critical Care, 18*(2), 141–148.

51. Perkins, J. G., Cap, A. P., Weiss, B. M., Reid, T. J., & Bolan, C. D. (2008). Massive transfusion and nonsurgical hemostatic agents. *Critical Care Medicine, 36*(Suppl), S325–S339.

52. O'Connell, N. M., Perry, D. J., Hodgson, A. J., et al. (2003). Recombinant FVIIa in the management of uncontrolled hemorrhage. *Transfusion, 43*(12), 1649–1651.

53. Sumner, M. (2005). *Important drug warning.* Retrieved from http://www.fda.gov/downloads/Safety/MedWatch/SafetyInformation/SafetyAlertsforHumanMedicalProducts/UCM164108.pdf

54. Hsia, C. C., Chin-Yee, I. H., & McAlister, V. C. (2008). Use of recombinant activated factor VII in patients without hemophilia: A meta-analysis of randomized control trials. *Annals of Surgery, 248*(1), 61–68.

55. Franchini, M., Franchi, M., Bergamini, V., & Montagnana, M. (2010). The use of recombinant activated FVII in postpartum hemorrhage. *Clinical Obstetrics and Gynecology, 53*(1), 219–227.

56. Xanodyne Pharmaceuticals, Inc. (2009). *Lysteda prescribing information.* Retrieved from http://www.accessdata.fda.gov/drugsatfda_docs/label/2009/022430lbl.pdf

57. Society of Thoracic Surgeons Blood Conservation Guideline Task Force, Ferraris, V. A., Ferraris, S. P., Saha, S. P., Hessel, E. A. 2nd., Haan, C. K., Royston, B. D., and Body, S. (2007). Perioperative blood transfusion and blood conservation in cardiac surgery: The Society of Thoracic Surgeons and The Society of Cardiovascular Anesthesiologists Clinical Practice Guideline. *The Annals of Thoracic Surgery, 83,* S27–S86.

58. Roberts, I. G., & Olayemi, O. (2009-2015). *Tranexamic acid for the treatment of postpartum haemorrhage: An international randomised, double blind, placebo controlled trial.* ClinicalTrials.gov Identifier: NCT00872469: London School of Hygiene and Tropical Medicine and Indian Council of Medical Research: University College Hospital, Ibadan, Nigeria.

59. Waters, J. H., Biscotti, C., Potter, P. S., & Phillipson, E. (2000). Amniotic fluid removal during cell salvage in the cesarean section patient. *Anesthesiology, 92*(6), 1531–1536.

60. Bernstein, H. H., Rosenblatt, M. A., Gettes, M., & Lockwood, C. (1997). The ability of the Haemonetics 4 Cell Saver System to remove tissue factor from blood contaminated with amniotic fluid. *Anesthesia and Analgesia, 85*(4), 831–834.

61. Rebarber, A., Lonser, R., Jackson, S., Copel, J. A., & Sipes, S. (1998). The safety of intraoperative autologous blood collection and autotransfusion during cesarean section. *American Journal of Obstetrics and Gynecology, 179*(3 Pt 1), 715–720.

62. Singla, A. K., Lapinski, R. H., Berkowitz, R. L., & Saphier, C. J. (2001). Are women who are Jehovah's Witnesses at risk of maternal death? *American Journal of Obstetrics and Gynecology, 185*(4), 893–895.

63. Merion, R. M. (2006). Organ preservation. In M. W. Mulholland, K. D. Lillemoe, G. M. Doherty, R. V. Maier, & G. R. Upchurch (Eds.), *Greenfield's surgery: Scientific principles and practice* (4th ed., pp. 566–567). Philadelphia: Lippincott William & Wilkins.

64. Rosengart, M. R., & Billiar, T. R. (2006). Inflammation. In M. W. Mulholland, K. D. Lillemoe, G. M. Doherty, R. V. Maier, & G. R. Upchurch (Eds.), *Greenfield's surgery: Scientific principles and practice* (4th ed., pp. 124–163). Philadelphia: Lippincott William & Wilkins.

65. Clark, E. A., Fisher, J., Arafeh, J., & Druzin, M. (2010). Team training/simulation. *Clinical Obstetrics and Gynecology, 53*(1), 265–277.

66. Dildy, G. A. (2002). Postpartum hemorrhage: New management options. *Clinical Obstetrics and Gynecology, 45*(2), 330–344.

67. Oyelese, Y., & Ananth, C. V. (2010). Postpartum hemorrhage: Epidemiology, risk factors, and causes. *Clinical Obstetrics and Gynecology, 53*(1), 147–156.

68. Monarch Pharmaceuticals. (2004). *Pitocin (Oxytocin Injection, USP) Synthetic.* Bristol, TN: Author.

69. Breathnach, F., & Geary, M. (2009). Uterine atony: Definition, prevention, nonsurgical management, and uterine tamponade. *Seminars in Perinatology, 33*(2), 82–87.

70. Rivers, E. P., & Amponsah, D. (2010). Shock. In A. B. Wolfson, G. W. Hendey, L. J. Ling, & C. L. Rosen (Eds.), *Harwood-Nuss' clinical practice of emergency medicine* (5th ed. pp. 37–43). Philadelphia: Lippincott Williams & Wilkins.

71. American Association of Blood Banks, American Red Cross America's Blood Centers, Armed Services Blood Program. (2009). *Circular of information for the use of human blood and blood components: AABB* (pp. 1–38). Bethesda, MD: Author.

72. Spinella, P. C. (2008). Warm fresh whole blood transfusion for severe hemorrhage: U.S. military and potential civilian applications. *Critical Care Medicine, 36*(7 Suppl), S340–S345.

73. Spinella, P. C., Perkins, J. G., Grathwohl, K. W., Beekley, A. C., Holcomb, J. B. (2009). Warm fresh whole blood is independently associated with improved survival for patients with combat-related traumatic injuries. *The Journal of Trauma, 66*(Suppl. 4), S69–S76.

74. New York State Council on Human Blood and Transfusion Services and New York State Board for Nursing. (2008). *Transfusion reaction fact sheets: A companion reference to guidelines for monitoring transfusion recipients* (pp. 6B–15B). Albany, NY: New York State Department of Health.

75. Wallis, J. P. (2008). Red cell transfusion triggers. *Transfusion and Apheresis Science, 39*(2), 151–154.

76. Stevenson, H. (2007). *Canadian blood services clinical guide to transfusion* (pp. 14–33). Toronto, ON: Canadian Blood Services.

77. Ridley, S., Taylor, B., & Gunning, K. (2007). *Medical management of bleeding in critically ill patients: Desmopressin.* Retrieved from http://www.medscape.com/viewarticle/563820_3

78. Maslovitz, S., Barkai, G., Lessing, J. B., Ziv, A., & Many, A. (2007). Recurrent obstetric management mistakes identified by simulation. *Obstetrics and Gynecology, 109*(6), 1295–1300.

79. Lombaard, H., & Pattinson, R. C. (2009). Common errors and remedies in managing postpartum haemorrhage. *Best Practice and Research Clinical obstetrics and gynaecology, 23*(3), 317–326.

80. Gruen, R. L., Jurkovich, G. J., Mcintyre, L. K., Foy, H. M., & Maier, R. V. (2006). Patterns of errors contributing to trauma mortality: Lessons learned from 2,594 deaths. *Annals of Surgery, 244*(3), 371–380.

CHAPTER 16

Disseminated Intravascular Coagulation in Pregnancy

Melissa C. Sisson and Marcy M. Mann

For the past 50 years, disseminated intravascular coagulation (DIC) has been described in the obstetric literature because of its tendency to accompany certain obstetrical conditions. The clinical presentation and prognostic course of DIC are diverse and make the diagnosis and management of the disease a significant clinical challenge.

The subcommittee on DIC of the International Society on Thrombosis and Hemostasis defined DIC as:

> an acquired syndrome characterized by the intravascular activation of coagulation with loss of localization arising from different causes. It can originate from and cause damage to the microvasculature which if sufficiently severe can produce organ dysfunction.[1]

DIC is not a separate clinical entity; rather it is an effect of other disease processes. Therefore, the treatment of DIC is focused on identification and removal of the causative agent or insult while supporting the cardiopulmonary status of the mother. DIC represents a derangement of the balance between the procoagulant and fibrinolytic systems that occurs when normal hematologic regulatory mechanisms fail.

The incidence of DIC in pregnancy varies and is dependent on the underlying obstetric complication. For example, in cases of complete placental abruption accompanied by intrauterine fetal demise (IUFD) and hemorrhage, DIC is common.[2] In contrast, DIC associated with IUFD without placental abruption is quite rare except when products of conception are retained beyond 5 weeks.[3] The incidence of DIC associated with hemolysis, elevated liver enzymes, and low platelets (HELLP syndrome) has been reported to be 15 percent, but in preeclampsia without HELLP syndrome or placental abruption, frank DIC is almost never seen.[3–4] A consumptive coagulopathy is more common in the obstetric patient than acute, fulminant DIC.[1] All pregnant women may be at greater risk for DIC because of the complications unique to pregnancy that are associated with this syndrome.[3] Conditions associated with DIC in pregnancy are listed in Box 16-1.

Although acute coagulopathy during pregnancy is a rare event, it is associated with profound consequences that increase morbidity and mortality for both the mother and fetus. It is therefore important for health care providers of pregnant women to be knowledgeable about DIC, to facilitate early detection, and to optimize outcome.

NORMAL COAGULATION

Hemostasis is the process by which blood is maintained in a liquid state within vessels and bleeding from a damaged vessel is arrested. The primary components of hemostasis include the vascular endothelium, circulating platelets, and circulating blood proteins.

Disruption of the endothelium as a result of vascular damage sets into motion the three phases of hemostasis: formation of a temporary platelet plug, activation of the coagulation cascade to produce a fibrin clot, and activation of the fibrinolytic system to break down the clot. The endothelium provides a physical barrier to keep blood inside the vessels and prevents clotting by secreting nitric oxide (NO) and prostacyclin, which inhibit platelet activity.[5] Exposure of subendothelial collagen stops the secretion of NO and prostacyclin and initially produces localized vasoconstriction that assists in reduction of blood flow and loss. Release of histamine and serotonin further promote vasoconstriction.

Platelets, formed in the bone marrow from megakaryocytes, circulate in the blood and play the vital role of first responders when blood loss is detected. When platelets come into contact with the collagen underlying the damaged endothelium, they swell and assume irregular shapes. Their contractile proteins contract forcefully and release granules that contain multiple active factors that cause them to adhere to each other and to collagen.[6] von Willebrand factor (vWF) is found in one type of these granules and in circulating blood

Box 16-1. OBSTETRIC CONDITIONS ASSOCIATED WITH DIC

- Placental abruption
- HELLP syndrome
- Massive blood transfusions
- Septic or saline abortion
- Amniotic fluid embolus
- Acute fatty liver of pregnancy
- Retained IUFD
- Demise of second twin

and contributes to platelet activation. In addition, vWF mediates adhesion of platelets to subendothelial surfaces.[7]

Platelets secrete adenosine diphosphate (ADP), and their enzymes form thromboxane A_2, which causes further platelet aggregation.[7]

Glycoproteins on the platelet surface repulse adherence to normal endothelium but cause adherence to injured areas of the vessel wall.[8] The platelet membrane contains large amounts of phospholipids that activate many stages of blood coagulation.[6] Platelets have prothrombin receptors that attract prothrombin, which eventually is converted to thrombin, to the site of injury. They also play a role in clot retraction. The role of platelets in hemostasis is summarized in Table 16-1.

The second phase of hemostasis involves local activation of the coagulation cascade, which results in thrombin production and eventual formation of a fibrin clot. Circulating blood proteins, the third component of hemostasis, include those of the coagulation system, the fibrinolytic system, the kinin system, and the complement system. These systems work collectively to provide a complex system of checks and balances that regulate clot formation.

The blood proteins in the coagulation system, traditionally referred to as clotting factors, are manufactured in the liver and can be functionally divided into enzymes and cofactors.[5] Enzymes are activated clotting factors, whereas cofactors are substances that accelerate the rate of substrate activation by enzymes. The coagulation system is a series of self-amplifying substrate-to-enzyme interactions, activated by three types of injuries: trauma to tissue, trauma to vascular endothelium, and trauma to red blood cells (RBCs) or platelets.[7]

When one or more of these injuries occurs, thrombin is generated via the intrinsic pathway (contact system) or extrinsic pathway (tissue factor). The intrinsic pathway is activated when factor XII (Hageman factor) is altered due to trauma to the blood vessel or exposure to vascular wall collagen.[6] The extrinsic pathway is activated by tissue thromboplastin (tissue factor), which alters factor VII.[6] The final stages of clot formation begin with the activation of factor X, the first step in a converging pathway that brings the intrinsic and extrinsic pathways together. This process is represented in Figure 17-1, in Chapter 17. An important difference between the pathways is that the extrinsic pathway is activated very rapidly, most often within seconds, whereas the intrinsic pathway is more slowly activated, with clot formation complete within 1 to 6 minutes.[6]

The activation of factor X begins the final common pathway and leads to the conversion of circulating prothrombin to thrombin. Thrombin acts as a proteolytic enzyme and cleaves fibrinopeptides A and B from fibrinogen, a large circulating plasma protein. Fibrin monomers are formed as a result of this cleavage and are

TABLE 16-1

Role of Platelets in Hemostasis

Platelet Adhesion	Platelet Activation	Platelet Aggregation
• Injury occurs • Platelets come in contact with subendothelium (injured tissue) • Mediated by vWF in microvasculature • Mediated by fibrinogen in central circulation • Platelets bind with the subendothelium	• Once adhered to injured vessel, platelets activate • Platelets change shape and activate receptors on their surface • Platelets make and release thromboxane A_2 and platelet activating factor (PAF) • Thromboxane A_2 and PAF are agonists for platelet aggregation • Thromboxane A_2 and PAF are also vasoconstrictors • Localized vasoconstriction occurs at the site of injury	• Platelet agonists activate and attract more platelets • Activated platelets combine with adhered platelets • Thrombin (which is made via the clotting cascade) further enhances the process • Fibrinogen and vWF meditate platelet aggregation • Platelet plug formed and bleeding initially stops

then joined by activating factor XIII, and a stable clot is produced.[6]

Three major regulatory mechanisms control coagulation: the fibrinolytic system, antithrombin III (AT III), and protein C. These systems, aided by rapid blood flow and removal of activated clotting factor by the reticuloendothelial system, localize clot formation and maintain the liquid state of blood.

In the final phase of hemostasis, the fibrinolytic system begins the breakdown of fibrin when the clot is formed. This is illustrated in Figure 17-2 in Chapter 17. Plasminogen is incorporated into the fibrin clot and when activated is converted to plasmin, which systematically lyses fibrin. Four major fragments called fibrin degradation products (FDPs), also referred to as fibrin split products (FSPs), are liberated: X, Y, D, and E. The FDPs have anticoagulant properties which include disruption of fibrin polymerization, coating of platelets, and formation of soluble fibrin monomer complexes (SFMCs).[6] FDPs exert their anticoagulant effect when they cannot be adequately cleared because of excess fibrin formation. The pathophysiological effect of FDPs in obstetrics is especially significant because they decrease myometrial contractility and can worsen uterine atony.[3]

Antihrombin III (AT III) is the central physiologic antagonist to coagulation. It is a glycoprotein that binds to activated factors XII, XI, IX, and X and slowly inactivates thrombin. AT III inactivates thrombin by forming a 1:1 molecular complex with it, and the presence of these thrombin-antithrombin (TAT) complexes confirms the presence of thrombin.[9] When AT III combines with heparin, thrombin inactivation is accelerated.[3]

Protein C is a vitamin K–dependent proenzyme that is found in plasma. When activated by thrombin, protein C degrades activated cofactors V and VIII. Protein C then exerts an anticoagulant effect by inhibiting a portion of the coagulation cascade. Thrombomodulin and protein S serve as cofactors for protein C.[3]

COAGULATION IN PREGNANCY

Pregnancy has been referred to as a hypercoagulable state. Normal changes in the hemostatic system during pregnancy are presented in Box 16-2.[10] All coagulation factors are elevated with the exception of factors XI and XIII, which are believed to decrease.[3] In addition, fibrinolytic activity appears to be decreased during pregnancy, probably due to an increase in plasminogen activator inhibitor.[11] Levels of AT III remain unchanged, as do levels of protein C. Protein S, which potentiates the action of protein C, is also decreased.[10] Alterations in the hemostatic mechanism are believed to occur in order to maintain the pregnancy and to protect from blood loss at delivery.

Box 16-2. HEMOSTATIC ALTERATIONS IN PREGNANCY

- Increase in factors V, VII, VIII, IX, X, XII, prothrombin
- Increased fibrinogen 200–400 mg/dL to 400–600 mg/dL
- Decrease in factors IX and XIII
- No effect on protein C, antithrombin III
- Decrease in protein S
- Decreased fibrinolysis

PATHOPHYSIOLOGY OF DIC

In DIC, there is a loss of localization of coagulation due to the initial generation of thrombin by exposure to tissue factor (extrinsic pathway), the amplification of thrombin formation through the intrinsic pathway, the parallel activation of the inflammatory pathway, and the loss of adequate hemostatic and endothelial responses.[12] This results in the following pathological consequences:[10,12]

- disseminated fibrin thrombi, which results in obstruction of blood flow that produces end-organ ischemia and necrosis
- activation of the kinin system, which causes vascular permeability, hypotension, and shock
- activation of the complement system, which results in red cell and platelet lysis, increased vascular permeability, and shock
- release of cytokines, including interleukins (IL) 1 and 6, and tumor necrosis factor (TNF)
- plasmin-induced lysis of fibrin, liberation of FDPs, and further deletion of coagulation factors, which results in hemorrhage and shock.

The process is a self-perpetuating cycle of excessive clot formation and hemorrhage. Activation of the systemic inflammatory response can amplify coagulation through proinflammatory mediators, and likewise, DIC can amplify the inflammatory response and worsen the cycle.[12] DIC secondary to obstetric complications linked to endothelial dysfunction may give rise to systemic inflammatory response syndrome (SIRS), which may result in multiple organ dysfunction syndrome (MODS).

Predisposing Obstetric Conditions

In normal pregnancy, the coagulation and fibrinolytic systems appear to be in a hyperdynamic state with both increased production and turnover of several procoagulants.[3,13] It has therefore been suggested that pregnancy may represent a state in which there is an increased susceptibility to DIC. The intrapartum activation of coagulation—as evidenced by increases in FPA, activated Hageman factor (XIIa), SFMCs, and activation of fibrinolysis, indicated by increased FDPs—implies that normal parturition may actually represent a low-grade DIC.[13] Hypothetically, a pregnant woman exposed to a specific stimulus, such as release of tissue thromboplastin during placental abruption, may be at far greater risk for overt coagulopathy than her nonpregnant counterpart. There is to date no scientific evidence to support this theory. The obstetric conditions more commonly associated with DIC and related coagulation abnormalities are described in Box 16-1. Changes that occur in the hemostatic system during normal pregnancy are presented in Box 16-2.

Placental abruption, which complicates approximately 1 percent of deliveries, is considered a common obstetric cause of DIC.[2] Up to 10 percent of patients with a clinically significant abruption may have a coagulopathy, with postpartum hemorrhage the most frequent cause of death.[13] Severe coagulation defects occur most often when the abruption results in IUFD.[14] When the abruption is severe, the coagulopathy is related to systemic consumption of clotting factors and activation of fibrinolysis, rather than local consumption of clotting factors as occurs with retroplacental clot formation.[14] The trophoblast contains the highest concentration of tissue thromboplastin, and the continued release of thromboplastin from the site of the abruption into the systemic circulation results in disseminated consumption of clotting factors and secondary fibrinolysis.[3] Thromboplastins activate the coagulation system through the extrinsic pathway by binding factor VII.[3] The degree of thrombocytopenia, AT III consumption, hypofibrinogenemia, and D-dimer elevation correlates with the clinical severity of the abruption, and with the time interval between placental separation and delivery.[3] Postpartum hemorrhage is the most common cause of maternal morbidity secondary to placental abruption. It is likely that this is related to an increase in FDPs that lead to uterine atony.[3]

Preeclampsia or eclampsia may initially produce thrombocytopenia due to platelet consumption but rarely causes overt coagulopathy. It is the endothelial damage related to preeclampsia or eclampsia that causes a low-grade compensated DIC. A number of coagulation abnormalities have been observed in preeclampsia. AT III, which is unaltered in normal pregnancy, is reduced. Levels of D-dimer are elevated. Factor VIII consumption and FPA concentration are increased, reflecting the conversion of fibrinogen to fibrin.

Frank DIC in preeclampsia or eclampsia is rarely seen in the absence of placental abruption or HELLP syndrome.[15–16] An international multicenter study found the frequency of DIC in HELLP syndrome to be 6 percent and in severe preeclampsia to be 1 percent.[17] When eclampsia occurs, the incidence of DIC rises to 7 to 10 percent.[18] Although many women with preeclampsia demonstrate a subclinical coagulopathy, those who experience another complication such as placental abruption or HELLP syndrome are at significantly greater risk for mortality.

Amniotic fluid embolus (AFE), also referred to as anaphylactoid syndrome of pregnancy, is a rare obstetric complication characterized by profound hypotension, hypoxia, cardiovascular collapse, and coagulopathy. Maternal mortality associated with this condition is reported to be 60 to 80 percent.[19] Of those who survive, only 15 percent are neurologically intact. Should the initial cardiopulmonary insults be survived, the patient may die from the ensuing coagulopathy.[20] A thorough discussion of this condition is presented in Chapter 19 of this text.

The etiology of the coagulopathy in AFE is controversial. Although amniotic fluid is known to have a procoagulant effect, its role in the syndrome remains inconclusive.[20] Laboratory abnormalities include marked hypofibrinogenemia. Clark and colleagues postulated that the coagulopathy in both placental abruption and AFE is due to activation of the clotting cascade after exposure of the maternal circulation to fetal antigens with thromboplastin-like effects.[19] Noting similarities in the pathophysiology of DIC, septic shock, and anaphylactic shock, these authors suggested that AFE be renamed "anaphylactoid syndrome of pregnancy."[19]

Diagnosis of AFE is largely clinical, since histologic findings are neither sensitive nor specific.[20] Initial therapy includes administration of oxygen in high concentration, volume expansion, inotropic support, and blood and blood component therapy.

Acute fatty liver of pregnancy (AFLP) another rare and potentially fatal disorder is characterized by fulminant liver failure, hypoglycemia, and severe reduction in clotting factors. DIC and a significant depression of AT III are hallmarks of this condition.[3]

The pathophysiology of AFLP is poorly understood, and current research is focused on maternal and fetal free fatty acid enzyme deficiencies.[21] Fetuses with a deficiency of the enzyme long chain 3 hydroxy acyl-coenzyme A dehydrogenase (LCAAD) accumulate fatty acids that have not been oxidized and are hepatotoxic to the mother.[21] Delivery is a cornerstone of treatment, and liver enzymes usually return to normal within a few days.[21]

CLINICAL PRESENTATION

As outlined previously, the patient with DIC may present with a diverse clinical picture. Signs and symptoms may be as innocuous as epistaxis or as profound as massive hemorrhage. A fulminant overt DIC is most often associated with severe placental abruption, AFE, or both, while a chronic non-overt DIC occurs more often in women with preeclampsia or eclampsia. Patients with a clinical presentation of non-overt DIC are at increased risk for overt DIC.

Although bleeding is the presenting sign of DIC, it is always preceded by thrombosis which varies with the organs affected. Patients may have clinical signs of thrombosis, which may include peripheral cyanosis, renal impairment, drowsiness, confusion, coma, and cardiorespiratory failure.[1] Large- and small-vessel thrombosis, with impairment of blood flow, ischemia, and end-organ damage, usually lead to "irreversible morbidity and mortality."[16] There is a high probability that dysfunction will occur in cardiac, pulmonary, renal, hepatic, and central nervous systems.[16]

Most commonly, the patient with DIC bleeds from at least three unrelated sites.[1,14] Blood may ooze from venipuncture sites as well as other sites of trauma. Epistaxis, ecchymosis, purpura, petechiae, and other abnormal integumentary manifestations are common.[16] Large subcutaneous hematomas and deep tissue bleeding can also be seen.[16] Hypotension due to hemorrhage and activation of the kinin system almost always accompanies DIC.[16]

DIAGNOSIS OF DIC

In the obstetric patient presenting with massive hemorrhage, the collection of specimens for analysis of laboratory data may prove academic due to the obvious need for expedient clinical intervention. However, as a screening tool and guide for therapy, assessment of laboratory data is essential. There are both global and specific molecular marker laboratory tests available to measure changes in coagulation, but no gold standard test exists for confirming the diagnosis of DIC.[22]

The more common and available tests for coagulation assessment include platelet count, serum fibrinogen, prothrombin time (PT), and activated partial thromboplastin time (aPTT) (Table 16-2). The PT, which reflects extrinsic coagulation, is generally prolonged in the patient with DIC, as is aPTT, which measures intrinsic coagulation. PT and aPTT are limited in diagnostic value because 50 percent of patients with DIC have a normal PT and aPTT, as compared to fibrinogen and platelets, which are decreased in most all patients with DIC.[3]

FDPs are elevated in 85 to 100 percent of patients with DIC.[16] However, the presence of FDPs is non-specific, and they can be elevated as a result of other medical conditions.[3] D-dimer is a unique fibrin degradation fragment liberated when plasmin lyses cross-linked fibrin clots.[1] FDPs appear earlier in the coagulation

TABLE 16-2	
Laboratory Abnormalities in DIC	
Platelet count	Decreased
Fibrinogen	Decreased
Antihrombin III	Decreased
Protein C	Decreased
Prothrombin time	Prolonged
Partial thromboplastin time	Prolonged
Fibrin degradation products (fibrin split products)	Increased
Fibrinopeptide A	Increased
Prothrombin fragment 1 and 2	Increased
Thrombin–antithrombin complex	Increased
Platelet factor 4	Increased

cascade, prior to cross-linking of fibrin, and are associated with clot breakdown.[1] D-dimer indicates the presence of thrombin (clot formation) and plasmin (clot breakdown).[3] D-dimer seems to be one of the most reliable of common tests available for diagnosis of DIC in the nonobstetric population.[1,16] Unfortunately, because D-dimer is present in pregnancy and increased toward term, its usefulness in pregnancy has not been established. Less widely available molecular markers for coagulation include plasma FPA, prothrombin fragments 1 and 2 (PF 1 and 2), AT III, thrombin–antithrombin (TAT) complex, protein C, and platelet factor 4.[16] The presence of PF 1 and 2 and TAT complexes is sensitive and specific for thrombin generation.[9]

Baktiari and colleagues found that the presence of an abnormal aPTT waveform correlated with the presence of DIC.[9] An automated coagulation analyzer uses a photo-optical detection system that can quantify changes in light transmission when plasma clots alter activation and recalcification.[9] An abnormal biphasic waveform occurs in an aPTT and reportedly is a good detector of DIC. The more severe the biphasic waveform, the better the prediction of DIC.[12] In their study of 331 intensive care patients, Dempfle and colleagues found that a biphasic waveform showed high specificity for the diagnosis of overt DIC.[23]

Recently, DIC scoring systems have been proposed to assist in diagnosis of the condition based on objective clinical data and laboratory parameters.[24] The leading scoring algorithms for DIC from the Japanese Ministry of Health and Welfare (JMHW) and the International Society of Thrombosis and Hemostasis (ISTH) utilize similar clinical and laboratory criteria that include commonly available global coagulation studies.[24] The ISTH score adds optional molecular markers and biphasic aPTT waveform analysis.[22] A third scoring system by the Japanese Academy of Acute Medicine (JAAM) recognizes the link between coagulation and inflammation, and adds SIRS as one of its criteria for diagnosing DIC.[24] The JAAM scoring system also adds rate of decline in platelet count.[24] In their study, Gando and colleagues found that fibrinogen level had no impact on predicted outcome, and it subsequently was eliminated from the JAAM scoring criteria.[24] In their prospective multi-center study, these authors demonstrated that the JAAM DIC criteria facilitated earlier diagnosis ($p < .001$) than the two prior systems.[24] On the day of DIC diagnosis, 67.4 percent of patients met the JAAM scoring criteria.[24]

CLINICAL MANAGEMENT OF DIC

Therapy for DIC is predicated on the degree to which the underlying mechanism can be identified and eliminated. For example, in patients with DIC associated with conditions such as preeclampsia, superimposed hypertension, placental abruption, or sepsis secondary to intrauterine infection, removal of the products of conception typically facilitates resolution of the process. However, of equal importance is timely initiation of appropriate interventions that address secondary complications that place the patient at risk for serious sequelae, morbidity, and mortality.

The broad goal of such clinical management strategies and interventions is to optimize hemodynamic function and oxygen transport in an attempt to improve overall tissue oxygenation, reduce the risk of end-organ dysfunction and failure, and reduce the risk of morbidity and mortality. A detailed presentation of concepts related to hemodynamic function, oxygen transport physiology, clinical assessment methods, and specific management strategies to achieve these goals is found in Chapter 4 of this text.

A chronic subclinical DIC that may occur secondary to IUFD or death of one fetus in a multiple gestation may require delivery to facilitate resolution of the disease process. Once the stimulus for coagulopathy is eliminated, serial monitoring of clotting studies, volume replacement, and astute clinical evaluation are usually sufficient.

An acute, fulminant DIC mandates a more aggressive approach. Acute hemorrhage accompanied by hypovolemic shock can rapidly result in inadequate cardiac output and oxygen delivery to tissues, with ultimate progression to cell injury and death. Blood component administration is essential to achieving a successful outcome. A thorough discussion of concepts related to hemorrhage, shock, and blood component therapy is presented in Chapter 15 of this text.

In the actively bleeding patient with hypovolemic shock, transfusion of PRBCs is required. This will improve oxygen-carrying capacity and oxygen delivery to the tissues. Transfusion of PRBCs is not intended to expand plasma volume. The restoration of tissue perfusion and oxygenation are critical to the resolution of the shock state.

Platelet transfusion is indicated in the actively bleeding patient with a platelet count of 50,000 mm^3 or in the preoperative patient with a count under 50,000 mm^3.[25] Prophylactic transfusion of platelets in the patient without active bleeding has largely been discontinued. If spontaneous vaginal delivery is anticipated, a platelet count of 20,000 mm^3 is the threshold for transfusion.[3] The typical dose of platelets is 5 to 7 units.[25] Platelets may be obtained from single or multiple donors. Platelets obtained by platelet pheresis can yield larger amounts of platelets than from a single unit of whole blood.[26] Platelet concentrate prepared from platelet pheresis and from 4 units of whole blood yield similar numbers of platelets but there is less donor exposure via platelet pheresis.[26–27]

The use of fresh frozen plasma (FFP) is indicated in patients bleeding due to clotting factor deficiency. FFP is indicated when PT and aPTT are prolonged and International Normalized Ratio (INR) is increased.[3] FFP contains AT III, fibrinogen, and clotting factors V, XI, and XII.[28] DIC leads to depletion of fibrinogen, factor V, and factor VIII.[3] The usual dose of FFP in fulminant DIC is 4 to 6 units.[3] Transfusion of FFP may facilitate volume replacement because each unit contains 250 milliliters, but it should not be used exclusively for this purpose.[28]

Optimization of preload by administration of intravascular fluid volume is crucial to the successful management of the bleeding patient with DIC. The challenge inherent in fluid replacement is to promote prompt restoration of circulatory volume without causing volume overload. This concept is based on the Frank-Starling relationship between preload and cardiac output, explained more fully in Chapter 4 of this text. Isotonic crystalloid solutions are recognized universally as the primary fluid for acute intravascular volume expansion.[28] A practical approach to acute blood loss is to first restore volume with crystalloid and then to infuse PRBCs if tachycardia, hypotension, and tachypnea persist.[23] For most patients, the use of crystalloids with the addition of blood products is adequate for volume resuscitation.

Also supportive in the treatment of the actively bleeding patient with DIC is optimization of oxygenation. Restoration of adequate cardiac output and improvement of oxygen-carrying capacity by optimization of hemoglobin are clinical management strategies to improve the patient's oxygenation status. It may also be necessary in certain patients to consider endotracheal intubation and mechanical ventilation. Mechanical ventilation in pregnancy, including criteria for considering intubation and mechanical ventilatory support, is described in Chapter 5 of this text. Administration of pharmacologic agents may be indicated for maintenance of blood pressure, once adequate blood volume has been achieved with crystalloid infusion. Such pharmacologic support may include administration of drugs to enhance inotropic response of the ventricles. Administration of vasopressors may also be indicated for select patients. A thorough presentation of pharmacologic agents that may be used in the care of critically ill obstetric patients is found in Chapter 6 of this text.

Because DIC is a condition of excessive coagulation, the idea of treating the disease with an anticoagulant has been studied. At this time, heparin is not a generally accepted treatment for obstetric causes of DIC. Heparin acts to neutralize thrombin by accelerating the activity of AT III. Since AT III levels are depleted in acute DIC, heparin therapy may not be efficacious. Heparin should be limited to low-dose heparin administration only in patients with intact vascular systems, no evidence of bleeding, and with a prolonged triggering mechanism such as IUFD.[3]

The following treatment strategies for DIC are currently under investigation, but not approved by the U. S. Food and Drug Administration (FDA) for use during pregnancy. AT III concentrate is available and is effective in treatment of obstetric causes of DIC. AT III is a natural inhibitor of coagulation, and patients with DIC are deficient in AT III. In obstetrics, the use of AT III has resulted in decreased levels of FDPs and increases in fibrinogen and platelets.[3] High-dose AT III for treatment of sepsis and DIC is currently in clinical trials.[29]

Factor VIIa enhances the thrombin burst that converts fibrinogen to a fibrin clot and has been used in nonpregnant patients to reverse or control DIC.[30] Pepas, Arif-Adib, and Kadir reported on 17 cases of puerperal hemorrhage with DIC treated with recombinant factor VIIa.[29] In all 17 cases, hemostasis was achieved successfully. Other case studies have reported successful treatment of DIC in pregnant women with recombinant factor VIIa for AFE and postpartum hemorrhage following Cesarean section.[31,32] Although there are increasing obstetric case reports of factor VIIa successfully used in DIC, it remains a very expensive treatment and concern has been raised about the apparent risk of thromboembolic events following its use.[33]

The synthetic serum protease inhibitors gabexate mesilate and nafamostat mesilate block thrombin generation and increase fibrinolysis, and in other countries they have been used to treat DIC in obstetrics.[3] Unlike heparin, they exert their impact independent of ATIII.[3]

Protein C is a naturally occurring anticoagulant protein that inhibits factors Va and VIIIa and activates the fibrinolytic system.[3] Recombinant human activated protein C (APC) may also exert anti-inflammatory effects.[1] Intravenous infusions of protein C for obstetric DIC have been reported; however, safety for use during pregnancy has not been established.[1,3] In a large randomized double-blind study, septic patients with evidence of end-organ dysfunction, including coagulopathy treated with APC, experienced a 6.1 percent absolute risk reduction in 28-day mortality rate (P = 0.005).[12]

Recently, the American College of Obstetricians and Gynecologists (ACOG) has advocated medical emergency preparedness for DIC that includes establishment of early warning systems, designation of first responders, and performance of practice drills.[34] A review of maternal mortality data in the United Kingdom concluded that hemorrhage drills serve to keep both labor and delivery and blood bank staff prepared and should be performed regularly.[25] Interdisciplinary practice drills for obstetric complications such as obstetric hemorrhage are becoming commonplace in hospitals.

General Clinical Management Principles

The initial goal in clinical management of the patient with DIC is early detection of coagulopathy and recognition of the potential for significant sequelae. A physiologic emergency, such as DIC, is often preceded by a period of instability during which timely intervention may make a difference in patient outcome.[33] The need for professional collaboration between nurses and physicians cannot be overemphasized.

The detection of abnormal coagulation requires assessment of both clinical and laboratory data. Laboratory screening includes a baseline hemoglobin, hematocrit, serum fibrinogen, platelet count, PT, aPTT, FDPs, and/or D-dimer. The frequency of blood collection for further assessment of laboratory data is determined by the presence of abnormalities. Physical assessment includes specific attention to the presence of petechiae, ecchymosis, hematoma formation, vaginal bleeding, gingival bleeding, hematuria, and conjunctival hemorrhage. If DIC is suspected, trauma such as venipuncture, intramuscular injection, central venous access, and arterial puncture should be carefully considered.

In the actively bleeding patient, blood loss should be quantified when possible. Blood component replacement is often necessary and has been described previously. Early risks of blood administration include transfusion reaction, transmission of infectious disease, and circulatory overload. The onset of a transfusion reaction is characteristically rapid, and signs and symptoms may include chills, chest and flank pain, cardiovascular collapse, and DIC.[26] Major hemolytic reactions frequently occur in the first 10 to 15 minutes after initiation of a blood transfusion; thus, the patient should be closely assessed for evidence of a reaction.[25] If an adverse reaction occurs, the transfusion should be stopped immediately, the intravenous tubing flushed with normal saline, and the patient managed empirically. Late transfusion risks also include late immunologic and non-immunologic complications, including bacterial contamination and infectious disease.[26] Transfusion-related acute lung injury (TRALI) is an additional risk of transfusion that has an unknown cause and is treated with aggressive management of ventilation and oxygenation.[26]

Strict adherence to procedures for patient identification when administering blood products is critical. The most common cause of fatal hemolytic transfusion reaction continues to be transfusion of ABO-incompatible PRBCs.[23] The American Association of Blood Banks (AABB) has defined the process of patient identification for each step of the process from specimen collection to immediately prior to transfusion.[25]

Rapid administration of blood products may be inhibited by their viscosity and by the internal lumen size of the intravenous catheter. Concurrent administration of other fluids or medications is prohibited. Hypotonic solutions may cause hemolysis; therefore, blood products should be administered through a primed intravenous line of normal saline.[25] Warming of blood products protects the patient from hypothermia, and will increase the flow rate up to 2.5 times.[28] Administration of cold blood products at a rate exceeding 100 mL/min can alter conduction of the sino-atrial node and result in cardiac arrest.[25] Standard blood administration sets contain filters sufficiently small to trap blood clots, fibrin strands, and other debris.[25] Blood filters add resistance, but it can be minimized by replacing them after every 3 to 4 units of blood product or by using microaggregate filters when multiple transfusions are anticipated.[25]

Fluid volume deficit accompanies hemorrhage and is responsible for significant morbidity in cases of DIC. The need for fluid replacement may be assessed by measurement of urine specific gravity, hematocrit/hemoglobin, pulmonary capillary wedge pressure, and intake and output.

Many factors influence the effectiveness of fluid administration, including the size of the intravenous catheter and tubing, the viscosity of the fluid, and infusion techniques. As large a catheter as possible should be placed, because flow rate is a function of the radius of the catheter and the length of the tubing. Multilumen catheter extension sets, Y-connectors, and piggyback devices have the potential to sacrifice flow. Pressure bags increase the flow rate over baseline gravity flow, but should be used with caution since they can cause hemolysis of PRBCs.

The amount and rate of fluid replacement therapy vary, depending on the severity of the deficit. Replacement of volume with isotonic crystalloid is usually a 3:1 ratio to estimated blood loss.[25] The best indication that fluid therapy is successful is the resolution

of the clinical signs and symptoms of shock, the return of normal oxygen delivery and consumption, and the normalization of maternal arterial blood gases.[26]

Impaired fetal gas exchange may occur as a consequence of decreased uteroplacental perfusion due to maternal hemorrhage and shock. The systemic nature of DIC can precipitate impairment of the cardiovascular, renal, liver, and central nervous systems and pulmonary function, particularly when blood loss is great. Goals of patient care focus on astute physical assessment of the patient, interpretation of clinical assessment findings, and evaluation of laboratory data. Timely identification of adverse changes in the patient's status is crucial, in order to reduce the risk of compromise to major organ systems.

In addition to assessment of maternal vital signs, urine output should be assessed hourly. A urine output of greater than 25 mL/hr generally coincides with adequate perfusion of the kidneys.[26] Serum creatinine and blood urea nitrogen (BUN) should also be assessed for elevations consistent with renal involvement. Liver function tests should be assessed serially with attention to elevation of SGOT, SGPT, and bilirubin. Nausea, vomiting, and right upper quadrant or shoulder pain suggest liver involvement. Close assessment of mental status is necessary because an alteration may be an early expression of cerebral hemorrhage or thrombosis due to DIC. Pulmonary involvement may represent an iatrogenic cardiogenic pulmonary edema or ventricular failure from fluid overload. Assessment findings such as dyspnea, tachypnea, adventitious breath sounds, and cyanosis are common in the patient with pulmonary edema. Pulse oximetry and measurement of arterial blood gases may also prove useful.

CASE EXCERPT

These concepts are represented in the following excerpt from an intrapartum clinical case study of a woman who developed DIC. The case involved a 27-year-old gravida 1 at 26 1/7 weeks gestation. Her prenatal history was significant for three days of "spotting" and mild cramping at 18 weeks gestation. She subsequently exhibited signs and symptoms of preeclampsia unresponsive to outpatient management, and required hospital admission. Her blood pressure at that time ranged from 138 to 150 mmHg systolic and 78 to 104 mmHg diastolic. Qualitative urine assessment by dipstick revealed 2+ proteinuria. Complete blood count (CBC) and liver function tests (LFT) were normal except for a slightly low hemoglobin (Hgb) of 11.3 g/dL. Evaluation of a full DIC panel was deferred due to the presence of normal initial laboratory results. Within 48 hours of admission, the patient's blood pressure had normalized without episodic elevations. Evaluation of a 24-hour urine collection revealed less than 300 mg of protein and normal creatinine clearance. The decision was

TABLE 16-3

Case Study Excerpt: Vital Signs

Vital Signs	Admission	20 min After Admission		60 min Later		4 hours Later
BP (mmHg)	80/32 (MAP, 48)	64/20 (MAP, 35)	**Transfusions Moved to OR Intubation/ventilation Vassopressors Warming blanket/ bed**	90/54 (MAP, 66)	**Insulin Drip in Process**	110/64 (MAP, 79)
HR/min	126	144		135		107
Resp/min	24	38		20 vent		18 vent
T – F°(C°)	97.8 (36.6)			98.0 (36.1)		99.1 (37.3)
SaO₂ (%)	97	92		100		97

BP = blood pressure, HR = heart rate, MAP = mean arterial pressure, OR = operating room, min = minutes, Resp = respirations, SaO_2 = arterial oxygen saturation of hemoglobin by pulse oximetry, T = temperature, vent = ventilator breaths per minute.

made to discharge the patient home. Instructions included limiting activities to strict bedrest and notifying her prenatal care provider if abnormal symptoms developed or she had any questions. An outpatient follow-up appointment was also made.

Six days after discharge, the patient was admitted to the hospital secondary to complaints of severe abdominal pain, vaginal bleeding with two "plum-sized" clots noted, and sudden onset of vomiting. Vital signs at the time of initial presentation to labor and delivery are presented in Table 16-3. Intravenous (IV) access was established, blood samples were obtained, and fluid resuscitation was started with normal saline. The fetal heart rate could not be obtained by auscultation, and a bedside ultrasound was performed, which confirmed an IUFD. A vaginal exam was performed and revealed the patient's cervix to be 7 cm dilated, 90 percent effaced, and vertex fetal presentation at +1 station. Bleeding was observed at the IV site, and vaginal bleeding was noted to have increased. A second IV site was accessed with a 14 gauge catheter in the opposite arm. A blood sample was obtained for assessment of clotting function. Updated vital signs and laboratory data are presented in Table 16-4. They are abnormal and express the severity of the patient's consumptive coagulopathy. The following blood products were ordered: 4 units of uncrossmatched O-negative PRBCs, 4 units FFP, 10 units of cryoprecipitate (Cryo), and 2 platelet pheresis packs. The blood bank personnel were advised of the hemorrhage and DIC and continued to type and crossmatch additional blood products based on the institution's protocol for obstetric hemorrhage.

Spontaneous vaginal delivery occurred followed by immediate placental expulsion. Uterine atony ensued. The patient's vital signs and other clinical assessment findings were consistent with shock. Volume resuscitation with normal saline was continued, and transfusion of 4 units of O-negative PRBCs was initiated. Blood warmers were used during transfusion of all blood

products. The patient was moved to the operating room, and the decision was made to proceed with endotracheal intubation and ventilatory support secondary to respiratory distress. Immediate goals were to improve oxygen delivery to end-organs and initiate interventions to resolve uterine atony and abate active bleeding.

Over the following 2 hours, 6 additional units of PRBCs were transfused to improve oxygen-carrying capacity by optimizing the hemoglobin level. Seven units of FFP, 1 platelet pheresis pack and 10 units of pooled Cryo were also administered to correct the coagulopathy. The patient's bleeding continued, and surgery for uterine hemostatsis (B-Lynch suturing technique) was started. Follow-up laboratory data are displayed in Table 16-4.

The 60-minute laboratory data in Table 16-4 demonstrate modest improvements in PT, aPTT and fibrinogen, but the fibrin split products remained grossly abnormal. Interventions to improve the patient's coagulopathy and optimize her hemoglobin were aggressively continued. Within an hour, the surgery was completed and the uterus was replaced in the abdomen.

Approximately 4 hours after admission, the following blood products had been transfused: 10 additional units PRBCs, 13 units FFP, 1 platelet pheresis pack, and 10 units of pooled Cryo. The patient's DIC laboratory values improved, compared to those obtained at hourly intervals prior to surgical hemostasis, and are shown in Table 16-4. Hemoglobin increased, which subsequently improved delivery of oxygen to the tissues and end-organs. Clotting studies (PT, aPTT, and fibrinogen) also improved, although PT and aPTT remained abnormal, indicating a need for further infusion of Cryo or FFP. Since the platelet count was greater than 50,000 and there was no active bleeding, the decision was made that immediate platelet transfusion was not warranted, unless further surgery became necessary or the platelet count decreased.

During the first 4 hours following admission, acute volume resuscitation and replacement of blood products

TABLE 16-4

Case Study Excerpt: Laboratory Data

	Admission	60 minutes Later*	4 hours Later†	Normal Values‡
Hgb (g/dL)	6.2	5.9	12.7	12–16
HCT (%)	18.0	17.4	36.5	38–48
Platelets (K/µL)	48	35	78	150–450
PT (sec)	44	30.9	23.1	11.5–15.0
PTT (sec)	>180	146	49.8	22.9–26.8
Fibrinogen (mg/dL)	80	126	211	205–483
Fibrin split products (mg/dL)	>20	>20	>20	<5
Smear/comments	platelets large forms/ clumps, rbc fragments	schistocytes, anisocytosis	schistocytes, anisocytosis, ovalocytes	(no comments)

Hgb = hemoglobin, HCT = hematocrit, PT = prothrombin time, PTT = partial thromboplastin time, FSP = fibrin split products, Smear/Comments = annotations from blood smear.

*Data obtained approximately 60 minutes later, following transfusion of approximately 6 units packed red blood cells (PRBCs), 7 units fresh frozen plasma (FFP), 1 platelet pheresis pack (PltPhres), and 10 units cryoprecipitate (Cryo).

†Data obtained approximately 4 hours later, following additional transfusion of approximately 10 units PRBC, 13 units FFP, 1 PltPhres pack, and 10 units Cryo.

‡Normal reference values for lab (nonpregnant).

required IV administration of a total of 18,300 mL of fluid (crystalloid and blood components). Estimated blood loss was 8,000 mL, and total urine output for the time period was 110 mL. Subsequently, the patient no longer required vasopressors for blood pressure support and there was no further bleeding. In addition, mechanical ventilation settings were adjusted. The fraction of inspired oxygen (FiO_2) and positive end-expiratory pressure (PEEP) were decreased, peak pressures were low to normal, and the SaO_2 remained at 95 percent or greater. Such findings suggested that left ventricular function was adequate and there were no clinical signs or symptoms or pulmonary edema.

Assessment of fluid balance is critical in any patient with DIC, since administration of a diuretic or vasodilator may have been indicated if, after the coagulopathy resolved, pulmonary edema developed. During the active resuscitation period, loop diuretics were not used due to the potential for exacerbating hypovolemia and/or nephron damage in the hypoxic kidney.

Further, initiation of an IV insulin infusion to regulate the patient's blood glucose level (a mainstay in adult critical care because of the reduced morbidity and mortality rates in patients with normalized blood glucose levels) was started in the operating room. Although the optimum blood glucose level for the best outcome had not been established at the time, the goal was to maintain the patient's glucose level between 85 and 110 mg/L.

During the course of the next 24 hours, DIC labs were normalized by targeted administration of blood products. On the second hospital day, the patient developed azotemia and oliguric acute kidney injury (AKI). The pathophysiology and management of AKI are presented in detail in Chapter 13 of this text. Secondary to oliguric AKI, invasive central hemodynamic monitoring was initiated. Short term hemofiltration with dialysis was initiated, to which the patient responded well. She was discharged 14 days following delivery with normal coagulation and renal function. Grief counseling and support were initiated while the patient was hospitalized, and additional supportive resources were discussed with the patient and her family following discharge.

SUMMARY

Certain complications unique to pregnancy and the intrapartum period may increase the susceptibility of the woman to DIC. The clinical presentation and prognostic course of DIC is diverse, ranging from a mild consumptive coagulopathy to death from shock or multiple organ system failure. Therefore, laboratory and clinical assessment are essential in order to guide clinical decisions. The plan of patient care includes focus on elimination of the underlying mechanism, initiation of appropriate and adequate blood component therapy, and hemodynamic and oxygenation support, in order to decrease the risk of devastating maternal or fetal consequences.

REFERENCES

1. Taylor, F. B., & Toh, C. H. (2001). Toward a definition, clinical and laboratory criteria and a scoring system for DIC. *Thrombosis and Haemostasis, 86,* 1327–1330.

2. Hladky, K., Yankowitz, U., & Hansen, W. F. (2002). Placental abruption. *Obstetrical and Gynecological Survey, 57,* 299–305.

3. Pachelo, L. D., Van Hook, J. W., & Gei, A. F. (2004). Disseminated intravascular coagulation. In G. A. Dildy, M. A. Belfort, G. R. Saade, et al. (Eds.), *Critical care obstetrics* (4th ed.). (pp. 394–407). Hoboken, NJ: Wiley-Blackwell.

4. Sibai, B. M. (2004). Diagnosis, controversies and management of the syndrome of HELLP. *Obstetrics and Gynecology, 103,* 981–991.

5. Stokol, T. (2010). *Hemostasis. Cornell University College of Veterinary Medicine.* [Online]. Retrieved from http://ahdc.vet.cornell.edu/clinpath/modules/coags/coag.htm

6. Guyton, A. C., & Hall, V. C. (2006). Hemostasis and coagulation. In A. C. Guyton & V. C. Hall (Eds.), *Textbook of medical physiology* (11th ed., pp. 457–468). Philadelphia: W.B. Saunders Company.

7. S. Robert, R. S. Porter, J. L. Kaplan & M. H. Beers (Eds.) (2007). *Hemostasis. Merck manual for healthcare professionals.* [Online]. Retrieved from http://www. merckmanuals.com/professional/sec11/ch134/ch134a.html

8. Pettker, C. M., & Lockwood, C. V. (2007). Thromboembolic disorders. In S. G. Gabbe, V. R. Niebyl, J. L. Simpson, et al. (Eds.), *Obstetrics: Normal and problem pregnancies* (5th ed., pp. 1064–1079). Philadelphia: Churchill Livingstone.

9. Baktiari, K., Meijers, J. C., deJonge, E., & Levi, M. (2004). Prospective validation of International Society of Thrombosis and Hemostasis scoring system for disseminated intravascular coagulation. *Critical Care Medicine, 33*(12), 2416–2421.

10. Gordon, M. C. (2007). Maternal physiology. In S. G. Gabbe, V. R. Niebyl, J. L. Simpson, et al. (Eds.), *Obstetrics: Normal and problem pregnancies* (5th ed., pp. 55–84). Philadelphia: Churchill Livingstone.

11. Norwitz, E. R., Robinson, J. N., & Malone, F. D. (2004). Pregnancy induced physiologic alterations. In G. A. Dildy, M. A. Belfort, G. R. Saade, et al. (Eds.), *Critical care obstetrics* (4th ed., pp. 19–42). Hoboken, NJ: Wiley-Blackwell.

12. Toh, C., & Downey, C. (2005). Back to the future: Testing in disseminated intravascular coagulation. *Blood Coagulation and Fibrinolysis, 16,* 535–542.

13. Letsky, E. A. (2000). Disseminated intravascular coagulation, best practice and research. *Clinical Obstetrics and Gynecology, 1,* 623–644.

14. Oyelese, Y., & Arbath, C. V. (2006). Placental abruption. *Obstetrics and Gynecology, 108,* 1005–1016.

15. Baxter, V. K., & Weinstein, L. (2004). HELLP syndrome: State of the art. *Obstetrical and Gynecological Survey, 59,* 838–845.

16. Bick, R. L. (2004). Disseminated intravascular coagulation: current concepts of etiology, pathophysiology, diagnosis and treatment. *Hematology Oncology Clinics of North America, 17,* 149–176.

17. Faridi, A., Heyl, W., & Rath, W. (2000). Preliminary results of an international multicenter trial. *International Journal and Obstetrics and Gynecology, 69,* 279–280.

18. Sibai, B. M. (2005). Diagnosis, prevention and management of eclampsia. *Obstetrics and Gynecology, 105,* 402–410.

19. Clark, S. L, Hankins, G. D. V., Dudley, D. A., Dildy, G. A., & Porter, T. F. (1995). Amniotic fluid embolism: Analysis of the national registry. *American Journal of Obstetrics and Gynecology, 172*(4), 1158.

20. Dildy, G. A., & Clark, S. L. (2004). Anaphylactoid syndrome of pregnancy (amniotic fluid embolism). In G. A. Dildy, M. A. Belfort, G. R. Saade, et al. (Eds.), *Critical care obstetrics* (4th ed., pp. 463–471). Hoboken, NJ: Wiley-Blackwell.

21. Gunterpalli, M. D., & Steingrub, J. (2005). Hepatic disease and pregnancy: An overview of diagnosis and management. *Critical Care Medicine, 33*(Suppl. 10), S323–S339.

22. Woodside, K. J., & Hunter, G. C. (2006). Disseminated intravascular coagulation scoring system in the critically ill. *Critical Care Medicine, 34,* 899–900.

23. Dempfle, C. E., Lorenz, S., Smolinski, M., Wurst, M., West, S., Houdijk, W. P., et al. (2004). Utility of activated partial thromboplastin time waveform analysis for identification of sepsis and disseminated intravascular coagulation in patients admitted to a surgical intensive care unit. *Critical Care Medicine, 32,* 520–524.

24. Gando, S., Iba, T., Ohtomo, Y., Ohtomo, Y., Okamoto, K., Koseki, K., et al. Japanese Association for Acute Medicine Disseminated Intravascular Coagulation (JAAM DIC) Study Group. (2006). A multicenter prospective validation of disseminated intravascular coagulation diagnostic criteria for critically ill patients: Comparing current criteria. *Critical Care Medicine, 34,* 625–631.

25. Sacks, D. A. (2004). Blood component replacement therapy. In G. A. Dildy, M. A. Belfort, G. R. Saade, et al. (Eds.), *Critical care obstetrics* (4th ed., pp. 162–183). Hoboken, NJ: Wiley-Blackwell.

26. Smeltzer, S. C., Bare, B. G., Hinkle, J. L., & Cheever, K. H. (Eds.). (2008). Assessment and management of patients with hematologic disorders. *Brunner & Suddarth's textbook of medical-surgical nursing, volume I* (11th ed., pp. 1035–1117). Philadelphia: Lippincott Williams & Wilkins.

27. British Committee for Standards in Haematology, Blood Transfusion Task Force. (2003). Guidelines for the use of platelet transfusions. *British Journal of Hematology, 122*(1), 10–23.

28. Franciois, K. E., & Foley, M. R. (2007). Antepartum and postpartum hemorrhage. In S. G. Gabbe, J. R. Niebyl, & J. L. Simpson (Eds.), *Obstetrics: normal and problem pregnancies* (5th ed., pp. 456–485). Philadelphia: Churchill Livingstone.

29. Zeelander, S., Hack, C. E., & Wuillemin, W. A. (2005). Disseminated intravascular coagulation in sepsis. *Chest, 128,* 2864–2875.

30. Pepas, C. P., Anif-Adib, M., & Kadir, R. (2006). Factor VIIa in puerperal hemorrhage with disseminated intravascular coagulation. *Obstetrics and Gynecology, 108,* 757–761.

31. Moscardo, F., Perez, F., de la Rubia, J., et al. (2001). Successful treatment of severe intra-abdominal bleeding associated with intravascular coagulation using recombinant activated factor VII. *British Journal of Haematology, 113,* 174–176.

32. Prosper, S. C., Goudge, C. S., & Lupo, V. R. (2007). Recombinant factor VIIa to successfully manage disseminated intravascular coagulation from amniotic fluid embolism. *Obstetrics and Gynecology, 109,* 524–525.

33. American College of Obstetrics and Gynecologists (ACOG) (2006). Postpartum Hemorrhage. *ACOG Practice Bulletin No. 76.*

34. American College of Obstetrics and Gynecologists (ACOG) (2006). Medical Emergency Preparedness. *ACOG Committee Opinion No. 353.*

CHAPTER 17

Venous Thromboembolism in Pregnancy

Patricia M. Witcher and Lewis Hamner

Venous thromboembolism (VTE) is a disease process that collectively refers to deep vein thrombosis (DVT) and pulmonary embolism (PE). While the incidence of VTE during pregnancy is unknown, there is a general belief that pregnancy predisposes women to VTE because of changes in the coagulation system during pregnancy. Events and procedures commonly performed during pregnancy have a propensity for thrombogenesis. An understanding of the significance of VTE, physiology of coagulation, and predisposing risk factors facilitates the medical provider and the professional nurse in the identification of women at risk so that appropriate evaluation and treatment can be employed.

INCIDENCE AND SIGNIFICANCE

As many as 30 to 50 percent of DVTs are unrecognized and, if untreated, DVT may progress to PE in about 15 to 25 percent of patients.[1-3] DVT occurs with the same or higher frequency during the antepartum period as the postpartum period.[4-6] The risk for PE is greatest during the postpartum period.[3,6,7] PE is of ultimate concern because of the mortality risk. It remains one of the leading causes of death in pregnant women.[8] Morbidities associated with VTE include pulmonary hypertension (following recovery from an acute PE event), recurrence of VTE, and increased risk for venous insufficiency from compromised blood flow to the affected limb.[9,10]

The incidence of VTE in pregnant women is estimated to be 0.5 to 3 per 1,000 pregnancies across all reproductive ages.[4,11-15] This incidence is somewhat higher than what is reported for the general population, which is estimated to be about 1 to 1.45 per 1,000 adults each year.[16,17] The incidence of VTE in the general population varies based upon ethnicity. Individuals of Asian Pacific or Hispanic descent have a 2.3- to 4-fold lower risk than Caucasians and African Americans.[16] The true incidence of VTE in pregnant women is unknown, but

there is a general belief that pregnancy is associated with as much as a two- to sixfold increase in VTE risk.[3,4,18,19] Vascular and hemostatic changes of pregnancy may account for a potentially increased risk.

PHYSIOLOGY OF COAGULATION

Normal coagulation requires a balance between procoagulants and anticoagulants. Anticoagulants usually exceed procoagulants in the circulation until a triggering mechanism, such as vascular or tissue injury, activates coagulation.[20] The complex system of coagulation relies upon further interaction of anticoagulants and procoagulants so that excessive coagulation does not occur. Typically, injury to the vessel wall or to the red blood cells initially results in vasoconstriction to minimize the surface area that requires clotting and platelet activation. Following platelet activation, platelets adhere to the damaged vessel wall and secrete multiple substances that perpetuate further platelet adherence, platelet aggregation, and activation of clotting factors.[21] What ensues is a complicated sequence of activation of clotting factors with the end result being formation of a stable clot. Figure 17-1 illustrates normal coagulation.

Vascular or tissue trauma, or trauma to the blood itself, may initiate the clotting cascade by what has been referred to as the intrinsic and extrinsic pathways. The intrinsic pathway begins with activation of factor XII. Activated factor XII (XIIa) then activates factor XI (XIa), which cleaves factor IX to form activated factor IX (IXa), which, in turn, activates factor VIII (VIIIa). Factor X becomes activated (Xa) by factor VIIIa as well as from activated factor VII (VIIa) along with the cofactor, tissue thromboplastin, which propagates coagulation via the extrinsic pathway. The extrinsic pathway is also stimulated by vascular or extravascular tissue injury and begins with tissue thromboplastin (factor III). Both the intrinsic and extrinsic pathways converge to the

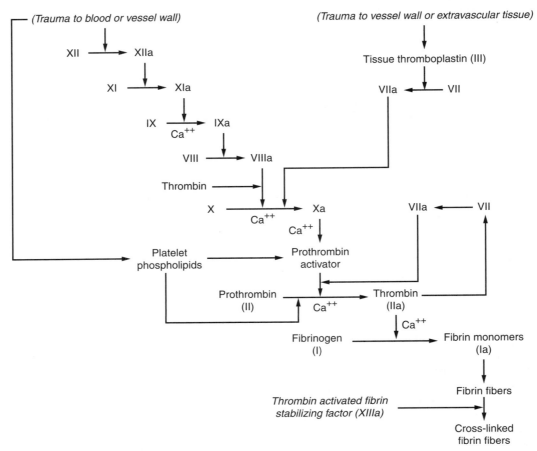

FIGURE 17-1   Coagulation cascade. Adapted from Dizon-Townsend, D., Shah, S. S., & Phelan, J. P. (2004). Thromboembolic disease. In G. A. Dildy, M. A. Belfort, G. R. Saade, et al. (Eds.), *Critical care obstetrics* (4th ed. pp. 275–291). Hoboken, NJ: Wiley-Blackwell; and Guyton, A. C., & Hall, J. E. (2006). *Textbook of medical physiology* (11th ed. pp. 451–468). Philadelphia: Elsevier Saunders.

common pathway, which begins with the activation of factor X (Xa). Prothrombin activator enzymatically cleaves prothrombin into thrombin. Thrombin facilitates further activation of factors V, VIII and XIII and cleaves fibrinogen into fibrin, which combines with other fibrin monomers to form fibrin fibers. Thrombin activates fibrin stabilizing factor (XIIIa), which is released from platelets that are entrapped in the fibrin clot, in order to promote a stable clot by promotion of cross-linkages with and between other fibrin fibers.[20]

Several clotting inhibitors are stimulated by certain clotting factors in an effort to regulate thrombus formation. Figure 17-2 depicts the process responsible for regulation of coagulation. A deficiency or impaired activity in these inhibitors results in excessive clotting. Thrombin that does not absorb to fibrin fibers combines with antithrombin (AT III). In addition to inactivating thrombin, AT III further blocks the activation of fibrinogen. When heparin, which normally exists in low concentrations in the blood, increases in the circulation (i.e., pharmacologic administration) it combines with AT III and removes thrombin as well as activated factors XII, XI, IX and X.[20] Plasminogen activator gradually becomes activated by factor XIIa and converts plasminogen—which is trapped inside the clot—into plasmin, which in turn promotes lysis of the clot. The digestion of fibrin by plasmin yields fibrin degradation products (FDPs), also known as fibrin split products (FSPs), measurement of which provides some evidence of fibrinolysis.[21] Plasmin assists in the regulation of coagulation by digesting coagulation factors XII, VIII, V, and prothrombin.[20] Thrombomodulin, a protein normally bound to the endothelial membrane that specifically binds to thrombin, is another mechanism that prevents further extension of the clot beyond what is required in order to promote hemostasis at the site of vascular injury. The thrombomodulin–thrombin complex, along with protein S, activates protein C, resulting in activated protein C (APC). APC, along with cofactor

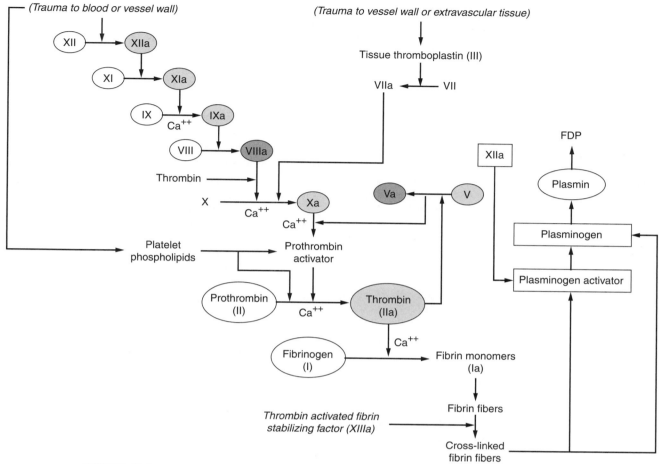

FIGURE 17-2 Regulation of the coagulation cascade. Plasmin digests factors XII, VIII, and V; prothrombin; and fibrinogen. AT III and heparin complex removes thrombin and activated factors XII, XI, X, and IX. Activated protein C along with cofactor, protein S inactivates activated Factors VIII and V. Adapted from Dizon-Townsend, D., Shah, S. S., & Phelan, J. P. (2004). Thromboembolic disease. In G. A. Dildy, M. A. Belfort, G. R. Saade, et al. (Eds.), *Critical care obstetrics* (4th ed. pp. 275–291). Hoboken, NJ: Wiley-Blackwell; and Guyton, A. C., & Hall, J. E. (2006). *Textbook of medical physiology* (11th ed. pp. 451–468). Philadelphia: Elsevier Saunders.

protein S, inactivates factors VIII and V to promote anticoagulation and perpetuate the balance between procoagulants and anticoagulants.

HEMOSTATIC CHANGES DURING PREGNANCY

Rudolf Virchow, a German pathologist, identified three primary mechanisms (Virchow's triad) that lead to thrombosis. These are illustrated in Figure 17-3 and include endothelial damage, venous stasis, and hypercoagulability.

Some degree of vascular damage may occur during vaginal delivery or Cesarean section. Endothelial damage promotes exposure of blood to tissue thromboplastin and activation of the components of the coagulation cascade, although this plays less of a role than the hormonal and hemostatic changes of pregnancy in promoting thrombosis.[16,22] Hormonal and hemodynamic changes of pregnancy contribute to venous stasis because of the increase in circulating blood volume combined with hormonally mediated venous distention and increased blood capacity in the periphery.[3,4,9,22] Venous return is further obstructed by the gravid uterus.[2,3] Reduction in the velocity of blood flow occurs in the lower extremities, starting early in the first trimester and continuing throughout pregnancy and the postpartum period. The decreased blood velocity is more pronounced in the left leg than the right and is thought to result from increased

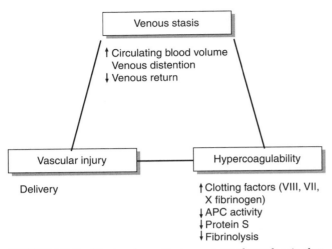

FIGURE 17-3 Mechanisms that promote thrombosis during pregnancy.

compression of the left common iliac vein by the right iliac artery, which crosses on the left side only.[3-4,9] Venous stasis is believed to predispose to thrombus formation because blood stasis reduces clearance of activated clotting factors, thus allowing them to deposit in muscular venous network or in the valve cusp pockets of the deep veins.[6,23] The interaction between the procoagulants and anticoagulants further determines if any thrombus that has formed extends.

Pregnancy-related changes in the coagulation system promote a hypercoagulable state with increases in clotting factors such as factors VIII, VII, X and fibrinogen and decreases in inhibitors of clotting.[3-5,11,22,24,25] These changes are summarized in Figure 17-4. Thrombin generation therefore increases. There are decreases in protein S and increased resistance to activated protein C which contribute to hypercoagulability.[3,5,9,14,22,24,25] Fibrinolysis is

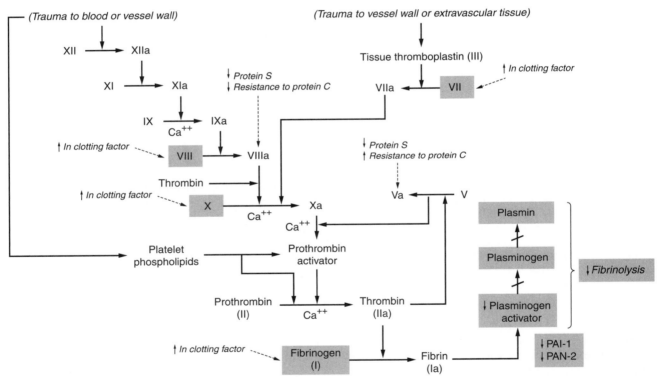

FIGURE 17-4 Pregnancy-related changes in coagulation factors. Pregnancy-related changes are indicated in green. Adapted from Bates, S. M., & Ginsberg, J. S. (2001). Pregnancy and deep vein thrombosis. *Seminars in Vascular Medicine, 1*(1), 97–104; Bloomenthal, D., Delisle, M. F., Tessier, F., & Tsang, P. (2002). Obstetric implications of the factor V Leiden mutation: A review. *American Journal of Perinatology, 19*(1), 37–47; Bowles, L., & Cohen, H. (2003). Inherited thrombophilias and anticoagulation in pregnancy. *Best Practice and Research Clinical Obstetrics and Gynaecology, 17*(3), 471–489; Hague, W. M., & Dekker, G. A. (2003). Risk factors for thrombosis in pregnancy. *Best Practice and Research Clinical Haematology, 16*(2), 197–210; James, A. H., Brancazio, L. R., & Ortel, T. L. (2005). Thrombosis, thrombophilia, and thromboprophylaxis in pregnancy. *Clinical Advances in Hematology and Oncology, 3*(3), 187–97; Rai, R., & Regan, L. (2000). Thrombophilia and adverse pregnancy outcome. *Seminars in Reproductive Medicine, 18*(4), 369–77; and Stone, S. E., & Morris, T. A. (2005). Pulmonary embolism during and after pregnancy. *Critical Care Medicine, 33*(Suppl. 10), S294–S300.

TABLE 17-1

Inherited Thrombophilias in Pregnancy

Highest Risk for VTE	*Modest Risk for VTE*	*Low Risk for VTE*
• Homozygous Factor V Leiden mutation (FVL) • Homozygous prothrombin G20210A mutation • Antithrombin III deficiency • Compound heterozygous FVL and prothrombin G20210A mutation **Acquired** • Antiphospholipid antibodies • Lupus anticoagulant • Anticardiolipin antibody	• Heterozygous FVL • Heterozygous prothrombin G20210A mutation • Activated protein C resistance • Protein S deficiency • 4G/4G Type-1 plasminogen activator inhibitor mutation (PAI-1)	• Methylenetetrahydrofolate reductase (MTHFR C677T) mutation

also reduced, perhaps secondary to a reduction in the activation of plasminogen activator which occurs as a result of decreases in plasminogen activator inhibitors 1 and 2 (PAI-1 and PAI -2).[3–5,14,22,25] The latter is derived from the placenta.[4]

RISK FACTORS FOR VTE

VTE during pregnancy is multifactorial and arises from a complex interaction between the hemostatic changes of pregnancy, underlying thrombophilia, and additional acquired risk factors. In general, women at highest risk for VTE are those with an inherited thrombophilic condition and a prior history of VTE. Thrombophilia may be inherited or acquired; the prevalence of the different thrombophilias varies with regard to ethnicity and thrombogenic potential as well as the predisposition to adverse pregnancy events.[26] The most common acquired thrombophilia is antiphospholipid antibody syndrome (APS), which is characterized by the presence of antiphospholipid antibodies, lupus anticoagulant (LAC), and anticardiolipin antibody (ACLA) with arterial and/or venous thrombosis. There are multiple inherited thrombophilias with varying propensities for thrombosis based upon the specific abnormality. These are listed in Table 17-1. In general, the thrombophilias associated with the highest incidence of VTE are the least common during pregnancy. The thrombophilias that are considered to be the most thrombogenic without a personal or family history of VTE are compound heterozygous factor V Leiden and prothrombin G20210A mutation (inheritance of both thrombophilias), homozygous factor V Leiden mutation, the homozygous form of prothrombin G20210A mutation, and AT III deficiency.[9,26,27]

Women with a previous VTE are considered to be at increased risk for recurrence of VTE during a subsequent pregnancy; the risk for recurrence often depends upon the particular risk factor(s) involved (Table 17-2). In general, women with a history of prior VTE associated with an idiopathic risk factor (i.e., VTE during previous pregnancy, oral contraceptives, or evidence of inherited thrombophilia) are at increased risk for recurrence of VTE compared to women with prior VTE that was associated with a nonrecurrent or transient risk factor (i.e.,

TABLE 17-2

Risk Factors for Venous Thromboembolism During Pregnancy

Risk Factors with Significant Predisposition	• Previous VTE • Personal or family history of VTE • Thrombophilia, acquired or inherited • Age greater than 35 years • Obesity (BMI >30.0) • Cesarean section
Other Risk Factors	• Operative delivery or instrumentation • Major pelvic or abdominal surgery at time of Cesarean section • Higher parity • Prolonged immobility • Active infection or inflammatory process • Dehydration • Gross varicose veins • Chronic disease process (such as nephrotic syndrome, sickle cell disease, heart disease)

BMI = body mass index, VTE = venous thromboembolism

prolonged immobility or surgery).[27,28] Additionally, those women with a family history of VTE in a first-degree relative (i.e., parent or sibling) before age 50 may also be at increased risk for VTE during pregnancy.[27]

Other risk factors, with or without underlying thrombophilia, contribute to thrombogenesis, again emphasizing that VTE is a multifactorial process. The risk factors, other than personal or family history of VTE or thrombophilia, that carry the greatest predisposition to VTE during pregnancy include increasing age, obesity, and mode of delivery, primarily Cesarean section.[2,9,10,12,13,16,9,29–32] Increasing age and obesity may contribute to the risk of VTE secondary to disturbed blood flow, increase in clotting factors, or impaired fibrinolytic activity.[16] The risk for VTE in the general population varies based upon type of surgical procedure as well as the presence of other comorbid conditions, with the greatest risk occurring in orthopedic surgery or surgery for malignancies. Surgical procedures, such as laparotomy, may present less risk for VTE because of reduced tissue damage from the surgical procedure and/or better mobilization following surgery.[16] Although Cesarean section may be considered a relatively low-risk surgical procedure (i.e., early mobilization following delivery and short duration of surgery), it is believed to increase the risk for VTE two- to tenfold over vaginal delivery, possibly from endothelial or vascular damage during delivery.[7,12] The majority of postpartum PE is most strongly associated with Cesarean section over other modes of delivery.[13] Emergency Cesarean section is more hazardous than elective Cesarean section.[2,33] Obesity, while an independent risk factor for VTE, also presents additional predisposition at the time of Cesarean section for VTE. These include a higher risk of blood loss from delivery, prolonged operating time, increased use of uterotonics, and postpartum wound infection or endometritis.[30]

The presence of multiple risk factors, with or without Cesarean section, increases the risk for VTE. These include operative vaginal delivery, major pelvic or abdominal surgery at the time of Cesarean section, higher parity, prolonged immobility, inflammatory process or active infection, dehydration, gross varicose veins, or chronic disease such as nephrotic syndrome, sickle cell disease, or heart disease.[7,9,10,13,14,22,34,35] The presence of multiple risk factors, rather than a single risk factor, is probably of greater concern regarding the overall risk for VTE. Consensus is lacking as to which risk factors necessitate thromboprophylaxis.[27,36–38] The decision to administer anticoagulants for either prophylaxis or treatment versus no pharmacologic treatment during the antpartum and postpartum periods is individualized based upon the physician's assessment of the patient's VTE history, thrombogenecity of the inherited thrombophilia, and presence of additional risk factors.

In general, postpartum anticoagulant dosages should be equivalent or greater to the dosages prescribed during the antepartum period.[27]

THROMBOPHILIAS

Antithrombin Deficiency

AT deficiency arises from multiple possible mutations that result in either reduction in circulating AT III or decreased AT III activity. The deficiency promotes increased thrombosis because of reduction in or impaired removal of thrombin and activated factor X (Xa). Regulation of coagulation is further hindered by the deficiency in AT because the in-activation of factors XIIa, XIa, and IXa is blocked. Inheritance of AT deficiency is typically by autosomal dominance and almost always presents in the heterozygous state. Homozygous manifestation of AT deficiency is extremely rare and is usually lethal early in life through neonatal thrombosis.[39] AT deficiency is the rarest thrombophilia.

Factor V Leiden Mutation

Factor V Leiden mutation (FVL) manifests functionally as resistance to activated protein C and involves a mutation in the factor V gene, rendering it resistant to cleavage by activated protein C. Activated protein C resistance (APCR) hinders the breakdown of factor Va, creating a hypercoagulable state as a result of increased generation of thrombin.[9,11,23,25] APCR is the most common cause of VTE; more than 95 percent of APCR is caused by FVL.[11] FVL is more prevalent in Western Europeans and Caucasians compared to a low incidence in those of African American or Asian descent.[9,11,26] FVL mutation occurs in heterozygous (expression on one allele) and homozygous (expression on both alleles) forms. Homozygous FVL, which is less prevalent than the heterozygous form, confers a much higher risk for VTE compared to the risk with the heterozygous form.[11,26,40]

Prothrombin Gene (G20210A) Mutation

Prothrombin gene G20210A mutation, named accordingly due to the location of the mutation on the prothrombin gene, promotes VTE as a result of an increase in circulating levels of prothrombin. Like FVL, it demonstrates homozygosity and heterozygosity. Homozygosity for the prothrombin mutation presents a much higher risk of VTE, similar to that with homozygous FVL or AT deficiency. Heterozygous prothrombin gene G20210A mutation, while more prevalent, carries a lower risk for VTE in comparison to the homozygous form. Compound heterozygotes for FVL and prothrombin G20210A mutation (possessing one allele from each variant) are at higher risk for VTE compared to heterozygotes for FVL or the prothrombin gene mutation.

Deficiencies in Protein C and Protein S

Protein C and S deficiencies propagate VTE from either decreased circulating levels or impaired activity of protein C or protein S. Although relatively rare, their ability to promote thrombosis is high, similar to the VTE risk associated with FVL and the prothrombin gene mutation.[26]

Methylenetetrahydrofolate Reductase C677T Mutation

A mutation in the enzyme methylenetetrahydrofolate reductase (MTHFR C677T) interferes with normal metabolism of homocysteine to methionine, an essential amino acid. Elevation in homocysteine levels is further exacerbated by folic acid deficiency. Hyperhomocysteinemia, along with a deficiency in folic acid, has been noted in women whose children were born with neural tube defects.[41] Severe hyperhomocysteinemia, although rare, also predisposes individuals to significant neurologic abnormalities, premature atherosclerosis, and VTE.[26] Venous thromboembolism is not linked directly to the MTHFR mutation, but predisposes individuals with this genetic variant to VTE when there is a concomitant vitamin B deficiency (vitamin B_{12} and folic acid). While a risk for non-pregnant individuals, this mutation does not appear to increase the risk for VTE in pregnant women, probably as a result of a normal physiologic reduction in homocysteine levels and/or folic supplementation during pregnancy directed at reducing the risk of neural tube defects in the fetus.[9] Although the risk for VTE is low, women with hyperhomocysteinemia are predisposed to adverse pregnancy outcomes such as early pregnancy loss or severe preeclampsia.[40] This warrants educating the woman about the importance of daily folic acid and vitamin B supplements.

Antiphospholipid Syndrome

Antiphospholipid syndrome (APS) is an autoimmune disorder characterized by systemic abnormalities that arise from vascular thrombosis (venous and arterial), elevated circulating levels of anticardiolipin antibody (ACL), and lupus anticoagulant (LA). It is the most common cause of acquired thrombophilia during pregnancy and has significant maternal–fetal implications.[19,42] The antiphospholipid antibodies (APLAs) anticardiolipin (ACL) and lupus anticoagulant (LA) are closely related autoantibodies that have been associated with arterial or venous thromboses secondary to their reaction with phospholipid components of cellular membranes.[26,42]

Thromboses from APLAs may occlude any blood vessel throughout the body. Arterial thrombosis may lead to stroke, which is the most common consequence of arterial thrombosis, or other neurologic insults. Other sites of arterial thrombosis include retinal, subclavian, digital or brachial arteries. Venous thrombosis leads most often to lower extremity VTE with progression to PE.[26] While thrombosis remains the most problematic of complications, APLAs also account for adverse pregnancy outcomes, including recurrent pregnancy loss, preeclampsia, and intrauterine fetal growth restriction.[19,42]

Screening for Thrombophilia

Laboratory screening for the presence of inherited thrombophilias appears to offer a logical strategy for the prevention of VTE. Despite the strong association between thrombophilia and thrombosis, however, the presence of a thrombophilic condition, by itself, does not necessarily result in a thrombotic event during pregnancy, despite the hypercoagulable state of pregnancy.[27,36] Additionally, although an association has been proposed between thrombophilic conditions and adverse pregnancy outcomes—such as fetal loss, placental abruption, intrauterine growth restriction, and preeclampsia[9,11,43]—a definitive link has not been established.[27,44] Routine laboratory screening for thrombophilia is therefore controversial, and probably of little value.[27,36] Laboratory screening for thrombophilias may be useful if detection of a particular thrombophilia would lead to the decision to proceed with prophylaxis during pregnancy or postpartum even in the absence of an indication for anticoagulant administration.[27]

Laboratory screening during pregnancy, if it is determined to be indicated, is problematic because the hemostatic changes in pregnancy necessitate adaptation of cutoff values for interpretation.[9,22] Thus, screening is often deferred until after the initial postpartum period. Whenever possible, laboratory testing for thrombophilia is generally performed while the patient is not pregnant, not on anticoagulant therapy or prophylaxis, and remote from the VTE event (after 6 weeks).[27] Identification of genetic mutations, such as FVL or prothrombin G20210A mutation, is not altered by pregnancy and can be tested during pregnancy. However, many providers may choose to defer laboratory screening until complete evaluation can be performed.

DEEP VEIN THROMBOSIS

Clinical Manifestations

DVT may manifest as leg swelling with or without pain or tenderness. However, signs and symptoms are clinically

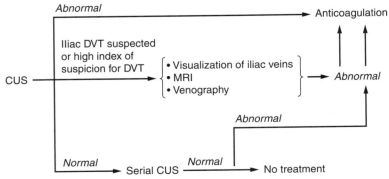

FIGURE 17-5 Diagnosis of deep vein thrombosis. Adapted from Dizon-Townsend, D., Shah, S. S., & Phelan, J. P. (2004). Thromboembolic disease. In G. A. Dildy, M. A. Belfort, G. R. Saade, et al. (Eds.), *Critical care obstetrics* (4th ed. pp. 275–291). Hoboken, NJ: Wiley-Blackwell; Laros, R. K. (2004). Thromboembolic disease. In R. K. Creasy, R. Resnik, & J. D. Iams (Eds.), *Maternal-fetal medicine. Principles and practice* (5th ed. pp. 845–858). Philadelphia: W.B. Saunders Company; Ginsberg, J. S., & Bates, S. M. (2003). Management of venous thromboembolism during pregnancy. *Journal of Thrombosis and Haemostasis, 1*(7), 1435–1442; and Stone, S. E., & Morris, T. A. (2005). Pulmonary embolism during and after pregnancy. *Critical Care Medicine, 33*(Suppl. 10), S294–S300.

unreliable; fewer than 50 percent of suspected cases of DVT are confirmed with objective testing.[4,22] Objective diagnostic evaluation is often warranted in order to reduce unnecessary exposure to therapeutic anticoagulation. Many of the diagnostic tests available to nonobstetric providers provide less reliable confirmation in the obstetric population or are less desirable in obstetrics due to concern for fetal radiation exposure. Furthermore, the diagnostic tests have not been rigorously researched in the obstetric population; interpretation of test results in women during pregnancy and the postpartum period often requires modification of the plan of care that follows.

In the pregnant woman, DVT usually occurs more often in the proximal leg veins.[45] Initial evaluation includes collection of detailed data that may indicate DVT. Pain, tenderness, and/or swelling are unilateral. The affected leg is considered to be edematous when there is a greater than 2 cm difference in the circumference between the leg with a DVT and the leg without a DVT. Swelling may or may not be accompanied by pain or tenderness. Homans' sign is positive when passive dorsiflexion of the foot of the relaxed affected leg produces pain, typically in the calf or popliteal areas.[21] Iliac DVT may be suspected when the entire leg is edematous and back pain is present.[18] Findings of marked edema, cyanosis or pallor, or a cold extremity are less common; their presence may indicate obstruction from ileofemoral thrombosis, which is rare.[21]

Clinical diagnosis of DVT is often difficult. The vast majority of women with leg swelling or pain do not have DVT. While every woman with this complaint does not require diagnostic testing, other findings that strengthen the suspicion of DVT during the initial evaluation may lead the obstetric provider to perform objective diagnostic testing. Risk factors, such as personal or family history of VTE, prolonged bedrest, or a recent surgical procedure may warrant diagnostic testing. Additionally, the majority of DVT during pregnancy occur in the left leg.[3,4,9,18,45] The etiology is attributed to increased compression of the left common iliac vein by the right iliac artery, which only crosses on the left side.[3,4,9,18] Presence of symptoms in the left leg may prompt further diagnostic evaluation as well.

Diagnostic Evaluation

In general, diagnostic evaluation begins with noninvasive tests (Fig. 17-5). Compression ultrasound (CUS) including Doppler is sensitive and specific for the diagnosis of proximal DVT in symptomatic, non-pregnant individuals. Although it has not been meticulously evaluated in the obstetric population, it is the method of choice for initial evaluation of DVT symptoms because there is no radiation exposure and no known risks.[4,18,21,22,38] CUS utilizes an ultrasound transducer placed over the vein that detects changes in sound frequency that characterize venous flow and allows evaluation of the venous anatomy. Maneuvers such as voluntary contraction of the calf muscles, Valsalva's maneuver, direct compression of the veins with the ultrasound probe, and, to some extent, direct visualization of a mass in the vessel lumen, enable the examiner to identify filling defects of the lumen, which may indicate thrombosis as well as other etiologies producing pain and swelling.[21,38] Alone, CUS is less accurate for isolated calf thrombosis; therefore, serial CUS is employed in order to exclude possibility of extension of a calf vein thrombosis.[21] The care providers reinforce with the woman that CUS is typically repeated within a few days to a week of the initial exam to exclude the possibility of DVT.[18,21,38] CUS is also unreliable for the detection of isolated iliac DVT, because inferior vena cava compression by the gravid uterus may obscure the ability to visualize the iliac vessels. Further diagnostic testing may be necessary if iliac DVT is suspected.[4,21]

Limited venography, in which the abdomen is shielded with a lead apron, may be required to diagnose calf DVT when initial noninvasive tests are equivocal or a high index of suspicion continues despite negative CUS. Complete venography without a lead apron or MRI may be considered when iliac DVT is suspected and cannot be ruled out with initial tests.[18] Visualization of filling defects aided by the injection of contrast dye in more than one radiographic view identifies a DVT.[21] While it remains the gold standard for diagnosis of DVT during pregnancy, venography has considerable limitations.[4,18,21,38] Fetal radiation exposure, while a concern in general, is less than 1.0 rads (0.01 Gy). This level is well below the minimum level that would be considered teratogenic and below the level associated with development of childhood cancers, which is 5 to 10 rads (0.05 to 0.1 Gy).[4,21] Abdominal shielding reduces exposure further to less than 0.05 rads (0.0005 Gy).[4] Despite the reassurance that fetal radiation exposure is reduced, other limitations remain. Results may be unreliable because of incomplete filling of the iliac and femoral veins due to their large diameter. Accurate results are also dependent upon the examiner's technique, site of selection for injection of the contrast dye, positioning of the patient, muscular contraction, or other pathology, such as a hematoma, cellulitis, edema, or muscle rupture. Additionally, venography is associated with phlebitis from the contrast dye. This risk can be reduced by a lower concentration of the contrast medium, heparinized saline flush after dye injection, and use of corticosteroids.[21] Contrast dye is excreted by the kidneys, and some media are nephrotoxic; the patient is encouraged to maintain adequate fluid intake in order to promote dilution of the dye and its elimination.

Magnetic resonance imaging (MRI) of the lower extremities has the potential for use during pregnancy. It appears to be sensitive for isolated iliac DVT and femoral-popliteal DVT without radiation exposure, but has not yet been incorporated into management guidelines for diagnosis of DVT during pregnancy.[3,4,18,21,38]

Other methods used to diagnose DVT in the nonobstetric population, such us impedance plethysmography (IPG) and D-dimer testing, are not typically incorporated into the evaluation scheme for DVT during pregnancy. IPG diagnoses DVT through the detection of venous flow by electrical impedance. Inflation of a thigh cuff occludes venous return; thereby increasing the volume in the calf veins. In the absence of thrombosis, abrupt release of thigh cuff pressure induces rapid venous flow which increases the electrical resistance to flow in the calf. Thrombosis is implicated when the venous flow is decreased as a result of venous obstruction.[21,38] Compression of the inferior vena cava by the gravid uterus can produce false positive results; its utility in pregnancy is unclear.[21,38] However, if selected as a method for diagnosis of DVT, like CUS, serial testing is recommended when it is negative for DVT.[14] D-dimer measures fibrin degradation in the circulation as a result of fibrin generation during clotting. A negative D-dimer excludes DVT in the nonobstetric population; a positive assay indicates further objective diagnostic evaluation. D-dimer testing for DVT has not been evaluated in pregnancy and is of limited value during pregnancy. A negative result is unlikely, due to a progressive increase in D-dimer levels as normal pregnancy advances. Additionally, elevated D-dimer levels may also be associated with preterm labor, placental abruption, and hypertensive disorders of pregnancy.[3,4]

PULMONARY EMBOLISM

Clinical Manifestations

When DVT progresses to pulmonary embolism (PE), it often does so without any signs or symptoms until the individual presents with cardiopulmonary compromise.[38] Signs and symptoms of PE are nonspecific.[14] Dyspnea and tachypnea are the most common symptoms that prompt further evaluation. Clinical presentation with complaints of shortness of breath and/or chest pain prompt the provider to evaluate vital signs along with arterial oxygen saturation (SaO$_2$) while collecting further data that will facilitate medical diagnosis and the treatment course. Although absent in many individuals with PE, other signs and symptoms include pleuritic chest pain, cough, hemoptysis, and friction rub. Chest pain, tachycardia, hypotension, atelectatic crackles, diaphoresis, cyanosis, and syncope are more significant signs and symptoms that suggest possible massive PE, defined as 50 percent or greater occlusion of the pulmonary artery circulation. These manifestations may also initially implicate myocardial infarction in the differential diagnoses.[21,38] Prompt recognition and expeditious physician notification are warranted because of the potential for cardiopulmonary compromise. The medical provider is optimally informed of tachycardia, tachypnea, and/or hypotension as well as SaO$_2$ of less than 90 percent on room air. Interventions, such as lateral positioning, intravenous volume expansion, and/or initiation of pharmacotherapy are directed at restoring hemodynamic stability. Continued decrease in SaO_2 despite administration of supplemental oxygen may necessitate intubation and mechanical ventilation in order to restore adequate oxygenation. The care providers can anticipate that laboratory and further clinical evaluation will accompany stabilization measures and initiation of heparin therapy.

Initial laboratory studies include electrocardiogram (ECG), arterial blood gas analysis, and possibly a chest radiograph (X-ray). Tachycardia is the most common cardiac arrhythmia. Some women may exhibit nonspecific T-wave inversion and ECG changes indicative of right-sided strain or axis shift.[38] Unless the woman is significantly compromised in her pulmonary status, an arterial blood gas analysis is usually obtained while the woman is breathing room air. An arterial partial pressure of oxygen (PaO_2) greater than 80 to 85 mmHg may rule out PE in some circumstances. However, additional diagnostic studies may be needed to avoid consequences stemming from thrombosis.[21,38] A chest X-ray often reveals some abnormality nonspecific to PE; its utility lies in excluding other causes of pulmonary signs and symptoms.[21]

Diagnostic Evaluation

Therapeutic heparin is usually initiated as soon as PE is suspected and continued until diagnostic studies exclude PE.[38] Initial diagnostic studies usually commence with ventilation-perfusion (V/Q) scan or spiral computed tomography (CT) scan; both are noninvasive. The V/Q scan provides visualization of perfusion and air distribution in the lungs using a radiographic tracer that is injected intravenously (perfusion) and inhaled (ventilation), with radiographic views in multiple positions in order to detect a perfusion defect, indicative of obstructed blood flow from the thrombus in the pulmonary circulation. The amount of radiation exposure varies with the radioisotopes used and is within the safe range of 0.006 to 0.018 rads (0.6^{-4} to 0.18^{-4} Gy) for the perfusion scan and 0.001 and 0.035 rads (0.1^{-4} to 0.35^{-4} Gy) for the ventilation scan.[3] The results from V/Q scanning can be described as normal (normal perfusion and ventilation), low probability, high probability (perfusion defect with normal ventilation), and nondiagnostic or intermediate.[18,38] A normal V/Q scan indicates the absence of perfusion and ventilation abnormalities and excludes the diagnosis of PE. A high probability scan, especially if coupled with high pre-test probability or clinical manifestations suggestive of PE, may be considered sufficient to proceed with therapeutic anticoagulation for PE. Because other

pulmonary abnormalities such as pneumonia, atelectasis, effusion, or a mass can produce perfusion defects, further objective testing may be warranted before confirming the diagnosis of PE. Similarly, low probability scans are interpreted in light of the clinical likelihood of PE based upon presenting symptoms.[3,21,38] The majority of V/Q scans fall in the nondiagnostic or intermediate category, neither excluding nor confirming PE.[21] Therefore, further diagnostic studies may be incorporated into the medical plan of care.

Spiral CT is an alternative to the V/Q scan and is gaining popularity for the diagnosis of PE. Some institutions have replaced V/Q scanning with spiral CT in their diagnostic algorithm for PE.[38] Spiral CT requires intravenous injection of contrast dye in order to provide views of the pulmonary circulation; the fetal radiation exposure is comparable to V/Q scanning.[3,21] A summary of diagnostic studies for the confirmation of PE is provided in Figure 17-6.

Pulmonary arteriography remains the definitive method for confirming the diagnosis of PE. Injection of contrast dye selectively into the lobar or segmental branches of the pulmonary artery allows for visualization of filling defects or termination of vessels which may indicate thrombosis.[21] Although the gold standard, this study is typically reserved for individuals in whom PE cannot be diagnosed or excluded or in those rare individuals in whom initiation of thrombolytic therapy (i.e., tissue plasminogen activator) or surgical intervention (i.e., pulmonary embolectomy) is contemplated as a life-preserving measure.[21,38] Pulmonary arteriography has been largely replaced by noninvasive studies. Another approach is to follow nondiagnostic V/Q scans or V/Q scans with low clinical suspicion for PE, with bilateral CUS. If CUS is abnormal, PE may be confirmed. If CUS is normal, then progression to pulmonary arteriography or serial CUS while initiating therapeutic heparin may be considered to confirm or rule out the diagnosis of PE.[18]

PROPHYLAXIS AND TREATMENT DURING THE ANTEPARTUM PERIOD

Consideration of VTE prophylaxis in women at low to moderate risk for VTE is based upon expert opinion, extrapolated from nonobstetric studies.[26,38] Anticoagulation is indicated for the prevention and treatment of thrombosis in women at high risk and very high risk for VTE. Unfractionated heparin or low-molecular-weight heparin (LMWH) are the most commonly used pharmacologic agents. When directed at prophylaxis, small doses of anticoagulants are able to inhibit the initiation of the clotting cascade. However, once thrombin

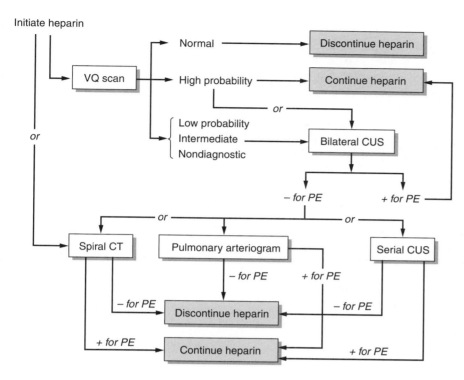

Initiate heparin

FIGURE 17-6   Diagnosis of pulmonary embolism. Adapted from Dizon-Townsend, D., Shah, S. S., & Phelan, J. P. (2004). Thromboembolic disease. In G. A. Dildy, M. A. Belfort, G. R. Saade, et al. (Eds.), *Critical care obstetrics* (4th ed. pp. 275–291). Malden, MA: Blackwell Publishing; Laros, R.K. (2004). Thromboembolic disease. In R. K. Creasy, R. Resnik, & J. D. Iams (Eds.), *Maternal-fetal medicine: Principles and practice* (5th ed. pp. 845–858). Philadelphia: W.B. Saunders Company; Ginsberg, J. S., & Bates, S. M. (2003). Management of venous thromboembolism during pregnancy. *Journal of Thrombosis and Haemostasis, 1*(7), 1435–1442; and Stone, S. E., & Morris, T. A. (2005). Pulmonary embolism during and after pregnancy. *Critical Care Medicine, 33*(10 Suppl), S294–S300.

has formed, higher doses are required to restrict further extension of a clot.[21]

Heparin

Heparin does not cross the placenta due to its large molecular size and does not predispose the fetus to the risk of hemorrhage or teratogenesis.[3,4] Heparin inhibits clotting by binding to antithrombin III. Once bound to AT III, the complex primarily facilitates binding and neutralization of activated factor X (Xa) and thrombin. Heparin is not absorbed by the gastrointestinal tract, therefore parenteral administration is required. It may be administered subcutaneously or intravenously; intramuscular administration is inadvisable due to the potential for hematoma formation as well as unpredictable absorption rates by this route.[21] When heparin is selected for the treatment of VTE, therapeutic doses of heparin by the intravenous route are conventionally employed in order to ensure more predictable absorption. The intravenous loading dose is usually within the range of 70 to 100 units/kg,[8,21,24,46] or 5,000 to 10,000 units with a minimum loading dose of 5,000 units.[18,21,24] Higher loading doses up to 150 units/kg or 15,000 units may be required for acute PE.[21] Following the loading dose, maintenance infusion may be initiated at a rate of 15 to 25 units/kg/hour and titrated every 4 to 6 hours to achieve an aPTT of 1.5 to 2.5 times control values or about 60 to 80 seconds.[14,18,21,38,46] Anticoagulation is therapeutic within this range; an aPTT level of less than

1.5 times control is associated with thrombus extension and an aPTT level that exceeds 2.5 times the control is associated with increased risk for bleeding episodes.[38] Spontaneous hemorrhage is associated with an aPTT greater than 135 seconds for longer than 12 hours, necessitating interruption of heparin therapy and administration of protamine sulfate.

Duration of intravenous heparin therapy is continued until symptoms resolve and there is no evidence of recurrence of thrombus formation before transitioning to subcutaneous heparin or LMWH in therapeutic doses—about 5 to 7 days for acute PE or 3 to 5 days for DVT.[3,21,38] Table 17-3 summarizes intravenous heparin infusion for VTE and dosing parameters based upon aPTT levels. Following initial treatment, subcutaneous administration of either heparin or LMWH is begun and continued for 3 to 6 months up to 6 to 12 weeks postpartum; the duration and dosage depend upon the VTE event and predisposing risk factor(s).[4,14,38] The medical provider will typically also consider the risk factors and VTE event that require conversion to prophylactic doses or continuation of therapy at an adjusted dosage for the remainder of the pregnancy and postpartum period. Adjusted-dose heparin incorporates similar dosing schedules as described for intravenous administration and is titrated to achieve a therapeutic aPTT of 1.5 to 2.5 times control. Subsequent pregnancies or future surgical procedures that predispose the woman to an increased risk of VTE will typically necessitate prophylaxis again, depending upon the particular risk factors.

TABLE 17-3

Intravenous Heparin Infusion

IV loading dose **(Minimum 5000 units IV)**	70 to 100 units/kg OR 5,000–10,000 units (Acute PE: up to 150 units/kg or 15,000 units)
Maintenance infusion	Initial dose/rate: 30,000 units/24 hr = 1250 units/hr OR 15 to 25 units/kg

Obtain aPTT 4–6 hours after loading dose

aPTT (seconds)	Dosage	Laboratory Evaluation
<50	Re-bolus. **AND (increase infusion rate as ordered)** ↑ 120 units/hr (↑ 1–2 units/kg/hr as ordered)	aPTT in 4–6 hr
50–59	↑ 120 units/hour (↑ 1–2 units/kg/hr as ordered)	aPTT in 4–6 hr
60–85	No change	aPTT in AM
86–95	↓ 80 units/hr (↓ 1–2 units/kg/hr as ordered)	aPTT in AM
96–120	Hold infusion for 30 min **AND** ↓ 80 units/hr	aPTT in 4–6 hr
>120	Hold infusion for 60 min **AND** ↓ 160 units/hr (↓ 2–3 units/kg/hr as ordered)	aPTT in 4–6 hr

Adapted from Dizon-Townsend, D., Shah, S. S., & Phelan, J. P. (2004). Thromboembolic disease. In G. A. Dildy, M. A. Belfort, G. R. Saade, et al. (Eds.), *Critical care obstetrics* (4th ed. pp. 275–291). Malden, MA: Blackwell Publishing.

Prophylactic dosing regimens for heparin during pregnancy include administration of 5,000 units subcutaneously every 12 hours throughout pregnancy or progressive increases in the dose with advancing gestation: 5,000 to 7,500 units subcutaneously every 12 hours in the first trimester, 7,500 to 10,000 units subcutaneously every 12 hours in the second trimester, and 10,000 units subcutaneously every 12 hours during the third trimester.[21,27,38] See Table 17-4 for a summary of dosages. Certain women will require an adjusted anticoagulation dosage if they are at exceptionally high risk for recurrent VTE. Dosages are directed at achieving a therapeutic aPTT. Heparin requirements may increase in pregnancy due to increased circulating proteins that bind to heparin, increased clearance of heparin by the kidneys secondary to increased glomerular filtration rate and/or increased placental degradation of heparin.[3] Additionally, anticoagulation protocols have been derived from literature focused on the nonobstetric population. Therefore, aPTT is usually monitored every 1 to 2 weeks in order to determine heparin requirements as pregnancy advances.[4]

Complications From Heparin
Although uncommon, potential maternal complications with heparin therapy include bleeding, osteoporosis,

and immune-mediated reactions. The risk for bleeding is approximately 2 percent, similar to the risk in the nonobstetric population; the risk for spontaneous hemorrhage increases significantly when the aPTT exceeds 135 seconds for longer than 12 hours.[4] When bleeding occurs or aPTT levels are significantly above therapeutic control, the nurse can anticipate orders for the administration of protamine sulfate. One milligram of protamine sulfate is required to neutralize 100 units of a heparin. Protamine sulfate, while given to neutralize heparin, possesses mild anticoagulant properties. Therefore, no more than 50 mg of protamine sulfate should be administered during a 10-minute period because of the risk of further bleeding.[38]

Long-term heparin therapy is associated with osteopenic fractures due to decreases in bone density with doses that exceed 15,000 units per day for more than 6 months.[38] Bone density changes are partially reversible; the risk for osteoporosis can be reduced by administering calcium and vitamin D.[4,24,38] Other less severe reactions include hypotension, alopecia, allergic reactions, pain at the injection site, and thrombocytopenia.[38] Thrombocytopenia may be attributed to either heparin-associated platelet agglutination or aggregation, which is mild and self-limited, or to heparin-

TABLE 17-4

Subcutaneous Anticoagulant Dosing During Pregnancy

Prophylactic Doses
    Heparin
- First trimester: 5,000–7,500 units every 12 hours
- Second trimester: 7,500–10,000 units every 12 hours
- Third trimester: 10,000 units every 12 hours unless aPTT is elevated
  OR
- Minidose: 5,000 every 12 hours
  5000–10,000 units every 12 hours throughout pregnancy

**   *Low-Molecular-Weight Heparins (LMWH)***

enoxaparin	40 mg once daily
dalteparin	5,000 units once or twice daily
tinzaparin	4,500 units once daily (may require dosage modification for extremes of body weight)

Intermediate-Dose LMWH

enoxaparin	40 mg every 12 hours
dalteparin	5,000 units every 12 hours

Adjusted-Dose Therapy

May target an anti-Xa level of 0.6 to 1.0 units/mL for twice daily dosing or slightly higher for once-daily dosing

    Heparin   More than 10,000 units every 12 hours adjusted for aPTT 1.5 to 2.5 times control (60–80 seconds) 6 hours after injection

**   *LMWH***

enoxaparin	1 mg/kg every 12 hours
dalteparin	200 units/kg once daily or every 12 hours
tinzaparin	175 units/kg once daily

Adapted from American College of Obstetricians and Gynecologists. (2010). Inherited thrombophilias in pregnancy. Practice Bulletin Number 113. *Obstetrics and Gynecology, 116,* 212–222.

induced thrombocytopenia (HIT), which is associated with more significant complications.[38] HIT involves an immune-mediated thrombocytopenia from IgG anti-platelet antibodies resulting in platelet activation and extension of venous thrombosis or development of new arterial thrombus.[3,24,46] The incidence of HIT is about 1 to 3 percent, with a 30 percent risk of mortality and a 20 percent risk of amputation of the affected limb in the nonobstetric population.[24]

HIT is suspected when platelets fall by 50 percent from the baseline within 5 to 15 days of initiating heparin. Heparin is discontinued while alternate anticoagulant therapy is considered by the medical provider. Platelet transfusion is relatively contraindicated; a prescriptive plan that includes non-heparin anticoagulants such as heparinoids like danaparoid, direct thrombin inhibitors such as lepirudin, or a direct factor Xa inhibitor such as fondaparinux[46,47] typically occurs only after consultation with a hematologist.[24]

The initial platelet count is reviewed prior to initiating heparin, with additional evaluation of platelet count within 5 to 15 days after initiating heparin. The nurse informs the medical provider of decreased platelet count and withholds the next dose of heparin if platelet count is less than 50,000 until further directed by the medical provider. The nurse also monitors for signs of increased bleeding. Increased bruising, particularly at the injection sites, may indicate faulty injection as well as propensity for bleeding; the nurse reviews intramuscular injection technique with the woman who self-administers heparin outpatient.

Low-Molecular-Weight Heparins

LMWHs do not cross the placenta and are considered a safe alternative to heparin during pregnancy.[3,4] They are produced by chemical cleavage of heparin, thereby yielding a smaller molecular chain. Because of the smaller chain, LMWHs preferentially inactivate factor X without acting on thrombin; thereby exerting anticoagulant effects with significantly less risk for bleeding than heparin. They also carry a lower incidence of severe thrombocytopenia and osteoporosis.[38] LMWHs have less variable absorption rates and therefore do not require monitoring in the non-pregnant population.[24] LMWHs are less protein-bound compared to heparin, but increased renal clearance and placental degradation may decrease the effectiveness of the dose typically provided for non-pregnant individuals. Monitoring anti-Xa activity [3,4,38] as well as dose adjustments during pregnancy may be necessary; however, recommendations by experts differ.[28,48,49–51] When given during pregnancy, the dosage of LMWHs is adjusted based upon maternal weight. Should monitoring be desired, anti-Xa activity levels are obtained mid-dose (i.e., 6 hours after the morning dose of every 12 hour schedule of enoxaparin).[18] The target range is 0.15 to 0.3 international units (IU)/mL when given for prophylaxis and between 0.5 and 1.0 IU/mL when given for treatment of VTE or in women at very high risk for recurrent VTE.[24,28] Anti-Xa monitoring is not routinely available in most hospitals; a laboratory external to the admitting hospital may be required. LMWHs are more expensive than heparin; this disadvantage is overcome by the lack of requirement for monitoring in non-pregnant individuals. The decision to monitor only adds to the cost of therapy, which may reduce its attractiveness in some settings. There are three LMWHs currently available in the United States: enoxaparin (Lovenox), tinzaparin (Innohep), and dalteparin (Fragmin). Medical providers have most experience with enoxaparin during pregnancy. Dosage schedules are summarized in Table 17-4.[18,27]

Warfarin

Warfarin (Coumadin) is typically reserved for administration during the postpartum period because it crosses the placenta and is associated with embryopathy if there is exposure during the first 6 to 12 weeks of pregnancy.[4,24] Exposure later in pregnancy increases the risk of fetal bleeding; the fetal liver is immature, and vitamin K–dependent clotting factors in the fetal circulation are low.[35] The risk for spontaneous abortion or stillbirth is also increased from placental hemorrhage.[38] Antepartum administration following counseling regarding the risks of warfarin during pregnancy is confined to women who may require the better prophylaxis offered by warfarin, such as those with mechanical heart valves or AT deficiency with prior VTE. For those women who consent to warfarin therapy during pregnancy, heparin is typically administered for the first 14 weeks of pregnancy before transitioning to warfarin for the remainder of the pregnancy.[38] Warfarin is addressed further with discussion of postpartum management later in this chapter.

Mechanical Prophylaxis

Intermittent compression of the leg muscles with pneumatic or sequential compression devices counteracts venous stasis by promoting blood flow during bedrest or general anesthesia.[7] Although data are limited, it is suggested that women undergoing Cesarean birth are at higher risk for VTE, especially if emergency Cesarean

section is required. Additional accompanying risk factors as described earlier in this chapter may further increase the risk. Women at moderate risk for VTE may benefit from mechanical prophylaxis during Cesarean birth; the recommendation for pneumatic compression during and after Cesarean birth is based upon expert opinion and data are limited.[15,34,37] Additionally, there are no data as to which compression sleeve, such as a boot, calf sleeve, or calf-to-thigh sleeve provides the most adequate prophylaxis. Therefore, the decision to implement mechanical prophylaxis for antepartum patients or those women undergoing Cesarean birth is individualized based upon physician discretion and institutional guidelines. Pneumatic compression, if implemented, is probably most beneficial if applied prior to Cesarean delivery and continued postpartum until the woman is fully ambulatory. This may not be feasible in women undergoing unanticipated or emergency Cesarean birth, as a delay in emergency birth may ensue due to placement of the compression sleeves. In these situations, mechanical compression is implemented following delivery in the recovery room whenever possible.

INTRAPARTUM CONSIDERATIONS

The risk of hemorrhage during labor and birth requires consideration as to timing and selection of anticoagulation. Cesarean birth is associated with a higher risk for hemorrhage; the risk for hemorrhage from vaginal birth increases if there is thrombocytopenia or uterine atony.[21] Heparin or LMWH is generally discontinued 24 hours prior to induction of labor or as soon as spontaneous labor begins.[18] Elevated, or therapeutic, aPTT levels may persist for up to 28 hours, necessitating discontinuation of heparin earlier than 24 hours in women on higher doses of heparin. Intravenous heparin may be required in these women who are at especially high risk for VTE (i.e., artificial heart valves, recent PE, or recent ileofemoral thrombosis) during labor with efforts to discontinue heparin 4 to 6 hours before anticipated delivery; this timeframe is based upon the premise that aPTT levels would more than likely be within normal range at the time of delivery.[18,38] Therapeutic anticoagulation, especially with LMWHs, may predispose the woman to spinal or epidural hematoma with regional anesthesia. The option of regional anesthesia is preserved whenever possible because of the risks of general anesthesia in the obstetric population. Many providers elect to convert women from LMWH to heparin as early as 36 to 38 weeks gestation with discontinuation of heparin before induction or onset of spontaneous labor to preserve the option of regional anesthesia for labor and/or Cesarean birth.[40] A shortened timeframe from discontinuation of anticoagulants to onset of labor (less than 12 to 24 hours) may prohibit regional anesthesia, but this is controversial.[18,24] Although there are no data in pregnant women, up to 5,000 units of heparin does not appear to present a significant risk for epidural or spinal hematoma. The American Society of Regional Anesthesia recommends that regional anesthesia be delayed for 24 hours after the last dose of LMWH if adjusted-dose therapy was employed during the antepartum period. Needle insertion is delayed for at least 12 to 24 hours after the last dose of LMWH when lower doses or prophylactic doses have been administered.[18,24] Regional anesthesia may similarly be delayed after the last dose of heparin in most clinical settings as well. Laboratory monitoring, even of anti Xa levels, probably does not adequately predict the risk for bleeding.

Additional precautions are often required for those few women who require warfarin during the antepartum period because it may take anywhere from 3 to 14 days for the fetal effects from anticoagulation to abate, which significantly increases the risk for fetal hemorrhage as well as maternal hemorrhage. Obstetric and anesthesia providers should be informed of the last dose of warfarin administration prior to admission for childbirth. The order for 5 mg of oral or subcutaneous vitamin K may be anticipated in order to normalize the PT within 6 hours. The newborn may also be administered 1 mg vitamin K intramuscularly immediately after delivery. Because difficult or instrumental delivery cannot be anticipated in many circumstances, it may be prudent to thaw fresh frozen plasma (FFP) within about 40 to 60 minutes prior to the anticipated time of delivery to manage any additional maternal or fetal bleeding that may be encountered; FFP is more likely to be required for a newborn at 35 weeks gestation or less.[38]

POSTPARTUM MANAGEMENT

Following delivery, re-initiation or new initiation of heparin or LMWH is typically delayed for 12 to 24 hours after the last epidural dose or catheter removal providing the woman is stable.[18] Pneumatic compression devices are continued until the woman is ambulatory unless otherwise ordered by the obstetric provider. Heparin or LMWH resumption with conversion to warfarin during hospitalization is ideal in order to ensure adequate laboratory monitoring. Along with resumption of dosage schedule administered for heparin or LMWH during the antepartum period, warfarin may be initiated in doses of 10 to 15 mg orally once daily.[21] Heparin is generally continued until the international normalized ratio (INR) is sustained between 2.0 and 3.0 for 2 consecutive days or 3.0 to 4.0 if VTE prophylaxis is indicated for a mechanical heart valve.[40] Warfarin is then continued for 4 to 6 weeks postpartum or up to a minimum of 3 months total duration for VTE in the index pregnancy.[3,4] Warfarin is considered to be safe in breast-feeding women, but this is somewhat controversial.[38]

SUMMARY

The risk factors for thrombogenesis as well as how pregnancy influences the risk for VTE are primarily based upon expert opinion in the literature rather than randomized clinical trials that have focused specifically on the pregnant population. Therefore, the decision to incorporate mechanical and/or pharmacologic prophylactic measures into best practice guidelines is determined and individualized by each health care institution. During pregnancy, women present additional challenges that often require consideration when generating and applying such guidelines. The clinical presentation may be obscured by normal pregnancy complaints often necessitating objective diagnostic testing. Selection of tests is based upon potential maternal–fetal risks as well as reliability in identifying DVT and/or PE in the obstetric population. Finally, selection and administration of anticoagulants during pregnancy and the postpartum period often requires adjustments in order to achieve adequate therapeutic levels while minimizing the risks to the woman and her developing fetus and newborn. The plan of care for women at risk for VTE or who experience a VTE event is interdisciplinary with collaboration from obstetricians, anesthesiologists, and obstetric nurses. Consultation with medical, surgical, or hematologic specialists may also be helpful.

REFERENCES

1. Bick R. L., & Kaplan, B. L. (2004). Thromboprophylaxis in surgical patients. *European Journal of Medical Research*, 9(3), 104–111.
2. Eldor, A. (2001). Unexplored territories in the nonsurgical patient: A look at pregnancy. *Seminars in Hematology*, 39(2 Suppl. 5), 39–48.
3. Stone, S. E., & Morris, T. A. (2005). Pulmonary embolism during and after pregnancy. *Critical Care Medicine*, 33(Suppl. 10), S294–S300.
4. Bates, S. M., & Ginsberg, J. S. (2001). Pregnancy and deep vein thrombosis. *Seminars Vascular Medicine*, 1(1), 97–104.
5. Hague, W. M., & Dekker, G. A. (2003). Risk factors for thrombosis in pregnancy. *Best Practice and Research Clinical Haematology*, 16(2), 197–210.
6. Helt, J. A., Kobbervig, C. E., James, A. H., Petterson, T. M., Bailey, K. R., & Melton, L. J. 3rd. (2005). Trends in the incidence of venous thromboembolism during pregnancy or postpartum: A 30-year population-based study. *Annals of Internal Medicine*, 143(10), 697–706.
7. Samama, C. M., Albaladejo, P., Benhamou, D., Bertin-Maghit, M., Bruder, N., Doublet, J. D., et al. Committee for

Good Practice Standards of the French Society for Anaesthesiology and Intensive Care (SFAR). (2006). Venous thromboembolism prevention in surgery and obstetrics: Clinical practice guidelines. *European Journal of Anaesthesiology, 23*(2), 95–116.

8. Berg, C. J., Chang, J., Callaghan, W. M., & Whitehead, S. J. (2003). Pregnancy-related mortality in the United States, 1991–1997. *Obstetrics and Gynecology, 101*(2), 289–286.

9. Greer, I. A. (2004). Prevention of venous thromboembolism in pregnancy. *European Journal of Medical Research, 9*(3), 135–145.

10. Gates, S., Brocklehurst, P., & Davis, L. J. (2002). Prophylaxis for venous thromboembolic disease in pregnancy and the early postnatal period. *The Cochrane Database of Systematic Reviews, 2,* CD001689.

11. Bloomenthal, D., Delisle, M. F., Tessier, F., & Tsang, P. (2002). Obstetric implications of the factor V Leiden mutation: A review. *American Journal of Perinatology, 19*(1), 37–47.

12. Casele, H., & Grobman, W. A. (2006). Cost-effectiveness of thromboprophylaxis with intermittent pneumatic compression at cesarean delivery. *Obstetrics and Gynecology, 108*(3 Part 1), 535–540.

13. Gates, S. (2000). Thromboembolic disease in pregnancy. *Current Opinion in Obstetrics and Gynecology, 12*(2),117–122.

14. Kent, N., Leduc, L., Crane, J., Farine, D., Hodges, S., Reid, G. J., et al. (2000). Prevention and treatment of venous thromboembolism (VTE) in obstetrics. *JSOGC, 22*(9), 736–749.

15. Quinones, J. N., James, D. N., Stamilio, D. M., Cleary, K. L., & Macones, G. A. (2005). Thromboprophylaxis after cesarean delivery: A decision analysis. *Obstetrics and Gynecology, 106*(4), 733–740.

16. Ageno, W., Squizzato, A., Garcia, D., & Imberti, D. (2006). Epidemiology and risk factors of venous thromboembolism. *Seminars in Thrombosis and Hemostasis, 32*(7), 651–658.

17. Spyropoulos, A. C. (2005). Emerging strategies in the prevention of venous thromboembolism in hospitalized medical patients. *Chest, 128*(2), 958–969.

18. Ginsberg, J. S., & Bates, S. M. (2003). Management of venous thromboembolism during pregnancy. *Journal of Thrombosis and Haemostasis, 1*(7), 1435–1442.

19. Porter, T. F., & Scott, J. R. (2005). Evidence-based care of recurrent miscarriage. *Best Practice & Research Clinical Obstetrics & Gynaecology, 19*(1), 85–101.

20. Guyton, A. C., & Hall, J. E. (2006). *Textbook of medical physiology* (11th ed., pp. 451–468). Philadelphia: Elsevier Saunders.

21. Dizon-Townsend, D., Shah, S. S., & Phelan, J. P. (2004). Thromboembolic disease. In G. A. Dildy, M. A. Belfort, G. R. Saade, et al. (Eds.), *Critical care obstetrics* (4th ed., pp. 275–291). Malden, MA: Blackwell Publishing.

22. James, A. H., Brancazio, L. R., & Ortel, T. L. (2005). Thrombosis, thrombophilia, and thromboprophylaxis in pregnancy. *Clinical Advances in Hematology and Oncology, 3*(3), 187–197.

23. Weitz, J. I., Hirsh, J., & Samama, M. M. (2004). New anticoagulant drugs: The seventh ACCP conference on antithrombotic and thrombolytic therapy. *Chest, 126*(Suppl. 3), 265S–286S.

24. Bowles, L., & Cohen, H. (2003). Inherited thrombophilias and anticoagulation in pregnancy. *Best Practice & Research Clinical Obstetrics & Gynaecology, 17*(3), 471–489.

25. Rai, R., & Regan, L. (2000). Thrombophilia and adverse pregnancy outcome. *Seminars in Reproductive Medicine, 18*(4), 369–377.

26. Lockwood, C. J., & Silver, R. (2004). Thrombophilias in pregnancy. In R. K. Creasy, R. Resnik, & J. D. Iams (Eds.), *Maternal-fetal medicine: Principles and practice* (5th ed., pp. 1005–1021). Philadelphia: W.B. Saunders Company.

27. American College of Obstetricians and Gynecologists. (2010). Inherited thrombophilias in pregnancy. Practice Bulletin Number 113. *Obstetrics and Gynecology, 116,* 212–222.

28. Weitz, J. I. (2009). Prevention and treatment of venous thromboembolism during pregnancy. *Catheterization and Cardiovascular Interventions, 74*(Suppl. 1), S22–S26.

29. Greer, I. A. (2006). Anticoagulants in pregnancy. *Journal of Thrombosis and Thrombolysis, 21*(1), 57–65.

30. Andreasen, K. R., Andersen, M. L., & Schantz, A. L. (2004). Obesity and pregnancy. *Acta Obstetricia Et Gynecologica Scandinavica, 83*(11), 1022–1029.

31. Jacobsen, A. F., Drolsum, A., Klow, N. E., Dahl, G. F., Qvigstad, E., & Sandset, P. M. (2004). Deep vein thrombosis after elective cesarean section. *Thrombosis Research, 113*(5), 283–288.

32. Porreco, R. P., Adelberg, A. M., Lindsay, L. G., & Holdt, D. G. (2007). Cesarean birth in the morbidly obese woman: A report of 3 cases. *Journal of Reproductive Medicine, 52*(3), 231–234.

33. Jackson, N., & Paterson-Brown, S. (2001). Physical sequelae of caesarean section. *Best Practice & Research Clinical Obstetrics & Gynaecology, 15*(1), 49–61.

34. Gidiri, M., Sant, M., Philips, K., & Lindow, S. W. (2004). Thromboprophylaxis for caesarean section: How can update and coverage be improved? *Journal of Obstetrics and Gynaecology, 24*(4), 392–394.

35. Greer, I. A. (2003). Prevention of venous thromboembolism in pregnancy. *Best Practice and Research Clinical Haematology, 16*(2), 261–278.

36. Simioni, P. (2009). Thrombophilia and gestational VTE. *Thrombosis Research, 123*(Suppl. 2), S41–S44.

37. Bates, S. M., Greer, I. A., Hirsh, J., & Ginsberg, J. S. (2004). Use of antithrombotic agents during pregnancy: The seventh ACCP conference on antithrombotic and thrombolytic therapy. *Chest, 126*(Suppl. 3), 627S–644S.

38. Laros, R. K. (2004). Thromboembolic disease. In R. K. Creasy, R. Resnik, & J. D. Iams (Eds.), *Maternal-fetal medicine: Principles and practice* (5th ed., pp. 845–858). Philadelphia: W.B. Saunders Company.

39. Kobayashi, T. (2005). Antithrombin abnormalities and perinatal management. *Current Drug Targets, 6*(5), 559–566.

40. Wu, O., Robertson, L., Twaddle, S., Lowe, G. D., Clark, P., Greaves, M., et al. (2006). Screening for thrombophilia in high-risk situations: Systematic review and cost-effectiveness analysis. The Thrombosis: Risk and Economic Assessment of Thrombophilia Screening (TREATS) study. *Health Technology Assessment, 10*(11), 1–110.

41. Nussbaum, R. L., McInnes, R. R., & Willard, H. F. (Eds.). (2001). *Thompson and Thompson genetics in medicine* (6th ed. pp. 289–310). Philadelphia: W.B. Saunders Company.

42. Khare, M., & Nelson-Piercy, C. (2003). Acquired thrombophilias and pregnancy. *Best Practice & Research Clinical Obstetrics & Gynaecology, 17*(3), 491–507.

43. Said, J. M., Higgins, J. R., Moses, E. K., Walker, S. P., Borg, A. J., Monagle, P. T., et al. (2010). Inherited thrombophilia polymorphisms and pregnancy outcomes in nulliparous women. *Obstetrics and Gynecology, 115*(1), 5–13.

44. Silver, R. M., Zhao, Y., Spong, C. Y., Sibai, B., Wendel, G. Jr., Wenstrom, K., et al. Eunice Kennedy Shriver National Institute of Child Health and Human Development Maternal-Fetal Medicine Units (NICHD MFMU) Network. (2010). Prothrombin Gene G20210A mutation and obstetric complications. *Obstetrics and Gynecology, 115*(1), 14–20.

45. Wee-Shian, C., Spencer, F. A., & Ginsberg, J. S. (2010). Anatomic distribution of deep vein thrombosis in pregnancy. *CMAJ, 182*(7), 657–660.

46. Gibson, P. S., & Powrie, R. (2009). Anticoagulants and pregnancy: When are they safe? *Cleveland Clinic Journal of Medicine, 76*(2), 113–127.

47. Hirsh, J., Guyatt, G., Albers, G. W., Harrington, R., & Schünemann, H. J. (2008). Executive summary: American College of Chest Physicians evidence-based clinical practice guidelines (8th ed.). *Chest, 133,* 71S–109S.

48. Bombeli, T., Raddatz Mueller, P., & Fehr, J. (2001). Evaluation of an optimal dose of low-molecular-weight heparin for thromboprophylaxis in pregnant women at risk of thrombosis using coagulation-activation markers. *Haemostasis, 31*(2), 90–98.

49. Norris, L. A., Bonnar, J., Smith, M. P., Steer, P. J., & Savidge, G. (2004). Low molecular weight heparin (tinzaparin) therapy for moderate risk thromboprophylaxis during pregnancy: A pharmacokinetic study. *Thrombosis and Haemostasis, 92*(4), 791–796.

50. Ellison, J., Walker, I. D., & Greer, I. A. (2000). Antenatal use of enoxaparin for prevention and treatment of thromboembolism in pregnancy. *BJOG, 107*(9), 1116–1121.

51. Kher, A., Bauersachs, R., & Nielsen, J. D. (2007). The management of thrombosis in pregnancy: Role of low-molecular-weight heparin. *Thrombosis and Haemostasis, 97*(4), 505–513.

CHAPTER 18

Sepsis in Pregnancy

Julie M. R. Arafeh and Bonnie K. Dwyer

The systemic response to infection can evoke a spectrum of disease states generally and collectively referred to as sepsis. Sepsis is a long-standing leading cause of death in adult intensive care units (ICUs); and, according to the most recent data published by the National Institutes of Health (NIH), is one of the leading causes of death in the United States.[1,2] Although the incidence of one sepsis-related disease state, specifically septic shock, during pregnancy is rare, it remains a major contributor to maternal mortality.[3]

Standardized terminology was described and adopted in 1992 that encompassed a range of illnesses called *sepsis*. A consensus, with respect to terminology, provided a framework from which subsequent research has drawn to refine both diagnostic and clinical management strategies. Based on this research, a series of time-sensitive clinical management goals were identified and grouped into *bundled protocols*. The purpose of these protocols is to foster early recognition and treatment of severe sepsis. Inherent in these protocols is provision of patient care in an intensive care environment where appropriate resources are available, and collaboration may be facilitated.

This chapter reviews the epidemiology and primary etiologies of sepsis, specifically sepsis in an obstetric population. Sepsis-related definitions and critical pathophysiologic concepts are presented. Significant complications related to sepsis are reviewed, and clinical management strategies are described, including the critical role of collaboration.

EPIDEMIOLOGY

Several large population-based studies have examined the incidence of sepsis and its associated mortality. Dombrovsky and colleagues conducted a trend analysis from the years 1993 to 2003 that studied hospitalization rates for patients with severe sepsis, and subsequent mortality and case fatality rates.[1] Data were collected by the Nationwide Inpatient Sample (NIS), a 20% stratified

sample of all United States community hospitals. Analysis of data revealed that hospital admissions for patients with severe sepsis nearly doubled from 1993 to 2003. The mortality rate from the same time period also significantly increased. Despite the overall increase in the number of cases, a decrease was seen in the case fatality rate. Hospitalization and mortality rates were higher for men compared with women; but, interestingly, the case fatality rate was higher for women. The most common site of infection was the respiratory tract.

An observational cohort pan-European study was subsequently conducted regarding the incidence of sepsis in ICUs in 24 European countries, and used the same operational definitions as the study by Dombrovsky.[4] Over 3,000 patients, admitted with a diagnosis of sepsis over a two-week study period, were included in the study. The diagnosis of sepsis was noted in more than 35% of patients admitted to an ICU. In units with a high incidence of admissions secondary to sepsis, a higher mortality rate was also noted. Variables associated with a higher mortality rate included: a more severe degree of organ failure, advanced age, and other medical conditions such as cirrhosis or an excessive positive fluid balance. The responsible microorganism was identified in only 60% of patients in the study. Gram-negative and gram-positive microorganisms were found in cultures with similar frequency. As in the study by Dombrovsky, the most frequent site of infection was the lung.

INCIDENCE IN PREGNANCY

Multiple studies have addressed sepsis during pregnancy. Mabie and colleagues reported results from their study of a series of 18 pregnant women diagnosed with sepsis collected over a ten-year period.[3] They estimated the incidence to be 1 in 8,338 deliveries. In their series, the causes of sepsis were pyelonephritis (6), chorioamnionitis (3), toxic shock (2), postpartum endometritis (2), septic abortion (1), ruptured appendix (1), ruptured ovarian abscess

TABLE 18-1

Consensus Conference Definitions of Sepsis: 1992

Term	Definition
Infection	Microbial phenomenon characterized by an inflammatory response to the presence of microorganisms or the invasion of normally sterile host tissue by those organisms.
Bacteremia	The presence of viable bacteria in the blood.
Systemic inflammatory response syndrome/SIRS	The systemic inflammatory response to a variety of severe clinical insults including: trauma, burns, pancreatitis, and infection.
Sepsis	The systemic response to infection.
Severe sepsis	Sepsis associated with organ dysfunction, hypoperfusion, or hypotension. Hypoperfusion and perfusion abnormalities may include, but are not limited to, lactic acidosis, oliguria, or an acute alteration in mental status.
Septic shock	Sepsis with hypotension, despite adequate fluid resuscitation, along with the presence of perfusion abnormalities that may include, but are not limited to, lactic acidosis, oliguria, or an acute alteration in mental status. Patients who are on inotropic or vasopressor agents may not be hypotensive at the time that perfusion abnormalities are measured.
Hypotension	A systolic BP <90 mmHg or a reduction of >40 mmHg from baseline in the absence of other causes for hypotension.
Multiple organ dysfunction syndrome/MODS	Presence of altered organ function in an acutely ill patient such that homeostasis cannot be maintained without intervention.

*Lower limits of normal systolic blood pressures of obstetric patients have yet to be established. Although patients may have a systolic pressure <90 mmHg and are able to maintain perfusion pressures, the threshold for inadequate pressure may only be slightly below 90 mmHg. Therefore, obstetric patients with lower than normal systolic blood pressure or MAPs may require alternative methods to identify hypotension of sepsis.

Data from Members of the American College of Chest Physicians/Society of Critical Care Medicine Consensus Conference Committee. American College of Chest Physicians/Society of Critical Care Medicine Consensus Conference: Definitions for sepsis and organ failure and guidelines for the use of innovative therapies in sepsis. (1992). *Critical Care Medicine, 20,* 864–874.

(1), necrotizing fasciitis (1), and bacterial endocarditis (1). The mortality rate was 28%. *Escherichia coli,* group A beta-hemolytic *Streptococcus,* and group B *Streptococcus* were the organisms most often identified. In 2003, Kankuri and colleagues reported results from a study of pregnant women with sepsis which included 43,483 deliveries that occurred between the years 1990 and 1998.[5] They calculated the incidence of sepsis with bacteremia to be 1 in 1,060. Variables most often associated with sepsis, in the setting of documented bacteremia, included obesity, primiparous status, preterm delivery, and Cesarean delivery. Of the 41 women who had sepsis with bacteremia, 1 developed septic shock. No deaths were reported.

A review article on sepsis in pregnancy by Fernandez-Perez and colleagues reported that sepsis in pregnancy was a rare event; the incidence of sepsis in their review declined from 0.6% in 1979 to 0.3% in 2000.[6] However, they concluded that when sepsis did occur in pregnancy, the potential for maternal mortality was significant. Such trend analyses are possible in part because of international consensus on the definition of *sepsis.*

DEFINITIONS

In 1992, a consensus committee from the American College of Chest Physicians (ACCP) and the Society of Critical Care Medicine (SCCM) published definitions of infection, bacteremia, systemic inflammatory response system (SIRS), sepsis, severe sepsis, and septic shock.[7] Definitions described by this committee are presented in Table 18-1. These definitions were revised in 2001, during an International Sepsis Definitions Conference that included representation from the SCCM, the European Society of Intensive Care Medicine, the ACCP, the American Thoracic Society, and the Surgical Infection Society.[8] The goal of the conference was to make revisions that more clearly defined the clinical criteria for SIRS and sepsis, in order to facilitate diagnosis. The revised criteria are presented in Table 18-2. Although the revised criteria can provide a useful framework from which early diagnosis may be facilitated, they are not necessarily specific to SIRS or sepsis. Future understanding of the pathophysiology of sepsis, with respect to its triggers and mediators, may provide better tools for early identification and diagnosis. For example, when the role of inflammatory mediators in the systemic response to infection is better understood, these mediators may be useful as biochemical markers for SIRS and sepsis.[8]

PATHOPHYSIOLOGY

The pathophysiology of sepsis, the role of the immune system in sepsis, and the individual response of the

TABLE 18-2

Signs of Systemic Inflammation in Response to Suspected or Documented Infection and Normal Changes in Pregnancy that Mimic Systemic Inflammation

Parameter	Nonpregnant: SSC Findings Consistent with Presumptive Sepsis	Pregnant or Postpartum: Normal Alterations that Mimic Sepsis
General Findings		
Fever	Core temperature >38.3°C	
Hypothermia	Core temperature <36°C	Both magnesium sulfate therapy and epidural anesthesia may lower temperature.
Heart rate (HR)	>90 beats per minute or >2 σ above normal for age	HR increased in pregnancy; further increases in labor; further increases secondary to number of fetuses.
Tachypnea	Respiratory rate greater than normal	
Altered mental status		
Significant edema or positive fluid balance	>20 mL/kg over 24 hours	• Decreased COP predisposes to generalized edema, pulmonary edema, and dependent edema. • Preeclampsia may cause nonseptic endothelial damage, causing proteinacious extravascular fluid leakage.
Hyperglycemia in the absence of diabetes	Plasma glucose >120 mg/dL or 7.7 mmol/L	
Inflammatory Findings		
Leukocytosis	WBC count >12,000 μL	OB patients ↑ WBC counts • normal in pregnancy: 5000–12,000/uL • average in labor: up to 14,000–16,000/uL • late labor and postpartum: up to 25,000/uL • post Cesarean section: up to 30,000/uL
Leukopenia	WBC count <4000 μL	
Normal white blood cell (WBC) count	With >10% immature forms	Immature forms of WBC increase with contractions, delivery, and postpartum
Plasma C-reactive protein	>2 σ above the normal value	The validity of relying on elevated C-reactive protein (CRP) in the diagnosis of sepsis in obstetric patients remains unknown. In normal pregnancy, CRP increases early in pregnancy and may remain elevated long after delivery of the infant. Elevated CRP is also found in pregnant patients (independent of BMI) at risk for type 2 diabetes mellitus.
Plasma procalcitonin	>2 σ above the normal value	Procalcitonin (PCT) levels in pregnancy have been shown to be elevated in patients with PROM without evidence of clinical infection. The usefulness of PCT levels in the diagnosis of sepsis in obstetric patients is unknown at this time.
Hemodynamic Findings		
Arterial hypotension	SBP <90 mmHg, MAP <70 mmHg, or an SBP decrease >40 mmHg or <2 σ below normal for age	• MAP at 36–38 weeks gestation: 85 mmHg to 95 mmHg • Normal MAP postpartum: 69 mmHg to 94 mmHg
SvO$_2$	>70%	Normally elevated during labor, delivery, and immediately postpartum
Cardiac index	>3.5 L/min/m^2	Cardiac output (CO) in pregnancy significantly increases and is further increased during labor, delivery, and operative delivery. • CO at 20–28 weeks: +32% • CO at 36–38 weeks: +43% • Term: 6–7 L/min (at rest) • Term labor: ↑ 40%–50%

TABLE 18-2 (Continued)

Signs of Systemic Inflammation in Response to Suspected or Documented Infection and Normal Changes in Pregnancy that Mimic Systemic Inflammation

Parameter	Nonpregnant: SSC Findings Consistent with Presumptive Sepsis	Pregnant or Postpartum: Normal Alterations that Mimic Sepsis
Organ Dysfunction Findings		
Arterial hypoxemia	PaO_2/FiO_2 <300	Since values for pregnancy have not been determined, these parameters may be used as a guideline for diagnosis
Acute oliguria	Urine output <0.5 mL·kg·hr or 45 mmol/L for at least 2 hrs	
Creatinine increase	>0.5 mg/dL	
Coagulation abnormalities	INR >1.5 or aPTT >60 secs	
Ileus	Absent bowel sounds	
Thrombocytopenia	Platelet count <100,000 µL	
Hyperbilirubinemia	Plasma total bilirubin >4 mg/dL or 70 mmol/L	
Tissue Perfusion Findings		
Hyperlactatemia	>1 mmol/L	• Maternal serum lactate increases during labor and delivery. The increase is related to the duration of labor, pushing, and delivery. • Elevation of serum lactate has also been reported in nonlabor patients on beta-mimetic therapy for preterm labor.
Decreased capillary refill or mottling		

σ = standard deviation; aPTT = activated partial thromboplastin time; BMI = body mass index; INR = international normalized ratio; PROM = prolonged rupture of the membranes; SBP = systolic blood pressure.

Data from Cano, A., Martínez, P., Parrilla, J. J., & Abad, L. (1985). Effects of intravenous ritodrine on lactate and pyruvate levels: Role of glycemia and anaerobiosis. *Obstetrics and Gynecology, 66*(2):207–210; Levy, M. M., Fink, M. P., Marshall, J. C., Abraham, E., Angus, D., Cook, D., et al. SCCM/ESICM/ACCP/ATS/SIS (2003). SCCM/ESICM/ ACCP/ATS/SIS International Sepsis Definitions Conference. *Critical Care Medicine, 31*, 1250–1256; Qiu, C., Sorensen, T. K., Luthy, D. A., & Williams, M. A. (2004). A prospective study of maternal serum C-reactive protein (CRP) concentrations and risk of gestational diabetes mellitus. *Paediatric and Perinatal Epidemiology, 18*, 377–384; and Torbé, A. (2007). Maternal plasma procalcitonin concentrations in pregnancy complicated by preterm premature rupture of membranes. *Mediators of Inflammation*, Article ID 35782, pp. 1–5. Retrieved from http://www.hindawi.com/journals/mi/2007/035782/abs

host are not completely understood. These concepts are the focus of research and continue to generate debate. Historically, antimicrobial therapy was the mainstay for treatment of sepsis. However, despite the widespread use of antibiotics and pharmacologic advances, mortality rates have remained essentially unchanged. The lack of a favorable impact of antibiotics on mortality rates has prompted further study into the role of the immune system in sepsis. A prevalent hypothesis attributes the pathophysiologic alterations of sepsis to immune system dysfunction or maladaptation. The degree of immune dysfunction is likely related to multiple factors, including the virility of the pathogen, the health status of the host, the genetic response of the host to infection, and the severity of the infection.[9]

THE IMMUNE SYSTEM

A thorough discussion of the immune system is beyond the scope of this chapter; however, a review of key concepts is presented in order to facilitate understanding of the pathogenesis of sepsis. The goals of the immune system are to prevent and fight infection; however, the process is not completely understood. In addition, the ability of an individual's immune system to respond to pathogens may be unique and subsequently play a role in the course infection takes in that person.

After epithelial penetration, the first line of immune defense is white blood cells such as granulocytes, macrophages, and monocytes. Surface receptors called *toll-like receptors* (TLRs), located on antigen-presenting

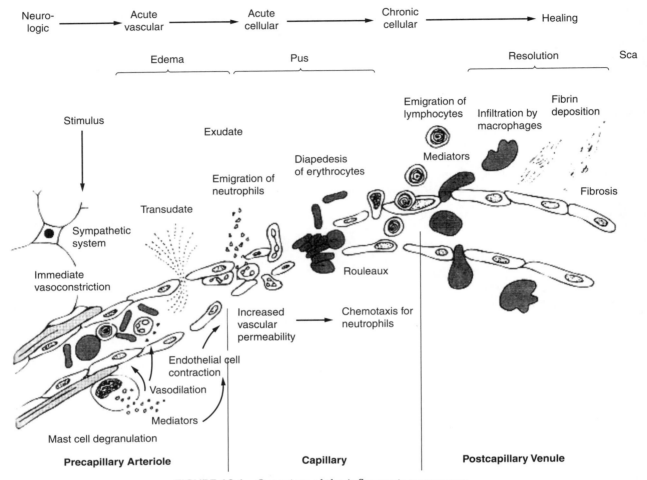

FIGURE 18-1   Overview of the inflammatory process.

cells including granulocytes, macrophages, and monocytes, recognize specific patterns on the surface of microorganisms (pathogen-associated molecular patterns or PAMPs). TLRs react with the pathogen and release substances that activate the immune system.[10] Specific TLRs recognize specific groups of microorganisms. For example, TLR4 recognizes the lipopolysaccharide of gram-negative bacteria, while TLR3 recognizes viruses. As a group, TLRs provide early detection and response to invading pathogens. However, the specific activation of individual TLRs may in part explain the variety of courses different infections often take. Further study may reveal methods to measure TLR response, which may facilitate identification of the pathogen, enhance prediction of complications, and determine treatment to optimize the immune response, especially in cases where the individual response is either too aggressive or absent.[11]

If these immune mechanisms are insufficient to control the pathogen, a second form of immunity, called *adaptive immunity*, is activated. Adaptive immunity is triggered by a specific antigen and has memory for that antigen; this permits rapid response following subsequent exposures. This response is mediated by the release of signaling molecules called *cytokines*. Cytokines mediate the processes of inflammation, including but not limited to vasodilation, vasopermeability, activation of adhesion molecules, and coagulation. An overview of the inflammatory response is depicted in Figure 18-1. Cytokine release can lead to damage of healthy endothelium, resulting in pathologic vasodilation and vasopermeability. This may also include activation of the coagulation cascade and depression of fibrinolysis. Increased vasopermeability and vasodilation ultimately lead to the clinical syndrome termed *distributive shock*, manifested by hypotension and decreased systemic vascular resistance (SVR). Subsequently, oxygen transport is impaired and the risk of end-organ dysfunction or failure is increased. Activation of the coagulation cascade results in the formation of thrombi in the microcirculation, which results in the mechanical obstruction of oxyhemoglobin reaching distal capillaries. This further interferes with oxygen delivery to tissues.[9]

Although dysfunction or maladaptation of the immune system likely facilitates pathophysiologic changes associated with sepsis, therapies developed to counteract pro-inflammatory mediators have yielded mixed results in clinical trials. It is clear that the cascade of inflammatory mediators involved in the development of sepsis is complex. In the future, purposeful manipulation of cytokine activity may be therapeutic; however, the physiologic effects of cytokines must first be better understood.[12,13]

Genetic polymorphism also likely plays a role in an individual's inflammatory response and susceptibility to infection. A polymorphism is a common variation in a gene or DNA sequence. These alterations may or may not have a noticeable effect on gene function. Polymorphisms of cytokine or cytokine receptor genes can, however, result in an imbalance in the anti-inflammatory and pro-inflammatory responses to microorganisms. Inflammatory maladaptation may decrease survival in patients with sepsis. Polymorphisms that affect the ability of immune cells to identify specific microorganisms may also alter the disease course. Continued research may provide evidence regarding why different patients with sepsis have different systemic responses, under what seem to be similar clinical circumstances.[14]

ALTERATIONS IN HEMODYNAMIC FUNCTION

The pathophysiologic events described above lead to alterations in hemodynamic function.[15] A thorough discussion of clinical concepts related to hemodynamic and oxygen transport, including critical concepts related to interpretation of data obtained via invasive central hemodynamic monitoring during pregnancy, is presented in Chapter 4 of this text. Select concepts will be presented in the description of treatment strategies for the patient with sepsis.

The Surviving Sepsis Campaign (SSC) divides sepsis into three stages; each stage is described in the portion of their document that includes definitions.[16] However, sepsis has generally been divided into two stages—early and late—largely distinguished by the patient's cardiovascular function. This conceptual framework may facilitate clinical decision-making. In the early stage of sepsis, inflammatory mediators produce endothelial damage. This causes capillary damage and subsequent increased vascular permeability. In turn, colloid osmotic pressure (COP) values decrease; a result of the loss of serum proteins across capillary membranes. Subsequently, interstitial fluid volume increases while intravascular volume decreases. Hemodynamic alterations during this stage include central hypovolemia; specifically, decreased preload that refers to a reduction in ventricular end-diastolic volume. When preload decreases, the potential for decreased cardiac output and oxygen transport increases. Compensatory mechanisms to these hemodynamic alterations include increased ventricular contractility and increased heart rate. Selective vasoconstriction may also occur, in order to increase perfusion of available blood, oxygen, and nutrients to the most essential organ systems. If central mixed-venous oxygen saturation (SvO_2) via a fiberoptic pulmonary artery catheter (PAC) is continually assessed, or a central mixed-venous blood gas sample is intermittently obtained, the SvO_2 values may be increased above pregnancy baseline. This is because compensatory mechanisms result in increased cardiac output and oxygen transport; thus, more oxygenated blood is returned to the pulmonary vasculature. However, SvO_2 values may be decreased because cellular ability to effectively extract oxygen from hemoglobin, in response to the increased need for oxygen at the tissue level, may be intact during the early stage of disease.

As sepsis progresses in severity, compensatory mechanisms may become inadequate, leading to decreased cardiac output and oxygen delivery. Specific hemodynamic alterations associated with worsening of the disease process may include loss of various compensatory mechanisms: ventricular contractility may decrease or fail; hypotension caused by loss of vascular tone may occur; and maternal heart rate may decrease and include the presence of significant cardiac arrhythmias. Ultimately, these adverse changes cause cardiac output and oxygen transport to significantly decrease, leading to an increased risk of end-organ dysfunction or failure. SvO_2 values during this stage may decrease significantly. This is because decreased cardiac output causes less oxygenated blood to be made available to tissues; thus, less oxygenated blood is returned to the pulmonary vasculature. To compound these adverse events, the cell's ability to extract and use oxygen is impaired. For this reason, SvO_2 values may actually increase significantly, indicating the inability of cells to effectively extract oxygen. Cellular mitochondria become unable to utilize available oxygen, resulting in further damage to the cell.

In the setting of hypoxemia, cellular hibernation is known to occur in myocardial cells. In hibernation, the cell reduces function to the most elemental level to retain viability. Autopsy findings demonstrate that cells also hibernate in the setting of sepsis.[17] However, in contrast to other hypoxemic conditions, in the case of sepsis, cells do not appear to be able to reverse hibernation when adequate oxygen delivery is returned.

Tissue hypoxia and cellular damage eventually lead to multiple organ system dysfunction and failure, a hallmark of severe sepsis and septic shock.[18] The pregnant woman may be particularly vulnerable to secondary complications from sepsis.[6] Specifically, the lungs during pregnancy are more susceptible to pulmonary edema secondary to decreased COP.[6] The hypercoagulable state during pregnancy further contributes to the potential for development of disseminated intravascular coagulation (DIC) and microvascular thrombosis in the presence of sepsis.[6] A detailed discussion of these complications can be found in other chapters of this text.

DIAGNOSIS

The SSC emphasizes early identification of clinical signs of sepsis and organ dysfunction, in order to promote initiation of treatment as soon as possible.[16] Knowledge of risk factors may help to identify the subset of patients most likely to develop sepsis. The more commonly cited risk factors relevant to the obstetric population are presented in Box 18-1. Sepsis has been reported to occur three times more frequently in preterm versus term births and three times more frequently in Cesarean versus vaginal deliveries.[5] The bedside care provider may be the first to recognize signs and symptoms associated with sepsis in an at-risk patient.[9]

Box 18-1. RISK FACTORS FOR SEPSIS IN THE OBSTETRIC POPULATION

Existing infection
• Pyelonephritis
• Pneumonia
• Necrotizing fasciitis
• Chorioamnionitis

Preterm birth
Cesarean birth
Primiparity
Obesity

Data from Fernandez-Perez, E. R., Salman, S., Pendam, S., & Farmer, C. (2005). Sepsis during pregnancy. *Critical Care Medicine, 33*(Suppl.), S286–S293; Kankuri, E., Kurki, T., Carlson, P., & Hiilesmaa, V. (2003). Incidence, treatment and outcome of peripartum sepsis. *Acta Obstetricia Et Gynecologica Scandinavica, 82,* 730–735; Mabie, W. C., Barton, J. R., & Sibai, B. (1997). Septic shock in pregnancy. *Obstetrics and Gynecology, 90,* 553–561; Martin, S. & Foley, M. (2006). Intensive care in obstetrics: An evidence-based review. *American Journal of Obstetrics and Gynecology, 1195,* 673–689; and Shapiro, J. M. (2006). Critical care of the obstetric patient. *Journal Intensive Care Medicine, 21,* 278–286.

Early diagnosis of sepsis relies on astute patient assessment and appropriate interpretation of assessment findings. While assessment of some parameters requires use of invasive monitoring techniques, other signs and symptoms may be detected by assessing trends in routine clinical assessment findings such as temperature, blood pressure, heart rate, respiratory rate and effort, breath sounds, arterial oxygen saturation (SaO_2), and urine output. In addition, assessment of a patient's level of consciousness, mentation, and skin perfusion may also reveal changes in clinical status compatible with sepsis. Fetal status should also be assessed, depending on the estimated gestational age, as fetal compromise may be an early indicator of an adverse change in maternal status.

Models to assist with identification of critically ill nonobstetric populations have emerged, such as Sequential Organ Failure Assessment (SOFA), Acute Physiology and Chronic Health Evaluation (APACHE) II, and Simplified Acute Physiology Score (SAPS).[19–21] Consistent use of a particular model among clinicians within a given institution has been recommended, in order to facilitate communication among care providers regarding changes in patient status.[6,9] However, superiority of one model over another has not been determined in the nonobstetric patient population, and none of these models incorporates the significant physiologic changes that normally occur during pregnancy. It is not surprising that recent investigation of the validity of the APACHE II and SAPS scores in pregnancy have reported that the scoring systems both over-predict and under-predict maternal death in the ICU.[22–24]

Once the diagnosis of sepsis has been made, a physical exam should be performed and the patient's history reviewed to facilitate identification of the source(s) of infection. Likely infectious sources differ, depending on the clinical situation such as an antepartum patient versus a postpartum patient or an outpatient versus a hospitalized patient. A systematic evaluation such as a "head to toe" assessment may be useful. Infectious sources are numerous and include: meningitis, sinusitis (especially if a nasogastric tube is in place); pharyngitis/oral ulcers/oral abscess; intravascular line sepsis; mastitis; endocarditis; pneumonia; abdominal sepsis (e.g., gallbladder, appendicitis, and abscess); endometritis/uterine abscess/chorioamnionitis; pyelonephritis; septic pelvic thrombosis; and cellulitis/fasciitis/soft tissue abscess. Both history and physical exam assist to narrow the differential diagnosis so that subsequent laboratory testing may be targeted appropriately.

Laboratory evaluation includes a complete blood count and white blood cell count with differential. An arterial blood gas and serum lactate level may help to evaluate tissue perfusion. Blood and urine cultures are also evaluated. Cultures of other fluids (including amniotic fluid), ultrasound/CT imaging, and chest x-ray, may also be helpful with identification of an infectious source. Laboratory assessment of renal function, liver function, and coagulation profile are useful for assessment of end-organ function. Fetal well being should also be assessed using techniques appropriate for gestational age.[25]

Collaboration between health care providers, including subspecialty consultation as indicated, facilitates timely and effective clinical management, once sepsis is suspected and/or diagnosed. Effective communication and collaboration promotes efficient clinical decision-making, including anticipated level of clinical care, patient location, fetal surveillance, and timing of delivery. Such communication also facilitates preparation for maternal and neonatal special care needs. Ideally, appropriate resources and an expected plan of care have been identified and are in place before a patient is diagnosed. Consideration of the physiologic impact of pregnancy on sepsis facilitates a more rapid and targeted response when such a patient is identified. Often, collaboration between the bedside and unit-based staffs (e.g., nurses and resident physicians) and/or private practice or faculty physicians is responsible for timely diagnosis, mobilization of appropriate resources, promotion of clear communication among disciplines, and an efficient decision-making process regarding initial treatment and patient location.

TREATMENT

The general principal of critical care in pregnancy is to stabilize the mother first. Maternal stabilization generally is beneficial to the fetus. A goal of clinical treatment of a patient with sepsis is to optimize cardiac output and oxygen transport while avoiding multi-organ system failure and death.

It should be recalled that cardiac output is determined by preload, afterload, contractility, and heart rate. Oxygen delivery (DO_2) is determined by cardiac output and arterial oxygen content (CaO_2). (Refer to Chapter 4 of this text for a thorough discussion of these parameters.) *Preload* refers to the tension or load on a muscle as it begins to contract. In the context of the cardiovascular system, preload is the length of the ventricular muscle fiber at end-diastole. The principal determinant of muscle fiber length is the amount of blood in the ventricles at the point of maximal filling. Preload may be low, secondary to decreased intravascular volume caused by endothelial damage, discussed previously in this chapter. Compression of the vena cava and aorta by the gravid uterus may also decrease preload by compromising venous return and ventricular filling.

Interventions to increase preload include maternal positioning to laterally displace the uterus and administration of intravenous crystalloid fluid. If the patient requires intubation and mechanical ventilation, the head of the bed should also be elevated to prevent ventilator-associated pneumonia (VAP). The degree of elevation is 30 to 45 degrees. Dependent on the patient's hemoglobin level, administration of packed red blood cells (PRBCs) may also be considered. However, if left-ventricular contractility is impaired secondary to worsening of sepsis, preload may be high. Administration of a positive inotrope (e.g., dobutamine) is considered in such cases in order to improve left-ventricular contractility, normalize preload, and improve cardiac output. *Afterload* refers to the resistance or load that opposes ventricular ejection of blood during systole. Systemic vascular resistance (SVR) is afterload applied against the left ventricle. SVR is a hemodynamic parameter mathematically derived from mean arterial blood pressure and cardiac output. For this reason, in the absence of invasive hemodynamic monitoring via a PAC, blood pressure is often used as a parameter to estimate or reflect SVR. Hypotension and low SVR in the patient with sepsis may be an indication of worsening of the disease process. In such cases, optimization of preload is the first-line treatment followed by inotrope administration if left-ventricular contractility is impaired. In the event these measures are not effective, administration of a vasopressor may be considered. Conversely, if preload is low, compensatory catecholamine release may result in vasoconstriction and increased SVR. The goal of treatment in such cases is optimization of preload.

Particular care should be exercised when interpreting these hemodynamic parameters in the pregnant woman, since physiologic changes of pregnancy are significant and dynamic. The processes of labor and delivery of the fetus, along with peripartum events, further affect these hemodynamic values in normal pregnancy.

DELIVERY

In some circumstances, it may not be possible to stabilize the mother. In such cases, delivery may be considered, in order to improve maternal status. However, delivery of the fetus is associated with significant blood loss; therefore, arterial oxygen content (CaO_2) and oxygen delivery (DO_2) are decreased. The autotransfusion of blood that normally occurs following delivery of the fetus and placenta significantly alters preload and cardiac output. These alterations may worsen the status of an unstable pregnant woman with sepsis. For these reasons, a decision regarding timing of delivery should be carefully considered with multidisciplinary input.

SURVIVING SEPSIS CAMPAIGN

Because sepsis is uncommon in pregnancy, no randomized controlled trials are available to guide care. Therefore, treatment in pregnancy may be similar to that in other patient populations. However, care should be taken to integrate significant physiologic alterations known to accompany pregnancy when providing clinical care to the pregnant woman with sepsis. This is especially important with respect to hemodynamic and oxygen transport dynamics, as well as pulmonary physiology and related assessment parameters.

In 2004, the SSC published international guidelines for treatment of the more severe forms of sepsis, based on the best available evidence. The original guidelines were updated in 2008 by over 50 internationally recognized experts on sepsis. This campaign resulted in the development of management strategies that are time sensitive. The strategies are divided into two groups: (1) Initial resuscitation within the first 6 hours of diagnosis, and (2) Continuing therapy after the first 6 hours. The strategies are further divided into *recommendations* and *suggestions*, based on the strength of the supporting evidence. Information regarding the quality of evidence considered and the review process that led to development of the guidelines was published in 2008.[16]

INITIAL RESUSCITATION

"Early goal-directed therapy" or initial resuscitation is the recommended approach for the treatment of sepsis in nonpregnant patients. Diagnosis or suspicion of severe sepsis, including documentation of parameters such as hypotension and elevated serum lactate greater than 4 mmol/L, mark the beginning of the 6-hour initial resuscitation period.[16]

Rivers and colleagues conducted a randomized controlled trial in which nonpregnant patients with severe sepsis were randomized to "early goal-directed therapy" or conventional therapy in the first 6 hours after diagnosis.[26] Outcomes were statistically significantly better in patients in the "early goal-directed therapy" group. Specific outcomes included: (1) improved mean arterial blood pressures; (2) decreased end-organ damage; (3) decreased mortality in-hospital (59% vs. 38%), at 28 days (61% vs, 40%), and 60 days (70% vs. 50%); and (4) decreased duration of hospital stay in patients who survived (18.4 days vs. 14.6 days).

The work of Rivers and others was analyzed by the SSC and resulted in recommendation of a specific *bundled protocol*. Crystalloid is given to maintain an adequate preload. In the nonobstetric patient population, the central venous pressure (CVP) is used to assess preload with a recommended goal between 8 and 12 mmHg. Vasopressors are recommended if the mean arterial pressure (MAP) is still less than 65 mmHg or the urine output is less than 0.5 mL/kg/hour, after preload has been optimized. After these adjustments, if the central venous oxygenation saturation is less than 70%, red cells are transfused to keep the hematocrit greater than 30. (Central venous oxygenation is measured at the level of the right atrium or the superior vena cava, as opposed to mixed venous oxygen saturation, which is measured with a PAC.) The ionotrope dobutamine is recommended if the CVP or PCWP, MAP, and hematocrit are optimized (according to the protocol) and the central venous oxygenation is still less than 70%. If optimal hemodynamics cannot be achieved, patients are mechanically ventilated and sedated to decrease oxygen consumption.[16,26] Significant issues that should be considered when caring for the septic obstetric patient are presented in Boxes 18-2 and 18-3.

Shorr and colleagues conducted a study to analyze outcomes following implementation of an early treatment protocol similar to the one described above. They compared 60 patients treated prior to implementation of the protocol with 60 patients treated according to the protocol. Their results demonstrated lower mortality and lower costs after protocol implementation.[27] Similar protocols have not been developed and studied in the obstetric population.

It should be noted that controversy exists regarding guidelines recommended by the SSC.[28] Whereas most of the medical community received the guidelines with enthusiasm, criticisms were made public just after their publication. Three major limitations have been identified and include: (1) sepsis as a public health issue; (2) the weight of the evidence behind the recommendations; and (3) the absence of recommendations related to the prevention of sepsis. Support of the project from the pharmaceutical and medical equipment industries has also been a source of criticism. It has been suggested that new guidelines be developed based on solid evidence without interference from pharmaceutical or medical equipment industries.[28]

BROAD-SPECTRUM ANTIBIOTICS

In patients with sepsis, the infectious source is not usually known at the time of initial presentation. The most common sources in parturients are pyelonephritis, chorioamnionitis, and endometritis.[29] Broad-spectrum antibiotics should cover gram-positive microorganisms (including groups A and B streptococci and *Staphylococcus aureus*), gram-negative microorganisms (including *Escherichia coli* and *Klebsiella* species) and

Box 18-2. RECOMMENDATIONS AND SUGGESTIONS FOR INITIAL RESUSCITATION

Recommendations:
- Initial resuscitation measures begun *without delay* regardless of patient location
- Clinical goals:
  - Optimize preload to improve left ventricular contractility
    - In nonpregnant patients, CVP 8–12 mmHg (12–15 mmHg if ↓ ventricular compliance or if on mechanical ventilation)
    - In pregnant patients, some practitioners prefer to use a PCWP to assess preload rather than a CVP. If this is chosen, a PAC should be placed. The PCWP goal is 10–12 mmHg. (12–14 mmHg if on mechanical ventilation).
  - MAP ≥65 mmHg
  - Urine output ≥0.5 mL/kg/hr
  - Support oxygen transport
    - In nonpregnant patients: Central venous (superior vena cava location) O_2 saturation ≥70% or mixed venous ≥65%
    - In pregnant patients: Mixed venous O_2 saturation (SvO_2) ≥65–70%
- Cultures before antibiotic therapy (do not delay antibiotics if cultures cannot be obtained quickly):
  - Blood cultures (1–2 with at least one drawn percutaneously)
  - Within 48 hours, one blood culture from each vascular access site/device
  - Culture all clinically relevant sites

- Utilize imaging to facilitate infection location and sampling
- Target antibiotic administration in first hour after recognition of severe sepsis or septic shock:
  - One to two broad-spectrum drugs for most likely microbes that will infiltrate presumed/known site
  - Reassess daily for most appropriate drug therapy
  - Duration of antibiotics depends on clinical response and situation
  - Discontinue promptly if etiology determined noninfectious
- Localization of infection:
  - Ideally within first 6 hours
  - Develop and implement plan of care to address infection based on type and location
  - Selected treatment plan for infection should have highest efficacy with least negative patient sequelae
  - Discontinue invasive devices if infection suspected

Suggestions:
- Considerations if venous O_2 saturation level not obtained with above measures:
  - Additional fluid administration
  - Transfusion to hematocrit of ≥30%
  - Dobutamine infusion (max 20 µg/kg/min)
- Consider combination therapies with *Pseudomonas* or in neutropenic patients
  - Continue combination therapy up to 3–5 days
  - De-escalate following susceptibilities

Data from Dellinger, R. P., Levy, M. M., Carlet, J. M., Bion, J., Parker, M. M., Jaeschke, R., et al. (2008). Surviving Sepsis Campaign: International guidelines for management of severe sepsis and septic shock. *Intensive Care Medicine, 34*, 17–60.

anaerobic microorganisms. The increasing prevalence of methicillin-resistant *Staphylococcus aureus*, highly resistant gram-negative bacilli, and fungal organisms should be considered in a patient who has previously been hospitalized.[25,29] Once an infectious source has been identified, the antibiotic spectrum should be narrowed in order to avoid the emergence of antibiotic resistance.

MECHANICAL VENTILATION

If noncardiogenic pulmonary edema (also called acute lung injury [ALI] or acute respiratory distress syndrome [ARDS]) is present with sepsis, mechanical ventilation with low tidal volumes may be considered. This includes tidal volumes between 4 and 6 mL/kg ideal body weight, keeping plateau pressure under 30 cm H_2O. This type of ventilation has been shown to decrease mortality (39.8% vs. 31%) in nonpregnant

patients with sepsis-related ARDS.[30] In some cases, low tidal volume ventilation can result in respiratory acidemia. This may be corrected by increasing the rate of breaths per minute delivered by the ventilator. In a study by the ARDS Network, if the arterial blood gas indicated a pH of less than 7.15, despite respiratory rate increases, bicarbonate was given.[30] This type of mechanical ventilation has not been studied in pregnant patients. In pregnancy, ideal prepregnancy body weight, and thus tidal volumes, may be difficult to calculate. Keeping the plateau pressure under 30 cm H_2O may be a helpful guideline. Arterial blood gases (ABGs) are monitored periodically, as well as other oxygenation indices, in order to assess the patient's pulmonary status. Whereas a mild respiratory acidemia may be tolerated in nonpregnant individuals, the effect on maternal and fetal status is not known.

Significant physiologic changes occur during pregnancy that impact the pregnant woman's pulmonary and respiratory function. Significant changes are

Box 18-3. RECOMMENDATIONS AND SUGGESTIONS FOR CONTINUING THERAPY

Fluid Therapy
Recommendations
- Crystalloids or colloids for resuscitation
- Invasive monitoring:
  - Nonpregnant: CVP target: ≥8 mmHg; for mechanically ventilated ≥12 mmHg
  - Pregnant: Some practitioners would consider placing a PAC to evaluate the PCWP. To optimize cardiac output, a goal PCWP is 8–10 mmHg (12–14 mmHg if on mechanical ventilation).
- Fluid challenges can be used when associated with optimization of hemodynamics:
  - Nonpregnant: Crystalloid challenge: 1,000 mL over 30 minutes; colloid challenge: 300–500 mL over 30 minutes; more volume may be needed in cases of tissue hypoperfusion
  - Pregnant: Crystalloid challenge: 250 to 1,000 mL over 15 to 20 minutes. May repeat boluses for hypoperfusion. If >2,000 mL required, consider placing PAC to follow PCWP, CO, SvO$_2$, and oxygen transport parameters.
  - If cardiac filling pressures increase, without improvement in cardiac output, reduce fluids

Vasopressor and Inotropic Therapy
Recommendations
- MAP ≥65 mmHg
- Initial vasopressor should be either norepinephrine or dopamine given by central venous access
- Renal or low-dose dopamine for renal perfusion is no longer recommended
- Insert arterial line as soon as possible if vasopressor is utilized
- Dobutamine for myocardial dysfunction with increased cardiac filling pressures and low cardiac output
- Avoid elevating cardiac index to predetermined supranormal levels

Suggestions
- Do not use epinephrine, phenylephrine, or vasopressin as first-line drug
  - Consider use of vasopressin 0.03 units/min with norepinephrine; expect similar effect to use of norepinephrine alone
- If poor response to first-line agents, consider epinephrine as first alternative agent

Steroid Therapy
Recommendations
- Hydrocortisone dose ≤300 mg/day
- Do not use to treat sepsis in absence of shock unless indicated by endocrine status or corticosteroid history

Suggestions
- Consider IV hydrocortisone when hypotension is not responsive to adequate fluid resuscitation and vasopressor

- ACTH stimulation test not recommended in adults with septic shock
- Hydrocortisone preferred to dexamethasone
- If alternative to hydrocortisone is being given that does not have significant mineralocorticoid effect, may add fludrocortisone at 50 µg po daily; fludrocortisone optional if hydrocortisone used
- When vasopressors are discontinued, corticosteroids can be weaned

Blood Component Therapy
Recommendations
- Use packed red blood cells to maintain hemoglobin between 7.0–9.0 g/dL
  - Certain clinical conditions will require higher hemoglobin levels, such as severe hypoxemia, hemorrhage, lactic acidosis, cyanotic heart disease, myocardial ischemia
  - Higher hemoglobin levels in pregnancy may also be required to maintain adequate oxygen delivery
- Do not use erythropoietin to treat low hemoglobin due to sepsis
  - May be used for other indications
- Give platelets for:
  - Level <5,000/mm^3 whether bleeding or not
  - Serious risk of bleeding with counts of 5,000 to 30,000 mm^3
  - If surgery or invasive procedure planned, counts should be ≥50,000/mm^3
  - If vaginal delivery planned, counts should be >35,000–40,000/mm^3
  - If cesarean section planned, counts should be ≥50,000
- Do not use fresh frozen plasma to treat laboratory coagulation values unless clinical evidence of bleeding or invasive procedure

Suggestions
- Do not use antithrombin therapy

Ventilation Therapy for Sepsis-Induced Lung Injury
Recommendations
- Tidal volume goal of 6 mL/kg predicted body weight (if pregnant, use prepregnant ideal body weight)
- Beginning upper limit plateau pressure ≤30 cm H$_2$O
- Permissive hypercarbia
- Nonpregnant: allow elevation of PaCO$_2$ above normal as needed to decrease plateau pressures and tidal volumes
- Pregnant: determine with obstetric providers/intensivists maximum levels of PaCO$_2$ if fetus viable
- Avoid lung collapse with positive end-expiratory pressure
- Semi-recumbent position with head of bed at 30°–45° with mechanical ventilation unless contraindicated (if pregnant, laterally tilt pelvis to avoid vena cava syndrome)
- Evaluate routinely for discontinuation of mechanical ventilation (use weaning protocol)

Box 18-3. RECOMMENDATIONS AND SUGGESTIONS FOR CONTINUING THERAPY (Continued)

- Do not use PAC for routine monitoring
- Consider using PAC in obstetric patients
- If no signs of tissue hypoperfusion use conservative fluid management

Suggestions
- Ventilation:
  - Nonobstetric: patients with mild respiratory failure may be candidates for noninvasive ventilation
  - Obstetric: avoid using noninvasive ventilation
  - In patients who require high levels of FiO_2 or plateau pressure, consider use of prone position if patient can tolerate position change. (There are no studies of prone positioning during pregnancy. If indicated, adapt positioning devices to prevent compression of the uterus from maternal weight.)

Sedation, Analgesia, and Neuromuscular Blockade Therapies
Recommendations
- Use same sedation protocol and goals as used for critically ill mechanically ventilated patients
- Use continuous infusion or intermittent bolus sedation protocols with sedation scales and daily interruption/lightening for awakening
- Avoid neuromuscular blockade when possible, with continuous infusion; monitor depth with train of four

Insulin Therapy
Recommendations
- After stabilization, use insulin to treat hyperglycemia
- Maintain blood glucose at <150 mg/dL using a validated protocol (nonpregnant)
- For pregnant patients, consult with obstetric, maternal-fetal medicine providers for preferred range of maternal blood glucose.
- Monitor blood glucose levels every 1–2 hours when giving IV insulin and provide glucose calorie source
- Point-of-care tests revealing low blood glucose levels should be cautiously interpreted, as arterial or plasma glucose levels may be overestimated

Renal Replacement Therapy
Suggestions
- Intermittent hemodialysis and continuous veno-venous hemofiltration (CVVH) are equal
- CVVH allows for easier management of hemodynamically unstable patients
- For pregnant patients, consult with maternal–fetal medicine or obstetric providers to develop plan to prevent maternal hypotension during dialysis (or CVVH, continuous veno-venous hemodialysis [CVVHD], etc.) and need for fetal surveillance during procedure.

Bicarbonate Therapy
Recommendations
- Do not use to improve hemodynamics or reduce need for vasopressor with lactic acidosis attributed to hypoperfusion (pH ≥7.15)

Deep Vein Thrombosis Prophylaxis Therapy
Recommendations
- Either low-dose unfractionated heparin or low-molecular-weight heparin can be used if contraindications do not exist
- If heparin is contraindicated, use compression stockings or mechanical compression device

Suggestions
- Mechanical and pharmacologic therapies may both be used for high-risk patients
- Utilize low-molecular-weight heparin over unfractionated heparin for patients at very high risk

Stress Ulcer Prophylaxis Therapy
Recommendations
- H_2 blocker or proton pump inhibitor can be used for prophylaxis
  - Benefit of prevention of upper GI bleed should be compared with potential risk of VAP

Limitation of Support
Recommendations
- Include patient and family in plan of care using probable outcomes and setting reasonable expectations

Data from Dellinger, R. P., Levy, M. M., Carlet, J. M., Bion, J., Parker, M. M., Jaeschke, R., et al. (2008). Surviving Sepsis Campaign: International guidelines for management of severe sepsis and septic shock. *Intensive Care Medicine, 34,* 17–60.

discussed at length in Chapter 9 of this text. These changes alter maternal ABGs; specifically, normal ABGs during pregnancy result in a compensated respiratory alkalemia. There is also a right shift in the maternal oxyhemoglobin dissociation curve, and a left shift in the fetal oxyhemoglobin dissociation curve, during pregnancy. These alterations facilitate normal maternal-fetal gas exchange. It is essential that these issues be integrated into the plan of care for the pregnant woman who requires mechanical ventilation. Mechanical ventilation

during pregnancy is discussed at length in Chapter 5 of this text.

AREAS OF CURRENT RESEARCH

Directed Corticosteroid Therapy

The use of corticosteroids to help manage sepsis has been contemplated for many years. Studies have shown conflicting outcomes. The use of early high-dose steroids in patients with severe sepsis has not been shown in randomized controlled trials to alter outcome.[25,31] However, a recent study by Annane and colleagues demonstrated a durable mortality benefit and decreased vasopressor use in a subgroup of patients with sepsis with relative adrenal insufficiency (e.g., those who were not responsive to corticotrophin stimulation).[31]

For now, the use of corticosteroid in the treatment of sepsis in nonpregnant patients remains controversial. Its use, however, may be considered in patients with relative adrenal insufficiency. Adverse effects of steroids include decreased immunity, poor wound healing, and hyperglycemia. Additionally, corticosteroid use in pregnancy is also associated with varying levels of increased serum glucose, and an impediment to wound healing.[6] This topic has not been studied in septic pregnant patients. Therefore, the risks and benefits of corticosteroids should be carefully considered before they are used.

Activated Protein C (APC)

Activated protein C (APC) is an anticoagulant that has been studied for the treatment of sepsis. The mechanism by which it may be useful for sepsis is unclear. It has been shown in a randomized trial to decrease mortality from 30.8% to 24.7% in patients with severe septic shock. Its greatest benefit may be in patients thought *a priori* to have the highest mortality risk. Another study of its use in septic patients with a low mortality risk showed no benefit.[25]

APC is an anticoagulant; therefore, hemorrhage is the biggest concern with its use. It is contraindicated in patients at high risk for hemorrhage (e.g., trauma or surgery in the last 12 hours, platelets less than 30,000, or concurrent anticoagulation). It is not contraindicated in pregnancy.[25]

Pregnancy results in many procoagulant effects. Thus, the effectiveness of APC in a pregnant septic patient may be different than in a nonpregnant patient. Its effect on the fetal-placental unit is unknown.[29]

Tight Glycemic Control (Insulin Therapy)

Intensive insulin therapy in critically ill *surgical* patients has been shown in a randomized trial to reduce mortality. However, in a randomized trial by the same group, there was no mortality benefit in a group of critically ill *medical* patients (not necessarily septic patients). Tight glycemic control has not been studied well in septic patients or pregnant patients.[25]

SUMMARY

In the absence of cardiovascular disease states, sepsis and septic shock are the number one cause of mortality in ICUs throughout North America. It is no surprise that sepsis and septic shock in pregnancy, although rare, are serious and potentially lethal complications with high rates of maternal, fetal, and neonatal morbidity and mortality. In an attempt to decrease deaths from sepsis and septic shock throughout the world, the SSC was established to guide providers with standardized tools to identify and manage patients at risk and diagnosed with septic shock. Unfortunately, the SSC does not address the unique challenges in providing care to septic obstetric patients, nor does it provide guidance in the difficult process of adapting the current recommendations. Therefore, obstetric providers continue to base clinical decisions on the tenets of obstetrical critical care, which center on the support and optimization of oxygen transport parameters.

Until more data exist that address specific questions of appropriateness of SSC recommendations in the obstetric population, it is recommended that providers target supportive measures that have been shown to optimize maternal and fetal outcomes. Additionally, providers should remain attentive to future research in the SSC and be ready to integrate multidisciplinary guidelines of practice that are shown to improve patient outcomes.

REFERENCES

1. Dombrovsky, V. Y., Martin, A. A., Sunderram, J., & Paz, H. L. (2007). Rapid increase in hospitalization and mortality rates for severe sepsis in the United States: A trend analysis from 1993 to 2003. *Critical Care Medicine, 35*, 1244–1250.
2. Miniño, A. M., Heron, M. P., Murphy, S. L., & Kochanek, K. D. (2007). Deaths: Final data for 2004. *National Vital Statistics Reports, 55*(19), 1–120.
3. Mabie, W. C., Barton, J. R., & Sibai, B. (1997). Septic shock in pregnancy. *Obstetrics and Gynecology, 90*, 553–561.
4. Vincent, J. L., Sakr, Y., Sprung, C. L., Ranieri, V. M., Reinhart, K., Gerlach, H., et al. Sepsis Occurrence in Acutely Ill Patients Investigators. (2006). Sepsis in European intensive care units: Results of the SOAP study. *Critical Care Medicine, 34*, 344–353.
5. Kankuri, E., Kurki, T., Carlson, P., & Hiilesmaa, V. (2003). Incidence, treatment and outcome of peripartum sepsis. *Acta Obstetricia Et Gynecologica Scandinavica, 82*, 730–735.
6. Fernandez-Perez, E. R., Salman, S., Pendam, S., & Farmer, C. (2005). Sepsis during pregnancy. *Critical Care Medicine, 33*(Suppl.), S286–S293.
7. Members of the American College of Chest Physicians/ Society of Critical Care Medicine Consensus Conference Committee. American College of Chest Physicians/Society of Critical Care Medicine Consensus Conference: Definitions for sepsis and organ failure and guidelines for the use of innovative therapies in sepsis. (1992). *Critical Care Medicine, 20*, 864–874.
8. Levy, M. M., Fink, M. P., Marshall, J. C., Abraham, E., Angus, D., Cook, D., et al. SCCM/ESICM/ACCP/ATS/SIS (2003). SCCM/ESICM/ ACCP/ATS/SIS International Sepsis Definitions Conference. *Critical Care Medicine, 31*, 1250–1256.

9. Kleinpell, R. M., Graves, B. T., & Ackerman, M. H. (2006). Incidence, pathogenesis and management of sepsis. *AACN Advanced Critical Care, 17*, 385–393.

10. Kaufmann, S. H. E., & Kabelitz, D. (2002). *Introduction: The immune response to infectious agents in methods of microbiology* (Vol. 32). Amsterdam: Elsevier Science.

11. Leaver, S. K., Finney, S. J., Burke-Gaffney, A., & Evans, T. W. (2007). Sepsis since the discovery of Toll-like receptors: Disease concepts and therapeutic opportunities. *Critical Care Medicine, 35*, 1404–1410.

12. Osuchowski, M. F., Welch, K., Sidiqui, J., & Remick, D. G. (2006). Circulating cytokine/inhibitor profiles reshape the understanding of the SIRA/CARS continuum in sepsis and predict mortality. *Journal of Immunology, 177*, 1967–1974.

13. Hotchkiss, R. S., & Karl, I. E. (2003). The pathophysiology and treatment of sepsis. *NEJM, 348*, 138–150.

14. Papathanassoglou, E. D. E., Giannakopoulou, M. D., & Bozas, E. (2006). Genomic variations and susceptibility to sepsis. *AACN Advanced Critical Care, 17*, 394–422.

15. Ahrens, T. (2006). Hemodynamics in sepsis. *AACN Advanced Critical Care, 17*, 435–445.

16. Dellinger, R. P., Levy, M. M., Carlet, J. M., Bion, J., Parker, M. M., Jaeschke, R., et al. (2008). Surviving Sepsis Campaign: International guidelines for management of severe sepsis and septic shock. *Intensive Care Medicine, 34*, 17–60.

17. Hotchkiss, R., Swanson, P., Freeman, B., Tinsley, K. W., Cobb, J. P., Matuschak, G. M. (1999). Apoptic cell death in patients with sepsis, shock and multiple organ dysfunction. *Critical Care Medicine, 27*, 1230–1251.

18. Uchino, S., Kellum, J. A., Bellomo, R., Doig, G. S., Morimatsu, H., Morgera, S., et al. Beginning and Ending Supportive Therapy for the Kidney (BEST Kidney) Investigators. (2005). Acute renal failure in critically ill patients: A multinational multicenter study. *JAMA, 294*, 813–818.

19. Giuliano, K. K. (2007). Physiological monitoring for critically ill patients: Testing a predictive model for the early detection of sepsis. *American Journal of Critical Care, 16*, 122–131.

20. Rivers, E. P., McIntyre, L., Morrow, D. C., & Rivers, K. K. (2005). Early and innovative interventions for severe sepsis and septic shock: Taking advantage of a window of opportunity. *CMAJ, 173*, 1054–1065.

21. Ely, E. W., Kleinpell, R. M., & Goyette, R. E. (2003). Advances in the understanding of clinical manifestations and therapy of severe sepsis: An update for critical care nurses. *American Journal of Critical Care, 12*, 120–135.

22. Gilbert, T. T., Smulian, J. C., Martin, A. A., Ananth, C. V., Scorza, W., Scardella, A. T. et al. Critical Care Obstetric Team. (2003). Obstetric admissions to the intensive care unit: Outcomes and severity of illness. *Obstetrics and Gynecology, 102*(5 Pt 1), 897–903.

23. Karnad, D. R., Lapsia, V., Krishnan, A., & Salvi, V. S. (2004). Prognostic factors in obstetric patients admitted to an Indian intensive care unit. *Critical Care Medicine, 32*(6), 1418–1419.

24. Stevens, T. A., Carroll, M. A., Promecene, P. A., Seibel, M., & Monga, M. (2006). Utility of Acute Physiology, Age, and Chronic Health Evaluation (APACHE II) score in maternal admissions to the intensive care unit. *American Journal of Obstetrics and Gynecology, 194*(5), 13–15.

25. Russell, J. (2006). Management of sepsis. *NEJM, 355*(16), 1699–1713.

26. Rivers, E., Nguygen, B., Havstad, S., Ressler, J., Muzzin, A., Knoblich, B., et al. Early Goal-Directed Therapy Collaborative Group. (2001). Early goal directed therapy in the treatment of severe sepsis and septic shock. *NEJM, 345*(19), 1368–1377.

27. Shorr, A. F., Micek, S. T., Jackson, W. L Jr., & Kollef, M. H.(2007). Economic implications of an evidence-based sepsis protocol: Can we improve outcomes and lower costs? *Critical Care Medicine, 35*, 1257–1262.

28. Salluh, J. I. F., Bozza, P. T., & Bozza, F. (2008). Surviving sepsis campaign: A critical reappraisal. *Shock, 30*(Suppl.1), 70–72.

29. Martin, S., & Foley, M. (2006). Intensive care in obstetrics: An evidence-based review. *American Journal of Obstetrics and Gynecology, 1195*, 673–689.

30. ARDS Network. (2000). Ventilation with lower tidal volumes as compared with traditional tidal volumes for acute lung injury and the acute respiratory distress syndrome. *NEJM, 342*, 1301–1308.

31. Annane, D., Sebille, V., Charpentier, C., Bollaert, P. E., François, B., Korach, J. M., et al. (2002). Effect of treatment with low doses of hydrocortisone and fludrocortisone on mortality in patients with septic shock. *JAMA, 288*, 862–871.

CHAPTER 19

Amniotic Fluid Embolus (Anaphylactoid Syndrome of Pregnancy)

Renee' Jones and Steven L. Clark

Amniotic fluid embolus (AFE), also referred to as anaphylactoid syndrome of pregnancy, is an extremely rare and catastrophic event that occurs when amniotic fluid gains entrance into the maternal circulation, causing potentially life-threatening maternal reactions.[1] This enigmatic phenomenon is classically characterized by hypoxia, hypotension, cardiovascular collapse, and coagulopathy. It has been documented worldwide, with an estimated incidence of 1 in 8,000 to 1 in 83,000 deliveries.[2] The incidence in the United States is estimated between 1 in 8,000 and 1 in 30,000 deliveries.[2] A population-based study of over one million deliveries in California during 1994–1995 reported an incidence of 1 in 20,000 deliveries.[3] However, it is important to note that the true incidence of AFE is not known, because of the difficulty in confirming the diagnosis and inconsistent reporting of nonfatal cases. The maternal mortality rate from AFE is between 61% and 86%, and makes it a leading cause of death in Western industrialized countries.[2] Many women with suspected AFE die within the first hour after the onset of classic symptoms. Only 15% of patients who survive are neurologically intact. The fetal mortality rate is 21%, and, of the neonates who survive, 50% experience neurologic injury.[4] AFE continues to be the most lethal maternal complication in obstetrics and remains both unpreventable and unpredictable. Nevertheless, several significant advances have produced a better understanding of this complex condition.

This chapter provides an overview of essential concepts related to AFE. It presents an historical perspective that briefly chronicles early experience with this disorder, and describes The National Registry for Amniotic Fluid Embolus, from which data analysis has yielded valuable information. Issues that provide the framework for care are addressed, including description and etiology of the disorder, pathophysiology, clinical presentation, diagnostic criteria, and clinical management strategies, along with the inherent need for professional collaboration, communication, and teamwork in the clinical setting.

HISTORICAL PERSPECTIVE

The first published case report of AFE is attributed to Meyer in 1926.[5] However, the first anatomic description of what may have been an AFE was provided by Baillie in 1789, as he described a case of uterine rupture.[6] In 1941, this condition became widely recognized when Steiner and Lushbaugh published their work.[7] They described autopsy findings in eight pregnant women with sudden shock and pulmonary edema that occurred during labor. In all cases, they found emboli in small pulmonary vessels that contained fat-positive aggregates and squamous epithelial cells, presumably of fetal origin. This concept is depicted in Figure 19-1 (A and B). Each figure illustrates the presence of squamous cells within the pulmonary artery vasculature at autopsy in women who died from AFE.

In a follow-up report by Liban and Raz in 1969, they described the presence of cellular debris throughout the kidneys, liver, spleen, pancreas, and brain of fourteen women who died from AFE.[8] Attwood and Rome published a report in 1975 in which they described the presence of incomplete uterine tears in cases diagnosed as AFE. They postulated that such tears may provide a point of entrance for amniotic fluid or other debris into the maternal system.[6] It was not until 1976 that Resnik reported the presence of mucin and fetal squamous cells in blood aspirated from a central venous catheter in a woman who survived a suspected AFE.[9] Similar

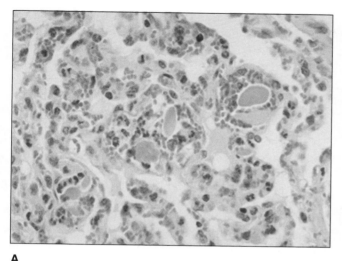

A

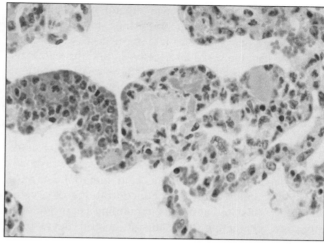

B

FIGURE 19-1   (**A** and **B**) Squamous cells within the pulmonary artery vasculature at autopsy of a woman who died secondary to AFE.

findings have also been documented in cases where there was no evidence suggestive of AFE. Figure 19-2 illustrates the presence of squamous cells identified in a buffy-coat preparation of blood aspirated from a pulmonary artery catheter in a woman with no signs or symptoms of AFE.

Since the initial description of AFE, more than 300 case reports have appeared in the literature.[1] Although most cases reportedly occurred during labor, sudden death in pregnancy has been attributed to AFE under a wide variety of circumstances. In 1948, Eastman cautioned that the diagnosis of AFE should not be a wastebasket for cases of unexplained maternal death in labor.[10] Subsequent efforts to better understand the syndrome of AFE make such errors less likely today.

THE NATIONAL REGISTRY

A National Registry for Amniotic Fluid Embolus was formed in 1995 by Clark and colleagues.[4] Data for the registry were collected between 1983 and 1993 and yielded sixty-nine cases. Data analysis indicated that exposure of the maternal circulation to small amounts of amniotic fluid initiated a syndrome similar to that of anaphylaxis and/or septic shock. Amniotic fluid acts as a foreign substance, similar to that of bacterial endotoxin or a specific antigen, and subsequently stimulates the release of several primary and secondary endogenous mediators. Included in this response is the release of histamine, bradykinin, cytokines, prostaglandins, leukotrienes, thromboxane, and arachidonic acid metabolites into the maternal circulation. It is postulated that the release of these mediators is responsible for development of the severe physiologic sequelae associated

with AFE. These include profound hypoxia, myocardial depression, decreased cardiac output, pulmonary hypertension, and disseminated intravascular coagulation (DIC). Based on analysis of data from the registry, the authors suggested that the term "amniotic fluid embolism" be discarded and the syndrome of acute peripartum hypoxia, hemodynamic collapse, and coagulopathy should be designated in a more descriptive manner, as "anaphylactoid syndrome of pregnancy."[4]

The U.K. Obstetric Surveillance System, in 2005, conducted a population-based cohort study to estimate the incidence of AFE and to investigate risk factors, management, and mortality.[2] The findings showed that the risk

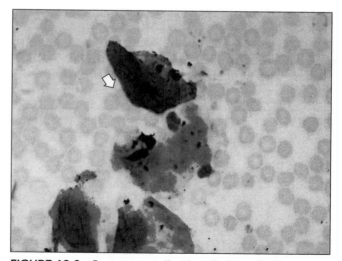

FIGURE 19-2   Squamous cells identified in a buffy-coat preparation of blood aspirated from a pulmonary artery catheter in a woman with no evidence of compromise. (Photo courtesy of Gary D.V. Hankins, MD.)

of amniotic fluid embolism was greater in induction of labor, multiple pregnancies, and ethnic minority women over 35 years of age. Almost half of the cases of amniotic fluid embolism occurred after delivery, and three fourths of the time, the woman had delivered by Cesarean section.

DESCRIPTION AND ETIOLOGY

Amniotic fluid is made up of maternal extracellular fluid, fetal urine, fetal squamous cells, lanugo, vernix caseosa, mucin, meconium, arachidonic acid metabolites, and, late in pregnancy, increased concentrations of prostaglandins.[11] This fluid and the surrounding sac provide an important protective mechanism for the developing fetus. Prior to labor, amniotic fluid does not normally enter the maternal circulation, because it is sealed within the amniotic sac. It has been postulated that amniotic fluid may enter the maternal circulation in one of three ways: 1) through the endocervix following rupture of amniotic membranes; 2) at the site of placental separation; or 3) at the site of uterine trauma, often in the form of lacerations that occur during the course of normal labor, fetal descent, and delivery.[12] In addition, introduction of amniotic fluid may also result from placental abruption and the accompanying clinical or subclinical disruption of fetal membranes. Once this barrier or membrane is ruptured, alteration of the pressure gradient may allow amniotic fluid to enter the uterine vessels and maternal venous circulation.[13] Another potential site for amniotic fluid entry is through small tears in the lower uterine segment and endocervical vessels.[11]

Early anecdotal reports suggested a possible causal relationship between hypertonic uterine contractions or administration of oxytocin and AFE. The historical anecdotal association between hypertonic uterine contractions and the onset of symptoms of AFE was addressed by analysis of data from the National Registry.[4] These data demonstrated that the hypertonic contractions commonly seen in association with AFE appear to be a result of the release of catecholamines into the circulation and part of the initial human hemodynamic response to any massive physiologic insult.[4] Under such circumstances, norepinephrine, in particular, acts as a potent uterotonic agent.[4,14] While the association of hypertonic uterine contractions and AFE appears to be valid, it is the physiologic response to AFE that causes the hypertonic contractions rather than the converse. In fact, there is complete cessation of uterine blood flow in the presence of even moderate contractions; thus, a hypertonic contraction is the least likely time during the labor process for any exchange between maternal and fetal compartments.[1,15] Analysis of National Registry data also revealed that oxytocin was not used with greater frequency in patients who

suffered AFE compared with the general population, nor did oxytocin-induced uterine hyperstimulation commonly precede AFE.[4] Thus, a causal relationship has been refuted both on statistical and physiologic bases.

PATHOPHYSIOLOGY

The pathophysiology of AFE remains incompletely understood. Given the fact that almost universal exchange between maternal and fetal compartments occurs around the time of birth, it is unclear why specific antigens within amniotic fluid, when introduced into the maternal circulation prior to birth, cause an intense pathophysiologic reaction in some women but are benign for most pregnant women. Further, there are no reliable risk factors or warning signs that predict or prevent this catastrophic event. It has been suggested that the amount of fetal debris or the specific type of debris may be significant variables responsible for the anaphylactoid maternal reaction to amniotic fluid.[1] Arachidonic acid metabolites have been implicated in the inflammatory response involved in sepsis and anaphylaxis and may be at least partly responsible for similar responses in cases of AFE.[16] The ability of arachidonic acid metabolites to cause similar physiologic and hemodynamic changes in animal models as those observed in human AFE has been noted.[16] Further, in the animal model of AFE, pretreatment with an inhibitor of leukotriene synthesis has been shown to prevent death.[11] There are several clinical findings frequently seen in sepsis and anaphylaxis that are also present in cases of AFE. These include coagulopathy, DIC, left-ventricular failure, and hemodynamic compromise. Clearly, the clinical manifestations of AFE are not identical; fever is unique to septic shock, and cutaneous manifestations are more common in anaphylaxis. Nonetheless, marked similarities exist, which suggest similar pathophysiologic mechanisms. This concept is depicted in Figure 19-3.[4] A detailed description of pathophysiologic concepts related to sepsis and septic shock is presented in Chapter 18 of this text. The presence of metabolites symbolizes a humoral mechanism.[17] These pathways invoke a proinflammatory response with subsequent release of cytokines and arachidonic acid in AFE.[18] This complex inflammatory cascade with mediator release leads to a systemic inflammatory response and subsequently multiple organ system dysfunction or failure.

CLINICAL PRESENTATION

The onset of signs and symptoms of AFE most commonly occurs during labor or immediately following delivery. Clinical signs and symptoms noted in patients

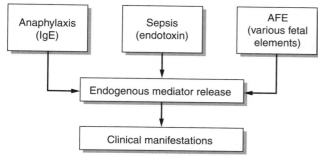

FIGURE 19-3 Proposed pathophysiologic relation between AFE, anaphylaxis, and sepsis. IgE, immunoglobulin E; AFE, amniotic fluid embolus. (Reproduced with permission from Clark, S. L., Hankins, G. D. V., Dudley, D. A., Dildy, G. A., & Porter, T. F. (1995). Amniotic fluid embolism: Analysis of the national registry. *American Journal of Obstetrics and Gynecology, 172*, 1158–1169.

TABLE 19-1

Signs and Symptoms Noted in Patients with Amniotic Fluid Embolus

Sign or Symptom	Number of Patients (%)
Hypotension	43 (100)
Nonreassuring FHR findings*	30 (100)
Pulmonary edema or ARDS[†]	28 (93)
Cardiopulmonary arrest	40 (87)
Cyanosis	38 (83)
Coagulopathy[‡]	38 (83)
Dyspnea[§]	22 (49)
Seizure	22 (48)
Atony	11 (23)
Bronchospasm[¶]	7 (15)
Transient hypertension	5 (11)
Cough	3 (7)
Headache	3 (7)
Chest pain	1 (2)

*Includes all live fetuses in utero at time of event

[†]Eighteen patients did not survive long enough for these diagnoses to be confirmed.

[‡]Eight patients did not survive long enough for this diagnosis to be confirmed.

[§]One patient was intubated at the time of the event and could not be assessed.

[¶]Difficult ventilation was noted during cardiac arrest in six patients, and wheezes were auscultated in one patient.

Reproduced with permission from Clark, S. L., Hankins, G. D. V., Dudley, D. A., Dildy, G. A., & Porter, T. F. (1995). Amniotic fluid embolism: Analysis of the national registry. *American Journal of Obstetrics and Gynecology, 172*(4), 1158–1169.

with AFE are described in Table 19-1.[4] In its classic form, the woman experiences the acute onset of hypoxia and hypotension followed by cardiopulmonary arrest. The initial episode often is complicated by development of DIC. The cardinal findings of AFE are hypoxia, hypotension with shock, altered mental status, and consumptive DIC.

The clinical course of AFE typically involves three phases. These phases are presented in Table 19-2. The first phase involves respiratory distress caused by pulmonary vasospasm, which results in acute hypoxia and myocardial dysfunction.[4] In some women, seizure or seizure-like activity may be the presenting symptom. Other possible symptoms include fetal bradycardia, cough, cyanosis, pulmonary edema, anxiety, vomiting, and chills. Rapid deterioration and death often ensue. A second phase, in patients who survive the initial insult, involves left heart failure and decreased cardiac output. Finally, a third phase may ensue, involving tissue hypoxia, shock, and consumptive coagulopathy, with subsequent multiple organ system failure.[4] Mortality

TABLE 19-2

Three Phases Associated with Amniotic Fluid Embolus

Phase	Pathophysiology	Signs and Symptoms

Phase One	• Amniotic fluid enters maternal pulmonary vasculature	• Hypoxemia/respiratory acidemia/cyanosis
		  • Dyspnea
		  • Cough
		  • Bronchospasm
		  • Pulmonary edema
		  • Respiratory Distress

Phase Two	• Release of inflammatory mediators • Myocardial depression • Lung injury • Neurologic compromise	• Acute renal failure/hypotension/shock • Cardiac failure/left-ventricular impairment/arrhythmias • Seizures/altered mentation
Phase Three	• Immunologic activation of coagulation pathway	• Intravascular congestion/bleeding/DIC

can be as high as 50% during this phase.[19] Some cases of AFE have been reported in which DIC was the only presenting symptom.[20] It must be emphasized that in any individual patient, any of the three principal phases may either be dominant or entirely absent.[4] Such clinical variations in this syndrome may be related to variations in the nature of either the antigenic exposure or the maternal response.

Hypoxia

Hypoxia associated with AFE varies throughout the event and is related to obstructive, cardiogenic, and inflammatory sources. In 93% of patients, hypoxia had an early onset and occurred as part of the initial presentation of respiratory arrest and cyanosis.[4] This initial hypoxia is likely due to severe ventilation and perfusion mismatching secondary to the embolic event. Another reason for the hypoxia may be cardiogenic pulmonary edema, which develops as a result of severe left-ventricular cardiac dysfunction. Patients who survive the initial insult may subsequently develop noncardiogenic pulmonary edema. This is secondary to pulmonary vascular damage, which permits leakage of proteinacious fluid across the capillary membrane into extravascular spaces within the lungs. This noncardiogenic pulmonary edema leads to acute respiratory distress syndrome (ARDS) and is associated with severe, secondary sequelae. In both phases of AFE, hypoxia is responsible for the potential development of widespread neurologic injury or death.

Hemodynamic Dysfunction

During the first phase of AFE, hypotension and shock develop. The etiology of shock is most likely cardiogenic secondary to left-ventricular failure, decreased cardiac output, and concomitant decreased oxygen transport. A detailed description of concepts regarding hemodynamic and oxygen transport physiology, including data interpretation, is found in Chapter 4 of this text. Later in the process, hypovolemia associated with DIC may also contribute to shock. The presence of left-ventricular dysfunction has been documented via data collected following pulmonary artery catheterization and by echocardiography. This concept is illustrated in Figure 19-4. The left heart filling pressures are elevated, with increases in pulmonary artery and pulmonary artery occlusion pressures coupled with decreased myocardial contractility. Cardiac arrhythmias such as bradycardia, asystole, ventricular fibrillation, and pulseless electrical activity (PEA) may ensue. Women who survive the initial phase may subsequently develop noncardiogenic pulmonary edema.[21] In addition to the pulmonary edema,

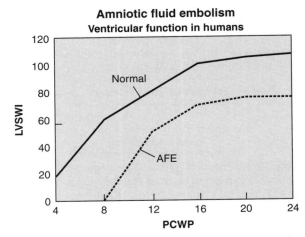

FIGURE 19-4 The relationship between left-ventricular contractility (LVSWI) and left-ventricular filling pressure (PCWP) in women with amniotic fluid embolism. LVSWI, left ventricular stroke work index; PCWP, pulmonary capillary wedge pressure; AFE, amniotic fluid embolus.

patients tend to develop symptoms similar to those of septic shock due to inflammatory processes.

Coagulopathy

Patients who survive the initial phase of AFE may later succumb to a secondary coagulopathy.[22] DIC is seen in up to 83% of patients with AFE who survive long enough to present with the associated signs and symptoms; and 50% of these women develop DIC within the first 4 hours of initial presentation.[23] The presenting manifestation is profound hemorrhage. The coagulopathy associated with AFE is a consumptive coagulopathy.[22] The etiology of DIC associated with AFE is undetermined, but amniotic fluid is known to have a direct factor X-activating property as well as a thromboplastin effect.[21] Amniotic fluid also contains a substantial amount of tissue factor, which may initiate the extrinsic clotting pathway. Phosphotidylserine, a phospholipid and thrombin activatable fibrinolysis inhibitor (TAFI) present in amniotic fluid, contributes to DIC.[21] Laboratory evidence of consumptive coagulopathy includes decreased fibrinogen, elevated D-dimer, elevated fibrin degradation products, and prolonged prothrombin and partial thromboplastin times. In some patients, DIC may be the dominant or only significant recognizable clinical factor. A thorough description of significant concepts related to DIC in pregnancy is found in Chapter 16 of this text.

Altered Mental Status

Encephalopathy occurs secondary to decreased oxygen delivery caused by low cardiac output secondary to left-ventricular failure and subsequent global hypoxia.

Seizure activity is present in 50% of patients with AFE.[4] Seizure activity may also exacerbate neurologic injury.

Abnormal Fetal Heart Rate Findings

Nonreassuring fetal heart rate (FHR) findings commonly precede or accompany maternal signs and symptoms of AFE. These may be the result of decreased uterine perfusion associated with maternal hypotension. In some cases, the absence of immediate maternal hypotension may reflect a compensatory adrenergic response to a systemic insult, with shunting of blood from the uterine circulation to maintain perfusion of maternal vital organs. Fetal capacity to compensate for this decrease in oxygenation may be depleted.[24] Thus, Category II or III FHR patterns may precede the onset of discernable clinical signs in the mother. FHR findings associated with a case of maternal AFE are presented in Figure 19-5 (A and B). Fetal intrauterine support may include administration of maternal oxygen, volume resuscitation, and lateral displacement of the uterus. Preparation for expeditious delivery of the fetus should also be considered.

DIAGNOSIS

Prompt recognition of clinical signs and symptoms associated with AFE is important to facilitate improved maternal and fetal outcomes. In the past, histologic confirmation of the clinical syndrome of AFE was often sought by the detection of cellular debris of presumed fetal origin either in the distal port of the pulmonary artery catheter or at autopsy.[1,22] However, as described previously in this chapter, this debris has been reported in blood samples obtained from normal pregnant women, and is not always detectable in women with AFE.[1] In analysis of data from the National Registry of AFE, fetal elements were found in approximately 50% of cases in which pulmonary artery catheter aspirate was analyzed, and in approximately 75% of cases in which autopsies were performed.[4] The frequency with which such findings are encountered varies with the number of histologic sections obtained. In addition, multiple special stains often are required to document such debris.[22] For example, focal interstitial hemorrhages in the kidneys, left ventricle, and the interventricular septum have been reported at the time of autopsy of women who died secondary to AFE. Use of Alcian Blue Periodic Acid–Schiff (PAS) stain yielded positive findings for mucin in the vasculature and Oil Red O stain for lipid was positive in the lungs.[25] Kobayashi and colleagues used antibody TKH-2, which reacts with meconium and the mucin derived from amniotic fluid, to stain the lung tissue of women with suspected AFE.[26] Their report suggested that TKH-2 immunostaining may be a sensitive method of detecting mucin in the lungs of women suspected of having an AFE.

Although supportive, the finding of fetal debris in the central maternal circulation is neither sensitive nor specific for the diagnosis of AFE. Rather, the diagnosis of AFE remains a clinical one, and should be strongly suspected in the woman who, during the peripartum period, acutely develops profound shock and cardiovascular collapse associated with severe respiratory distress or DIC. A list of differential diagnoses that should be considered is presented in Box 19-1.

CLINICAL MANAGEMENT

AFE is a clinical emergency and requires collaboration, effective communication, and teamwork from all members of the health care team. The obstetric nurse who provides direct patient care during the peripartum period should recognize clinical symptoms associated with AFE, initiate nursing interventions, and effectively communicate adverse changes in patient status to the physician. This emergency produces remarkably rapid deterioration in maternal and fetal status. Thus, care providers should work collaboratively to provide prompt, appropriate interventions when AFE is suspected.

The broad goal of clinical management is to optimize hemodynamic function, cardiac output, and oxygen transport, in an attempt to improve overall tissue oxygenation, reduce the risk of end-organ failure, and reduce morbidity and mortality. A detailed presentation related to hemodynamic function, oxygen transport physiology, clinical assessment methods, and specific management strategies to achieve these goals is found in Chapter 4 of this text. These goals and management strategies are summarized in Box 19-2.[1] Select strategies to achieve these goals are briefly described below.

Oxygenation

Oxygen transport is dependent on cardiac output and arterial oxygen content. Thus, optimization of cardiac output is a critical intervention to improve oxygenation. Arterial oxygen content (CaO_2) is dependent on the amount of oxygen chemically bound to hemoglobin, and to the amount of oxygen dissolved under pressure in plasma. A significantly disproportionate amount of oxygen is available bound to hemoglobin versus that which is dissolved in plasma. Thus, correction of maternal anemia and optimization of hemoglobin are valid strategies to improving oxygen delivery. Transfusion of packed red blood cells (PRBCs) may be considered in order to accomplish this goal.

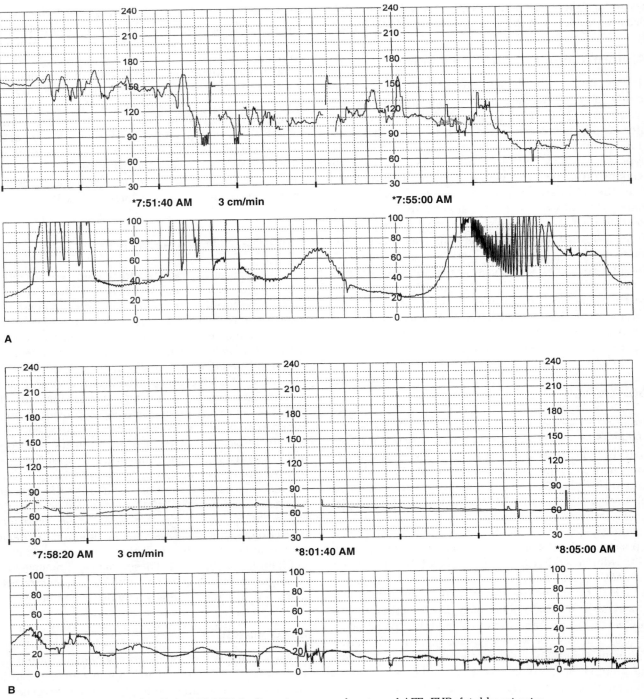

FIGURE 19-5   (**A** and **B**) FHR findings in a case of maternal AFE. FHR, fetal heart rate; AFE, amniotic fluid embolus.

If spontaneous respirations are present in a patient with a suspected AFE, supplemental oxygen should be initiated immediately. Oxygen may be administered by mask, if the airway is patent. Endotracheal intubation and subsequent support of ventilation and oxygenation may be necessary. Mechanical ventilation during pregnancy is addressed in Chapter 5 of this text and includes indications for intubation and mechanical ventilation, modes, adjuncts, settings, and clinical management strategies. The initial goal of oxygenation therapy when AFE is suspected is an arterial oxygen saturation (SaO_2) greater than or equal to 95% and an

Box 19-1. DIFFERENTIAL DIAGNOSES

Pulmonary thromboembolus
Air embolus
Hemorrhage
Aspiration
Anesthetic complications
Sepsis
Myocardial infarction
Cardiomyopathy
Eclampsia
Placental abruption
Ruptured uterus

Box 19-2. GOALS OF THERAPY AND CLINICAL MANAGEMENT STRATEGIES

Goals of Therapy
- Optimize hemodynamic function, cardiac output, and oxygen transport
- Maintain systolic BP ≥90 mmHg, urine output ≥30 mL/hr, SaO_2 ≥95%, and arterial pO_2 ≥60 mmHg
- Correct coagulation abnormalities

Clinical Management Strategies
- Initiate cardiopulmonary resuscitation (if indicated).
- Administer oxygen at high concentration. If spontaneous respirations are absent, ventilate the patient via bag, valve and mask, or endotracheal tube, and administer 100% oxygen (FiO_2 of 1.0).
- Assess fetal status. If nonreassuring FHR findings are present, initiate intrauterine support. Dependent on maternal status, consider delivery.
- Optimize preload. If left-ventricular contractility is decreased, inotropic support should be considered. Administration of a vasopressor may be indicated to correct hypotension refractory to volume resuscitation and inotropic support.
- Pulmonary artery catheterization provides data regarding hemodynamic function and oxygen transport status, and should be considered in order to guide specific hemodynamic management.
- Treat DIC. Administer blood and component therapy.
- Obtain consultations as indicated.
- Consider hydrocortisone 500 mg IV every 6 hours (two doses)
  - Assess critical laboratory values: Arterial blood gases, complete blood count, platelet count, fibrinogen, fibrin split products, prothrombin time, and partial thromboplastin time

arterial partial pressure of oxygen (PaO_2) greater than or equal to 60 mmHg.

In patients with AFE or other complications with complement system activation and/or DIC, tissue oxygenation may be further impaired by a decrease in oxygen delivery secondary to alterations in oxygen affinity. Oxygen affinity describes the relationship of hemoglobin and oxygen binding and unbinding in vitro. Factors present in anaphylaxis, septic shock, and probably AFE may reduce the ability of hemoglobin to release oxygen to organ systems during profound tissue hypoxia Thus, although total oxygen delivery may be improved, tissues may continue to experience ischemia due to the impaired ability to extract or utilize available oxygen. This mechanism may help explain why women who are successfully resuscitated after AFE continue to have significant neurologic sequelae.

Circulation

As previously described, oxygen transport is dependent on cardiac output. In turn, cardiac output is dependent on preload, afterload, contractility, and heart rate. Interventions to optimize preload include intravenous fluid resuscitation with isotonic crystalloid solution, and repositioning the patient to maximize venous return of blood to the heart. Inotropic support may be necessary to improve left-ventricular function and increase cardiac output. Initiation of central hemodynamic monitoring via pulmonary artery catheterization may be helpful in identification of additional interventions to correct specific hemodynamic abnormalities. Administration of other vasoactive medications may be indicated, dependent on patient response to initial interventions. Chapter 6 of this text provides a description of drugs commonly used in acute care of the pregnant woman, and includes indications for administration, method of action, dosage guidelines, and implications for clinical assessment of patient response to therapy.

In the event of maternal cardiopulmonary arrest in cases where AFE is suspected, the most common cardiac rhythm is pulseless electrical activity (PEA). Immediate initiation of maternal resuscitation, in accordance with current American Heart Association guidelines, is indicated. Cardiopulmonary resuscitation in pregnancy is described in Chapter 14, including interventions, modifications during pregnancy, and algorithms for pulseless cardiac rhythms.

Blood Component Therapy

Administration of blood component therapy is indicated to treat the consumptive coagulopathy that frequently accompanies AFE. A thorough description of DIC, including strategies to correct the coagulopathy, is presented in Chapter 16. Hemorrhage is a common complication included in this emergency syndrome. Significant concepts related to obstetric hemorrhage, including causes, secondary complications, clinical assessment, and management strategies, are described in depth in Chapter 15 of this text.

Delivery

In antepartum cases of suspected AFE, careful assessment of fetal status is indicated. If the mother is hemodynamically unstable but has not yet experienced cardiopulmonary arrest, consideration of efforts to stabilize the maternal status is appropriate and may result in improvement of fetal status as well. The decision to subject an unstable mother to major abdominal surgery is a difficult one, and each case must be individualized by the health care providers on the scene.[1] The process of making such a decision clearly represents one of many clinical and ethical challenges associated with care of the compromised or critically ill pregnant woman. Chapter 3 of this text explores this subject in detail.

In cases where the mother with a suspected AFE has progressed to cardiopulmonary arrest, the situation is different. Intact maternal survival is extremely unlikely, regardless of the therapy rendered. It is highly unlikely that performance of a Cesarean section would alter maternal outcome. Even properly performed cardiopulmonary resuscitation of the pregnant woman provides only a maximum of 30% of normal cardiac output during pregnancy. Thus, oxygen delivery is severely diminished. Under these circumstances, it is fair to assume that the proportion of blood shunted to the uterus and other splanchnic distribution approaches zero.[1] Thus, for practical purposes, the fetus most likely will be anoxic for the duration of the maternal cardiopulmonary arrest. Because the interval from maternal arrest to delivery of the fetus is directly correlated with newborn outcome, immediate perimortem Cesarean section should be initiated upon diagnosis of maternal cardiopulmonary arrest in cases where there is a high suspicion of AFE.[1]

Neonatal outcome in cases of maternal AFE is poor. If the event occurs prior to delivery, the neonatal survival rate is approximately 80%; however, only half of these fetuses survive neurologically intact.[4] Fetuses who survive to the time of delivery, following maternal cardiac arrest, generally demonstrate profound respiratory and/or metabolic acidemia. Although at the present time no form of therapy appears to be associated with improved maternal outcome, there is a clear relationship between neonatal outcome and timing of delivery in those women suffering cardiac arrest.[4]

SUMMARY

AFE or anaphylactoid syndrome of pregnancy remains an enigmatic phenomenon, despite many advances in the understanding of this complex condition. It also remains both unpreventable and unpredictable. It is anticipated that new insight into the pathophysiology of AFE, suggested by analysis of data from the United States National Registry of Amniotic Fluid Embolus, may facilitate further advances in the understanding and treatment of this catastrophic condition. Initiation of a National Registry of Amniotic Fluid Embolus in the United Kingdom should also provide further understanding of this obstetric complication.[27]

REFERENCES

1. Dildy, G. A., & Clark, S. L. (2004). Anaphylactoid syndrome of pregnancy (amniotic fluid embolism). In G. A. Dildy, M. A. Belfort, G. R. Saade, et al. (Eds.), *Critical care obstetrics* (4th ed., pp. 463–471). Boston: Blackwell Science.
2. Tuffnell, D. J. (2005). United Kingdom amniotic fluid embolism register. *British Journal of Obstetrics and Gynecology, 112,* 1625–1629.
3. Gilbert, W. M., & Danielsen, B. (1999). Amniotic fluid embolism: Decreased mortality in a population-based study. *Obstetrics and Gynecology, 93,* 973–977.
4. Clark, S. L., Hankins, G. D. V., Dudley, D. A., Dildy, G. A., & Porter, T. F. (1995). Amniotic fluid embolism: Analysis of the national registry. *American Journal of Obstetrics and Gynecology, 172*(4), 1158–1169.
5. Meyer, J. R. (1926). Embolia pulmonary amniocaseosa. *Bras/Med, 2,* 301–303.
6. Attwood, H. D., & Matthew, B. (1979). A possible early description of amniotic fluid embolism. *Australian/New Zealand Journal Obstetrics and Gynecology, 19,* 176–177.
7. Steiner, P. E., & Lushbaugh, C. C. (1941). Maternal pulmonary embolism by amniotic fluid. *Journal of American Medical Association, 117,* 1245.
8. Liban, E., & Raz, S. (1969). A clinicopathologic study of fourteen cases of amniotic fluid embolism. *American Journal of Clinical Pathology, 51,* 477–486.
9. Resnik, R., Swartz, W. H., Plumer, M. H., Benirschke, K., & Stratthaus, M. E. (1976). Amniotic fluid embolism with survival. *Obstetrics and Gynecology, 47,* 295–298.
10. Eastman, N. J. (1948). Editorial comment. *Obstetrical and Gynecological Survey, 3,* 35.
11. Moore, J., & Baldisseri, M. R. (2005). Amniotic fluid embolism. *Critical Care Medicine, 33*(10), S279–S285.
12. Abenhaim, H. A., Azoulay, L., Kramer, M. S., & Leduc, L. (2008). Incidence and risk factors of amniotic fluid embolism: A population based study on 3 million births in the United States. *American Journal of Obstetrics and Gynecology, 199,* 49.e1-8.
13. Kretzschmar, M., Zahm, D. M., Remmier, K., Pfeiffer, L., Victor, L., & Schirmeister, W. (2003). Pathophysiological and therapeutic aspects of amniotic fluid embolism (anaphylactoid syndrome of pregnancy): Case report with lethal outcome and overview. *Anesthesia, 52,* 419–426.
14. Conde-Agudelo, A., & Romero, R. (2009). Amniotic fluid embolism: An evidence based review. *American Journal of Obstetrics and Gynecology, 201,* 445 e1-445.e13.
15. Towell, M. E. (1976). Fetal acid-base physiology and intra-uterine asphyxia. In J. W. Goodwin, J. O. Golden, & G. W. Chance (Eds.), *Perinatal medicine* (p. 200). Baltimore: Williams and Wilkins.
16. Clark, S. L., Montz, F. J., & Phelan, J. P. (1985). Hemodynamic alterations associated with amniotic fluid embolism: A

reprisal. *American Journal of Obstetrics and Gynecology, 151*, 617–621.

17. Aurangzeb, I., George, L., & Raoof, S. (2004). Amniotic fluid embolism. *Critical Care Clinics, 20*, 643–650.

18. Davies, S. (2001). Amniotic fluid embolism: A review of the literature. *Canadian Journal of Anesthesia, 48*, 88–98.

19. Fletcher, S. J., & Parr, M. (2000). Amniotic fluid embolism: A case report and review. *Resuscitation, 43*, 141–146.

20. Gei, G., & Hankins, G. D. V. (2000). Amniotic fluid embolism: An update. *Contemporary OB/Gyn, 45*(1), 53–66.

21. Uszynski, M., & Uszynski, W. (2011). Coagulation and fibrinolysis in amniotic fluid: Physiology and observations on amniotic fluid embolism, preterm fetal membrane rupture, and pre-eclampsia. *Seminars in Thrombosis & Hemostasis. Hemostatic Factors in the Etiology, Early Detection, Prevention, and Management of Pre-Eclampsia, 37*(2), 165–174.

22. Clark, S. L. (2010). Amniotic fluid embolism. *Clinical Obstetrics and Gynecology, 53*(2), 322–328.

23. Porter, T. F., Clark, S. L., Dildy, G. A., & Hankins, G. D. V. (1996). Isolated disseminated intravascular coagulation and amniotic fluid embolism. *American Journal of Obstetrics and Gynecology, 174*, 486.

24. Perozzi, K. J., & Englert, N. C. (2004). Amniotic fluid embolism: An obstetric emergency. *Critical Care Nurse, 24*(4), 54–61.

25. Marcus, B. J., Collins, K. A., & Harley, R. A. (2005). Ancillary studies in amniotic fluid embolism: A case report and review of the literature. *American Journal of Forensic Medicine and Pathology, 26*(1), 92–95.

26. Kobayashi, H., Ohi, H., & Terao, T. (1993). A simple, noninvasive, sensitive method for diagnosis of amniotic fluid embolism by monoclonal antibody TKH-2 that recognizes NeuAc alpha 2-6GalNAc. *American Journal of Obstetrics and Gynecology, 168*(3 Pt 1), 848–853.

27. Tuffnell, D. J., & Johnson, H. (2000). Amniotic fluid embolism: The UK register. *Hospital Medicine, 61*, 532–534.

CHAPTER 20

Perinatal Infection

Patrick Duff

This chapter focuses on the principal bacterial, viral, and protozoan infections that pose a serious threat to the health and safety of the pregnant woman and her fetus or newborn. The review includes a discussion of group B streptococcal infection, cytomegalovirus infection, viral hepatitis, herpes simplex infection, human immunodeficiency virus infection, parvovirus infection, rubella, syphilis, toxoplasmosis, and varicella. The discussion highlights the clinical manifestations, adverse maternal and fetal consequences, diagnosis, and perinatal management of each infection.

CYTOMEGALOVIRUS INFECTION

Cytomegalovirus (CMV) is a DNA virus that is a member of the herpes virus family. Like herpes simplex virus, CMV may remain latent in host cells after the initial infection. Recurrent infection is usually due to reactivation of an endogenous latent virus rather than reinfection with a new strain of virus.[1]

CMV is not highly contagious, and, therefore, close personal contact is required for infection to occur. Horizontal transmission may result from transplantation of an infected organ or transfusion of infected blood, sexual contact, or from contact with contaminated saliva or urine. Vertical transmission may occur as a result of transplacental infection, exposure to contaminated genital tract secretions during delivery, or breast-feeding. The incubation period of the virus ranges from 28 to 60 days.[2]

Among young children, the most important risk factor for infection is close contact with playmates. Most children who acquire CMV infection are asymptomatic.[3] When clinical manifestations are present, they include malaise, fever, lymphadenopathy and hepatosplenomegaly. Similarly, most immunocompetent adults with CMV infection are asymptomatic or have only mild symptoms suggestive of a flu-like illness.

The diagnosis of CMV infection can be confirmed by isolation of virus in tissue culture. The highest concentration of virus typically is in urine, seminal fluid, saliva, and breast milk. Polymerase chain reaction methodology permits identification of viral antigen within 24 hours.[1,2]

Serologic methods also are helpful in establishing the diagnosis of CMV infection. In the acute phase of infection, IgM antibody is present in serum. IgM titers usually decline rapidly over a period of 30 to 60 days, but they can remain elevated for many months. There is no absolute IgG titer that clearly differentiates acute from recurrent infection. However, a fourfold or greater change in the IgG titer is consistent with recent acute infection. In addition, detecting "low acidity" IgG also is indicative of recent infection.

As a result of exposure to either young children or an infected sex partner, approximately 50% to 80% of adult women in the United States have serologic evidence of past CMV infection. Unfortunately, the presence of antibody is not perfectly protective against either reinfection or vertical transmission. Therefore, pregnant women with both recurrent and primary infection pose a risk to their fetus.[4,5]

Antepartum (congenital) infection poses the greatest risk to the fetus and results from hematogenous dissemination of virus across the placenta. Dissemination may occur with both primary and recurrent infection, but it is much more likely in the former setting. In women who acquire primary CMV infection during pregnancy, approximately 40% to 50% of the fetuses will be infected. The overall risk of congenital infection is greatest when maternal infection occurs in the third trimester, but the probability of severe fetal injury is highest when maternal infection develops in the first trimester.[4,5]

Approximately 5% to 15% of infants who develop congenital CMV infection as a result of primary maternal infection will be symptomatic at birth. The most common clinical manifestations of severe neonatal infection are hepatosplenomegaly, intracranial calcifications, jaundice,

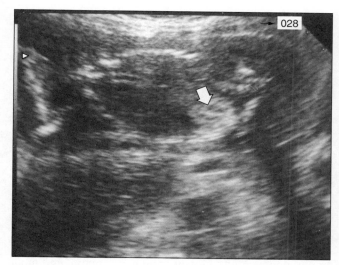

FIGURE 20-1   A longitudinal scan of the fetus shows echogenic bowel (*arrowhead*) characteristic of congenital CMV infection.

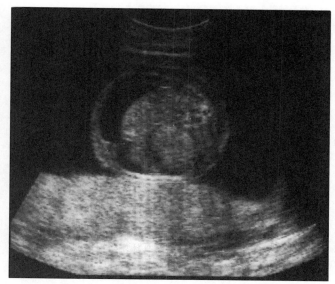

FIGURE 20-2   Isolated ascites is a possible manifestation of congenital CMV infection.

growth restriction, microcephaly, chorioretinitis, hearing loss, thrombocytopenia, hyperbilirubinemia, and elevated serum transaminase concentrations. Approximately 30% of severely infected infants die; 80% of survivors have major morbidity such as mental retardation, ocular abnormalities, or sensorineural hearing loss. Approximately 85% to 90% of infants with congenital CMV infection are asymptomatic at birth, and 10% to 15% subsequently develop hearing loss, chorioretinitis, or dental defects within the first two years of life.[1,4,5]

Pregnant women who experience recurrent or reactivated CMV infection are much less likely to transmit infection to their fetus. When recurrent infection develops in pregnancy, approximately 5% to 10% of infants will become infected; however, none of these neonates are symptomatic at birth. The most common sequelae are hearing loss, visual deficits, and mild developmental delays.[5]

Perinatal infection can occur during delivery as a result of exposure to infected genital tract secretions. Infection also may occur as a result of breast-feeding. However, infants infected by one of these mechanisms rarely have any serious injury.

Identification of CMV in amniotic fluid by either culture or polymerase chain reaction (PCR) is the most sensitive and specific test for diagnosing congenital infection.[6] However, mere identification of the virus does not necessarily delineate the severity of fetal injury. Fortunately, sonography is invaluable in providing information about severity of fetal impairment. The principal sonographic findings suggestive of serious fetal injury include microcephaly, ventriculomegaly, intracerebral calcification, fetal hydrops, growth restriction, and oligohydramnios. Less common findings include fetal heart block, intra-abdominal echodensities

(Figure 20-1), meconium peritonitis, renal dysplasia, and isolated serous effusions (Figure 20-2).

Until recently, no consistently effective therapy for congenital CMV infection was available. However, in 2005, Nigro and colleagues,[7] published an exciting report describing use of hyperimmune globulin as treatment and prophylaxis for congenital CMV infection. The authors performed a prospective cohort study at eight Italian medical centers. One hundred fifty-seven women had confirmed primary CMV infection. Of these, 148 were asymptomatic and were identified by routine serologic screening; eight had symptomatic viral infection, and one was identified because her fetus had abnormal ultrasound findings. Forty-five women had a primary infection more than 6 weeks before enrollment, underwent amniocentesis, and had CMV detected in amniotic fluid by PCR or culture. Thirty-one of these women received intravenous treatment with CMV-specific hyperimmune globulin (200 units, or mg, per kilogram of maternal body weight). Nine of the 31 received one or two additional infusions into either the amniotic fluid or umbilical cord because of persistent fetal abnormalities on ultrasonography. Fourteen women declined treatment; seven of them had infants who were acutely symptomatic at the time of delivery. In contrast, only one of the 31 treated women had an infant with clinical CMV disease at birth (adjusted odds ratio 0.02, p <.001).

In this investigation, 84 additional women did not undergo amniocentesis because their infection occurred within six weeks before enrollment, their gestational age was less than 20 weeks, or they declined amniocentesis. Thirty-seven of these women received 100 units of hyperimmune globulin per kilogram intravenously every month until delivery, and 47 declined treatment. Of the treated women, six delivered infected infants as compared with 19 of the untreated women (adjusted odds ratio 0.32, p = 0.04). No adverse effects of hyperimmune globulin were noted in either group receiving immunotherapy.

This intriguing report had several shortcomings.[8] The design of the study was neither randomized nor controlled. There are at least some biological reasons to question the remarkable success rates reported by the authors. Patients were not specifically stratified by presence or absence of major ultrasound abnormalities. Finally, the authors did not address the financial and logistic issues associated with screening large obstetric populations for CMV infection, triaging patients with inevitable false positive results, offering amniocentesis and targeted sonography to women who seroconvert, and then treating at risk patients with hyperimmune globulin. Nevertheless, the authors' observations are extremely interesting and promising and offer the best available therapy for this dangerous perinatal infection.

Ideally, preventive measures should be employed to ensure that women do not contract CMV infection during pregnancy. One simple measure is using CMV-negative blood products when transfusing pregnant women or fetuses. In addition, women should be encouraged to use careful handwashing techniques after handling infant diapers and toys.[1,8]

GROUP B STREPTOCOCCAL INFECTION

Streptococcus agalactiae is a gram-positive encapsulated bacterium that produces beta-hemolysis when grown on blood agar. On average, approximately 20% to 25% of pregnant women are colonized with group B streptococci in the lower genital tract and/or rectum. The group B *Streptococcus* is one of the most important causes of early-onset neonatal infection. The prevalence of neonatal group B streptococcal infection is approximately 0.5 per 1,000 live births, and approximately 10,000 cases of neonatal streptococcal septicemia occur each year in the United States.[9]

Approximately 80% to 85% of cases of neonatal group B streptococcal infection are early in onset, and these cases result almost exclusively from vertical transmission from a colonized mother to her infant. Early-onset infection typically presents as a severe pneumonia and/or overwhelming septicemia. In preterm infants, the mortality approaches 25%. In term infants, the mortality is lower, averaging approximately 5%.[9]

The major risk factors for early-onset infection include preterm labor, especially when complicated by preterm premature rupture of membranes; intrapartum maternal fever (due to chorioamnionitis); prolonged rupture of membranes (more than 18 hours); and previous delivery of an infected infant. Approximately 25% of pregnant women have at least one risk factor for early-onset group B streptococcal infection, and the presence of a risk factor dramatically affects the incidence of infection and the ultimate prognosis in infected neonates. For example, the neonatal attack rate in colonized patients is 40% to 50% when a risk factor is present and less than 5% in the absence of a risk factor. Moreover, in infected neonates, neonatal mortality approaches 30% to 35% when a maternal risk factor is present but is less than 5% when a risk factor is absent.[9]

At the present time, the gold standard for diagnosis of group B streptococcal infection is bacteriologic culture. The preferred medium is Todd-Hewitt broth or selective blood agar. The specimen for culture should be obtained from the lower vagina, perineum, and anus using a simple cotton swab.[10] Bergeron and colleagues recently reported exceptionally favorable results with a new PCR assay for group B streptococci.[11] In a series of 112 patients, the authors demonstrated a sensitivity of 97%, specificity of 100%, positive predictive value of 100%, and negative predictive value of 99%. This PCR assay now is commercially available and offers great promise as a rapid test for screening patients for group B streptococcal infection at the time that they are admitted to the labor and delivery unit. This test, and other nucleic acid amplification tests, are most effective when the laboratory specimen is allowed to incubate for 18 to 24 hours.[10]

The most effective strategy for prevention of early-onset neonatal group B streptococcal infection is based on guidelines published by the Centers for Disease Control and Prevention in 1996 and most recently modified in 2010.[12] The new guidelines recommend culturing select patients admitted to the hospital for assessment of preterm labor and/or preterm premature rupture of membranes. In addition, all patients should be cultured at 35 to 37 weeks. Patients who test positive should receive intrapartum antibiotic prophylaxis with one of the regimens outlined in Table 20-1. Women who previously delivered a baby who had group B streptococcal infection, women known to be colonized earlier in pregnancy, and women with prior group B streptococcal bacteriuria should not be routinely cultured at 35 to 37 weeks. They should be considered colonized and treated with prophylactic antibiotics intrapartum.

Ideally, antibiotics should be administered at least 4 hours prior to delivery. DeCueto and associates recently demonstrated that the rate of neonatal group B streptococcal infection was reduced significantly when patients were treated for at least this period of time.[13] Overall, if the guidelines outlined above are followed, the risk of neonatal infection should be reduced by approximately 80% in treated patients.[14]

TABLE 20-1

Intrapartum Prophylaxis for Group B
Streptococcal Infection

Drug	Dose
Ampicillin	2 g initially, then 1 g q4h
Penicillin	5 million units initially, then 2.5–3.0 million units q4h
Cefazolin*	1 g q8h
Clindamycin[†]	900 mg q8h
Vancomycin[†]	1 g q12h

*Cefazolin should be used in patients who have a non-life-threatening allergy to penicillin.

[†]These drugs should be used in patients who have a life-threatening allergy to penicillin. Clindamycin is preferred if the organism is known to be sensitive to the drug; however, up to 15% of strains are resistant. Vancomycin should be used if the organism is resistant to clindamycin or sensitivity tests are not available.

HEPATITIS

Hepatitis A

Hepatitis A, the second most common form of viral hepatitis in the United States, is caused by an RNA virus. The virus is transmitted by fecal–oral contact, and the incubation period varies from 15 to 50 days. Acute infections in children are usually asymptomatic; infections in adults are usually symptomatic. The diagnosis of acute infection is best confirmed by detection of IgM antibody specific for the hepatitis A virus. Hepatitis A does not cause a chronic carrier state. Perinatal transmission virtually never occurs, and, therefore, the infection does not pose a major risk to either the mother or the fetus unless the mother develops fulminant hepatitis and liver failure. Fortunately, this complication is extremely rare.[15]

Hepatitis A can be prevented by administration of an inactivated vaccine.[16] Standard immune globulin also provides reasonably effective passive immunization for hepatitis A if it is given within two weeks of exposure,

for example, in anticipation of travel to an area of the world where hepatitis A is endemic.

Hepatitis E

Hepatitis E is caused by an RNA virus, and the epidemiology of this infection is similar to that of hepatitis A. The disease is rare in the United States but is endemic in developing countries of the world. In these countries, maternal infection with hepatitis E has an alarmingly high mortality rate, in the range of 10% to 20%. This high mortality is due to the combined effect of hepatitis and poor nutrition, poor general health, and lack of access to modern medical care.[17,18]

The clinical presentation of acute hepatitis E is similar to that of hepatitis A. The most useful diagnostic test is serology. Hepatitis E does not cause a chronic carrier state, and perinatal transmission is extremely rare.[19,20]

Hepatitis B

Hepatitis B is caused by a DNA virus that is transmitted parenterally and by sexual contact. The virus also can be transmitted perinatally from an infected mother to her infant. Acute hepatitis B occurs in approximately 1 to 2 patients per 1,000 pregnancies in the United States; the chronic carrier state is present in 6 to 10 patients per 1,000 pregnancies.[15]

Approximately 90% of patients with hepatitis B mount an effective immunologic response to the virus and completely clear their infection. Less than 1% of infected patients develop fulminant hepatitis and die. Approximately 10% develop a chronic carrier state. The carrier state predisposes patients to severe chronic liver diseases such as chronic active or persistent hepatitis, cirrhosis, and hepatocellular carcinoma.[15]

The best method for diagnosing hepatitis B infection is serology. Table 20-2 demonstrates the possible results of serologic tests for hepatitis B virus. Clinicians should recognize that when the little e antigen is present in association with the surface antigen, viral replication is extensive and the patient is highly infectious.

TABLE 20-2

Serologic Diagnosis of Hepatitis B Infection

Condition	Surface Antigen	Antibody to Surface Antigen	Antibody to Core Antigen
Susceptible	Negative	Negative	Negative
Immune	Negative	Positive	Positive IgG
Acute infection	Positive	Negative	Positive IgM
Chronic infection	Positive	Negative	Positive IgG

PLEASE NOTE: Some acute and chronically infected patients may test positive for the e antigen. When this antigen is present, it denotes a particularly high level of infectivity.

Approximately 20% of pregnant women who are seropositive for hepatitis B surface antigen, but negative for the e antigen, will transmit infection to their neonates in the absence of intervention. Approximately 90% of mothers who are positive for both the surface antigen and e antigen will transmit infection.

Fortunately, excellent immunoprophylaxis for prevention of perinatal transmission of hepatitis B infection is now available. Infants delivered to seropositive mothers should receive hepatitis B immune globulin within 12 hours of birth. This passive immunization provides immediate protection against virus to which the infant is exposed during the birth process. Prior to discharge from the hospital, infants should begin the hepatitis B vaccination series. Active vaccination provides prolonged protection against hepatitis B. Infants delivered to mothers who are seronegative for hepatitis B require only the hepatitis B vaccine.[15,21]

Hepatitis D (Delta Virus Infection)

Hepatitis D is an RNA virus that depends upon coinfection with hepatitis B for replication. The epidemiology of hepatitis D is identical to that of hepatitis B. Patients who have both acute hepatitis B and hepatitis D are considered to have coinfection. These individuals typically clear both infections and have a very good long-term prognosis. Patients who have chronic hepatitis D infection superimposed upon chronic hepatitis B are considered to have a superinfection. These individuals are particularly likely to develop chronic liver disease.[22,23] The diagnosis of hepatitis D can be established by identifying the delta antigen in liver tissue or serum. However, the most useful diagnostic tests are detection of IgM and/or IgG antibody in serum.

As noted, hepatitis D can cause a chronic carrier state in conjunction with hepatitis B. Perinatal transmission of hepatitis D occurs, but it is uncommon because the immunoprophylaxis outlined above for hepatitis B is highly effective in preventing transmission of hepatitis D.[22,23]

Hepatitis C

Hepatitis C is caused by an RNA virus. Infection may be transmitted parenterally, via sexual contact, and perinatally.[24,25] Hepatitis C infection usually is asymptomatic. The diagnosis is confirmed by serologic testing. The initial screening test is an enzyme immunoassay (EIA), and the confirmatory test is a recombinant immunoblot assay (RIBA). The present generation of serologic tests does not consistently and precisely distinguish between IgM and IgG antibody.

In patients who have a low concentration of hepatitis C RNA and who do not have coexisting HIV infection,

the risk of perinatal transmission of infection is low — less than 5%. In patients who have a high serum concentration of hepatitis C RNA and/or have HIV infection, the perinatal transmission rate may approach 25%. Several non-randomized, uncontrolled cohort studies (level II evidence) support the role for an elective Cesarean delivery prior to the onset of labor and ruptured membranes in select women who have a high titer of hepatitis C virus RNA. For women who have undetectable serum concentrations of viral RNA, vaginal delivery is a reasonable plan of management. In addition, breast-feeding is acceptable and does not pose a significant risk of transmission of infection to the neonate.[26,27]

Hepatitis G

Hepatitis G is caused by an RNA virus that is related to the hepatitis C virus. Hepatitis G is more common than hepatitis C, but, fortunately, it is much less virulent. Many patients who have hepatitis G are coinfected with hepatitis A, B, and C, and with HIV.[28–30]

Most patients with hepatitis G are asymptomatic. The diagnosis is established by detection of virus by PCR and by identification of antibody by enzyme-linked immunosorbent assay (ELISA). Hepatitis G can cause a chronic carrier state, and perinatal transmission has been documented. However, the clinical effect of infection in the mother and baby is minimal.[28–30]

HERPES SIMPLEX VIRUS INFECTION

Herpes simplex virus (HSV) is a DNA virus that has two principal strains — HSV1 and HSV2. The former typically causes oral lesions, and the latter usually causes genital lesions. However, HSV1 can be responsible for ulcerated genital lesions, and HSV2 can be responsible for oral lesions. The infection is transmitted by intimate personal contact and is highly contagious.[31]

HSV2 is usually the organism of greatest concern to the perinatal and pediatric clinicians. HSV2 infections may be classified as primary, initial–non-primary, and recurrent, in accordance with the criteria listed in Table 20-3.

The characteristic lesion of HSV2 infection is a vesicle (Figure 20-3) that progresses, in sequence, to a pustule, then a shallow-based ulcer, then a crusted lesion. The duration of each of these lesions varies significantly, depending upon whether the infection is primary or recurrent, as noted in Table 20-4.

The most useful test for the clinical diagnosis of HSV infection is identification of the virus in the lesion by culture or PCR. When the lesion is in the vesicular stage, the frequency of viral isolation exceeds 90%. When the pustule is present, the frequency of viral isolation is

TABLE 20-3

Classification of Herpes Simplex Virus-2 Infections

Type of Infection	Criteria for Diagnosis	Usual Clinical Manifestations
Primary	• First clinical infection • No pre-existing antibody to either HSV-1 or HSV-2	• Systemic signs/symptoms such as malaise, fever, headache • Multiple painful vesicular lesions on external genitalia, vagina, and cervix
Initial, nonprimary	• No history of genital infection • Positive serology for HSV-1	• Minimal systemic signs • Fever, vesicular lesions
Recurrent	• Prior history of genital infection • Positive antibody for HSV-2	• No systemic signs/symptoms • Characteristic prodrome-paresthesias in area where vesicles later appear • Few vesicular lesions • Short period of viral shedding

approximately 85%. When the ulcer is present, the frequency of viral isolation is approximately 70%. When the lesions have crusted, the frequency of viral isolation declines to only 25%.[31]

HSV infection in pregnancy poses a risk to the fetus primarily at the time of delivery. Although the virus can be transmitted hematogenously across an intact placenta or transcervically across intact membranes, such transmission is extremely uncommon. The most likely mechanism of infection is exposure of the neonate to virus in the lower genital tract during the process of delivery. If a mother has a primary infection at the time of labor, and the infant delivers vaginally, the risk of infection is approximately 40%. In the era before the availability of acyclovir, at least half of these infants died, and most of the remainder had serious neurologic morbidity. If the mother has overt recurrent infection at the time of vaginal delivery, the risk of fetal infection is less than or equal to 5%. If the mother has a history of recurrent herpes but is simply asymptomatically shedding the virus at the time of delivery, the risk to the neonate is less than or equal to 1%.[32–35]

Neonatal HSV infection can take the form of a disseminated mucocutaneous eruption, central nervous system infection, or disseminated visceral infection. Approximately 30% of infants with disseminated disease die despite antiviral therapy and approximately 40% of survivors have severe neurologic damage.

At the time of the first prenatal appointment, every obstetric patient should be questioned in detail about a history of HSV infection. Patients with a positive history should be screened for all other STDs. If an initial episode of HSV develops during pregnancy, the diagnosis should be confirmed by culture or PCR. The diagnosis of subsequent episodes can be established on the basis of clinical examination.

Pregnant women with a severe primary infection should be treated with therapeutic doses of antiviral drugs. The most cost-effective treatment is acyclovir, 400 mg orally, 3 times daily, for 7 to 10 days. Although both famcyclovir and valacyclovir are highly effective against HSV, they are more expensive than generic acyclovir. Seriously ill, immunocompromised patients may require hospitalization and treatment with intravenous acyclovir.

Antiviral therapy also is indicated in pregnant patients who have a history of recurrent HSV infection. A recent systematic review confirmed major benefits of prophylactic use of oral acyclovir, 400 mg, 3 times daily, from 36 weeks until the time of delivery.[36] Patients who received prophylaxis had a markedly reduced risk of clinical recurrence (odds ratio 0.25), Cesarean delivery for recurrent infection (odds ratio 0.30), detection of HSV at the time of delivery (odds ratio 0.11), and frequency of asymptomatic shedding at the time of delivery (odds ratio 0.09) compared with women who received only placebo therapy.

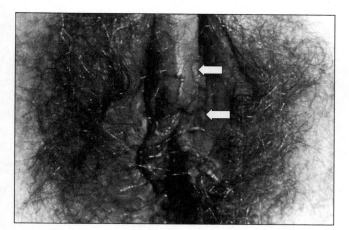

FIGURE 20-3 Shallow, painful ulcers (arrowheads) are the characteristic lesions of HSV infection.

TABLE 20-4

Usual Duration of Herpetic Lesions

Stage of Infection	Primary Infection (Days)	Recurrent Infection (Days)
Incubation period	2–10	1–2
Vesicle/pustule	6	2
Ulcer	6	3
Crust	8	5–7

At the time the patient is admitted in labor, she should be evaluated for the most appropriate method of delivery. If she has a prodrome or any visible lesion, she should have a Cesarean delivery regardless of whether or not the membranes are ruptured. If she has no prodromal symptoms and no visible lesions, she is a candidate for vaginal delivery, provided that there is no other indication for Cesarean delivery.[35]

HUMAN IMMUNODEFICIENCY VIRUS INFECTION

Human immunodeficiency virus (HIV) infection is caused by an RNA retrovirus. Two major strains of the virus have been identified—HIV1 and HIV2. Each major strain has several substrains. HIV1 is more widely prevalent throughout the world. HIV2 is endemic in certain parts of the world, such as sub-Saharan areas of Africa. HIV2 infection is rarely seen in the United States unless the patient traveled to an endemic area of the world or shared needles with or had sex with someone from an area of the world where HIV2 is prevalent.[37]

HIV infection is transmitted by three major mechanisms: sexual contact, intravenous drug use, and by perinatal transmission from an infected mother to her offspring. Previously, blood transfusion was an important mechanism of transmission, but, with the development of improved methods for screening the blood supply, this vector has become uncommon. Rare cases of HIV transmission have occurred as a result of organ donation and artificial insemination.

HIV infection typically evolves through four stages. The first stage of the infection is termed the acute retroviral illness. Within several weeks of exposure, the patient may develop a severe flu-like illness, characterized by malaise, poor appetite, weight loss, low-grade fever, and generalized lymphadenopathy.[38,39] Over a period of several weeks, this illness gradually resolves, and the patient enters the latent phase of infection. With appropriate antiretroviral therapy and supportive care, the latent phase of the illness may extend beyond 10 years in many patients. Ultimately, patients enter a symptomatic phase of the illness and, eventually, progress to AIDS.

Opportunistic diseases are the hallmark of HIV infection. The most common serious opportunistic disease in women is *Pneumocystis jiroveci* (formerly *carinii*) pneumonia. The second most common serious opportunistic disease is infection due to *Mycobacterium avium* complex (MAC). Kaposi's sarcoma, which is common in men with HIV infection, is rare in women. Other important opportunistic diseases include tuberculosis, toxoplasmosis, CMV infection, candidiasis, and non-Hodgkin's lymphoma.[40,41]

In the United States, the most common mechanism of transmission of HIV infection in women is now heterosexual contact with a high-risk male. Intravenous drug use also is an extremely important mechanism of transmission. Infection is more prevalent in African-American and Hispanic patients. The risk factors for sexual transmission of HIV infection are summarized in Box 20-1.[40,41]

The initial screening test for HIV infection is an enzyme immunoassay (EIA). If this test is positive, a confirmatory test such as the Western blot or the immunofluorescent assay (IFA) should be performed. If the confirmatory test also is positive, the diagnosis is established, and the probability of a false-positive sequence of reactions is less than 1 in 10,000.

The Centers for Disease Control and Prevention now recommend universal screening for HIV infection in pregnant women. The best strategy to ensure compliance

Box 20-1. RISK FACTORS FOR SEXUAL TRANSMISSION OF HIV INFECTION

- Multiple sex partners
- Receptive anal intercourse
- Unprotected intercourse
- Intravenous drug use
- Crack cocaine use
- Presence of ulcerated genital lesions
- Uncircumcised male partner
- Greater severity of illness in the index case
- Sex during menstruation
- Bleeding during intercourse (e.g., from trauma related to sexual assault)

Box 20-2. PRINCIPAL RISK FACTORS FOR PERINATAL TRANSMISSION OF HIV INFECTION

- History of previously affected infant
- Severe maternal disease
- Preterm delivery
- Intrapartum blood exposure
  - Vaginal lacerations
  - Episiotomy
  - Injury to infant's skin; e.g., from laceration due to forceps or vacuum extractor
- Rupture of membranes >4 hours
- Vaginal delivery (in select cases)
- Invasive antepartum procedures
  - Amniocentesis
  - Chorionic villus sampling
  - Cordocentesis
- Chorioamnionitis
- Concurrent sexually transmitted diseases

with screening is termed "opt out." With this strategy, HIV screening is considered a routine part of the prenatal laboratory test panel. Patients specifically have to decline the screening test; otherwise, it is routinely performed.

If a pregnant woman is HIV positive, and no treatment is administered, she has approximately a 25% risk of transmitting infection to her infant. Most cases of transmission occur at the time of delivery. Antenatal transmission is possible, usually as a result of invasive antepartum procedures. Postnatal transmission also can occur as a result of breast-feeding. With the appropriate interventions outlined below, the risk of perinatal transmission should be reduced from 25% to less than 2%. The principal risk factors for perinatal transmission of HIV infection are summarized in Box 20-2.[41]

If a pregnant woman is identified as HIV-positive, she should have a CD_4 count and viral load to assess her degree of immunosuppression, be screened for other sexually transmitted diseases, and be tested for tuberculosis. If the tuberculin skin test is positive, a chest x-ray should be performed to assess for active disease. Serologic tests for toxoplasmosis and cytomegalovirus infection should be obtained. She also should be vaccinated against several infections, including pneumococcal infection, influenza, hepatitis A, hepatitis B, and meningococcal meningitis.

In addition to the vaccines noted above, the patient also should receive prophylactic antibiotics against certain opportunistic pathogens.[42] If the patient's CD_4 count is below 200 cells per cubic millimeter and she previously has had an infection with pneumocystis, she should receive trimethoprim-

sulfamethoxazole—DS, one tablet daily. This medication also provides protection against toxoplasmosis infection. If the patient's tuberculin skin test is positive, and the chest x-ray shows no active disease, she should receive prophylaxis with isoniazid, 300 mg orally, daily, plus pyridoxine, 50 mg daily. The latter drug is administered to prevent peripheral neurotoxicity from isoniazid. If the patient's chest x-ray shows active tuberculosis, she must be treated with combination antibiotic therapy.

If the patient's CD_4 count falls to a range of 50 to 75 cells per cubic millimeter, she should receive prophylaxis against *Mycobacterium avium* complex. The appropriate prophylactic agent is azithromycin, 1,200 mg weekly. Patients who have recurrent candidiasis, should be treated with fluconazole, 150 mg orally, daily. If the patient's CD_4 count falls to a range of 50 cells per cubic millimeter or less, she also should receive prophylaxis with fluconazole to prevent cryptococcal infection. Patients who have recurrent herpes simplex virus infections should be treated with acyclovir, 400 mg, twice daily, for prophylaxis and three times daily for therapy.

The single most important intervention in pregnancy is treatment of the mother with highly active antiretroviral therapy.[41,43,44] The ACTG076 trial was the first to demonstrate that treatment of the pregnant woman with prophylactic zidovudine was extremely effective in reducing the rate of perinatal transmission of HIV infection.[44] In that trial, the rate of transmission was reduced from 26% in the placebo group to 8% in the group of patients who received zidovudine (level I evidence). Subsequent uncontrolled, retrospective studies (level II evidence) have shown that treatment of the mother with combination chemotherapy reduces the rate of perinatal transmission to less than 2%.[41]

The antiretroviral agents currently available are summarized in Table 20-5. One treatment regimen includes the four-drug regimen of zidovudine, lamivudine, ritonavir, and lopinavir. Zidovudine (300 mg) and lamivudine (150 mg) are administered as a single tablet, Combivir, twice daily. Lopinavir (400 mg) and ritonavir (100 mg) are administered as a single tablet of Kaletra, twice daily. The response to treatment should be evaluated by obtaining serial measurements of viral load. If a clear response to treatment has not occurred within 12 to 16 weeks, the patient should have viral genotyping to determine if she has a resistant organism. Poor response to treatment also may be due to noncompliance with prescribed therapy. Factors responsible for noncompliance include expense, drug intolerance, and failure to understand the treatment regimen.

If highly active antiretroviral therapy reduces the patient's viral load to less than 1,000 copies per milliliter, a vaginal delivery is appropriate, provided that

TABLE 20-5

Drugs for Treatment of HIV Infection

Agent	Usual Adult Dose	Major Adverse Effects
Nucleotide Analogue		
Tenofovir (Viread)	300 mg qd	GI irritation, elevation in transaminase concentrations, decrease in serum carnitine, and nephrotoxicity
Nucleoside Analogues		
Abacavir (Ziagen)	300 mg b.i.d.	Hypersensitivity reaction
Didanosine (DDI, Videx) or	200 mg b.i.d.	Pancreatitis and peripheral neuropathy
Videx EC	400 mg qd	
Emtricitabine (Emtriva)	200 mg qd	Headache, diarrhea, nausea, rash, hyperpigmentation, hepatitis
Lamivudine (3TC, Epivir)	150 mg b.i.d. or 300 mg qd	Marrow suppression
Stavudine (d4T, Zerit)	40 mg b.i.d.	Peripheral sensory neuropathy
Zalcitabine (ddC, Hivid)	0.75 mg q8h	Peripheral neuropathy, pancreatitis
Zidovudine (AZT, Retrovir)	300 mg b.i.d.	Marrow suppression
Combination Nucleoside Analogues		
Combivir (zidovudine + lamivudine)	1 tablet b.i.d.	Marrow suppression
Trizivir (zidovudine + lamivudine + abacavir)	1 tablet b.i.d.	Marrow suppression
Non-Nucleoside Reverse Transcriptase Inhibitors		
Delavirdine (Rescriptor)	400 mg t.i.d.	Rash, hepatitis
Efavirenz (Sustiva)	600 mg qd	Rash, CNS changes. Drug is teratogenic and should not be used in pregnancy.
Etravirine (Intelence)	200 mg b.i.d.	Rash, nausea, peripheral neuropathy, hepatitis
Nevirapine (Viramure)	200 mg b.i.d.	Rash, hepatitis
Unique Triple Combination		
Atripla (Efavirenz + emtricitabine + tenofovir)	Single daily dose 600 mg/200 mg/ 300 mg	Lactic acidosis, severe hepatomegaly, steatosis
Protease Inhibitors		
Amprenavir (Agenerase)	1200 mg b.i.d.	Rash and GI irritation
Atazanavir (Reyataz)	400 mg qd	Hyperbilirubinemia, prolonged Q-T interval, hyperlipidemia
Darunavir (Prezista) (Must be given with ritonavir)	600 mg/ 100 mg b.i.d.	Diarrhea, nausea, headache, increased transaminase activity, increased serum lipids
Indinavir (Crixivan)	800 mg t.i.d.	Nephrolithiasis, GI upset
Lopinavir/ritonavir (Kaletra)	3 gelatin capsules (133.3 mg/ 33.3 mg) b.i.d.	Diarrhea, nausea, fatigue, headache, asthenia
Nelfinavir (Viracept)	1250 mg b.i.d.	Diarrhea, fatigue, poor concentration
Ritonavir (Norvir)	100-400 mg b.i.d.	GI irritation, seizures, hepatitis, diabetes, marrow suppression
Tipranavir (Aptivus)—Must be given with ritonavir)	500 mg/200 mg b.i.d.	Hepatitis, diarrhea, nausea, vomiting, abdominal pain
Saquinavir Hard gel cap (Invirase) Soft gel cap (Fortovase)	400 or 1000 mg b.i.d. 1200 mg t.i.d.	GI irritation, peripheral neuropathy, headache, rash
Fusion Inhibitor		
Enfuvirtide (Fuzeon)	90 mg b.i.d.	GI irritation, rash, hypotension, injection site reaction
Integrase Inhibitor		
Raltegravir (Isentress)	400 mg b.i.d.	Diarrhea, nausea, headache
Viral Entry Inhibitor		
Maraviroc (Selzentry)	150–600 mg b.i.d.	Cough, fever, rash, abdominal pain, postural hypotension, MI, hepatotoxicity

CNS = central nervous system; MI = myocardial infarction.

there are no other indications for Cesarean delivery. However, if the patient does not have an optimal response to anti-retroviral therapy, she should be delivered by Cesarean at 38 weeks' gestation, prior to the onset of labor and ruptured membranes.[41,45–47] Regardless of the method of delivery, an infected patient should receive intravenous zidovudine during the delivery process.[43] For patients scheduled for Cesarean delivery, the zidovudine infusion should begin 4 hours prior to surgery. Infants delivered to infected mothers typically will be treated with antiviral agents for several weeks after delivery. If all of the interventions outlined above are successful, the risk of perinatal transmission of HIV infection should be less than 2%.[41,45–47]

PARVOVIRUS INFECTION

Parvovirus infection is a rare but potentially extremely serious perinatal complication. The infection is caused by a DNA organism, the B19 parvovirus. Infection is transmitted primarily by respiratory droplets and by infected blood products. Approximately 5% to 10% of school-age children have antibody to parvovirus. Seroprevalence increases progressively throughout childhood and young adult life to the point where approximately 50% to 60% of women of reproductive age have immunity.[48]

The incubation period for parvovirus is approximately 10 to 20 days. The most common clinical manifestation of infection is erythema infectiosum or fifth disease. Erythema infectiosum is manifested by low grade fever, malaise, myalgias, arthralgias, and a "slapped cheek" facial rash. An erythematous, lace-like rash also may extend onto the torso and upper extremities. The rash is neither pruritic nor painful. Erythema infectiosum often causes only mild symptoms in adults and children and, at times, is completely asymptomatic. In children, parvovirus infection also can cause transient aplastic crisis. This same disorder may occur in adults who have an underlying hemoglobinopathy.[49]

Parvovirus can cross the placenta and infect red cell progenitors in the fetal bone marrow, resulting in an aplastic anemia. The virus attaches to a particular antigen on the red cell stem cells. This same antigen, the i antigen, also is present on fetal myocardial cells, and, in some fetuses, cardiomyopathy may be present as well as aplastic anemia. The key manifestation of fetal infection is hydrops fetalis.[50]

The risk of fetal hydrops is directly related to the time in gestation that the maternal infection occurs. When maternal infection occurs in the first 12 weeks of gestation, the risk of hydrops fetalis varies from less than 5% to approximately 10%. When infection occurs in weeks 13 to 20 of gestation, the risk of infection declines to less than or equal to 5%. When maternal infection occurs beyond the 20th week of gestation, the risk of fetal hydrops is less than or equal to 1%.[50,51]

Aside from clinical examination, the best way to make the diagnosis of maternal parvovirus infection is through serologic testing.[49] Immediately after a documented exposure, the pregnant woman should have a test for IgM and IgG antibody. If the IgM antibody assay is negative and the IgG is positive, the patient is immune and should be reassured that there is no risk of fetal injury. If both the IgM and IgG assays are negative, the patient is susceptible, and she should be retested in approximately 3 weeks to determine if seroconversion has occurred. If the IgM assay is positive and the IgG is negative, the patient has an acute infection, indicating that she became infected within the past 3 to 7 days. If both the IgM and IgG assays are positive, then the patient has evidence of a subacute infection, indicating that the infection developed more than 7 days but less than 120 days ago.

Once maternal infection has been confirmed, the fetus must be evaluated for evidence of anemia. The best test for assessment of fetal anemia is ultrasound. Serial examinations should be performed for approximately 8 weeks after documentation of maternal infection, since the incubation period for fetal infections may extend up to 2 months. The most obvious ultrasound manifestation of fetal anemia is hydrops manifested by scalp edema, subcutaneous edema along the baby's trunk, pleural effusions, pericardial effusion, and ascites (Figure 20-4A and B). However, by the time the fetus has sonographic evidence of hydrops, its hematocrit may have declined to below 20 volumes percent. Therefore, a more precise way to detect evolving fetal anemia is to assess Doppler velocimetry in the middle cerebral artery.[52] Increases in peak systolic velocity in this vessel correlate extremely well with the fetal hematocrit. If middle cerebral artery velocimetry indicates fetal anemia, a cordocentesis should be performed to directly assess the fetal hematocrit. If anemia is demonstrated, an intrauterine blood transfusion should be performed.

At the present time, two retrospective studies (level II-2 evidence)[53,54] have demonstrated that intrauterine transfusion can be lifesaving in the setting of congenital parvovirus infection. The first study was published by Fairley and colleagues.[53] The authors' reviewed 66 cases of fetal hydrops due to congenital parvovirus infection. Twenty-six fetuses were dead at the time of diagnosis, and two were electively aborted. Twelve of 38 live fetuses had an intrauterine transfusion; 3 of the 12 died. Twenty-six fetuses did not receive an intrauterine transfusion, and 13 died. The odds ratio for fetal death in infants who received a transfusion was 0.14 (95% C.I. .02 to .96).

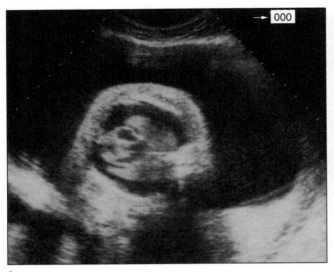

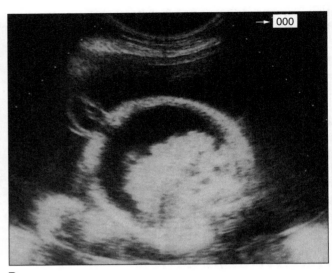

A   **B**

FIGURE 20-4   **A.** Fetal hydrops with bilateral pleural effusions and edema of the chest wall. **B.** Ascites and edema of the abdominal wall.

The second retrospective study was conducted by Rodis and associates.[54] The authors surveyed members of the Society for Maternal-Fetal Medicine and reported the outcomes of 460 cases of parvovirus infection. Twenty-seven of 164 fetuses who received an intrauterine transfusion died. One-hundred thirty-eight of 296 fetuses who did not receive an intrauterine transfusion died (P less than .001). Although cases of spontaneous resolution of fetal hydrops have been reported, the studies presented above clearly support a strong recommendation for intrauterine transfusion in the setting of fetal anemia due to congenital parvovirus infection.

Infants who survive intrauterine infection with parvovirus usually have an excellent long-term prognosis. Isolated case reports have been published documenting neurologic morbidity and prolonged, transfusion-dependent anemia, but these adverse sequelae are extremely rare.[55,56]

RUBELLA

Rubella (the three-day or German measles) is caused by an RNA virus. The infection is transmitted by respiratory droplets and is characterized by a diffuse, nonpruritic maculopapular skin rash. The disease primarily affects children. Since licensure of the first vaccine in 1969, the incidence of rubella has declined dramatically. However, approximately 10% of all women of reproductive age remain susceptible to rubella, either because they never were vaccinated as children or because their immunity has waned. Accordingly, clinicians still must be aware of the potential dangers of congenital rubella infection.[57]

Rubella is one of the most teratogenic of all viruses. If a mother is infected within the first 4 weeks following conception, there is a 50% probability that her infant will have findings of congenital rubella syndrome. When maternal infection occurs in the second 4 weeks after conception, the incidence of congenital rubella syndrome is 25%. When maternal infection occurs in the third month after conception, the incidence of congenital rubella declines to 10% and, when maternal infection occurs in the second or third trimester, the frequency of congenital rubella syndrome is less than or equal to 1%.[58,59]

The most common manifestations of congenital rubella syndrome are summarized in Table 20-6. The diagnosis of acute rubella infection in the mother is best established by clinical examination and by identification of IgM-specific antibody. The diagnosis of congenital rubella is best established by ultrasound examination. The key ultrasound findings that suggest congenital rubella syndrome are microcephaly, intrauterine growth restriction, and cardiac malformations.

TABLE 20-6

Most Common Manifestations of Congenital Rubella Syndrome

Anomaly	Percentage Affected
Deafness	60–75
Eye defects (cataracts, glaucoma)	10–30
CNS defects	10–25
Heart defects (PDA, pulmonic stenosis)	10–20

CNS = central nervous system; PDA = patent ductus arteriosus.

The prognosis for infants with congenital rubella is poor. Approximately 10% to 20% of affected infants die in the first year of life. Approximately 50% of children must attend schools for the hearing impaired. Only 25% are able to attend regular schools. In addition, children with congenital rubella syndrome may, later in life, develop diabetes. They also may develop an extremely serious neurologic condition, which is termed subacute sclerosing panencephalitis. This condition typically develops when an individual is 15 to 20 years of age. It is manifested by myoclonus and severe cognitive deterioration. Most affected individuals die within 6 months of the onset of symptoms.[60]

Interestingly, in individuals who have congenital rubella, antibody to the rubella virus typically disappears by age 4. As a result, these individuals then are susceptible to natural rubella infection.

All pregnant women should have a serologic test for rubella at the time of their first prenatal appointment. If the patient does not have a protective level of antibody, she should be counseled to avoid exposure to children with possible viral exanthems. If exposure occurs, and the patient develops acute rubella, she needs to be counseled about the risk of congenital rubella specific to her gestational age. She should be offered targeted ultrasound examination to assess for fetal injury and pregnancy termination, should serious fetal injury be documented.[61]

Ideally, women of reproductive age who are susceptible to rubella should be vaccinated prior to conception; alternatively, they should be vaccinated immediately postpartum. In addition, physicians should make certain that all workers in their office are immune to rubella and, therefore, do not pose a risk to susceptible patients.

The rubella vaccine is a live virus vaccine. It is available in a monovalent form, bivalent form (measles and rubella), and trivalent form (measles, mumps, rubella). The vaccine is usually very well tolerated. Approximately 10% of vaccinees develop arthralgias. Less than 1% develop frank arthritis. Mild constitutional symptoms occur in up to 25% of vaccine recipients. Vaccinees cannot transmit infection to susceptible contacts, and the vaccine may be administered to breast-feeding women.[62]

Following vaccination, a patient should be advised to use secure contraception for one month. Fortunately, there have been no reported cases of actual congenital rubella syndrome in patients who were inadvertently vaccinated during early pregnancy. The maximum theoretical risk of congenital rubella as a result of vaccination is 1% to 2%. Such a low risk certainly does not justify pregnancy termination should a patient be vaccinated early in gestation.[61,62]

SYPHILIS

The causative organism of syphilis is the spirochete, *Treponema pallidum*. Infection occurs primarily as a result of sexual contact. The organism readily penetrates mucosal barriers of the genital tract, and it is highly contagious. Infection develops in approximately 10% of sexual contacts after a single unprotected exposure and in 70% of contacts after multiple exposures. Syphilis also may be transmitted perinatally, and the consequences for the developing fetus can be devastating.[63,64]

Syphilis may be divided into four clinical categories: primary, secondary, tertiary, and neurosyphilis. In addition, the disease also may present as a latent infection, and, in fact, this is the most common presentation in obstetric patients. Latent syphilis is subdivided into early latent (less than 1 year duration) and late latent (greater than 1 year duration). The incubation period of syphilis ranges from 10 to 90 days. At the end of this period, the characteristic raised, painless chancre appears on the genitalia (Figure 20-5). In women, the chancre usually is on the cervix or vaginal wall and may not be apparent except on close inspection. In some patients, the chancre may be present in extragenital sites such as the fingers, oropharynx, nipples, or anus. The chancre usually heals in 3 to 6 weeks even without specific antimicrobial treatment.[63,64]

Patients who receive either no treatment, or inadequate treatment, may develop secondary syphilis 2 to 6 months after their primary infection. The principal clinical manifestation of this stage of infection is a generalized maculopapular rash that is most obvious on the palms of the hands and soles of the feet. This rash may be confused with disseminated gonococcal infection, measles, rubella, scabies, psoriasis, and a drug reaction. Other findings with secondary syphilis include

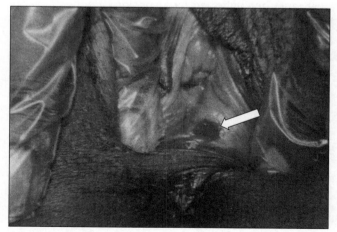

FIGURE 20-5   Characteristic chancre (arrowhead) of primary syphilis. (Photograph courtesy of Keith Stone, MD, University of Florida.)

mucus patches; shallow, painless ulcerations in the oropharynx; and condylomata lata, which are grayish, raised papules that appear near the anus and vulva. In addition, bone tenderness, iritis, alopecia, and generalized lymphadenopathy may be present. The lesions of secondary syphilis typically resolve in 3 to 6 weeks, even without treatment. Untreated patients then enter the latent phase of illness. In this phase, infected women pose only a small risk of horizontal transmission to their sex partner. However, vertical transmission to the fetus still may occur.[63,64]

Approximately one third of patients with untreated secondary disease ultimately develop tertiary syphilis after an interval of several years. Tertiary syphilis is characterized by three principal findings: gumma formation, cardiac lesions, and central nervous system abnormalities (neurosyphilis). The characteristic cardiac lesions are aortic insufficiency and dissecting aortic aneurysm. Neurologic manifestations include meningovascular syphilis, cranial nerve palsies, generalized paresis, tabes dorsalis, optic atrophy, uveitis, and Argyll-Robertson pupils. The Argyll-Robertson pupil is myotic and responds to accommodation but not to light. Four to nine percent of patients with untreated syphilis ultimately develop neurosyphilis. In some individuals, particularly those with concurrent HIV infection, neurologic manifestations may occur early in the course of the disease and may be responsible for severe morbidity.[63,64]

Treponema pallidum can be identified in overt lesions such as the chancre by dark field microscopy and fluorescent antibody staining. However, most cases of infection, particularly those in the latent stage, are diagnosed by serology. The initial screening test for syphilis should be a nontreponemal assay such as the Venereal Disease Research Laboratory test (VDRL) or the rapid plasma reagin (RPR) test. A positive screening test must be confirmed by a specific treponemal assay such as the fluorescent treponemal antibody absorption test (FTA-ABS) or the microhemagglutination assay (MHA-TP). Lumbar puncture is indicated when neurosyphilis is suspected and in all patients who are coinfected with syphilis and HIV. Cerebrospinal fluid abnormalities include a mononuclear pleocytosis (10 to 400 cells/cubic millimeter), elevated protein (greater than 45 mg/dL), and a positive VDRL.[63,64]

Congenital syphilis is an extremely serious perinatal infection. The organism can cross the placenta at any stage of gestation. Up to one third of fetuses with congenital syphilis are stillborn. The many possible clinical manifestations of congenital syphilis are summarized in Table 20-7. The frequency of vertical transmission varies specifically with the stage of maternal disease. In the primary and secondary stages of infection, the frequency of congenital infection is approximately 50%. In

---

TABLE 20-7

Principal Clinical Manifestations of Congenital Syphilis

Early Manifestations	Late Manifestations
Maculopapular rash	Dental defects
Syphilitic rhinitis ("snuffles")	Interstitial keratitis
	Deafness
Mucus patches	Depression of nasal bridge
Hepatosplenomegaly	Perioral fissures (rhagades)
Jaundice	Saber shins
Pneumonia	Hydrarthosis (Clutton joints)
Generalized lymphadenopathy	CNS abnormalities
	• Mental retardation
Osteochondritis	• Ventriculomegaly
Ocular abnormalities (iritis, chorioretinitis)	• Generalized paresis
	• Optic nerve atrophy

CNS = central nervous system.

---

the early latent stage of disease, the risk of congenital infection is approximately 40%. In late latent syphilis and tertiary syphilis, the risk of perinatal transmission decreases to less than or equal to 10%.[63,64]

The prenatal diagnostic test with the greatest potential for identifying the severely infected fetus is ultrasound. Ultrasound findings suggestive of in-utero infection include placentomegaly, intrauterine growth restriction, microcephaly, enlargement of the liver and spleen, and fetal hydrops.

The drug of choice for treatment of syphilis in pregnancy is penicillin.[65] Specific treatment regimens are summarized in Table 20-8. Patients who have a history of an allergic reaction to penicillin should be skin tested to determine if they are truly allergic. If allergy is confirmed, patients should be desensitized with either oral or intravenous regimens and then treated with penicillin.[66] Desensitization should be performed in consultation with an allergist and in an area of the hospital with immediate access to emergency resuscitative equipment. Alternative antibiotic regimens, such as ceftriaxone, tetracycline, and erythromycin, are not of proven value for prevention of congenital syphilis. They should be used only if desensitization is unsuccessful.

TOXOPLASMOSIS

Toxoplasmosis is caused by the protozoan, *Toxoplasma gondii*. The organism exists in three distinct life forms: trophozoite, cyst, and oocyst. Both cats and cows play an important role in the life cycle of the *Toxoplasma* organism. Cats, particularly those who spend most of their time outdoors, are the usual host for the oocyst,

TABLE 20-8

Treatment of Syphilis in Pregnancy

Stage of Syphilis	Treatment
Primary, secondary, and early latent	Benzathine penicillin G—2.4 million units I.M. in a single dose
Late latent or latent syphilis of unknown duration	Benzathine penicillin G—2.4 million units I.M. weekly × 3 doses
Tertiary syphilis (gumma or cardio-vascular disease)	Benzathine penicillin G—2.4 million units I.M. weekly × 3 doses
Neurosyphilis	Aqueous crystalline penicillin G—18–24 million units per day, administered as 3–4 million units I.V. q4h or by continuous infusion, for 10–14 days OR Procaine penicillin—2.4 million units I.M. once daily PLUS Probenecid—500 mg orally, q.i.d., both for 10–14 days

From Centers for Disease Control. (2010). Sexually transmitted diseases treatment guidelines. *MMWR, 59*, 1–110.

which forms in the feline intestine. The oocyst is excreted in feces, and then, subsequently, is ingested by grazing cattle. The oocyst is disrupted in the intestine of the cow, resulting in the release of the invasive trophozoite. This form of the organism disseminates throughout the cow's body, ultimately forming cysts in brain tissue and muscle. Human infection occurs when infected meat is ingested or when food has been contaminated by cat feces via flies, cockroaches, or fingers.[67,68]

As noted above, stray cats and domestic cats that eat raw meat are more likely to carry the parasite than cats that remain indoors most of the time. In point of fact, the most likely source of toxoplasmosis in the United States is ingestion of improperly cooked meat. The infectious organism is completely destroyed by thorough cooking of meat.

The frequency of seroconversion to toxoplasmosis during pregnancy is less than 5%, and the frequency of congenital infection is approximately 3 per 1,000 pregnancies. Most toxoplasmosis infections in immune competent adults are relatively asymptomatic. When symptoms are present, they typically mimic those of mononucleosis. In an immunocompromised host, toxoplasmosis can be a devastating infection that causes severe central nervous system injury.[67,68]

The best test for diagnosis of toxoplasmosis in the pregnant woman is serology. An acute infection is typically manifested by a positive IgM antibody assay, in combination with a negative IgG antibody assay. Interestingly, IgM antibody can persist for up to one year following an acute infection. Therefore, interpretation of toxoplasma serology can, in some instances, be problematic.[67,68]

When the mother develops a primary infection, there is approximately a 40% risk that her infant will be infected. Hematogenous dissemination across the placenta is most frequent when maternal infection occurs in the third trimester. However, the risk of fetal injury is most severe when maternal infection occurs in the first trimester.

The usual clinical manifestations of congenital toxoplasmosis infection include a purpuric rash, enlarged liver and spleen, ascites, and chorioretinitis. Other manifestations include periventricular calcifications, ventriculomegaly, seizures, uveitis, and mental retardation.

If a pregnant woman is found to have primary toxoplasmosis infection, her infant should be tested for evidence of congenital infection. The best diagnostic test is identification of toxoplasmic DNA by PCR in the amniotic fluid. The sensitivity of this test ranges from 64% to 100%, and the positive predictive value of the abnormal test approaches 100%.[69]

Once toxoplasmic DNA has been identified in the amniotic fluid, serial ultrasound examinations are indicated to assess for the extent of fetal injury. Possible abnormalities detected by ultrasound include ventriculomegaly, intracranial calcifications, microcephaly, ascites, hepatosplenomegaly, and intrauterine growth restriction.

A pregnant woman with a documented acute toxoplasmosis infection should be counseled about the potential risk for her baby. Two treatment options exist. First, she could be treated antenatally with sulfadiazine plus spiromycin.[70] In published reports, this combination regimen has been effective in treating congenital toxoplasmosis. Alternatively, treatment can be delayed until after delivery. In a recent report, the combination of pyrimethamine and sulfadiazine, combined with leucovorin, was highly effective in treating the neonate.[71]

The best approach to toxoplasmosis is prevention of the initial infection. Pregnant women with cats should be advised to have another family member change the cat litter. If this is not possible, the woman should change the cat litter daily, wear gloves when handling the litter, and wash her hands carefully afterward. In addition, patients should be advised to cook their meat thoroughly until the juices surrounding the meat are clear. In addition, they should be encouraged to wash fruits and vegetables carefully and to cleanse their hands thoroughly after handling food.

VARICELLA

The varicella zoster (V-Z) virus is a DNA organism that is a member of the herpes virus family. The organism is responsible for varicella (chickenpox) and herpes zoster infection (shingles). Varicella occurs in approximately 1 to 5 cases per 10,000 pregnancies.[72]

Transmission of varicella occurs primarily by respiratory droplets and, in some cases, by direct contact with active vesicular lesions. The organism has a short incubation period of 10 to 14 days and is highly contagious. The typical clinical manifestation is an intensely pruritic, disseminated vesicular rash. The lesions occur in crops and evolve in stepwise fashion from a vesicle to a pustule, eventually crusting over to form a dry scab. Although varicella is usually a relatively mild, self-limited infection in children, approximately 20% of infected adults develop pneumonia, and approximately 1% develop encephalitis. Both of these complications may be associated with serious morbidity and even mortality.[72]

All pregnant women should be questioned about prior varicella infection at the time of their first prenatal appointment. If they have a well-defined history of varicella, they should be reassured that second infections are extremely unlikely and that, should a second infection occur, the risk to the fetus is negligible. Women who are not certain of prior exposure should have a varicella zoster serology (IgG) at the time of the first prenatal appointment.[73] Approximately 75% of individuals who are unsure about their prior history have clear serologic evidence of immunity. Women who do not have antibody against varicella should be cautioned about the need to avoid exposure to individuals who have vesicular viral exanthems.

If a susceptible patient is exposed to another individual with varicella, she should be treated with one of two agents to prevent active infection. The most extensively tested regimen is varicella zoster immune globulin (VZIG), one vial per 10 kg of weight up to a maximum of five vials.[74] Unfortunately, the United States company that manufactured this agent recently discontinued its production. An alternative method of providing prophylaxis is to administer acyclovir (800 mg, 5 times daily for 7 days) or valacyclovir (1,000 mg, 3 times daily for 7 days).[75]

Pregnant women who develop varicella despite immunoprophylaxis should be treated with an antiviral agent such as oral acyclovir or valacyclovir.[76] The appropriate doses of these agents are listed above. Patients who have evidence of pneumonia, encephalitis, or disseminated infection and those who are immunosuppressed should be hospitalized and treated with intravenous acyclovir.[72] The appropriate intravenous dose of acyclovir is 5 to 10 mg/kg every 8 hours.

Varicella during pregnancy has been associated with spontaneous abortion, intrauterine fetal death, and congenital anomalies. Fortunately, however, these complications are rare. An investigation by Enders and associates showed that the frequency of fetal anomalies was less than 1% when maternal infection occurred in weeks 1 to 12 of pregnancy. The risk of fetal anomalies was 2% or less when maternal infection occurred in weeks 13 to 20 of gestation.[77,78]

The best test to diagnose fetal injury due to congenital varicella is targeted ultrasound examination. Possible ultrasound findings include intrauterine growth restriction, microcephaly, ventriculomegaly, echogenic foci in the fetal liver, and circular limb anomalies.

Another interesting sequelae of maternal varicella infection is neonatal varicella. This complication occurs when maternal infection develops in the period 5 days prior to, and 2 days after, delivery. When infection occurs in such close proximity to delivery, there is no opportunity for protective antibody to cross the placenta.[72] The manifestations of neonatal varicella include disseminated mucocutaneous infection, visceral infection (manifested by hepatitis and splenomegaly), pneumonia, and encephalitis. Prior to the availability of acyclovir, up to 30% of infected babies died of neonatal varicella.

Infants born during the window of time noted above must avoid contact with vesicular lesions on the mother's skin. Depending upon the severity and stage of the mother's illness, complete separation of mother and infant may be appropriate. These infants also should receive immunoprophylaxis with varicella zoster immune globulin (VZIG) or treatment with antiviral agents such as acyclovir.

The most important measure for prevention of infection during pregnancy is universal vaccination of all reproductive age women for varicella.[79] The varicella vaccine (Varivax) is a live virus vaccine. It produces seroconversion in approximately 90% of children and 70% to 80% of adults. Individuals ages 1 to 12 should receive one dose of the vaccine subcutaneously. Individuals older than 12 years of age require two subcutaneous doses of the vaccine, administered 4 to 6 weeks apart. Contraindications to the varicella vaccine include pregnancy, an immunodeficiency disorder, high-dose corticosteroid therapy, an allergy to neomycin, untreated tuberculosis, and a severe systemic illness.

REFERENCES

1. Duff, P. (1994). Cytomegalovirus infection in pregnancy. *Infectious Diseases in Obstetrics and Gynecology, 2,* 146–152.
2. Betts, R. F. (1983). Cytomegalovirus infection epidemiology and biology in adults. *Seminars in Perinatology, 7,* 22.
3. Adler, S. P. (1989). Cytomegalovirus and child day care. *The New England Journal of Medicine, 321,* 1290.
4. Stagno, S., Pass, R. F., Dworsky, M. E., et al. (1982). Congenital cytomegalovirus infection. *The New England Journal of Medicine, 306,* 945–949.

5. Fowler, K. B., Stagno, S., Pass, R. F., Britt, W. J., Boll, T. J., & Alford, C. A. (1992). The outcome of congenital cytomegalovirus infection in relation to maternal antibody status. *The New England Journal of Medicine, 326*, 663–667.

6. Donner, C., Liesnard, C., Content, J., Busine, A., Aderca, J., & Rodesch, F. (1993). Prenatal diagnosis of 52 pregnancies at risk for congenital cytomegalovirus infection. *Obstetrics and Gynecology, 82*, 481–486.

7. Nigro, G., Adler, S. P., LaTorre, R., & Best, A. M. (2005). Passive immunization during pregnancy for congenital cytomegalovirus infection. *The New England Journal of Medicine, 353*, 1350–1362.

8. Duff, P. (2005). Immunotherapy for congenital cytomegalovirus infection. *New England Journal of Medicine, 353*, 1402–1404.

9. American College of Obstetrics and Gynecologists. (1992). Group B streptococcal infections in pregnancy. *ACOG Technical Bulletin*, No. 170.

10. Jamie, W. E., Edwards, R. K., & Duff, P. (2004). Vaginal-perineal compared with vaginal-rectal cultures for identification of group B streptococci. *Obstetrics and Gynecology, 104*, 1058–1061.

11. Bergeron, M. G., Ke, D., Menard, C., Picard, F. J., Gagnon, M., Bernier, M., et al. (2000). Rapid detection of group B streptococci in pregnant women at delivery. *The New England Journal of Medicine, 343*, 175–179.

12. Centers for Disease Control. (2010). Prevention of perinatal group B streptococcal disease: Revised guidelines from the CDC. *MMWR, 59*(RR-10), 1–36.

13. DeCueto, M., Sanchez, M.-J., Sanpedro, A., Miranda, J. A., Herruzo, A. J., & Rosa-Fraile, M. (1998). Timing of intrapartum ampicillin and prevention of vertical transmission of group B streptococcus. *Obstetrics and Gynecology, 91*, 112–114.

14. Rosenstein, N. E., & Schuchat, A. (1997). Opportunities for prevention of perinatal group B streptococcal disease: A multistate surveillance analysis. *Obstetrics and Gynecology, 90*, 901.

15. Duff, P. (1998). Hepatitis in pregnancy. *Seminars in Perinatology, 22*, 277–283.

16. Duff, B., & Duff, P. (1998). Hepatitis A vaccine: Ready for prime time. *Obstetrics and Gynecology, 91*, 468.

17. Velazquez, O., Stetler, H. C., Avila, C., Ornelas, G., Alvarez, C., Hadler, S. C., et al. (1990). Epidemic transmission of enterically transmitted non-A, non-B hepatitis in Mexico, 1986-1987. *JAMA, 263*, 3281–3285.

18. Wong, D. C., Purcell, R. H., Sreenivasan, M. A., Prasad, S. R., & Pavri, K. M. (1980). Epidemic and endemic hepatitis in India: Evidence for a non-A, non-B hepatitis virus aetiology. *Lancet, 2*, 876.

19. Centers for Disease Control. (1993). Hepatitis E among U.S. travelers, 1989-1992. *MMWR, 42*, 1.

20. Khuroo, M. S., Kamili, S., & Jameel, S. (1995). Vertical transmission of hepatitis E virus. *Lancet, 345*, 1025.

21. Centers for Disease Control. (1991). Hepatitis B virus: A comprehensive strategy for eliminating transmission in the United States through universal vaccination: Recommendations of the Immunization Practices Advisory Committee (ACIP). *MMWR, 40*, 1.

22. Rizzetto, M. (1983). The delta agent. *Hepatology, 3*, 729.

23. Jacobson, I. M., Dienstag, J. L., Werner, B. G., Brettler, D. B., Levine, P. H., & Mushahwar, I. K. (1985). Epidemiology and clinical impact of hepatitis D virus (delta) infection. *Hepatology, 5*, 188–191.

24. Laver, G. M., & Walker, B. D. (2001). Hepatitis C virus infection. *The New England Journal of Medicine, 345*, 41–52.

25. Osmond, D. H., Padian, N. S., Sheppard, H. W., Glass, S., Shiboski, S. C., & Reingold, A. (1993). Risk factors for hepatitis C virus positivity in heterosexual couples. *JAMA, 269*, 361–365.

26. Gibb, D. M., Goodall, R. L., Dunn, D. T., Healy, M., Neave, P., Cafferkey, M., et al. (2000). Mother-to-child transmission of hepatitis C virus: Evidence for preventable transmission. *Lancet, 356*, 904–907.

27. European Paediatric Hepatitis C Virus Network. (2005). A significant sex—but not elective cesarean section—effect on mother-to-child transmission of hepatitis C virus infection. *Journal of Infectious Diseases, 192*, 1872–1879.

28. Alter, M. J., Gallagher, M., Morris, T. T., Moyer, L. A., Meeks, E. L., & Krawczynski, K., et al. (1997). Acute non-A-E hepatitis in the United States and the role of hepatitis G virus infection. *The New England Journal of Medicine, 336*, 741–746.

29. Alter, H. J., Nakasuji, Y., Melpolder, J., Wages, J., Wesley, R., Shih, J. W., et al. (1997). The incidence of transfusion-associated hepatitis G virus infection and its relation to liver disease. *The New England Journal of Medicine, 336*, 747–754.

30. Feucht, H. H., Zollner, B., Polywka, S., & Laufs, R. (1996). Vertical transmission of hepatitis G. *Lancet, 347*, 615.

31. Cook, C. R., & Gall, S. A. (1994). Herpes in pregnancy. *Infectious Diseases in Obstetrics and Gynecology, 1*, 298.

32. Brown, Z. A., Vontver, L. A., Benedetti, J., Critchlow, C. W., Sells, C. J., Berry, S., et al. (1987). Effects on infants of a first episode of genital herpes during pregnancy. *The New England Journal of Medicine, 317*, 1246–1251.

33. Whitley, R., Arvin, A., Prober, C., Corey, L., Burchett, S., Plotkin, S., (1991). Predictors of morbidity and mortality in neonates with herpes simplex virus infections. *The New England Journal of Medicine, 324*, 450–454.

34. Brown, Z. A., Benedetti, J., Ashley, R., Burchett, S., Selke, S., Berry, S., et al. (1991). Neonatal herpes simplex virus infection in relation to asymptomatic maternal infection at the time of labor. *The New England Journal of Medicine, 324*, 1247–1252.

35. Gibbs, R. S., & Mead, P. B. (1992). Preventing neonatal herpes—current strategies. *The New England Journal of Medicine, 326*, 946.

36. Sheffield, J. S., Hollier, L. M., Hill, J. B., Stuart, G. S., & Wendel, G. D. (2003). Acyclovir prophylaxis to prevent herpes simplex virus recurrence at delivery: A systematic review. *Obstetrics and Gynecology, 102*, 1396–1903.

37. O'Brien, T. R., George, J. R., & Holmberg, S. D. (1992). Human immunodeficiency virus type 2 infection in the United States. *JAMA, 267*, 2775.

38. Hammer, S. M. (2005). Management of newly diagnosed HIV infection. *The New England Journal of Medicine, 353*, 1702–1710.

39. Schacker, T., Collier, A. C., Hughes, J., Shea, T., & Corey L. (1996). Clinical and epidemiologic features of primary HIV infection. *Annals of Internal Medicine, 125*, 257.

40. Duff, P. (1996). HIV infection in women. *Primary Care Update OB/GYNs, 3*, 45.

41. Minkoff, H. (2003). Human immunodeficiency virus infection in pregnancy. *Obstetrics and Gynecology, 101*, 797–810.

42. Kovacs, J. A., & Masur, H. (2000). Prophylaxis against opportunistic infections in patients with human immunodeficiency virus infection. *The New England Journal of Medicine, 342*, 1416–1429.

43. ACOG Committee Opinion Number 304 (2004). Prenatal and perinatal human immunodeficiency virus testing:

Expanded recommendations. *Obstetrics and Gynecology, 104*(5 Pt 1), 1119–1124.

44. Connor, E. M., Sperling, R. S., Gelber, R., Kiselev, P., Scott, G., O'Sullivan, M. J., (1994). Reduction of maternal-infant transmission of human immunodeficiency virus type[1] with zidovudine treatment. *The New England Journal of Medicine, 331*, 1173–1180.

45. Mandlebrot, L., LeChanadec, J., Benebi, A., Bongain, A., Bénifla, J. L., Delfraissy, J. F., et al. (1998). Perinatal HIV-1 transmission. Interaction between zidovudine prophylaxis and mode of delivery in the French perinatal cohort. *JAMA, 280*, 55–60.

46. The international perinatal HIV group. (1999). The mode of delivery and the risk of vertical transmission of human immunodeficiency virus type 1. *The New England Journal of Medicine, 340*, 977.

47. Public Health Service Task Force Perinatal HIV Guidelines Working Group. (2002). Summary of the updated recommendations from the Public Health Service Task Force to reduce perinatal human immunodeficiency virus-1 transmission in the United States. *Obstetrics and Gynecology, 99*, 1117–1126.

48. Kumar, M. L. (1991). Human parvovirus B_{19} and its associated diseases. *Clinics in Perinatology, 18*, 209.

49. Centers for Disease Control. (1989). Risks associated with human parvovirus B_{19} infection. *MMWR, 38*, 81.

50. Rodis, J. F., Quinn, D. L., Gary, W., Anderson, L. J., Rosengren, S., Cartter, M. L., et al. (1990). Management and outcomes of pregnancies complicated by human B_{19} parvovirus infection: A prospective study. *American Journal of Obstetrics and Gynecology, 163*(4 Pt 1):1168-1171.

51. Public Health Laboratory Service Working Party on Fifth Disease. (1990). Prospective study of human parvovirus (B_{19}) infection in pregnancy. *BMJ, 300*, 1166.

52. Oepkes, D., Seaward, G., Vandenbussche, F. P. H. A., Windrim, R., Kingdom, J., Beyene, J., et al. DIAMOND Study Group. (2006). Doppler ultrasonography versus amniocentesis to predict fetal anemia. *The New England Journal of Medicine, 355*, 155–164.

53. Fairley, C. K., Smoleniec, J. S., Caul, O. E., & Miller, E. (1995). Observational study of effect of intrauterine transfusions on outcome of fetal hydrops after parvovirus B_{19} infection. *Lancet, 346*, 1335.

54. Rodis, J. F., Rodner, C., Hansen, A. A., Borgida, A. F., Deoliveira, I., & Shulman Rosengren, S. (1998). Long-term outcome of children following maternal human parvovirus B_{19} infection. *Obstetrics and Gynecology, 91*, 125–128.

55. Conry, J. A., Torok, T., & Andrews, I. (1993). Perinatal encephalopathy secondary to in utero human parvovirus B_{19} (HPV) infection, abstracted. *Neurology, 43*, A346.

56. Brown, K. E., Green, S. W., deMayolo, J. A., Bellanti, J. A., Smith, S. D., Smith, T. J., et al. (1994). Congenital anaemia after transplacental B_{19} parvovirus infection. *Lancet, 343*, 895–896.

57. Centers for Disease Control. (1994). Rubella and congenital rubella syndrome—United States, January 1, 1991–May 7, 1994. *MMWR, 43*, 391.

58. Miller, E., Cradock-Watson, J. E., & Pollock, T. M. (1982). Consequences of confirmed maternal rubella at successive stages of pregnancy. *Lancet, 2*, 781.

59. Munro, N. D., Smithells, R. W., Sheppard, S., Holzel, H., & Jones, G. (1987). Temporal relations between maternal rubella and congenital defects. *Lancet, 2*, 201.

60. McIntosh, E. D. G., & Menser, M. A. (1992). A fifty-year follow-up of congenital rubella. *Lancet, 340*, 414.

61. Centers for Disease Control. (1990). Rubella prevention: Recommendations of the Immunization Practices Advisory Committee (ACIP). *MMWR, 39*, 1.

62. Bart, S. W., Stetler, H. C., Preblud, S. R., Williams, N. M., Orenstein, W. A., Bart, K. J., et al. (1985). Fetal risk associated with rubella vaccine: An update. *Reviews of Infectious Diseases, 7*, S95–102.

63. Hook, E. W., & Marra, C. M. (1992). Acquired syphilis in adults. *New England Journal of Medicine, 326*, 1060.

64. Ricci, J. M., Fojaco, R. M., & O'Sullivan, M. J. (1989). Congenital syphilis: The University of Miami/Jackson Memorial Medical Center experience, 1986-1988. *Obstetrics and Gynecology, 74*, 687.

65. Centers for Disease Control. (2010). Sexually transmitted diseases treatment guidelines. *MMWR, 59*, 1–110.

66. Ziaya, P. R., Hankins, G. D. V., Gilstrap, L. C., & Halsey, A. B. (1986). Intravenous penicillin desensitization and treatment during pregnancy. *JAMA, 256*, 2561.

67. Beazley, D. M., & Egerman, R. S. (1998). Toxoplasmosis. *Seminars in Perinatology, 22*, 332–338.

68. Krick, J. A., & Remington, J. S. (1978). Toxoplasmosis in the adult—an overview. *The New England Journal of Medicine, 298*, 550.

69. Hohlfeld, P., Daffos, F., & Costa, J. M., Thulliez, P., Forestier, F., & Vidaud, M. (1994). Prenatal diagnosis of congenital toxoplasmosis with a polymerase-chain reaction test on amniotic fluid. *The New England Journal of Medicine, 331*, 695–699.

70. Daffos, F. (1998). Prenatal management of 746 pregnancies at risk for congenital toxoplasmosis. *The New England Journal of Medicine, 318*, 271.

71. Guerina, N. G., Hsu, H. W., Meissner, H. C., Maguire, J. H., Lynfield, R., Stechenberg, B, (1994). Neonatal serologic screening and early treatment for congenital Toxoplasma gondii infection. *The New England Journal of Medicine, 330*, 1858–1863.

72. Chapman, S., & Duff, P. (1993). Varicella in pregnancy. *Seminars in Perinatology, 17*, 403–409.

73. McGregor, J. A., Mark, S., Crawford, G. P., & Levin, M. J. (1987). Varicella zoster antibody testing in the care of pregnancy women exposed to varicella. *American Journal of Obstetrics and Gynecology, 157*, 281.

74. Centers for Disease Control. (1996). Prevention of varicella. Recommendations of the Advisory Committee on Immunization Practices (ACIP). *MMWR, 45*(Suppl.), 1.

75. Asano, Y., Yoshikawa, T., Suga, S., Kobayashi, I., Nakashima, T., Yazaki, T., et al. (1993). Postexposure prophylaxis of varicella in family contact by oral acyclovir. *Pediatrics, 92*, 219–222.

76. Wallace, M. R., Bowler, W. A., Murray, N. B., Brodine, S. K., & Oldfield, E. C. (1992). Treatment of adult varicella with oral acyclovir: A randomized, placebo-controlled trial. *Annals of Internal Medicine, 117*, 358.

77. Pastuszak, A. L., Levy, M., Schick, B., Zuber, C., Feldkamp, M., Gladstone, J., (1994). Outcome after maternal varicella infection in the first 20 weeks of pregnancy. *The New England Journal of Medicine, 330*, 901–905.

78. Enders, G., Miller, E., Cradock-Watson, J., Bolley, I., & Ridehalgh, M. (1994). Consequences of varicella and herpes zoster in pregnancy: Prospective study of 1,739 cases. *Lancet, 343*, 1548–1551.

79. Duff, P. (1996). Varicella vaccine. *Infectious Diseases in Obstetrics and Gynecology, 4*, 63–65.

CHAPTER 21

Trauma in Pregnancy

Donna Ruth and Richard S. Miller

Trauma is the most frequent cause of death in women 35 years of age or younger and is the leading cause of death among women of childbearing age. While most injuries that bring pregnant women to the hospital are relatively minor and have little or no adverse impact on the pregnancy outcome, 1 in 12 pregnant women sustains a significant traumatic injury, making trauma the leading cause of nonobstetric maternal death in the United States.[1,2] Fetal morbidity and mortality are also potential significant consequences of maternal traumatic injury. Fetal death rates, reported to be as high as 65%, are actually higher than maternal death rates secondary to trauma.[3] The magnitude of this issue has implications for both obstetric and trauma clinical health care providers.

The distribution of reported cases of maternal trauma increases as the pregnancy progresses. Approximately 10% to 15% of injuries occur in the first trimester, 32% to 40% occur in the second trimester, and approximately 50% to 54% occur in the third trimester.[4,5] The overall incidence of trauma in pregnant women is estimated to be 5% to 10%.[6] The nature of the injuries has been reported as follows: 55% from motor vehicle accidents (MVAs), 22% from falls, 22% from assaults, and 1% from burns.[7] Although often associated with minor injuries, MVAs cause death more frequently than any other source of maternal trauma.

Although most traumatic injuries during pregnancy are relatively minor in nature, health care providers should remember that even apparently minor injuries have the potential to cause significant maternal and fetal morbidity and mortality. The potential for both immediate and long-term adverse impact on fetal well being exists. An understanding of the impact of traumatic injury on both the mother and fetus, knowledge of the anatomic and physiologic changes of pregnancy, familiarity with maternal trauma assessment skills, and prompt initiation of clinical interventions and treatments, facilitate timely and appropriate care for pregnant trauma patients. These issues will be discussed in this chapter, including the inherent need for effective collaboration.

MATERNAL ADAPTATIONS AND RELEVANCE TO TRAUMA CARE

The mechanisms of maternal and fetal injury, gestational age of the fetus, and secondary complications determine the maternal–fetal response to trauma. Pregnancy causes both anatomic and physiologic changes that affect an individual's response to traumatic injury. These changes may mask serious derangements in maternal physical integrity and may also influence patterns of injury. The pregnant trauma patient's initial contact with medical and nursing personnel often occurs in the emergency department (ED), where lack of familiarity with obstetric principles and the normal changes associated with pregnancy is common. Conversely, medical and nursing obstetric personnel may be unfamiliar with principles of trauma stabilization and management. Therefore, provision of quality clinical care to pregnant trauma patients is facilitated when resources and interdisciplinary collaboration are available.

A comprehensive discussion of the extensive physiologic changes associated with normal pregnancy is beyond the scope of this chapter. However, the following provides an overview of significant physiologic changes that may affect trauma during pregnancy.

Cardiovascular Adaptations

Extensive changes occur in the maternal cardiovascular system during pregnancy. Plasma blood volume increases 50%. Red blood cell volume increases 30%. The maternal heart rate is increased by 10% to 15%, and maternal cardiac output is increased 30% to 50%. The end result of these adaptations is the ability to provide increased cardiac output, and oxygen and nutrient delivery, to the growing uterus and developing fetus. Any condition that causes a reduction in perfusion to the uterus is poorly tolerated by the fetus. Providers must be acutely aware that this increase in blood volume may initially mask a significant hemorrhage that may have significant consequences for both the mother and fetus. During pregnancy there is increased blood flow to the uterus. Every 8 to 11 minutes, the total circulating maternal blood volume flows through the uteroplacental bed, contributing to the potential for significant hemorrhage with any maternal abdominal trauma.

Pregnancy is considered a high-flow, low-resistance state. Under the influence of progesterone, the smooth muscles surrounding blood vessels are relaxed during pregnancy. This results in decreased systemic vascular resistance (SVR) and blood pressure that reaches its nadir in the second trimester. As the gestation progresses, SVR and maternal blood pressure gradually increase. Maternal blood pressure returns to prepregnancy levels by the end of the third trimester. During pregnancy the uteroplacental bed functions as a dilated, passive, low-resistance system. Perfusion pressure determines blood flow to the uterus and under normal circumstances there is no uteroplacental vasoconstriction to impede blood flow. Therefore, any condition that results in a decrease in maternal blood pressure, such as hemorrhage or hypovolemia, results in vasoconstriction of the uterine arteries and shunting of blood to the essential organs. This shunting of blood away from the uteroplacental bed has the compensatory effect of maintaining maternal blood pressure at the expense of the fetus. The increased blood volume of pregnancy and this physiologic shunting are what allow the maternal trauma patient to maintain relative physiologic stability until massive blood loss has occurred.[8] Once tachycardia and hypotension develop, considered hallmark symptoms of blood loss, the care provider may already be behind with respect to resuscitative efforts.[9] Therefore, tachycardia and hypotension in the pregnant trauma patient are clinically significant findings that require careful evaluation and should not be solely attributed to pregnancy.[10]

Additionally, maternal positioning has significant effects on maternal blood pressure and uterine blood flow. When the pregnant patient is placed in a supine position, the gravid uterus compresses the inferior vena cava. The end result of this compression is a decrease in venous return, a decrease in cardiac output, and a decrease in uterine blood flow, which can have profound effects on both normal and hemodynamically compromised patients. Thus, the supine position should be avoided. To avoid the supine position, providers may use a wedge or rolled blankets to tilt the spinal backboard in a 15 degree tilt.[11] If it is not possible to tilt the spinal backboard, then manual displacement of the uterus should be done. Care must be taken to ensure that the spine remains secure and aligned until a spinal injury is ruled out. These simple maneuvers are very effective in alleviating supine hypotension and its effect on uterine blood flow.

Pulmonary System Adaptations

The maternal pulmonary system also undergoes significant adaptations that may affect trauma management in the pregnant patient. These adaptations occur to ensure that the developing fetus has adequate oxygen delivery and are discussed in detail in Chapter 5 of this text. As a result of these changes, the pregnant patient normally has a chronic compensated respiratory alkalemia that is reflected in the arterial blood gases.

The pregnant patient has diminished oxygen reserve and decreased blood buffering capacity. When caring for pregnant trauma patients, any acid–base balance disturbances should be evaluated, keeping in mind that a primary normal change in acid–base balance already exists. This leaves the pregnant trauma patient vulnerable to hypoxemia and less able to compensate when acidemia ensues.

A significant anatomic adaptation is the change in the location of the maternal diaphragm. As the uterus grows, the maternal diaphragm is displaced 4 centimeters above its normal location. This change in location must be considered if placement of a chest tube is necessary, to avoid injury to the diaphragm. If placement of a chest tube is performed, a higher insertion point should be utilized. In pregnant patients this insertion point is usually between the third and fourth intercostal space.

Gastrointestinal System Changes

As the pregnancy progresses, the enlarging uterus causes compartmentalization and cephalad displacement of intra-abdominal organs.[12] The net result is that altered patterns of pain may occur with injury; therefore, upon physical examination, abdominal tenderness, rebound tenderness, or guarding may be absent, despite the presence of significant injury.

Secondary to the influence of progesterone and the relaxation of smooth muscle that occurs during pregnancy, there is a significant decrease in gastrointestinal motility. The result is delayed gastric emptying and laxity of the esophageal sphincter. This means the pregnant trauma patient is vulnerable to regurgitation of abdominal contents and pulmonary aspiration. Therefore, early placement of a nasogastric tube for gastric decompression is recommended. During bag and mask ventilation and/or initial intubation of the pregnant patient, cricoid pressure is commonly requested to prevent gastric insufflation and aspiration. However, cricoid pressure is contraindicated in the pregnant trauma patient until spinal instability and injury are assessed and determined to be absent.

Genitourinary System Adaptations

During pregnancy the bladder is displaced both anteriorly and superiorly by the growing uterus. The bladder essentially becomes an abdominal organ and much more vulnerable to injury. The renal pelvises and ureters are dilated secondary to relaxation of the smooth muscle and compression from the growing uterus. The gravid uterus may obstruct or impede urinary outflow. There is also an increase in renal blood flow, leading to an increase in glomerular filtration rate (GFR). This results in an increase in creatinine clearance during pregnancy. During pregnancy, a serum creatinine that would be considered normal in a nonpregnant patient may reflect seriously compromised renal function and requires further evaluation.[12]

Reproductive System Adaptations

The uterus increases dramatically in size as the pregnancy progresses. By 12 weeks gestation, the uterus moves out of the pelvis and becomes an abdominal organ, making it vulnerable to injury. In addition, because of the increased blood flow to the uterus during pregnancy, the likelihood of hemorrhage with any uterine injury or pelvic trauma is significantly increased.[13]

Secondary to these and other alterations during pregnancy, the potential for significant clinical problems exists in the pregnant trauma patient. A summary of these potential problems is presented in Box 21-1.

ASSESSMENT OF THE PREGNANT TRAUMA PATIENT

Trauma assessment begins during prehospital care and continues once the patient is transported to the ED. At the ED, the primary survey begins in order to identify any life-threatening conditions, initiate or continue resuscitative measures that began in the field, and initiate additional treatments as warranted. Once the primary survey is complete, the secondary survey begins. The secondary survey includes a detailed head-to-toe examination, management of non–life-threatening injuries, and continued reassessment of maternal and fetal condition. It is during the secondary survey that a more complete fetal evaluation occurs.

Box 21-1. POTENTIAL PROBLEMS RELATED TO THE PREGNANT TRAUMA PATIENT

Maternal Hemodynamic Instability
- Maternal hemorrhage and shock secondary to traumatic injury
- Maternal hemorrhage and shock secondary to uterine damage
- Maternal hemorrhage and shock secondary to placental abruption
- Maternal hemorrhage and shock secondary to penetrating trauma
- Decreased cardiac output related to vena cava compression by the enlarged uterus

Inadequate Maternal Pulmonary Function
- Venous stasis and pulmonary emboli related to hypercoagulability and immobility
- Impaired gas exchange related to pulmonary contusion
- Alteration in ventilation related to pleural space injuries
- Alteration in ventilation related to bony thoracic fractures

Fetal Compromise
- Fetal hypoxemia secondary to maternal shock
- Fetal hypoxemia secondary to uterine damage
- Fetal hypoxemia secondary to placental abruption
- Premature rupture of membranes
- Onset of preterm labor
- Direct fetal injury secondary to maternal trauma
- Fetal injury secondary to penetrating trauma
- Emergency delivery secondary to fetal compromise and/or uterine or placental injuries
- Alteration in uteroplacental perfusion related to cardiovascular compromise secondary to maternal positioning

Alteration in Psychosocial Well Being
- Maternal and family anxiety related to sudden and unexpected hospitalization during pregnancy
- Maternal and family anxiety related to pending surgical procedures and possible fetal injury or death
- Alteration in maternal–infant bonding related to patient's condition and fetal outcome
- Alteration in maternal–infant bonding related to maternal injuries and clinical condition

Prehospital Care

Initial prehospital care should include assessment of the clinical condition of the patient. If it is known that the patient is pregnant, transport to a level one trauma center with obstetric capabilities should be arranged, particularly if there is hemodynamic instability, loss of consciousness, or the fetus is viable. This assessment may not be possible if the patient is unable to communicate, is not visibly pregnant, or maternal obesity makes assessment of gestational age difficult.

Whenever possible, information related to the pregnancy should be sought by the initial responders and communicated to the accepting facility. This allows time for notification of both the obstetric and neonatal teams so that comprehensive, multidisciplinary care can begin immediately upon arrival at the trauma center. Vital signs should be obtained and symptoms assessed, with the knowledge that pregnant patients may not present in the same manner as nonpregnant patients.

If hemorrhage is suspected, two large bore (14 or 16 gauge) intravenous catheters should be placed and volume resuscitation initiated. Supplemental high flow oxygen via mask should be administered. When obstetric patients are placed on a spinal back board, a 15 degree lateral tilt should be maintained to avoid compression of the vena cava and aorta by the gravid uterus. Failure to properly position these patients can result in decreased uteroplacental perfusion as well as inadequate perfusion of other vital organs.

Primary Survey

The primary survey is the systematic evaluation of a trauma patient performed according to standard Advanced Trauma Life Support (ATLS) protocols.[14] This survey is accomplished within minutes and includes simultaneous assessment and interventions when significant, immediate, life-threatening injuries are present. Assessment and treatment priorities, in accordance with ATLS recommendations, are presented in Box 21-2.

The primary survey always begins with assessment of the patient's airway. This includes the basic "look, listen, and feel" for movement of air. For the conscious patient, airway assessment can be accomplished at a glance; that is to say, the patient who is talking or shouting has an open, intact airway. An unconscious patient requires close assessment and may require assistance to obtain or maintain an open airway.

Protection of the airway is of the utmost importance. Maintenance of a patent airway and establishment of adequate ventilation and oxygenation may require intervention. If fetal hypoxemia is to be avoided, early aggressive maternal ventilatory support may be required. High flow oxygen via mask, if not already initiated, should be administered, even if there are no visible signs of respiratory distress. Oxygen demands are increased during pregnancy and traumatic injury further increases these demands. Pregnant trauma patients who have a respiratory rate of less than 12 breaths per minute or greater than 25 breaths per minutes may need additional intervention and support.

If airway patency is in doubt, use of a simple device such as an oropharyngeal airway may be sufficient. However, complete control of the airway is often required, in order to ensure adequate maternal oxygenation; therefore, endotracheal intubation may be necessary. Nasal intubation should be avoided in pregnant patients, since the increased vascularity in the upper airway and nares predisposes pregnant women to significant bleeding during this potentially traumatic procedure.

If endotracheal intubation is required, pre-oxygenation is essential, since the pregnant patient is vulnerable to rapid oxygen desaturation surrounding the period of time endotracheal intubation is performed.[9] Placement of a pulse oximeter allows for assessment of arterial oxygen saturation (SaO_2) and detection of oxyhemoglobin desaturation. Since pregnant women are at increased risk for aspiration during intubation, placement of an oral or nasogastric tube for gastric decompression is an important safeguard. These measures, along with vigilant assessment and rapid intervention in the event of vomiting, may decrease the incidence of this very serious complication.

Assessment of bleeding and circulation are performed concurrently during the primary survey. Clinical parameters that are useful to assess circulation include heart rate, pulse quality, and capillary refill. These parameters reflect the adequacy of maternal perfusion. It is important to note that time-consuming traditional assessment of arterial blood pressure may not be necessary for patients who present with evidence of hypovolemic shock. For example, the presence of a palpable carotid artery pulse indicates a systolic arterial blood pressure of at least 60 mmHg, a palpable femoral pulse indicates a systolic pressure of at least 70 mmHg, and the presence of a palpable radial pulse indicates a systolic pressure of at least 80 mmHg. Traditional assessment of

Box 21-2. ADVANCED TRAUMA LIFE SUPPORT (ATLS) PRIMARY ASSESSMENT

Airway
- Assessment and maintenance (the importance of this step cannot be underestimated or minimized)

Bleeding
- Assessment of bleeding, including amount and source of bleeding

Circulation
- Assessment, including control of hemorrhage and treatment of hypovolemic shock

Disability and Displacement
- Assessment of neurologic function
- In pregnant women, displacement of the uterus to avoid uterine compression of the vena cava and aorta, as well as supine hypotension

Exposure
- Undress the patient to assess for injury
- Avoid hypothermia

arterial blood pressure should be performed for obstetric trauma patients as time permits.

When evaluating circulatory status, the physiologic changes of pregnancy cannot be ignored. The significant increase in maternal intravascular volume associated with normal pregnancy may mask hypovolemic shock, until significant blood loss has occurred. Care providers should assess for evidence of hemorrhage and initiate appropriate treatment when such evidence is present. Hypotension should be presumed to be secondary to hypovolemia, until proven otherwise.[15] Significant compromise in uterine blood flow may exist, even with a normal maternal arterial blood pressure, because of the physiologic shunting that occurs to preserve blood flow to the heart, lungs, brain, and kidneys.

If not already in place, two large bore (14 to 16 gauge) intravenous catheters should be inserted and 1 to 2 liters of warmed crystalloid solutions should be infused. Normal saline or lactated Ringer's solutions are the fluids of choice for volume resuscitation. In the face of continued hemorrhage and maternal instability, transfusion of O-negative blood should begin immediately, followed by type-specific or cross-matched packed red blood cells (PRBCs) and fresh frozen plasma as soon as it is available.

Shock may be exacerbated in the pregnant trauma patient by supine positioning. This may be avoided by tilting the spinal back board 15 degrees or by manual lateral displacement of the uterus. Appropriate positioning and uterine displacement should be considered for all obstetric trauma patients with an estimated fetal gestational age of greater than or equal to 20 weeks.

Generally, vasopressor medications do not have a role in the treatment of hypovolemic shock, and this axiom is especially true for pregnant trauma patients.[16] Judicious volume resuscitation is the treatment of choice. The goal of this therapy is to optimize preload and improve cardiac output. Vasopressor medications, especially if administered when preload is inadequate, may likely cause a significant reduction in uterine blood flow, resulting in decreased oxygen delivery to the fetus. In addition to decreased perfusion of the uteroplacental bed, decreased perfusion to other maternal end-organ systems is possible and the risk of end-organ dysfunction or failure is increased. Blood pressure should be supported with vasopressor medications as a last resort, since they treat only a symptom and do not address the cause of the hypovolemia. Blood flow to the uterus is best restored by replacement and maintenance of maternal circulating blood volume. Care providers should consider the potential sources of bleeding. Sources of significant blood loss in trauma patients are presented in Box 21-3.

The next assessment in the primary survey is for disability or displacement. A brief neurologic assessment is performed to reveal the patient's level of consciousness and sensorimotor function. Displacement of

Box 21-3. POTENTIAL SOURCES OF SIGNIFICANT BLOOD LOSS IN TRAUMA PATIENTS

- Chest
- Abdomen
- Retroperitoneal area
- Pelvis
- Long bones
- Skin
- Pregnant women: uteroplacental bed

the uterus should be addressed at this point in the survey, if the patient is known to be pregnant.

The Glasgow Coma Scale (GCS) is the accepted method for evaluation and monitoring of neurologic status. The GCS is presented in Table 21-1. This method relies on objective assessments and enhances continuity of care. Descriptive terms such as lethargic, obtunded, or vegetative may be interpreted differently by team members involved in patient care and should be avoided. Early assessment is important because establishment of a baseline assists in identification of signs of compromise. Scores are derived by selecting the numeric value for the best response in the three components of the evaluation and by calculating the total. A GCS of 8 or less may be indicative of significant ongoing neurologic pathology and requires emergent intubation.

Sensorimotor functions may be easily evaluated in the conscious patient. If the patient is unconscious, how she responds to painful stimuli is indicative of level of function. Withdrawal from or localization of pain indicates

TABLE 21-1

Glasgow Coma Scale (GCS)

Eyes	4	Open spontaneously
	3	Open to verbal command
	2	Open to pain
	1	No response
Best motor response		
To verbal command:	6	Obeys
To painful stimulus:	5	Localizes pain
	4	Flexion–withdrawal
	3	Flexion–decorticate
	2	Flexion–decerebrate
	1	No response
Best verbal response	5	Oriented, converses
	4	Disoriented, converses
	3	Inappropriate words
	2	Incomprehensible sounds
	1	No response

Total Score: 3–15.

intact sensorimotor function. Decorticate or decerebrate posturing accompanies deep cerebral hemispheric or upper brainstem injury. Spinal cord injury and any accompanying neurologic shock may be difficult to diagnose in the woman with an altered level of consciousness. A high index of suspicion of neurologic injury should be maintained in women with refractory hypotension, when there is no apparent source of bleeding, no tachycardia, and warm extremities.

The primary survey is completed by exposing the patient. This means the patient should be undressed from head to toe and carefully examined. Care should be taken to avoid hypothermia during this examination. Measures used to maintain body temperature include the use of warm blankets, use of convective air warmers, use of fluid-circulating heating blankets, use of reflective blankets, and use of warm intravenous fluids and blood products. During the exposure, assessment for any obvious injury should be done. At this point in the survey, the patient may have been identified as pregnant and preliminary assessment of the pregnancy should begin.

Initial maternal evaluation and resuscitation takes precedence over fetal evaluation. The leading cause of fetal death is maternal death. Early recognition of maternal compromise and rapid maternal resuscitation reduces maternal mortality. To enhance fetal survival, all efforts should be directed at maternal stabilization. Once this has occurred, further evaluation of fetal status should begin.

Secondary Survey

Once the primary survey and initial resuscitation measures have been completed, a more complete secondary survey commences. The secondary survey consists of a full assessment, system by system, using the "head to toe" approach. Some modifications to the secondary survey should be done related to the presence of a pregnancy. During the secondary survey, pregnancy-specific evaluation includes assessment for the presence of vaginal bleeding, ruptured amniotic membranes, uterine contractions, signs or symptoms compatible with placental abruption, direct fetal or uterine injury, and fetal compromise.

An abdominal assessment is an essential component of the secondary survey. Included in this assessment is a focused assessment with sonography for trauma (FAST) scan. The FAST scan provides a screening tool for intraperitoneal hemorrhage. An obstetric ultrasound may also be done at this time. The obstetric ultrasound should be done to assess gestational age, fetal heart motion, location of the placenta, amount of amniotic fluid, and fetal activity. The ultrasound may identify a placental abruption; however, ultrasound is not a very reliable diagnostic tool for placental abruption. Therefore, placental abruption should not be ruled out based on a negative ultrasound exam.

The secondary survey should also include a speculum exam. The purpose of this exam is to assess for vaginal bleeding, rupture of membranes, inspection of the cervix for dilation and effacement, identification of vaginal sidewall lacerations, and injuries that may be associated with pelvic fractures.

Abdominal and pelvic assessments assume greater significance in the pregnant trauma patient. Assessment of the uterus and fetus provides information related to fetal viability. Pelvic assessments identify maternal injuries, such as pelvic fractures, that may be more common in pregnant trauma patients. Specific fetal and uterine assessments will be discussed later in the chapter.

Pelvic bony structures should be evaluated both clinically and radiographically. The management of pelvic fractures is complicated and several modifications may be needed for pregnant patients. Both percutaneous and open fixation of pelvic fractures may be performed with good fetal and maternal outcomes.[17] With pelvic fractures, there is a significant risk of retroperitoneal bleeding and hemorrhage. It is also important to note that pelvic fractures have been associated with the highest risk of placental abruption, as well as maternal and fetal mortality.[18]

Ultrasound is a useful tool for imaging in the pregnant trauma patient, since it has no associated radiation exposure. However, such as with pelvic fractures and other injuries, radiographic diagnostic imaging studies may be necessary. Clinically necessary studies should not be deferred because of concerns related to fetal exposure to radiation. When such studies are necessary, the uterus should be shielded as much as possible to minimize exposure. The American College of Obstetricians and Gynecologists (ACOG) has published guidelines related to diagnostic imaging during pregnancy.[19] It is important to remember that if multiple radiographic studies are required, consultation with a radiologist or radiation specialist should take place, so that an accurate estimate of the cumulative exposure may be done.[20]

Genitourinary injuries are rare, but blood at the urinary meatus and labial hematomas may be indicative of injury. If these are present, placement of an indwelling urinary catheter should be deferred, until definitive studies can be done. If neither is observed, a urinary catheter should be inserted, to assess urinary output and rule out gross hematuria. If gross hematuria is present, the provider should consider and evaluate for bladder, urinary tract, or renal injury. This may be done either by computed tomography (CT) with contrast or by cystogram.

Blood may be drawn and sent for laboratory analysis during the secondary survey. Immediate assessments may include complete blood count, serum electrolytes, and serum glucose determinations. Clotting studies are indicated if a placental abruption is suspected, and provide a baseline in the event that disseminated intravascular coagulation (DIC) develops. The fibrinogen levels and several clotting factors, including factors VII, VIII, IX and X, are all increased during pregnancy. The provider should be aware that fibrinogen levels that are normal for a nonpregnant patient may be indicative of placental abruption and DIC in a pregnant patient.[12] This increase in fibrinogen and clotting factors provide some protection if hemorrhage occurs but also places the pregnant patient at risk for thromboembolic disease. Arterial blood gases should be evaluated when indicated. Care providers should remember the normal blood gases associated with normal pregnancy. Any evidence of maternal acidemia requires evaluation and intervention to correct this condition, as some evidence suggests that maternal acidemia may be linked to poor fetal outcomes.[21]

Testing for fetomaternal hemorrhage should be done on all pregnant patients, regardless of degree or severity of injury. The three techniques commonly used for confirmation and volume estimation of the bleed are flow cytometry, gel agglutination, and Kleihauer-Betke (acid elution). The most commonly used method is Kleihauer-Betke, or KB. The KB stain allows for diagnosis of fetomaternal hemorrhage by detecting the presence of fetal red blood cells in the maternal circulation. A positive KB test may also be an indication of the degree of disruption and help identify patients at risk for preterm labor.[22] An Rh negative pregnant woman with a positive KB test should be treated with Rh immune globulin (RhIG) within 72 hours of injury to prevent Rh isoimmunization. A single 300-microgram dose of RhIG protects against 15 milliliters of fetal blood. Even in the absence of detectable fetal cells in the Rh negative and previously nonimmunized trauma patient, administration of a single 300-microgram dose of RhIG should be considered, given the significant risk of fetomaternal hemorrhage in trauma patients.

Optimal care of the pregnant trauma patient is promoted by a psychosocial assessment and provision of emotional support that includes her family and/or support persons. Although trauma assessment and resuscitation demand strict attention to the patient's physical condition, as much time as possible should be spent in determining the patient's emotional status, extended support system, and in reassuring the patient that aggressive trauma care and resuscitation offer the fetus the best chance of survival. Extreme physical stress and fear are known to affect physiologic function and have been correlated with increased uterine activity.

The patient and her family should be kept informed of her condition, the status of the fetus, and should be allowed to express their fear and anxiety within a supportive milieu. Family members should be allowed to remain with the patient when possible.

Uterine Activity and Fetal Assessment

Assessment of uterine activity should be done for all pregnant trauma patients with an estimated fetal gestational age greater than 23 to 24 weeks. These assessments include: fundal height measurement, palpation of the uterus for tenderness or rigidity, palpation of the uterine resting tone, external uterine activity monitoring for the presence or absence of contractions, frequency of contractions, and duration of contractions. Fetal assessment includes auscultation of the fetal heart rate, if the estimated gestational age is less than 23 weeks. External electronic fetal heart rate monitoring should be initiated if the estimated fetal gestational age is greater than or equal to 23 weeks, which is generally considered the age of viability. If external electronic fetal heart rate monitoring is utilized, assessment should include: baseline fetal heart rate, variability, presence, or absence of accelerations or decelerations (e.g., late, variable, early, or prolonged decelerations).

Assessment for rupture of amniotic membranes should also be done as a component of the fetal environment. During the secondary survey, when the speculum exam is performed, the vagina should be visually inspected for "pooling" of amniotic fluid. If fluid is seen in the posterior vaginal fornix, or if fluid leakage from the cervix is confirmed, more definitive testing (e.g., pH analysis, fern test) should follow.

During initial maternal stabilization efforts, fetal assessment should be limited to the estimation of gestational age and evidence of fetal life. More extensive assessment should begin as soon as possible but should never take precedence over maternal resuscitation efforts. Medical and nursing personnel with expertise in obstetrics and fetal monitoring should be actively involved during the assessment process.

INJURIES UNIQUE TO PREGNANT TRAUMA PATIENTS

Fetal Morbidity and Mortality

The most common cause of fetal death in maternal trauma is maternal death. The second leading cause of fetal death is placental abruption. Pearlman and colleagues noted a 41% fetal mortality rate if the maternal injuries were life threatening and a 1.6% fetal mortality rate if the maternal injuries were not life threatening.[23]

Providers should be aware that, while it is not common, fetal death may occur even in the absence of significant maternal injury. Worsening maternal injury severity score, increasing maternal fluid requirements, and maternal hypoxia and acidemia may all be important predictors of fetal morbidity and mortality.

The fetus is generally well protected from direct injury, because the maternal soft tissue, uterus, placenta, and amniotic fluid all absorb and distribute the energy from a direct blow to the abdomen. In most cases of minor trauma the fetus survives intact. Direct fetal injury is more common in the third trimester when the uterine wall is thinned and there may be less amniotic fluid to absorb impact. Direct fetal injury is also more common with penetrating abdominal wounds, such as stabbing and gunshots, where the projectile hits the fetus.

During the third trimester, the fetal head may be engaged in the pelvis. If abdominal or pelvic trauma occurs, the fetal head impacts against the maternal bony pelvis, leaving the fetus vulnerable to skull fractures and brain injury.

Placental Abruption

Placental abruption is a common complication following both significant maternal injury and minor abdominal trauma. Placental abruption can be a devastating complication of maternal trauma, requiring aggressive maternal resuscitation and emergency delivery of the fetus. Hypovolemic shock, DIC, and fetal demise are all common complications of placental abruption. The incidence of placental abruption in cases of trauma during pregnancy ranges from 1% to 60%.[23] Diagnosis may be made based on presenting signs and symptoms, findings on physical exam, laboratory assessments that indicate bleeding, and ultrasound. It should be noted that the sensitivity of ultrasound for detection of placental abruption is approximately 50% and a negative ultrasound does not rule out abruption.

Placental abruption occurs most often after blunt trauma, such as motor vehicle accidents, falls, and assaults. The mechanism of injury is the rapid deceleration that occurs with blunt trauma. This causes a rapid compression, followed by expansion of the uterus. This produces shearing forces that tear an essentially rigid, nonelastic placenta from the more flexible uterine wall. This separation of the placenta from the uterine wall leads to bleeding and decreased blood flow to the placenta and fetus. Fetal death may rapidly ensue if the amount of separation is significant. With placental separation of greater than 50%, the fetal prognosis is extremely poor. Maternal complications include hemorrhage, DIC, and death. Thorough discussions of hemorrhage and DIC are presented in Chapters 15 and 16 of

this text. Treatments include administration of oxygen, aggressive fluid resuscitation with both crystalloids and blood products, and often emergency delivery of the fetus.

Physical exam may reveal the presence of uterine tenderness, abdominal pain on palpation, uterine contractions, a rigid abdomen, and vaginal bleeding. However, the absence of these findings does not exclude the presence of an abruption. Perhaps the most sensitive indicator of placental abruption is fetal heart rate abnormalities and the presence of uterine contractions with elevated uterine resting tone. Therefore, it is recommended that continuous electronic fetal heart rate and uterine activity monitoring should be initiated on patients with viable pregnancies as soon as possible after admission to the trauma center. Continuous monitoring is preferred over intermittent auscultation, since the latter only provides a fetal heart rate specific to the time of auscultation. Fetal heart rate changes that may accompany placental abruption include: fetal tachycardia, fetal bradycardia, absent variability, recurrent late decelerations, and a sinusoidal baseline pattern. If a fetal heart rate abnormality is present or regular uterine contractions are present, the patient should be monitored until these resolve or the fetus is delivered.

Uterine Rupture

Uterine rupture is rare, complicating less than 1% of all maternal trauma patients. Uterine rupture is associated almost universally with fetal mortality. Maternal mortality in cases of uterine rupture is approximately 30%.[24] Most cases of uterine rupture involve trauma to the uterine fundus and the risk increases with gestational age. It is more common in women who have had previous uterine surgery. In maternal trauma patients without previous uterine surgery, the rupture is more likely to occur on the posterior wall of the uterus, making detection more difficult.[25] Presenting signs and symptoms include: excruciating abdominal pain, asymmetric uterine shape, ability to palpate fetal parts through the abdominal wall, and profound maternal hypovolemic shock. Patients who experience a uterine rupture require immediate surgical intervention.

Perimortem Cesarean Delivery

When maternal cardiac arrest occurs and there is a potentially viable fetus, a perimortem Cesarean delivery may be done. The best fetal outcomes occur if the surgery is performed and the fetus delivered within 4 minutes of the maternal cardiac arrest.[26] A thorough discussion of cardiopulmonary resuscitation during pregnancy, including perimortem Cesarean delivery, is presented in Chapter 14 of this text. This procedure was

Trauma OB protocol

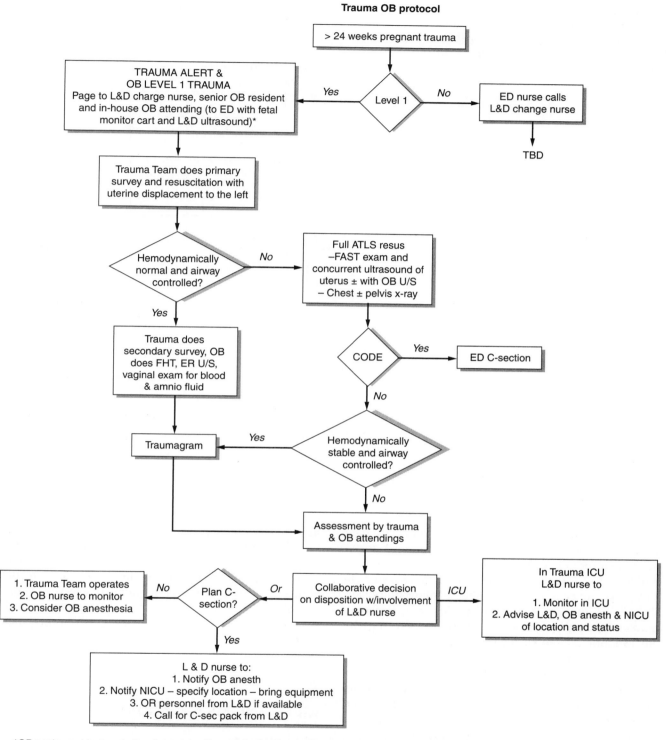

*OB senior resident and attending advise Trauma Scribe Nurse "OB Team here on standby." Remain on standby outside trauma bay awaiting direct communication with Trauma Team Leader and/or Trauma attending

FIGURE 21-1 Sample algorithm for care of the obstetric trauma patient. (For additional information: http://www.mc.vanderbilt.edu/surgery/trauma/mdprotocolstyle.htm).

FIGURE 21-2 Initial resuscitation of the pregnant trauma patient. *Source*: Van Hook, J. W., Gei, A. F., & Pacheco, L. D. (2004). Trauma in pregnancy. In G. A. Dildy, et al. (Eds.). *Critical care obstetrics* (4th ed.). Malden, MA: Blackwell Science.

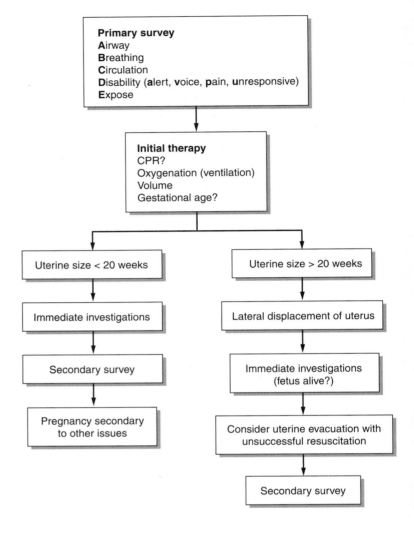

originally proposed by Katz in 1986, secondary to data that suggested that emptying the uterus relieves aortocaval compression, promotes venous return, increases cardiac output, and thus improves maternal survival. In 2005, Katz and colleagues published a follow-up review. They found that in 38 cases of perimortem Cesarean delivery there were 34 infants who survived initially and 13 mothers who survived. It was noted that these findings were most relevant when the cause of the maternal arrest was not related to trauma. In the 9 cases in which the procedure was performed for arrests related to maternal traumatic injury, only 3 infants and none of the mothers survived.[27] The effectiveness of this procedure remains an unresolved issue.

If the procedure is to be undertaken, several important factors should be considered. The gestational age of the fetus should be one of the factors, since survival prior to 23 weeks gestation is limited even under ideal circumstances. Delivery of a fetus at this gestational age may not improve venous return sufficiently to benefit the mother. The resources available at the hospital,

including neonatal intensive care providers and equipment, should also be an important consideration. If the procedure is performed, it should not be delayed to move the pregnant patient to the operating suite but should instead be done in the trauma bay by the trauma and obstetric teams.

An algorithm for the resuscitation of the pregnant trauma patient that addresses these issues is presented in Figures 21-1 and 21-2.

MECHANISMS OF INJURY

Blunt Trauma

Blunt trauma may be the result of motor vehicle accidents, falls, or physical assault. Since the growth of the uterus causes changes in the location of the abdominal organs, the pattern of injury with blunt abdominal injury may be altered from that of the nonpregnant patient. Also, injuries to the spleen and the liver are more common in pregnant trauma patients who experience blunt force abdominal trauma.

Motor vehicle accidents (MVAs) are the leading cause of fetal death related to maternal trauma.[28] Fetal death is the result of placental abruption in 50% to 70% of cases where the maternal injury is from an MVA.[29] Maternal ejection from the vehicle and the presence of head injuries are both predictive of poor maternal and fetal outcomes.

It is well known that wearing safety belts can lessen the risk of injury from an MVA. During pregnancy, specific recommendations exist regarding the use of safety belts. They are required by law and when worn correctly decrease the frequency of ejection from the vehicle, which is associated with poor maternal and fetal outcomes. Improper safety belt use increases the likelihood of excessive maternal bleeding and thus increases the risk of fetal death.[30]

It is imperative that providers discuss the importance of proper safety belt use early and often during prenatal care. Correct placement of both the lap belt and shoulder harness are important. The lap belt should be worn under the uterus and across the thighs. The shoulder harness should lie across the chest between the breasts. A safety belt that is improperly placed across the uterine fundus may result in deceleration injury and the result may be a potential placental abruption or uterine rupture. The properly placed three-point restraint system (lap belt and shoulder harness) may limit injury to the gravid uterus in sudden deceleration injuries.

The use of airbags during pregnancy remains controversial. Several studies have been performed to evaluate the effect of airbag deployment during pregnancy. The results of these studies have been conflicting. The potential for placental abruption, fetal injury, and uterine injury exists from airbag deployment, because of the proximity of the gravid uterus to the forceful, rapid expansion of the airbag. The National Highway Traffic Safety Administration does not consider pregnancy an indication for deactivation of airbags. They do recommend deactivation if the mother cannot position herself so that there is at least 10 inches of space between the uterine fundus/sternum and the center of the airbag cover.[31] Overall, it is felt that use of airbags, in conjunction with proper positioning of the mother and correctly placed three-point restraint systems, provides the best protection to the pregnant woman and her fetus.[15]

The process of evaluating the pregnant patient who presents with blunt abdominal trauma is similar to that of the nonpregnant patient. The presence of the gravid uterus may, however, alter the pattern of injury. Bowel injuries are less common but splenic and hepatic injuries are more common with any blunt abdominal trauma in the pregnant patient. Upper abdominal pain may be present. Referred shoulder pain is associated with splenic or hepatic injury when a significant subdiaphragmatic hematoma is present. A FAST scan may be used for identification of intraperitoneal fluid collections secondary to hemorrhage. Computed tomography (CT) scanning may facilitate diagnosis when the patient's condition is confounding.

The incidence of falls increases as the pregnancy advances because the change in the center of gravity in the pregnant women makes her more susceptible to falls. The extent of the injury is related to the specifics of the fall, including the distance and the body part that hits first. Women who fall and hit their abdomen/uterus are at increased risk for placental abruption and preterm labor because of the mechanism of injury in acceleration/deceleration accidents described previously. Women who fall should be carefully questioned regarding the details of the fall and assessment initiated for all who are at risk for placental abruption.

Blunt abdominal trauma may be one of the more common types of intimate partner violence during pregnancy. It is not uncommon for intimate partner violence to begin or escalate during pregnancy. The abuser tends to focus the attacks on the abdomen, breasts, and genitalia, the so called "swim suit" area. The effects of intimate partner violence may include placental abruption and uterine injury. The attacks may also become increasingly violent and include knife wounds, gunshot wounds, and homicide. In pregnant assault victims, increased rates of maternal mortality and uterine rupture from intimate partner violence have been noted.[32] If providers suspect that maternal injuries may be related to intimate partner violence, screening tools to evaluate for intimate partner violence are widely available and should be utilized as appropriate.[33] Additionally, if intimate partner violence is suspected as the cause of maternal injury, appropriate reporting and referrals should be initiated without delay.

Penetrating Abdominal Trauma

The two most common types of penetrating abdominal trauma are gunshot and stab wounds. Mortality rates following a gunshot and stab wound are lower in pregnant women than in their nonpregnant counterparts. This is because of the anatomic changes that occur related to the growing uterus. Maternal abdominal organs are displaced posteriorly and cephalad. The gravid uterus serves to shield other abdominal contents from the force of the penetrating projectiles when the impact is below the uterine fundus.[1] The fetal mortality rate ranges from 40% to 70% in cases of penetrating abdominal trauma and generally results from either direct fetal injury from the missile or from preterm delivery following the injury.[34,35]

The upper abdomen is the most frequent site of abdominal stab wounds. Small bowel involvement is more common with upper abdominal stab wounds. Because of the likelihood of small bowel injury and the potential for diaphragmatic injury, it is recommended that all pregnant women with this injury have surgical exploration. A complete evaluation may include: local wound exploration, FAST scan, CT scan, laparoscopy, or immediate surgical exploration.[12]

Pregnant women who are victims of gunshot wounds have become more common. Assessments should include: the pathway of the bullet(s), the locations of all ballistic injuries, radiographic studies to locate the bullet(s) and/or fragments, and the locations and types of proximal injuries. Generally, surgical exploration is performed for women with intra-abdominal gunshot wounds.

During surgical exploration, the uterus should be carefully inspected for injury. Traction or twisting of the uterus should be avoided as these maneuvers may decrease blood flow to the placenta. Delivery by Cesarean section during surgical exploration may be necessary if the gravid uterus prevents adequate exposure for repair of maternal injuries or there is evidence of nonreassuring fetal status.[12] The gestational age of the fetus, the presence of direct fetal injury from the bullet(s), maternal prognosis, and fetal prognosis are factors that should be considered when decisions related to the timing of delivery are made. Direct uterine injury to the fundus or body of the uterus may necessitate Cesarean delivery. If preterm labor is diagnosed, short-term use of magnesium sulfate is the drug of choice for tocolysis. Betasympathomimetic medications should be avoided because of their effects on maternal hemodynamics. Nonsteroidal anti-inflammatory medications should be avoided because of their effect on platelet function.

Women who experience penetrating abdominal trauma should be evaluated for and receive tetanus prophylaxis. If the patient has not previously been immunized, the toxoid is administered in conjunction with the tetanus immunoglobulin.[2]

Burns

Burns during pregnancy may be caused by exposure to a thermal, chemical, or electrical source. Maternal and perinatal morbidity and mortality increase as the total body surface area burned increases.[36] Pregnant women who experience major burns are subject to all the complications of burn victims, including cardiovascular instability, respiratory distress, sepsis, and renal and liver failure.[37] The best chance of fetal survival is maternal survival. Overall, the treatment of burn patients is unchanged by the presence of a pregnancy.

Initial management should be centered on airway protection, fluid replacement, and pain management. In calculating the percent of the burn, add 5% to the total score if the gravid abdomen is involved. Transport to a burn center is important and should be done when appropriate.

Again, the importance of airway management is essential. Endotracheal intubation may be required if inhalation injury is suspected or the patient is not able to adequately ventilate and oxygenate. Use of continuous pulse oximetry may be useful in assessing oxygenation status. Pulse oximetry, however, is not reliable in patients with carbon monoxide poisoning, because the technology cannot identify and measure the different forms of hemoglobin. Carboxyhemoglobin, the hemoglobin combined with carbon monoxide, is incorrectly measured by pulse oximetry as hemoglobin with 90% oxygen saturation. This falsely high SaO_2 value is displayed on the pulse oximeter when in fact the tissues do not have adequate oxygen, lactate levels increase, and metabolic acidosis ensues. When carbon monoxide poisoning is suspected, or when a patient has worsening acidemia, despite hemoglobin saturation values greater than 90%, an arterial blood gas sample is obtained and analyzed with a Co-oximeter, which accurately measures various types and amounts of hemoglobin in the blood. Carbon monoxide may have been inhaled in a closed fire and this substance freely crosses the placenta. Fetal hemoglobin has an increased affinity for binding with carbon monoxide, which may impede oxygen exchange and leave the fetus vulnerable to hypoxia. Oxygen is the treatment of choice and ventilation with 100% oxygen is recommended.

Fluid loss and fluid shifts may result in decreased blood flow to the uterus and placenta. This may lead to fetal hypoxemia and acidemia. The patient should be carefully assessed for hypovolemia, for which the treatment is aggressive fluid replacement. The pregnant burn patient requires additional fluid resuscitation beyond what the nonpregnant patient requires. Central invasive hemodynamic monitoring may be necessary to more accurately assess hemodynamic and oxygen transport status.

The risk of preterm labor increases as the total body surface burned is increased. The risk of preterm labor may decrease if hypotension, hypoxia, and sepsis are quickly reversed or avoided. External fetal monitoring may be done, with adequate maternal pain relief, even if the abdomen is burned. Monitoring equipment may be placed in sterile bags to help decrease the risk of infection. Ultrasound conduction gel should be used from a sterile or unopened container. Consultation with burn service colleagues to identify the best location for transducer placement is recommended to avoid further damage to injured tissue. Abdominal belts that secure the fetal monitoring transducers, if placed over burned tissue, should be as loose as possible. Again, adequate pain control is essential in pregnant burn victims and is managed the same as in nonpregnant patients. There are no data or reasons to withhold or decrease pain medications because the patient is pregnant. Decisions related to delivery should be made based on gestational age, fetal well-being, and maternal condition. Mode of delivery should be based on obstetric indications and women who have burn injuries may have a vaginal delivery.

SUMMARY

Pregnant trauma patients present specific challenges to the emergency, trauma, and obstetric personnel who provide care to them. Hospitals with specialized burn units should develop protocols that address the unique issues pregnant trauma patients present to the health care personnel who provide care in these units. These protocols should be developed with collaboration from nursing, medicine, and allied health teams. Protocols may include the teams who need to be involved, initial treatment and stabilization guidelines, assessment of fetal well-being, respiratory therapy, pharmacy services, pain services, physical therapy, occupational therapy, nutritional therapy, and others. Additionally, a collaborative plan that identifies the indications for delivery and perimortem Cesarean delivery is needed to coordinate care in the event maternal or fetal deterioration occurs.

Familiarity with the normal anatomic and physiologic changes of pregnancy, skill with trauma assessment and intervention, knowledge of the mechanisms of injury, and ability to accurately assess fetal well-being are essential to providing quality care to pregnant trauma patients. A collaborative, multidisciplinary team approach that includes nurses and physicians from emergency, trauma, and obstetric departments, who each bring specific abilities and knowledge to the care of these patients, promotes the best chance for both maternal and fetal survival.

REFERENCES

1. Laverly, J. P., & Staten-McCormick, M. (1995). Management of moderate to severe trauma in pregnancy. *Obstetrics and Gynecology Clinics of North America, 22*(1), 69–90.
2. Moise, K. J., & Belfort, M. (1997). Damage control for the obstetric patient. *Surgical Clinics of North America, 77*(2), 835–852.
3. Ali, J., Yeo, A., & Gant, T. (1997) Predictors of fetal mortality in pregnant trauma patients. *Journal of Trauma, 42*(5), 782–785.
4. Curet, M., Schermer, C., & Demarest, G. (2000). Predictors of outcome in trauma during pregnancy: Identification of patients who can be monitored for less than six hours. *Journal of Trauma, 49*(1), 18–25.
5. Fort, A., & Harlan, R. (1970). Pregnancy outcome after non-catastrophic maternal trauma during pregnancy. *Obstetrics and Gynecology, 35*(6), 912–915.
6. Mattox, K. L., & Goetzl, L. (2005). Trauma in pregnancy. *Critical Care Medicine, 33*(Suppl. 10), 385–389.
7. Connelly, A. M., Katz, V. L., & Bash, K. L. (1997). Trauma and pregnancy. *American Journal of Perinatology, 14*(6), 331–336.
8. Kuhlman, R. S., & Cruikshank, D. P. (1994). Maternal trauma during pregnancy. *Clinical Obstetrics and Gynecology, 37*(2), 274–293.
9. Tweddale, C. (2006). Trauma during pregnancy. *Critical Care Nursing Quarterly, 29*(1), 53–67.
10. Tsuei, B. (2005). Assessment of the pregnant trauma patient. *Injury, International Journal of the Care of the Injured, 37*(2), 367–373.
11. Vaizey, C. J., Jacobson, M. J., & Cross, F. W. (1994). Trauma in pregnancy. *British Journal of Surgery, 81*(4), 1406–1415.
12. Muench, M. V., & Canterino, J. C. (2007). Trauma in pregnancy. *Obstetrics and Gynecology Clinics of North America, 34*, 555–583.
13. Esposito, T. J. (1994). Trauma during pregnancy. *Emergency Medicine Clinics of North America, 12*(1), 167–199.
14. American College of Surgeons. (1999). *Committee on trauma: Resources for optimal care of the injured patient.* Chicago: Author.
15. Van Hook, J. W., Gei., & Pacheco, L. D. (2004). Trauma in pregnancy. In G. A. Dildy, et al. (Eds.), *Critical care obstetrics* (4th ed). Malden, MA: Blackwell Science.
16. Meroz, Y., Elchalal, U., & Ginosar, Y. (2007). Initial trauma management in advanced pregnancy. *International Anesthesiology Clinics, 25*, 117–129.
17. Leggon, R. E., Wood, G. C., & Indeck, M. C. (2002). Pelvic fractures in pregnancy: Factors influencing maternal and fetal outcomes. *Journal of Trauma, 53*(4), 796–804.
18. El Kady, D., Gilbert, W. M., Xing, G., & Smith, L. H. (2006). Associations of maternal fractures with adverse perinatal outcomes. *American Journal of Obstetrics and Gynecology, 195*(3), 711–716.
19. American College of Obstetricians and Gynecologists. (2004). *Committee opinion #299: Guidelines for diagnostic imaging during pregnancy. Obstetrics & Gynecology, 104*, 647–651.
20. Mattox, K. L., & Goetzl, L. (2005). Trauma in pregnancy. *Critical Care Medicine, 33*, 1–8.
21. Shah, K. H., Simons, R. K., Holbrook, T., Fortlage, D., Winchell, R. J., & Hoyt, D. B. (1998). Trauma in pregnancy: Maternal and fetal outcomes. *The Journal of Trauma, 45*, 83–86.
22. Muench, M. V., Baschat, A. A., Reddy, U. M., Mighty, H. E., Weiner, C. P., Scalea, T. M., et al. (2004). Kleihauer-Betke testing is important in all cases of maternal trauma. *The Journal of Trauma, 57*(5), 1094–1098.
23. Pearlman, M. D., Tininalli, J. E., & Lorenz, R. P. (1990). A prospective controlled study of outcome after trauma during pregnancy. *American Journal of Obstetrics and Gynecology, 163*, 1502–1507.
24. Pearlman, M. D., & Tininalli, J. E. (1993). Evaluation and treatment of the gravida and fetus following trauma during pregnancy. *Obstetrics and Gynecology Clinics of North America, 18*(2), 71–381.
25. Shah, A. J., & Kilcline, B. A. (2003). Trauma in pregnancy. *Emergency Medicine Clinics of North America, 21*(3), 615–629.

26. Katz, V. L., Dotters, D. J., & Droegemueller, W. (1986). Perimortem cesarean delivery. *Obstetrics and Gynecology, 68*(4), 571–576.

27. Katz, V. L., Balderston, K., & DeFreest, M. (2005). Perimortem cesarean delivery: Were our assumptions correct? *American Journal of Obstetrics and Gynecology, 192,* 1916–1921.

28. Weiss, H. B., Songer, T. J., & Fabio, A. (2001). Fetal deaths related to maternal injury. *JAMA, 286*(15), 1863–1868.

29. Weintraub, A. Y., Leron, E., & Mazur, M. (2006). The pathophysiology of trauma in pregnancy: A review. *Journal of Maternal Fetal Neonatal Medicine, 19*(10), 601–605.

30. Hyde, L. K., Cook, L. J., Olson, L. M., Weiss, H. B., & Dean, J. M. (2003). Effect of motor vehicle crashes on adverse fetal outcomes. *Obstetrics and Gynecology, 102*(2), 279–286.

31. National Highway Traffic Safety Administration. (1997). *National Conference on Medical Indications for Air Bag Disconnections: Final report. George Washington University Medical Center.* Washington, DC.

32. El Kady, D., Gilbert, W. M., Xing, G., & Smith, L. H. (2005). Maternal and neonatal outcomes of assaults during pregnancy. *Obstetrics and Gynecology, 105*(2), 357–363.

33. Chambliss, L. (2008). Intimate partner violence and its implication for pregnancy. *Clinical Obstetrics and Gynecology, 51*(2), 385–392.

34. Sandy, E. A., & Koerner, M. (1989). Self-inflicted gunshot wounds to the pregnant abdomen: Report of a case and review of the literature. *American Journal of Obstetrics and Gynecology, 6,* 30–31.

35. Sakala, E. P., & Kost, D. D. (1988). Management of stab wounds to the pregnant uterus: A case report and review of the literature. *Obstetrics and Gynecology, 43,* 319–324.

36. Polko, L. E., & McMahon, M. J. (1999). Burns in pregnancy. *Obstetrical and Gynecological Survey, 54,* 131–144.

37. Kennedy, B. B., Baird, S. M., & Troiano, N. H. (2008). Burn injuries and pregnancy. *Journal of Perinatal and Neonatal Nursing, 22*(1), 21–32

CHAPTER 22

Maternal Obesity: Effects on Pregnancy

Amy H. Picklesimer and Karen Dorman

The recognition of obesity as a major public health issue has only emerged in the past two decades, although overweight status and obesity have long been known to be significant causes of chronic disease. Some of the most common obesity-related health complications are hypertension, type II diabetes mellitus, osteoarthritis, sleep apnea and related respiratory disorders, dyslipidemia, coronary artery disease and stroke. Esophageal, colon, hepatic, renal, pancreatic, and endometrial cancers are more common in obese individuals who also, when compared with normal weight subjects are at a higher risk of death from cancer.[1-3] Women who are overweight or obese during their childbearing years are, therefore, at increased risk for pregnancy related complications and present management challenges for perinatal clinicians. This chapter focuses on the specific combination of obesity and pregnancy and delineates separate discussions of potential effects on the mother, fetus, and newborn.

Standard measurements for relating individual body weight to height are the basis for determining body mass index (BMI) which is calculated utilizing the standard formulas depicted in Table 22-1. This creates an objective measure of weight, scaled according to height, and is commonly used to categorize individuals into underweight (BMI <18.5), normal weight (BMI 18.5–24.9), overweight (BMI 25.0–29.9), and obese (BMI ≥30). Additionally, obese individuals are further subcategorized into Class I (BMI 30 to 34.9), Class II (BMI 35 to 39.9), and Class III or severe obesity (BMI greater than 40) (Table 22-2).[4] These categories are applied universally to adult men and women. Children and teenagers younger than age 20 are classified by a separate set of standards that are specific for both age and gender. Although BMI does not account for differences in body muscle mass, it provides a reasonably good approximation of population-level measures of fitness and has been used by the World Health Organization (WHO) and the National Institutes of Health (NIH) for this purpose.

The prevalence of obesity in the United States for adults of both sexes aged 20 to 74 years in 1962 was 13.4%. By 1994, the rate of obesity had more than doubled to 23.3%. This rate continues to increase, and was measured at 32.2% in the year 2004.[5,6] Not surprisingly, the obstetric population has seen an increase in the prevalence of obesity that parallels that seen in the general population. Data from 495,051 women in Utah documented the increase in rates of prepregnancy obesity (based on self-reported prepregnancy weights) from 25.1% in 1991 to 35.2% in 2001.[7] These rates are similar to the rates of 51.7% for overweight, 21.9% for obesity and 8.0% for extreme obesity found in a national survey of reproductive age women (age 20 to 39) in 2004.[5,8-11]

ANTEPARTUM COMPLICATIONS OF OBESITY DURING PREGNANCY

Several of the adverse health outcomes that affect non-pregnant obese individuals, like coronary artery disease or colon cancer, develop slowly and are more commonly seen outside of the reproductive years. Others, like hypertension and diabetes, are commonly seen in overweight or obese women who are of reproductive age. This population of women, as well as their fetuses and newborns, is at greater risk for medical and obstetric complications during and after pregnancy.

Maternal Complications

Hypertensive Disorders of Pregnancy

Hypertensive disorders of pregnancy include a spectrum that ranges from gestational hypertension, characterized by transient mild elevations in blood pressure, to pre-eclampsia and eclampsia, which are characterized by elevation of blood pressure and renal, hepatic and central nervous system end-organ involvement. See Chapter 7 for a complete discussion of hypertension in pregnancy.

TABLE 22-1

Calculation of Body Mass Index (BMI)

$BMI = \dfrac{Weight\ in\ Pounds \times 703}{Height\ in\ Inches^2}$	$BMI = \dfrac{Weight\ in\ Kilograms}{Height\ in\ Meters^2}$
Sample calculation:	Sample calculation:
Weight = 150 pounds	Weight = 68 kilograms
Height = 65 inches	Height = 1.65 meters
BMI = 150 × 703	BMI = 68.
65 × 65	1.65 × 1.65
BMI = 24.9 (normal weight)	BMI = 24.9 (normal weight)

Automated BMI calculators are widely available online. One is available free from the National Institutes of Health (in both metric and imperial) at this website: http://www.nhlbisupport.com/bmi/.

TABLE 22-2

Classification of Overweight and Obesity by BMI

Category	BMI Range
Underweight	<18.5
Normal weight	18.5 – 24.9
Overweight	25.0 – 29.9
Obesity, Class I	30.0 – 34.9
Obesity, Class II	35.0 – 39.9
Obesity, Class III	≥40

From National Heart, Lung, and Blood Institute. (1998). *Clinical Guidelines on the Identification, Evaluation, and Treatment of Overweight and Obesity in Adults.* National Institutes of Health Publication. 98–4083. Washington, DC: National Institutes of Health, p. xiv.

Multiple studies have documented an increased risk of hypertensive disorders of pregnancy in obese women. Bodnar and colleagues reported on a cohort of 38,188 pregnant women, 19% of whom were overweight or obese, in which they found a strong relationship between increasing prepregnancy BMI and increasing risk for both mild and severe preeclampsia (Figure 22-1). These authors found a twofold increase in risk for mild or severe preeclampsia for overweight women (BMI 25.0–25.9), approximately a threefold increase for obese women (BMI 30.0–34.9), and a fivefold increase in the risk for preeclampsia for severely obese women (BMI 35.0–39.9).[12] Similar findings were reported by Callaway and associates in a cohort of 11,252 Australian women, 34% of whom were overweight or obese, as well as by Cedergren and associates in a cohort of 621,221 Swedish women, 14% of whom were obese.[11,13]

Obese gravidas are not only at higher risk for developing hypertensive disorders of pregnancy, but also are more likely to begin pregnancy with a known diagnosis of chronic hypertension. It is well established that increasing BMI is strongly associated with an increased incidence of hypertension. Evidence from the Framingham Heart Study, a prospective population-based cohort study, demonstrated that hypertension and coronary artery disease were more common in obese and overweight individuals at all ages. Relative risk for hypertension in overweight adults was found to be 1.5 to 1.7, and 2.2 to 2.6 for obese adults, respectively. Additionally, population-attributable risk estimates from this cohort found that obesity or overweight status accounted for 34% of the risk in men and 62% in women.[14] The prevalence of chronic hypertension in the United States among all adults aged 18 to 39 years has been estimated at 7.2%, although almost half of hypertensive patients in this age group are not aware of

FIGURE 22-1 Association between prepregnancy BMI and the unadjusted prevalence of mild and severe preeclampsia by race/ethnicity. Curves were estimated by calculating predicted probabilities based on an unadjusted multinomial logistic regression model. Source: Bodnar, L. M., Catov, J. M., Klebanoff, M. A., Ness, R. B., & Roberts, J. M. (2007). Prepregnancy body mass index and the occurrence of severe hypertensive disorders of pregnancy. *Epidemiology, 18*(2), 234–239.

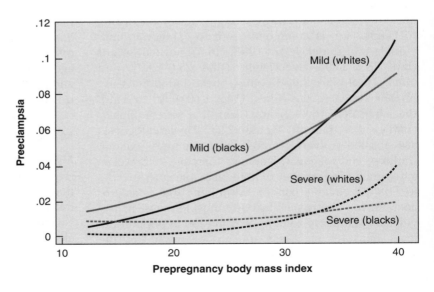

their diagnosis and fewer than one third are adequately treated for their disease.[15]

Management of the obese gravida is complicated by both the increased incidence of pre-existing hypertensive disease as well as the increased risk for development of hypertensive diseases of pregnancy. It is important to establish baseline blood pressure values in early pregnancy, and care should be taken to use properly sized blood pressure cuffs in order to ensure accurate measurements.[16] Additionally, evaluation of end-organ effects of hypertensive disease, such as heart failure or nephropathy, should be considered. Comprehensive evaluation of cardiac function may require electrocardiographic or echocardiographic testing. Renal function is commonly assessed by a 24-hour urine evaluation to measure total protein excretion. Establishing these parameters early in pregnancy will not only allow for optimal medical management during gestation, but also expedites identification of developing signs and symptoms of pregnancy-induced hypertensive disease and preeclampsia later in the pregnancy. Further discussion of blood pressure measurement and hypertensive disorders in pregnancy is found in Chapter 7.

Diabetes Mellitus

The second trimester of pregnancy is a physiologic state of insulin resistance. Hormones produced by the placenta lead to mild levels of maternal hyperglycemia in order to promote adequate fetal growth and development. Most gravidas adapt readily to this event. In some women, however, pancreatic insulin secretion is not adequate to counter the diabetogenic hormones. Women who have normal serum glucose levels prior to pregnancy demonstrate abnormally high postprandial and fasting serum glucose levels during pregnancy. This transient disease process is known as gestational diabetes. Although this condition resolves after delivery, untreated hyperglycemia in pregnancy is associated with a number of adverse maternal, fetal, and/or neonatal outcomes. These include: preeclampsia, disordered fetal growth, neonatal metabolic complications such as hyperbilirubinemia and hyperglycemia, and even fetal death.

The metabolic pathways in the development of obesity are complex, but adipocytes participate in several important signaling pathways that influence insulin sensitivity in the peripheral tissues.[17] As a result, obese women are at increased risk for developing gestational diabetes. Sebire and colleagues reported a retrospective study of 287,213 British women in which they found the relative risk of developing gestational diabetes in obese women (prepregnancy BMI 25 to 30) to be 1.68 (99% confidence interval [CI] 1.53 to 1.84) and severely obese women (prepregnancy BMI greater than 30) to be 3.6 (99% CI 3.25 to 3.98).[18] These findings were confirmed in a separate retrospective study of 1,644 American women

by Rudra and associates, in which obese women (BMI greater than 29) demonstrated a relative risk for developing gestational diabetes of 4.53 (95% CI 1.25 to 16.43). Additionally, these authors found that weight gain between the age of 18 years and the study pregnancy of greater than or equal to 10 kilograms conferred a relative risk of 3.43 (95% CI 1.60 to 7.37) when compared with women who had less than a 3-kilogram weight change over the same period.[19]

Obese gravidas are not only at higher risk for developing gestational diabetes, but also are more likely to begin pregnancy with a known diagnosis of pre-existing Type II diabetes. Evidence from the Nurses' Health Study, a prospective population-based cohort study of 43,581 women, demonstrated a linear relationship between increasing BMI and increasing incidence of diabetes. Even after adjusting for family history, levels of exercise, and dietary habits, the relative risk of future development of type II diabetes was 11.2 for women in the top tenth percentile of BMI when compared with women in the lowest tenth percentile.[20] In a prospective study by Rode and colleagues of 8,092 Danish women, the relative risk for a diagnosis of diabetes during pregnancy for overweight women (prepregnancy BMI 25 to 30) was found to be 3.4 (95% CI 1.7 to 6.8) and for severely obese women (prepregnancy BMI greater than 30) was found to be 15.3 (95% CI 8.2 to 28.6) when compared with normal weight women.[21]

Management of the obese gravida includes consideration of early screening for diabetes, rather than waiting for the traditional screening window for gestational diabetes of 24 to 28 weeks. A large number of obese women may in fact have undiagnosed Type II diabetes, which is manifest by abnormal glucose tolerance testing prior to 20 weeks of gestation. For obese women who develop gestational diabetes, promoting tight control of blood glucose values optimizes both maternal and fetal outcomes. The most successful management approaches are multidisciplinary and include physicians, nurse-educators, and dietitians. By strict adherence to diet, the incidence of fetal growth disorders, stillbirth, and maternal complications such as preeclampsia can be minimized. (Further discussion on diabetes in pregnancy can be found in Chapter 10.)

Nutrition and Weight Gain

Pregnancy is a period of rapid weight gain. Increases in blood volume, enlargement of the breasts and uterus, expansion of fat stores, as well as the weight of the fetus, placenta, and amniotic fluid all contribute to total weight gain during pregnancy. Current recommendations for weight gains in pregnancy are based on a report originally published by the Institute of Medicine (IOM) in 1990 and updated in 2009. These guidelines have been adopted by the American College of Obstetricians and Gynecologists (ACOG). These recommendations

TABLE 22-3

Recommended Gestational Weight Gain Based on Prepregnancy Body Mass Index (BMI)

Prepregnant BMI	Recommended Gain (lb)		Recommended Rate of Gain 2nd and 3rd Trimester*	
	Pounds	Kilograms	Pounds/Week	Kilograms/Week
Underweight BMI <18.5	28–40	12.5–18	0.5	1
Normal weight: BMI 18.5–24.9	25–35	11.5–16	0.4	1
Overweight BMI 25–29.9	15–25	7.0–11.5	0.3	0.6
Obese BMI ≥30	11–20	5–9	0.2	0.5

*Calculations assume a 0.5–2 kilogram (1.1–4.4 pound) weight gain in the first trimester.
Adapted from the Institute of Medicine (2009). *Weight gain during pregnancy: Reexamining the guidelines.* http://www.nap.edu/catalog/12584.html

are based on observational studies of prepregnancy weight, pregnancy weight gain, and birth outcomes. Using these data, the IOM categorized women by prepregnancy BMI with a different target weight gain for each category. (Table 22-3)[22] The 2009 updated recommendations also include an optimal rate of weight gain for each category of maternal BMI, which allows greater flexibility for counseling of patients who are already in their second or third trimester.

In a survey of 1,198 pregnant women, Stotland and associates found that those with a high prepregnancy BMI were more than four times as likely to report target gains above IOM guidelines.[23] A similar study of more than 7,000 pregnant women by Abrams and colleagues found that weight gains above the IOM recommendations were observed for 23% of the underweight women, 49% of the normal weight women, 70% of the overweight women, and 57% of the obese women.[24,25] Many women cite pregnancy as a cause of their obesity, which contributes to the widely held belief that childbearing leads to overweight status and obesity.[26,27] While several studies have found the average postpartum weight retention one year after delivery of approximately 0.5 kilograms, there is a wide variation in weight retention between individual women.[28,29] In a large Swedish study of 1,423 women using self-reported prepregnancy weights, 30% weighed less one year after delivery than they did before pregnancy, 56% gained 0 to 5 kilograms over the same time period, and 14% gained more than 5 kilograms.[29] Risk factors for postpartum weight retention in this study were excessive pregnancy weight gain, high prepregnancy BMI, and maternal age greater than 36 years.

From these data, it appears that overweight and obese women are at increased risk for excessive preg-

nancy weight gain and elevated postpartum weight retention. While pregnancy is not the ideal time for weight loss, adherence to a healthy diet will allow women to optimize pregnancy outcomes and decrease the risk for excessive weight gain. These goals can be achieved by providing specific weight gain goals in conjunction with nutritional guidance as necessary.

Fetal Complications

Macrosomia

Large for gestational age and fetal macrosomia are separate but overlapping descriptions of accelerated fetal growth that are associated with shoulder dystocia, birth trauma, and/or Cesarean delivery. Based on data from the National Center for Health Statistics, ACOG recommends using the term large for gestational age to describe an infant with a birth weight equal to or greater than the 90th percentile for any given gestational age. Their recommendation for the term fetal macrosomia, on the other hand, is that it should be reserved for those infants weighing more than 4,000 or 4,500 grams at birth.[30]

Factors that may predispose to fetal macrosomia include: pregestational or gestational diabetes, prepregnancy maternal obesity or overweight status, excessive weight gain during pregnancy, multiparity, male fetus, as well as constitutional factors such as ethnicity, maternal birth weight, and maternal height.[8,18,31,32] Many of these predisposing factors may coexist within a single pregnancy, confounding understanding of the relative importance of each factor. It appears, however, that increasing maternal weight is an independent variable for a macrosomic or large for gestational age infant. Cedergren and colleagues, in a study of more than

15,000 pregnant women with normal glucose tolerance testing, described odds ratios for large for gestational age infants to be increased for women with a BMI 29.1 to 35 OR 2.20 (95% CI 2.14 to 2.26), a BMI 35.1 to 40 OR 3.11 (95% CI 2.96 to 3.27), and women with a BMI greater than 40 OR 3.82 (3.56 to 4.16).[13]

CONGENITAL ANOMALIES

Population-based estimates for congenital anomalies, which include malformations, deformations, and chromosome anomalies present at birth, vary by organ system, but the overall incidence ranges from 2% to 4% of all pregnancies. The most common anomalies are neural tube defects, congenital cardiac malformations, orofacial clefts, and Trisomy 21, also known as Down syndrome.[33] These and other anomalies are one of the leading causes of infant mortality in the United States, and are indirectly or directly responsible for 21% of neonatal deaths and 18% of post-neonatal infant deaths.[34]

Obese women are at higher risk for having an infant with congenital cardiac defects, orofacial clefts, and neural tube defects.[35–37] Watkins and associates published a population-based case-control study of 645 women who gave birth to anomalous infants, excluding women with known diabetes. These authors found that obese women (BMI greater than or equal to 30) were more likely to have an infant with a neural tube defect (OR: 3.5, 95% CI: 1.2 to10.3), omphalocele (OR: 3.3; 95% CI: 1.0 to 10.3), heart defects (OR: 2.0; 95% CI: 1.2 to 3.4), or multiple anomalies (OR: 2.0; 95% CI: 1.0 to 3.8). Overweight women (BMI 25 to 29.9) also were more likely than average-weight women to have infants with heart defects (OR: 2.0; 95% CI: 1.2 to 3.1) and multiple anomalies (OR: 1.9; 95% CI: 1.1 to 3.4). Although these confidence intervals are wide, the authors discovered a dose-response relationship between increasing BMI and risk for birth defects such that every incremental increase in BMI conferred an additional 7% risk for congenital anomalies.[38]

The cause of this increased risk for birth defects in obese women is not clear. It is possible that some of these women have undiagnosed pregestational diabetes, which is known to confer additional risks of congenital anomalies to offspring. Additionally, increased BMI is associated with lower serum folate levels, which may contribute to the increased incidence of neural tube defects in obese women.[39] What is certain, however, is that obese women merit enhanced surveillance for birth defects. Unfortunately, prenatal screening tests such as ultrasound and maternal serum screening can be more difficult to interpret in obese women.[40,41]

A retrospective review by Hendler and colleagues of more than 11,000 pregnancies, in which 39% of women were obese, found that the rate of incomplete or suboptimal visualization of the fetal cardiac structures was as high as 37.3% in obese women, compared with only 18.7% in average-weight women. Similar findings were documented for craniospinal structures, with a suboptimal visualization rate of 42.8% compared with 29.5% in average-weight women.[42]

Fetal Demise

Pregnancy loss occurring prior to 20 weeks gestation is known as a spontaneous abortion or miscarriage, while pregnancy loss after 20 weeks is considered to be an intrauterine fetal death. This distinction is based on medico-legal reporting requirements established by the Center for Disease Control and Prevention's National Center for Health Statistics, in conjunction with the Department of Health and Human Services in individual states. The numerous factors that may contribute to intrauterine fetal demise can be grouped into three categories. Fetal problems, including congenital anomalies, account for 25% of antepartum fetal deaths. Maternal problems, including preeclampsia and diabetes, account for another 10%. Finally, placental or umbilical cord problems such as placental abruption or true knots in the umbilical cord account for 25% to 30% of intrauterine fetal deaths. However, no cause can be determined for the remaining 35% to 40% of intrauterine fetal deaths after 20 weeks gestation.[43]

Several studies have found that obesity is one of the maternal demographic factors associated with an increased risk for fetal death. A Swedish case-control study by Stephansson and associates of 649 women with antepartum stillbirths found the odds ratio of 2.7 (95% CI 1.5 to 5.0) for the risk of fetal death in overweight women (BMI 25.0 to 29.9), and 2.8 (95% CI, 1.3 to 6.0) for obese women (BMI greater than or equal to 30).[44] A Danish cohort study of 24,505 pregnancies, which included 112 stillbirths, found an odds ratio of 2.8 (95% CI: 1.5 to 5.3) for stillbirth in obese gravidas compared with women of normal weight.[45] This relationship persisted after controlling for maternal comorbidities such as diabetes and hypertension.

Childhood Obesity

Recent research indicates that the fetal environment likely plays a significant role in later health outcomes. Known as the Barker hypothesis, it describes the potential for programming of the adult phenotype based on prenatal exposures, such as maternal nutrition. It was first described in infants of undernourished pregnant women, whose children evidenced a "thrifty phenotype" of small size and lower metabolic rates. As a consequence, these infants were adapted for survival in an environment with limited resources. These same individuals, when exposed to rich diets later in life, were noted to be more likely to develop diabetes, hypertension, coronary artery disease, and obesity.[46–48]

Although it is difficult to control for all confounding factors, particularly behavioral decisions about diet and exercise that may be similar within a family unit, the association between prenatal exposures and adult disease has been described in diverse populations.[31] There is also a well-established link between maternal obesity and large for gestational age infants, who are also at increased risk for developing obesity later in life.[31,46,49] Proposed mechanisms for this relationship include dysregulation of central nervous system control of appetite regulation, peripheral changes in insulin sensitivity and alterations in pancreatic response to hyperglycemia.[46] Achieving the proper nutrition and weight gain during pregnancy is now known to be important not only for the health of the pregnant woman, but appears to have far-reaching consequences for the health of the fetus or infant as well.

INTRAPARTUM COMPLICATIONS OF OBESITY DURING PREGNANCY

Induction of Labor

Obese women undergo induction of labor more frequently because of a higher incidence of medical comorbidities such as hypertension and diabetes, as well as a higher incidence of post-dates pregnancy.[50] Robinson and colleagues reported rates for induction of labor in morbidly obese gravidas (weight greater than 120 kilograms at initiation of prenatal care) as 40%, which was significantly higher than the rates of 19% for women with normal weight (55 to 75 kilograms).[51] Additionally, these authors found that obese women demonstrate abnormalities in the second stage of labor more frequently, and require operative assistance due to soft tissue dystocia and poor maternal pushing efforts more frequently than women with normal BMI. Unfortunately, obese women are less likely to have a successful medical induction of labor and may require an operative delivery.[52] (Further discussion of induction of labor can be found in Chapter 12).

Cesarean Delivery

Rates of Cesarean birth are higher in obese women. Weiss and associates reported the results of a multicenter retrospective review of delivery data from 386 obese women (BMI 30 to 34.9) and 196 morbidly obese (BMI greater than or equal to 35) nulliparous women and demonstrated Cesarean delivery rates of 33.8% and 47.4%, respectively. These rates were significantly higher than the Cesarean delivery rate of 20.7% in nulliparous patients with normal BMI.[53] Similar findings have been reported by other authors.[18,50–51,53–55]

The technical aspects of Cesarean delivery are more complicated in obese women. Regular patient beds and operating room tables typically have a maximum weight limit of 500 pounds, and also may be too narrow to accommodate some extremely obese women.[56] Tables and beds that are specially designed to accommodate patients above these weight limits may need to be identified well in advance of their anticipated need.

Noninvasive measurement of arterial blood pressure in obese patients is a challenging aspect of care in general and during surgery. Blood pressures taken with an improperly sized cuff will give inaccurate readings. For obese women requiring Cesarean delivery, and particularly those with co-existing medical conditions, consideration should be given to placement of an arterial line for accurate assessment of hemodynamic status. This is particularly important since operative delivery is more complicated in the obese patient as operative times tend to be longer and blood loss greater.

Operative approaches in the obese gravida may also need to be modified depending on the size and location of any abdominal pannus. Although no randomized trials have been published, some authors recommend supra-umbilical incisions to decrease rates of wound separation and infectious morbidities.

Placement of a surgical drain in the subcutaneous layers has been advocated as a means to reduce wound seroma formation and subsequent infection. A Cochrane Review concluded that there were not enough data to recommend either for or against this technique.[57] A report by the U.S. Preventive Services Task Force published the same year, however, recommended using drains when the subcutaneous space was greater than or equal to 2 cm.[58]

Analgesia/Anesthesia for the Obese Gravida

Obesity is a risk factor for anesthesia-related maternal mortality.[59] Obese women are at increased risk of airway complications, cardiopulmonary dysfunction, perioperative morbidity and mortality, and also pose technical anesthesia challenges.[60]

Epidural analgesia can be successfully used in obese patients, but the placement of the epidural catheter may be complicated by improper positioning and difficulty identifying the midline in very obese women. This may lead to inadequate pain relief during labor, and may require replacement of the epidural catheter. Failure rates as high as 42% at initial placement have been reported, and up to 74% of women weighing more than 300 pounds will require more than one attempt at epidural catheter placement.[61] Additionally, even if the initial placement of the catheter tip is in the proper location, in obese women it is subject to the drag of maternal fat and can become dislodged by movement in bed.[60]

General endotracheal anesthesia carries additional risks for the obese gravida. Difficulty may be encountered with positioning on the operating room table, and important anatomic landmarks are often obscured. The incidence of difficult intubation in pregnant women over 300 pounds was reported in one retrospective case-control study to be as high as 35%, compared with 0% among normal-weight women.[62] Challenges that exist in caring for obese women under optimal clinical circumstances are only magnified during times of emergency. A multidisciplinary approach that includes obstetric, anesthesia, and nursing personnel allows anticipatory planning in case of an emergency in order to avoid unnecessary morbidities in this population of patients. (Further discussion related to anesthesia/analgesia is contained in Chapter 11.)

Vaginal Birth After Cesarean Delivery

For women with a history of a previous Cesarean delivery who elect to undergo trial of labor in a subsequent pregnancy, overall success rates are approximately 60% to 80%. Since this is such a wide range, clinicians have sought to identify clinical characteristics that are predictive of successful vaginal delivery. Multivariable regression analysis was performed on data gathered from a cohort of 7,660 women with a history of a previous Cesarean birth who underwent a subsequent trial of labor. Factors predictive of a successful VBAC include a nonrecurring indication for Cesarean delivery (breech presentation) and a history of a previous vaginal delivery. Advanced maternal age, non-White race and recurring indication for Cesarean section (failure to progress) were indicative of a lower chance of success. In this group, advancing BMI was also associated with a slightly decreased chance of successful trial of labor (OR 0.94, 95% CI 0.93 to 0.95).[63]

Other authors identified similar trends using weight-based groupings. Carroll and associates, in a case-control study with 70 patients in each arm, found a rate of 80% for successful trial of labor in women weighing less than 200 pounds, with rates decreasing to 57% for women weighing 200 to 300 pounds and a rate of vaginal delivery of only 13% in women weighing more than 300 pounds.[64]

Shoulder Dystocia

Shoulder dystocia results from a failure of delivery of the fetal shoulders using routine downward traction after delivery of the fetal head. It is caused by impaction of the fetal shoulder anteriorly against the pubic symphysis or posteriorly against the sacral promontory. Maneuvers required to dislodge and deliver the fetus may result in neurologic or orthopedic injury to the newborn. Additionally, maternal complications of shoulder dystocia include postpartum hemorrhage and significant soft tissue trauma. Fortunately, shoulder dystocia is a rare complication, occurring in approximately 0.5% to 1.5% of vaginal deliveries.[65]

Maternal obesity, because of its relationship with higher rates of fetal macrosomia and gestational diabetes, has consistently been found to be a predisposing factor for shoulder dystocia.[66–69] These rates may be somewhat inflated by challenges in adequately abducting the legs of obese women for placement in McRobert's or dorsal lithotomy position for delivery. Care should be taken to ensure that adequate personnel are available to provide assistance during vaginal delivery of an obese woman, particularly in the case in which a macrosomic infant is suspected.

Fetal Monitoring

Electronic monitoring, via external or internal methods, is routinely performed for more than 85% of women during labor as a means to assess for fetal well-being and to evaluate uterine activity.[70]

Proper placement of the transducers for fetal heart rate and maternal uterine activity assessment and/or maintenance of an adequate tracing may be difficult in women with central obesity and an unusually thick anterior abdominal wall or a large abdominal pannus. Challenges associated with external fetal heart rate monitoring for obese gravidas are magnified due to the increased incidence of medical complications of pregnancy, such as diabetes or hypertension, that often require frequent antenatal fetal surveillance. If it is not possible to maintain an adequate fetal heart rate tracing with an external fetal heart rate monitor, an ultrasonographic assessment with biophysical profile testing may be required.

During labor, there can be similar problems obtaining a continuous fetal heart rate tracing with external fetal heart rate monitors for very obese women. Internal fetal scalp electrodes should be considered if there is an inability to adequately document fetal well-being. Additionally, the complete inability to monitor the fetal heart rate tracing due to maternal obesity may be an indication for Cesarean delivery in some instances. This is a particularly important consideration for obese women requiring induction of labor, and the limitations of external fetal heart rate monitoring should be included in the informed consent process when induction agents such as prostaglandins or oxytocin are employed.

POSTPARTUM COMPLICATIONS OF OBESITY DURING PREGNANCY

Thromboembolism

Pregnancy is characterized by the presence of all three components of Virchow's triad: venous stasis, endothelial injury, and hypercoagulable state. As such, it is well recognized as a period during which all women are at increased risk for venous thromboembolic disease, including deep venous thrombosis and pulmonary embolism.

A complete discussion of thromboembolic disease in pregnancy and the postpartum period can be found in Chapter 17.

Obesity appears to be an independent risk factor for the development of thromboembolic disease in pregnancy. James and colleagues reviewed admission records of 14,335 women with pregnancy-associated thromboembolic events and found that obesity (BMI greater than 30) conferred an additional risk for thromboembolic events with an odds ratio of 4.4 (95% CI 3.4 to 5.7).[71] Simpson and associates, in a retrospective case-control study of 336 women with pregnancy-associated thromboembolic events, found that both overweight status (BMI 25–29.9) and obesity (BMI greater than 30) conferred an additional risk, with odds ratios 1.8 (95% CI 1.3 to 2.5) and 2.0 (95% CI 1.3 to 3.1).[72] Both authors found that more than half of all events occurred in these populations during the postpartum period.

Medical conditions that predispose to thromboemolic events during pregnancy include diabetes, hypertension, heart disease, antiphospholipid syndrome, lupus, sickle cell disease, inherited thrombophilias, and a history of a previous thromboembolic event.[71] Most of these, especially the presence of an inherited thrombophilia, confer significantly more risk than obesity as an independent risk factor. Many of these conditions, however, coexist in a single patient and therefore management must be individualized.

Currently, there is not enough evidence to recommend for or against thromboprophylaxis to pregnant women with obesity as their only risk factor for venous thromboembolism during pregnancy or the postpartum period.[44,57] These patients may benefit from nonpharmacologic interventions, such as pneumatic compression boots, hydration, and early postpartum ambulation.

Wound Disruption and Infection After Cesarean Delivery

Postpartum infectious complications are quite common; endometritis affects approximately 4% to 6% of delivered women and wound infection complicates 2% to 16%.[73,74] Patient characteristics that pose additional risk for surgical site complications have been well-studied and include many conditions more commonly found in obese gravidas such as prolonged labor, diabetes, anemia, smoking, and poor nutritional status.[75,76] Abdominal wall thickness greater than 3 cm, more frequently found in obese women, is associated with almost a three-fold increase in risk for postoperative wound infection.[77]

Placement of subcutaneous drains has been investigated as a strategy to decrease wound complications, particularly in obese gravidas. Unfortunately, the routine placement of subcutaneous drains has not been shown to prevent wound separation, wound infection, or wound seroma formation in several mulitcenter trials and in a meta-analysis from the Cochrane Review.[57,78]

Breast-Feeding

Successful initiation and continuation of breast-feeding depends upon not only complex physiologic changes in the postpartum period, but also on adequate social support for the nursing mother. Challenges that arise from the metabolic milieu of obesity, as well as social and behavioral factors that are independently associated with obesity, conspire to decrease rates of breast-feeding initiation, and to shorten the duration of breast-feeding for obese women.

By the second trimester of pregnancy, breast tissue has developed the capability to secrete colostrum. In the first few days following delivery, colostrum is the perfect low-volume, high-protein nutrition for the newborn. The drop in maternal serum progesterone levels following delivery, mediated by prolactin secretion, triggers mature milk production. For most women, this happens in the first 2 to 4 days postpartum, and is commonly described as the "milk coming in" or "dropping." Although the physiologic pathways are still poorly understood, obese women demonstrate blunted prolactin production in response to infant suckling in the first two days following delivery.[79] This results in a delay in the production of mature milk, which in turn requires more frequent or longer nursing periods.[79–81] Together, these represent an additional barrier to successful initiation of breast-feeding for the obese mother.

Obese women also experience difficulties with proper positioning and infant latch for nursing. Women with large breasts may have problems properly supporting both the infant and the breast while nursing. Additionally, large breasts may obstruct the view of the nipple and make it difficult to ensure a proper latch.[82] Hospital discharge policies that do not allow adequate time for obese women to learn breast-feeding techniques likely contribute to the lower rates of breast-feeding initiation and continuation in this population.

Most of the variation in breast-feeding rates is sociocultural, however, rather than biologic. Obese women are less likely to have been breast-fed themselves and report lower rates of intention to breast-feed.[83]

PREGNANCY AFTER BARIATRIC SURGERY

Bariatric surgery is indicated as a treatment for morbid obesity (BMI greater than 40) unresponsive to other weight-management therapies.[84] There are different types of surgical procedures employed to achieve weight loss. These include: establishing a state of chronic malabsorption (jejunal-ileal bypass; restricting capacity for food intake (gastric banding); or both (Roux-en-Y gastric bypass). More than 100,000 bariatric procedures were performed in the United States in 2003, and the number continues to rise.[85] The procedure is commonly performed in women of reproductive age, including adolescents.

Pregnancy following bariatric surgery is considered safe and infant outcomes are comparable to the overall obstetric population. In fact, pregnancy may be safer postoperatively for women who successfully decrease their BMI when compared with morbidly obese women.[86] The most significant risk is from macronutrient deficiencies such as iron or B-12, folate, and calcium, leading to anemia. There does not appear to be an increased risk of fetal growth disorders, diabetes, preeclampsia, or preterm labor.[87] Even in the first year following surgery, characterized by rapid weight loss and dramatic metabolic changes, pregnancy outcomes are favorable.[88]

SUMMARY

Caring for pregnant women who are either overweight or obese is clinically challenging. The incidence of overweight and obesity, with its associated medical comorbidities, is ever increasing in women of childbearing age. These women, as well as their infants, have a propensity for medical and obstetric complications during and after pregnancy. Weight loss prior to the pregnancy is the best way to decrease risk for both the mother and fetus. However, given that only a small minority of obese women will do so, it is up to the health care providers to be aware of the risks and complications that are associated with this population of pregnant women.

Pregnancy may be the first encounter with the health care system for many obese women. It is critical that these women, at greater risk for long-term complications, are given ample information to underscore the importance of initiating a weight loss program primarily in the postpartum period.

REFERENCES

1. Calle, E. E., Rodriquez, C., Walker-Thurmond, K., & Thun, M. J. (2003). Overweight, obesity, and mortality from cancer in a prospectively studied cohort of U.S. adults. *The New England Journal of Medicine, 348,* 1625–1638.
2. Calle, E. E., Thun, M. J., Petrelli, J. M., Rodriguez, C., & Heath, C. W. Jr. (1999). Body-mass index and mortality in a prospective cohort of U.S. adults. *The New England Journal of Medicine, 341,* 1097–1105.
3. Bray, G. A., & Bellanger, T. (2006). Epidemiology, trends, and morbidities of obesity and the metabolic syndrome. *Endocrine, 29,* 109–117.
4. National Heart, Lung, and Blood Institute. (1998). *Clinical Guidelines on the Identification, Evaluation, and Treatment of Overweight and Obesity in Adults.* National Institutes of Health Publication. 98–4083. Washington, DC: National Institutes of Health.
5. Ogden, C. L., Carroll, M. D., Curtin, L. R., et al. (2006). Prevalence of overweight and obesity in the United States, 1999–2004. *Journal of the American Medical Association, 295,* 1549–1555.
6. Kuczmarski, R. J., Flegal, K. M., Campbell, S. M., & Johnson, C. L. (1994). Increasing prevalence of overweight among US adults. The National Health and Nutrition Examination Surveys, 1960 to 1991. *Journal of the American Medical Association, 272,* 205–211.
7. LaCoursiere, D. Y., Bloebaum, L., Duncan, J. D., & Varner, M. W. (2005). Population-based trends and correlates of maternal overweight and obesity, Utah 1991–2001. *American Journal of Obstetrics and Gynecology, 192,* 832–839.
8. Baeten, J. M., Bukusi, E. A., & Lambe, M. (2001). Pregnancy complications and outcomes among overweight and obese nulliparous women. *American Journal of Public Health, 91,* 436–440.
9. Ehrenberg, H. M., Dierker, L., Milluzzi, C., & Mercer, B. M. (2002). Prevalence of maternal obesity in an urban center. *American Journal of Obstetrics and Gynecology, 187,* 1189–1193.
10. Lu, G. C., Rouse, D. J., DuBard, M., Cliver, S., Kimberlin, D., & Hauth, J. C. (2001). The effect of the increasing prevalence of maternal obesity on perinatal morbidity. *American Journal of Obstetrics and Gynecology, 185,* 845–849.
11. Callaway, L. K., Prins, J. B., Chang, A. M., & McIntyre, H. D. (2006). The prevalence and impact of overweight and obesity in an Australian obstetric population. *Medical Journal of Australia, 184,* 56–59.
12. Bodnar, L. M., Catov, J. M., Klebanoff, M. A., Ness, R. B., & Roberts, J. M. (2007). Prepregnancy body mass index and the occurrence of severe hypertensive disorders of pregnancy. *Epidemiology, 18*(2), 234–239.
13. Cedergren, M. I. (2004). Maternal morbid obesity and the risk of adverse pregnancy outcome. *Obstetrics and Gynecology, 103,* 219–224.
14. Wilson, P. W., D'Agostino, R. B., Sullivan, S., Parise, H., & Kannel, W. B. (2002). Overweight and obesity as determinants of cardiovascular risk: The Framingham experience. *Archives of Internal Medicine, 162,* 1867–1872.
15. Hajjar, I., & Kotchen, T. A. (2003). Trends in prevalence, awareness, treatment, and control of hypertension in the United States, 1988–2000. *Journal of the American Medical Association, 290,* 199–206.
16. Graves, J. W. (2001). Prevalence of blood pressure cuff sizes in a referral practice of 430 consecutive adult hypertensives. *Blood Pressure Monitor, 6,* 17–20.
17. Fruhbeck, G., Gomez-Ambrosi, J., Muruzabal, F. J., & Burrell, M. A. (2001). The adipocyte: A model for integration of endocrine and metabolic signaling in energy metabolism regulation. *American Journal of Physiology, Endocrinology and Metabolism, 280,* E827–E847.
18. Sebire, N. J., Jolly, M., Harris, J. P., Wadsworth, J., Joffe, M., & Beard, R. W., (2001). Maternal obesity and pregnancy outcome: A study of 287,213 pregnancies in London. *International Journal of Obesity Related Metabolic Disorders, 25,* 1175–1182.
19. Rudra, C. B., Sorensen, T. K., Leisenring, W. M., Dashow, E., & Williams, M. A. (2007). Weight characteristics and height in relation to risk of gestational diabetes mellitus. *American Journal of Epidemiology, 165,* 302–308.

20. Carey, V. J., Walters, E. E., Colditz, G. A., Solomon, C. G., Willett, W. C., Rosner, B. A., et al. (1997). Body fat distribution and risk of non-insulin-dependent diabetes mellitus in women. The Nurses' Health Study. *American Journal of Epidemiology, 145,* 614–619.

21. Rode, L., Nilas, L., Wøjdemann, K., & Tabor, A. (2005). Obesity-related complications in Danish single cephalic term pregnancies. *Obstetrics and Gynecology, 105,* 537–542.

22. Institute of Medicine. (2009). *Weight gain during pregnancy: Reexamining the guidelines.* Washington, DC: The National Academies Press.

23. Stotland, N. E., Haas, J. S., Brawarsky, P., Jackson, R. A., Fuentes-Afflick, E., & Escobar, G. J. (2005). Body mass index, provider advice, and target gestational weight gain. *Obstetrics and Gynecology, 105,* 633–638.

24. Abrams, B., Carmichael, S., & Selvin, S. (1995). Factors associated with the pattern of maternal weight gain during pregnancy. *Obstetrics and Gynecology, 86,* 170–176.

25. Carmichael, S., Abrams, B., & Selvin, S. (1997). The pattern of maternal weight gain in women with good pregnancy outcomes. *American Journal of Public Health, 87,* 1984–1988.

26. Rossner, S. (1999). Physical activity and prevention and treatment of weight gain associated with pregnancy: Current evidence and research issues. *Medicine and Science in Sports and Exercise, 31,* S560–S563.

27. Rossner, S., & Ohlin, A. (1995). Pregnancy as a risk factor for obesity: Lessons from the Stockholm Pregnancy and Weight Development Study. *Obesity Research, 3,* 267s–275s.

28. Gunderson, E. P., & Abrams, B. (2000). Epidemiology of gestational weight gain and body weight changes after pregnancy. *Epidemiology Review, 22,* 261–274.

29. Ohlin, A., & Rossner, S. (1990). Maternal body weight development after pregnancy. *International Journal of Obesity, 14,* 159–173.

30. American College of Obstetricians and Gynecologists. (2000). Fetal macrosomia. ACOG Technical Bulletin Number 22–November 2000. *Obstetrics and Gynecology, 96,* 341–345.

31. Ehrenberg, H. M., Mercer, B. M., & Catalano, P. M. (2004). The influence of obesity and diabetes on the prevalence of macrosomia. *American Journal of Obstetrics and Gynecology, 191,* 964–968.

32. Rosenberg, T. J., Garbers, S., Chavkin, W., & Chiasson, M. A. (2003). Prepregnancy weight and adverse perinatal outcomes in an ethnically diverse population. *Obstetrics and Gynecology, 102,* 1022–1027.

33. Centers for Disease Control. (2006). Improved national prevalence estimates for 18 selected major birth defects–United States, 1999–2001. *Morbidity and Mortality Weekly Report, 54,* 1301–1305.

34. Heron, M. P., & Smith, B. L. (2007). Deaths: Leading causes for 2003. *National Vital Statistics Report, 55,* 1–92.

35. Waller, D. K., Mills, J. L., Simpson, J. L., Cunningham, G. C., Conley, M. R., Lassman, M. R., et al. (1994). Are obese women at higher risk for producing malformed offspring? *American Journal of Obstetrics and Gynecology, 170,* 541–548.

36. Shaw, G. M., Todoroff, K., Schaffer, M., & Selvin, S. (2000). Maternal height and prepregnancy body mass index as risk factors for selected congenital anomalies. *Paediatric Perinatal Epidemiology, 14,* 234–239.

37. Queisser-Luft, A., Keininger-Baum, D., Menger, H., Stolz, G., Schlaefer, K., & Merz, E. (1998). Does maternal obesity increase the risk of fetal abnormalities? Analysis of 20,248 newborn infants of the Mainz Birth Register for detecting congenital abnormalities. *Ultraschall in der Medizin, 19,* 40–44.

38. Watkins, M. L., Rasmussen, S. A., Honein, M. A., Botto, L. D., & Moore, C. A. (2003). Maternal obesity and risk for birth defects. *Pediatrics, 111,* 1152–1158.

39. Mojtabai, R. (2004). Body mass index and serum folate in childbearing age women. *European Journal of Epidemiology, 19,* 1029–1036.

40. Drugan, A., Dvorin, E., Johnson, M. P., Uhlmann, W. R., & Evans, M. I. (1989). The inadequacy of the current correction for maternal weight in maternal serum alpha-fetoprotein interpretation. *Obstetrics and Gynecology, 74,* 698–701.

41. Wolfe, H. M., Sokol, R. J., Martin, S. M., & Zador, I. E. (1990). Maternal obesity: A potential source of error in sonographic prenatal diagnosis. *Obstetrics and Gynecology, 76,* 339–342.

42. Hendler, I., Blackwell, S. C., Bujold, E., Treadwell, M. C., Wolfe, H. M., Sokol, R. J., … Sorokin, Y. (2004). The impact of maternal obesity on midtrimester sonographic visualization of fetal cardiac and craniospinal structures. *International Journal of Obesity Related Metabolic Disorders, 28,* 1607–1611.

43. Eller, A. G., Branch D. W., & Byrne, J. L. (2006). Stillbirth at term. *Obstetrics and Gynecology, 108*(2), 442–447.

44. Stephansson, O., Dickman, P. W., Johansson, A., & Cnattingius, S. (2001). Maternal weight, pregnancy weight gain, and the risk of antepartum stillbirth. *American Journal of Obstetrics and Gynecology, 184,* 463–469.

45. Kristensen, J., Vestergaard, M., Wisborg, K., Kesmodel, U., & Secher, N. J. (2005). Pre-pregnancy weight and the risk of stillbirth and neonatal death. *British Journal of Obstetrics and Gynecology, 112,* 403–408.

46. Oken, E., & Gillman, M. W. (2003). Fetal origins of obesity. *Obesity Research, 11,* 496–506.

47. Barker, D. J. (1998). In utero programming of chronic disease. *Clinical Science, 95,* 115–128.

48. Godfrey, K. M., & Barker, D. J. (2000). Fetal nutrition and adult disease. *American Journal of Clinical Nutrition, 71,* 1344S–1352S.

49. Bianco, A. T., Smilen, S. W., Davis, Y., Lopez, S., Lapinski, R., & Lockwood, C. J. (1998). Pregnancy outcome and weight gain recommendations for the morbidly obese woman. *Obstetrics and Gynecology, 91,* 97–102.

50. Usha Kiran, T. S., Hemmadi, S., Bethel, J., & Evans, J. (2005). Outcome of pregnancy in a woman with an increased body mass index. *British Journal of Obstetrics and Gynecology, 112,* 768–772.

51. Robinson, H. E., O'Connell, C., Joseph, K. S., & McLeod, M. L. (2005). Maternal outcomes in pregnancies complicated by obesity. *Obstetrics and Gynecology, 106,* 1357–1364.

52. Kabiru, W., & Raynor, B. D. (2004). Obstetric outcomes associated with increase in BMI category during pregnancy. *American Journal of Obstetrics and Gynecology, 91,* 928–932.

53. Weiss, J. L., Malone, F. D., Emig, D., Ball, R. H., Nyberg, D. A., Comstock, C. H., et al. FASTER Research Consortium. (2004). Obesity, obstetric complications and cesarean delivery rate: a population-based screening study. *American Journal of Obstetrics and Gynecology, 190,* 1091–1097.

54. Ehrenberg, H. M., Durnwald, C. P., Catalano, P., & Mercer, B. M. (2004). The influence of obesity and diabetes on the risk of cesarean delivery. *American Journal of Obstetrics and Gynecology, 191,* 969–974.

55. Sheiner, E., Levy, A., Menes, T. S., Silverberg, D., Katz, M., & Mazor, M. (2004). Maternal obesity as an independent risk factor for caesarean delivery. *Paediatric Perinatal Epidemiology, 18,* 196–201.

56. Alexander, C. I., & Liston, W. A. (2006). Operating on the obese woman: A review. *British Journal of Obstetrics and Gynecology, 113*, 1167–1172.

57. Gates, S., & Anderson, E. R. (2005). Wound drainage for caesarean section. *Cochrane Database Systematic Review*, CD004549.

58. Berghella, V., Baxter, J. K., & Chauhan, S. P. (2005). Evidence-based surgery for cesarean delivery. *American Journal of Obstetrics and Gynecology, 193*, 1607–1617.

59. Endler, G. C., Mariona, F. G., Sokol, R. J., & Stevenson, L. B. (1988). Anesthesia-related maternal mortality in Michigan, 1972 to 1984. *American Journal of Obstetrics and Gynecology, 159*, 187–193.

60. Saravanakumar, K., Rao, S. G., & Cooper, G. M. (2006). Obesity and obstetric anaesthesia. *Anaesthesia, 61*, 36–48.

61. Perlow, J. H., & Morgan, M. A. (1994). Massive maternal obesity and perioperative cesarean morbidity. *American Journal of Obstetrics and Gynecology, 170*, 560–565.

62. Hood, D. D., & Dewan, D. M. (1993). Anesthetic and obstetric outcome in morbidly obese parturients. *Anesthesiology, 79*, 1210–1218.

63. Grobman, W. A., Lai, Y., Landon, M. B., Spong, C. Y., Leveno, K. J., Rouse, D. J., et al. National Institute of Child Health and Human Development (NICHD) Maternal-Fetal Medicine Units Network (MFMU). (2007). Development of a nomogram for prediction of vaginal birth after cesarean delivery. *Obstetrics and Gynecology, 109*(4), 806–812.

64. Carroll, C. S., Sr., Magann, E. F., Chauhan, S. P., Klauser, C. K., & Morrison, J. C. (2003). Vaginal birth after cesarean section versus elective repeat cesarean delivery: Weight-based outcomes. *American Journal of Obstetrics and Gynecology, 188*, 1516–1520.

65. American College of Obstetricians and Gynecologists (2002). ACOG practice bulletin. Clinical management guidelines for obstetrician-gynecologists. (202). Number 40. *Obstetrics and Gynecology, 100*, 1045–1050.

66. Jevitt, C. M. (2005). Shoulder dystocia: Etiology, common risk factors, and management. *Journal of Midwifery and Womens Health, 50*, 485–497.

67. Nocon, J. J., McKenzie, D., Thomas, L., & Hansell, R. S. (1993). Shoulder dystocia: An analysis of risks and obstetric maneuvers. *American Journal of Obstetrics and Gynecology, 168*, 1732–1737

68. Sheiner, E., Levy, A., Herskovitz, R., Hallak, M., Hammel, R. D., Katz, M., & Mazor, M. (2006). Determining factors associated with shoulder dystocia: A population-based study. *European Journal of Obstetrics, Gynecology and Reproductive Biology, 126*, 11–15.

69. Mazouni, C., Porcu, G., Cohen-Solal, E., Heckenroth, H., Guidicelli, B., Bonnier, P., et al. (2006). Maternal and anthropomorphic risk factors for shoulder dystocia. *Acta Obstetricia Et Gynecologica Scandinavica, 85*, 567–570.

70. American College of Obstetricians and Gynecologists. (2005). ACOG Practice Bulletin. Clinical management guidelines for obstetrician-gynecologists, Number 70, Intrapartum fetal heart rate monitoring. *Obstetrics and Gynecology, 106*, 1453–1460.

71. James, A. H., Jamison, M. G., Brancazio, L. R., & Myers, E. R. (2006). Venous thromboembolism during pregnancy and the postpartum period: Incidence, risk factors, and mortality. *American Journal of Obstetrics and Gynecology, 194*, 1311–1315.

72. Simpson, L. L. (2002). Maternal medical disease: Risk of antepartum fetal death. *Seminars in Perinatology, 26*, 42–50.

73. Parrott, T., Evans, A., Lowes, A., & Dennis, K. (1989). Infection following caesarean section. *Journal of Hospital Infection, 13*, 349–354.

74. Nielsen, T. F., & Hokegard, K. H. (1983). Postoperative cesarean section morbidity: A prospective study. *American Journal of Obstetrics and Gynecology, 146*, 911–916.

75. Schneid-Kofman, N., Sheiner, E., Levy, A., & Holcberg, G. (2005). Risk factors for wound infection following cesarean deliveries. *International Journal of Gynaecology and Obstetrics, 90*, 10–15.

76. Gould, D. (2007). Caesarean section, surgical site infection and wound management. *Nursing Standard, 21*, 57–58, 60, 62 passim.

77. Vermillion, S. T., Lamoutte, C., Soper, D. E., & Verdeja, A. (2000). Wound infection after cesarean: Effect of subcutaneous tissue thickness. *Obstetrics and Gynecology, 95*, 923–926.

78. Ramsey, P. S., White, A. M., Guinn, D. A., Lu, G. C., Ramin, S. M., Davies, J. K., et al. (2005). Subcutaneous tissue reapproximation, alone or in combination with drain, in obese women undergoing cesarean delivery. *Obstetrics and Gynecology, 105*, 967–973.

79. Rasmussen, K. M., & Kjolhede, C. L. (2004). Prepregnant overweight and obesity diminish the prolactin response to suckling in the first week postpartum. *Pediatrics, 113*, e465–e471.

80. Baker, J. L., Michaelsen, K. F., Sørensen, T. I., & Rasmussen, K. M. (2007). High prepregnant body mass index is associated with early termination of full and any breastfeeding in Danish women. *American Journal of Clinical Nutrition, 86*, 404–411.

81. Chapman, D. J., & Perez-Escamilla, R. (1999). Identification of risk factors for delayed onset of lactation. *Journal of the American Dietetic Association, 99*, 450–454.

82. Jevitt, C., Hernandez, I., & Groer, M. (2007). Lactation complicated by overweight and obesity: Supporting the mother and newborn. *Journal of Midwifery and Womens Health, 52*, 606–613.

83. Amir, L. H., & Donath, S. (2007). A systematic review of maternal obesity and breastfeeding intention, initiation and duration. *BioMed Central Pregnancy and Childbirth, 7*, 9.

84. Buchwald, H. (2005). Consensus conference statement bariatric surgery for morbid obesity: Health implications for patients, health professionals, and third-party payers. *Surgery for Obesity and Related Diseases, 1*, 371–381.

85. Santry, H. P., Gillen, D. L., & Lauderdale, D. S. (2005). Trends in bariatric surgical procedures. *Journal of the American Medical Association, 294*, 1909–1917.

86. Patel, J. A., Colella, J. J., Esaka, E., & Thomas, R. L. (2007). Improvement in infertility and pregnancy outcomes after weight loss surgery. *Medical Clinics of North America, 91*, 515–528.

87. Sheiner, E., Levy, A., Silverberg, D., Menes, T. S., Levy, I., Katz, M., et al. (2004). Pregnancy after bariatric surgery is not associated with adverse perinatal outcome. *American Journal of Obstetrics and Gynecology, 190*, 1335–1340.

88. Dao, T., Kuhn, J., Ehmer, D., Fisher, T., & McCarty, T. (2006). Pregnancy outcomes after gastric-bypass surgery. *American Journal of Surgery, 192*, 762–766.

PART IV

Clinical Care Guidelines

Nan Hess-Eggleston, Nan H. Troiano, Carol J. Harvey, and Bonnie Flood Chez

Guidelines for the Initial Assessment and Triage of Obstetric Patients

I. Policy

During the initial evaluation and triage of obstetric patients, qualified personnel collaborate to assess the patient, formulate medical and nursing diagnoses, identify actual or potential health problems, plan and implement care, and evaluate patient responses. Clinical actions from initial assessment to final disposition should be in accordance with EMTALA requirements.

II. General Guidelines

The initial assessment of obstetric patients, following presentation to a hospital setting, includes:

A. Maternal physical status
B. Fetal status
C. Labor status
D. Psychosocial status/patient and family teaching
E. Review of prenatal health records
F. Patient interview/history and physical examination

Further assessment is dependent on the patient's chief complaint and data gathered during the initial assessment. Triage guidelines for common chief complaints are outlined following the General Guidelines.

A. Maternal Physical Status

Assess and document the following:

1. The patient's chief complaint and the presence of symptoms
2. Date and time of arrival
3. Gravidity and parity (gravida, term, preterm, abortions, living)
4. Vital signs
5. Estimated date of delivery (EDD) as determined by dates and/or ultrasonography
6. Presence or absence of vaginal bleeding, including date and time of onset, duration, and associated events
7. Presence of "show" (pink, red, or brownish in color)
8. Pregnancy risk factors or known complications
9. Medical complications or health problems
10. Current medications
11. Known allergies
12. Psychosocial status (including evidence of domestic violence/intimate partner abuse)

B. Fetal Status

Assess and document the following:

1. Estimated gestational age (EGA) as determined by dates and/or ultrasonography
2. Presence/absence of fetal movement (as applicable/dependent on EGA)
3. Fetal heart rate (FHR) by auscultation or electronic fetal monitoring (EFM) (as applicable/dependent on EGA)

C. Labor Status

Assess and document the following:

1. Uterine activity
   a. Uterine contractions, including date and time of onset, frequency, intensity, and duration
   b. Uterine resting tone
2. Amniotic membranes
   a. Evidence of ruptured membranes (pH, fern, pool)
   b. Date and time membranes ruptured; color and characteristics of amniotic fluid
3. Cervical status (digital examination or speculum visualization)

a. Dilation, effacement, position
b. Fetal presentation and station

D. Psychosocial Status
Assess and document the following:
1. Support system
2. Situational stressors
3. Pre-existing stressors
4. Education level
5. Cultural and religious preferences
6. Substance use

III. **Triage Guidelines: Evaluation for Labor**
A. Maternal Status – (See *II. General Guidelines*)
B. Fetal Status – (See *II. General Guidelines*)
Further information to be obtained during initial evaluation includes:
1. Obtain a 20-minute electronic FHR tracing and assess baseline FHR and the presence or absence of periodic patterns. (See *Appendix B: Guidelines for Fetal Heart Rate Monitoring.*)
C. Labor Status (See *II. General Guidelines*)
Further information to be obtained during the initial evaluation includes:
1. Review prenatal health records for maternal and fetal history.
2. Palpate and inspect abdomen for the following:
   a. Tenderness, uterine contractions, and resting tone
   b. Scars
3. Obtain sample for fetal fibronection testing from women with indications.
4. Perform cervical examination, if no history of the following (unless specifically indicated/ordered and the rationale documented):
   a. Prematurity
   b. Rupture of membranes
   c. Vaginal bleeding
   d. Abnormal placentation
5. Encourage patient to ambulate or maintain an upright position following reassuring FHR monitor tracing (data compatible with Category I FHR criteria).
6. Repeat cervical examination (e.g., in approximately 1 hour) to assess for change in cervix.
D. Psychosocial Status – Patient/Family Teaching:
1. Signs and symptoms of labor
2. Fetal movement awareness
3. Interventions
4. Plan of care
5. Follow-up appointment with care provider

IV. **Guidelines for the Evaluation for Preterm Labor**
A. Maternal Status (See *II. General Guidelines*)
Further information to be obtained during initial evaluation includes:
1. Change in vaginal discharge
2. Presence/absence of report of low backache
3. Uterine cramping (menstrual-like cramps in abdomen or upper thighs)
4. Abdominal cramping (intestinal-like cramps with or without nausea, vomiting, or diarrhea)
5. Symptoms of urinary tract infection (UTI)
6. Symptoms of dehydration
7. Precipitating events
Further information to be obtained during initial evaluation may include assessment of fetal fibronectin.
B. Fetal Status (See *II. General Guidelines.*)*
1. <24 weeks gestation, auscultation may be performed.
2. ≥24 weeks gestation, obtain a 20-minute FHR tracing if possible and assess baseline FHR and the presence or absence of periodic patterns. (See *Appendix B: Guidelines for Fetal Heart Rate Monitoring.*)
3. Assess fetal presentation
C. Labor Status (See *II. General Guidelines*)
1. Obtain EFM tracing and assess for uterine contractions/activity.
D. Psychosocial Needs – Patient/Family Teaching:
1. Signs and symptoms of preterm labor
2. Precipitating events
3. Interventions
4. Fetal movement awareness
5. Plan of care
6. Follow-up appointment with care provider

V. **Guidelines for the Evaluation of Vaginal Bleeding**
A. Maternal Status (See *II. General Guidelines*)
Further information to be obtained during initial evaluation includes:
1. Onset and amount of bleeding
2. Previous episodes of bleeding
3. Precipitating events
B. Review prenatal health records (if available) to obtain information regarding:
1. Most recent ultrasound report (location of placenta)
2. Previous cervical exam
C. Obtain a 20-minute EFM tracing if possible to evaluate baseline FHR and the presence or

---

*Does not infer a national standard, but the collaborative agreed-upon age for intervention (at the individual institution).

absence of periodic patterns. (See *Appendix B: Guidelines for Fetal Heart Rate Monitoring.*)

D. Labor Status (See *II. General Guidelines*)

E. Psychosocial Needs – Patient/Family Teaching
1. Signs and symptoms of preterm/term labor
2. Signs of vaginal bleeding
3. Fetal movement awareness
4. Plan of care
5. Follow-up appointment with care provider

VI. **Guidelines for the Evaluation of Ruptured Membranes**

A. Maternal Status (See *II. General Guidelines*) Further information to be obtained during initial evaluation includes:
1. Time of suspected rupture of membranes
2. Description of fluid (color, odor)
3. Estimated volume of fluid

B. Fetal Status (See *II. General Guidelines*)
1. If no identified risk factors, intact amniotic membranes, and patient report of normal fetal movement, FHR may be evaluated by auscultation.
2. If risk factors are identified and/or patient reports decreased fetal movement, obtain a 20-minute electronic FHR tracing to evaluate baseline rate and the presence/absence of periodic patterns. (See *Guidelines for Fetal Heart Rate Monitoring.*)

C. Labor Status (See *II. General Guidelines*) Refer to *III. Triage Guidelines: Evaluation for Labor,* if applicable

D. Psychosocial Needs – Patient/Family Teaching
1. Signs and symptoms of preterm/term labor
2. Signs of ruptured membranes (color, odor, and volume of fluid)
3. Fetal movement awareness
4. Plan of care
5. Follow-up appointment with care provider

VII. **Guidelines for the Evaluation of Decreased Fetal Movement**

A. Maternal Status (See *II. General Guidelines*)

B. Fetal Status (See *II. General Guidelines.*)*
1. <24 weeks gestation, auscultation may be performed.
2. ≥24 weeks gestation, obtain a 20-minute EFM tracing if possible to evaluate baseline

and the presence/absence of periodic patterns. (See *Appendix B: Guidelines for Fetal Heart Rate Monitoring.*)

C. Labor Status (See *II. General Guidelines*) Refer to *III. Triage Guidelines: Evaluation for Labor,* if applicable

D. Psychosocial Needs – Patient/Family Teaching
1. Fetal movement awareness
2. Plan of care
3. Follow-up appointment with care provider

VIII. **Guidelines for the Evaluation of Preeclampsia**

A. Maternal Status (See *II. General Guidelines*) Further information to be obtained during initial evaluation includes:
1. History of elevated blood pressure
2. Signs and symptoms of preeclampsia (headache, vision changes, right upper quadrant pain, nausea, heartburn)
3. Review prenatal health records (if available) to obtain information regarding:
   a. Initial blood pressure (first trimester)
   b. Previous interventions to manage blood pressure
4. Assess patient for:
   a. Elevated blood pressure
   b. Proteinuria
   c. Baseline laboratory evaluation results
   d. Decreased urine output

B. Fetal Status (See *II. General Guidelines.*)*
1. <24 weeks gestation, auscultation may be performed.
2. ≥24 weeks gestation, obtain a 20-minute EFM tracing if possible and evaluate baseline rate and the presence/absence of periodic patterns. (See *Guidelines for Fetal Heart Rate Monitoring.*)

C. Labor Status (See *II. General Guidelines*) Refer to *III. Triage Guidelines: Evaluation for Labor,* if applicable

D. Psychosocial Needs – Patient/Family Teaching
1. Predisposing factors to preeclampsia
2. Signs and symptoms of preeclampsia
3. Interventions
4. Fetal movement awareness
5. Plan of care
6. Follow-up appointment with care provider

---

*Does not infer a national standard, but the collaborative agreed-upon age for intervention (at the individual institution).

Guidelines for Fetal Heart Rate Monitoring

I. **Methods of Assessment of Fetal Heart Rate (FHR)**

A. Auscultation – an intermittent assessment of fetal heart rate (FHR) with either Doppler ultrasound (US) or fetoscope (see AWHONN Practice Monograph 2009, Fetal Heart Rate Auscultation)

B. Electronic Fetal Monitoring (EFM) – an intermittent or continuous assessment of the FHR and/or uterine contractions with an electronic medical device. Devices (in general) measure maternal uterine activity and FHR. Data are recorded on timed printouts, and may be archived via digital electronic storage systems.

  1. External EFM Devices:

    a. Ultrasound Transducer – permits evaluation of baseline FHR variability (with third generation technology), and the presence or absence of periodic or episodic patterns (accelerations or decelerations) using Doppler technology.

    b. Tocodynamometer (toco) – permits evaluation of uterine contraction frequency and approximate duration. The intensity of the uterine contraction and resting tone are estimated by abdominal palpation.

  2. Internal EFM Devices:

    a. Fetal ECG (FECG) or Fetal scalp electrode (FSE) – permits direct monitoring of baseline FHR, variability, and presence or absence of periodic or episodic patterns (accelerations or decelerations)

    b. Intrauterine Pressure Catheter (IUPC) – permits direct evaluation of uterine contraction frequency, duration, intensity, and uterine resting tone via direct measurement of intrauterine pressure. Uterine activity may be quantified by calculation of Montevideo Units (MVU).

II. **Assessment Parameters**

A. Auscultation (intermittent)

  1. FHR assessment includes:

    a. Baseline rate

    b. Presence or absence of audible decelerations

  2. Uterine activity assessment includes abdominal palpation for contraction:

    a. Frequency

    b. Duration

    c. Intensity

    d. Uterine resting tone

B. Electronic Fetal Monitoring (intermittent or continuous)

  1. FHR assessment includes:

    a. Baseline rate

    b. Baseline variability

    c. Presence or absence of periodic or episodic patterns (accelerations or decelerations)

  2. Uterine activity assessment includes contraction:

    a. Frequency

    b. Duration

    c. Intensity (palpation if external toco)

    d. Uterine resting tone (palpation if external toco)

III. **Interpretation of Data**

A. Auscultation

  1. FHR characteristics that are considered normal:

    a. Normal baseline between 110 and 160 bpm

    b. Absence of audible decelerations

  2. FHR responses that are considered not normal:

    a. Abnormal baseline rate

    b. Audible decelerations

B. Electronic Fetal Monitoring

The National Institute of Child Health and Human Development (NICHD) guidelines divide EFM tracing characteristics (baseline rate, variability, accelerations, and decelerations) into three categories:

1. Category I: Normal

   This FHR tracing has the following characteristics and is almost always associated with normal fetal acid–base status at the time of observation:

   a. Baseline rate 110–160 bpm

   b. Moderate variability (6–25 bpm)

   c. Absence of late or variable decelerations

   d. Absence or presence of early decelerations

   e. Absence or presence of accelerations

2. Category II: Indeterminate

   Tracings in this category are not predictive of abnormal acid–base status, however, there are insufficient data to classify them as either Category I or Category III. These tracings may represent many tracings that are encountered in everyday clinical practice.

   A Category II tracing may show any of the following characteristics:

   a. Minimal variability

   b. Absent variability without recurrent decelerations

   c. Marked variability

   d. Absence of induced accelerations after fetal stimulation

   e. Recurrent variable decelerations with minimal to moderate variability

   f. Prolonged deceleration

   g. Recurrent late decelerations with moderate variability

   h. Variable decelerations with "slow return to baseline," "overshoots," or "shoulders"

3. Category III: Abnormal

   Tracings in this category are predictive of abnormal fetal acid–base status at the time of observation

   Tracings in this category demonstrate absent variability and any of the following:

   a. Bradycardia – baseline rate of <110 bpm for ≥10 minutes

   b. Recurrent variable decelerations – visually apparent abrupt decrease (onset to nadir is <30 seconds) in FHR below baseline. Decrease is ≥15 bpm. Duration is ≥15 seconds and <2 minutes.

   c. Recurrent late decelerations – visually apparent gradual decrease (onset to nadir is ≥30 seconds) in FHR below baseline.

   Generally, the onset, nadir, and recovery of the decelerations occur after the onset, peak, and recovery of the contraction, respectively.

   d. Sinusoidal pattern – An FHR pattern having a visually apparent, smooth, sine wave–like undulating pattern in the FHR baseline with a cycle frequency of 3–5 per minute that persists for 20 minutes.

IV. **Interventions**

A. Auscultation

   1. Normal FHR response

      a. No intervention; continue routine care

   2. Abnormal FHR response

      a. Initiate EFM

B. Electronic Fetal Monitoring

   1. Category I: Normal

      a. No intervention, continue routine care

   2. Category II: Indeterminate

      a. Are not predictive of abnormal fetal acid–base status; inadequate data at this time to classify as Category I or Category III.

      b. Evaluation and continued surveillance required, taking into account entire clinical circumstances.

      c. May initiate a plan to improve FHR tracing, including actions to promote fetal oxygenation, reduce uterine activity, alleviate umbilical cord compression, or correct maternal hypotension. Any actions should be individualized per clinical circumstances.

      Category II FHR tracings require evaluation and continued surveillance and reevaluation, taking into account the entire associated clinical circumstances.

   3. Category III: Abnormal

      Evaluation to identify the potential cause and initiate a plan to improve the FHR tracing, including actions to promote fetal oxygenation, reduce uterine activity, alleviate umbilical cord compression, or correct maternal hypotension:

      a. See Category II. Possible interventions (individualized per assessment) may include:

         i. Lateral positioning (either left or right)

         ii. Decrease/discontinue oxytocin, remove/withhold cervical ripening agent

         iii. Administer oxygen via non-rebreathing face mask at 10–12 L/min

         iv. Correct maternal hypotension

         v. Assess cervix for dilation or prolapsed cord

      vi. Modify pushing efforts (pushing with every other or every third contraction or discontinue pushing temporarily during second stage)

     vii. IV fluid bolus of lactated Ringer's solution or normal saline (isotonic solutions)

    viii. Tocolysis (i.e., terbutaline sulfate 0.25 mg subcutaneously for tachysystole)

      ix. Amnioinfusion during first stage labor for recurrent variable decelerations

       x. Acoustic stimulation or scalp stimulation (not clinically appropriate during decelerations)

      xi. Notify primary care provider and request evaluation of tracing

  b. Primary care provider to evaluate clinical situation and provide a plan of care, including potential decision regarding timing and route of delivery.

V.   Procedure for Antepartum Testing

A. Non-Stress Test (NST)

This test involves EFM to assess fetal biophysical capacity to elicit FHR accelerations within a specified period of time.

1. A *reactive test* implies that two or more fetal heart accelerations, each rising to ≥15 beats above the FHR baseline and lasting for a period of ≥15 seconds, occurring within a 20-minute time period for gestational age >32 weeks; for the fetus ≤32 weeks gestation, the criteria are modified to 10 bpm above baseline for ≥10 seconds.

2. A *nonreactive test* implies the fetus was unable to produce the desired amount of fetal heart accelerations within the allotted time period. (If the NST is nonreactive, the test may be continued for a second 20-minute segment if clinically appropriate.)

B. Contraction Stress Test (CST)

This test involves EFM to assess the ability of the fetus to tolerate reduced oxygen levels associated with normal uterine activity in labor. Contractions may be induced or spontaneous. Synonym: Oxytocin Challenge Test (OCT)

1. A *negative test* implies that no late decelerations occurred during three palpable contractions lasting ≥40 seconds in duration and occurring within a 10-minute time period.

2. A *positive test* implies that late decelerations occurred in response to 50% or more of the contractions within the allotted time period.

3. A *suspicious test* implies that at least one late deceleration occurred within the allotted time period.

4. An *unsatisfactory test* implies an inability to achieve the three required contractions within the 10-minute time period, or the monitor tracing was of poor quality and results could not be determined.

VI. Nursing Implications

Notify primary care provider in response to the following associated clinical findings:

A. Significant system findings

B. Blood pressure >140/90 or <80/40

C. Sustained maternal heart rate ≥120

D. Maternal temperature >100.4°F

E. Imminent delivery

F. Cord prolapse

G. The initial episode of a Category II tracing that does not change to a Category I tracing within 30 minutes.

H. Category III tracings

VII. Patient and Family Education

Inform patient and family regarding:

A. Orientation to facility hospital and unit

B. Plan of care

C. Purpose/method of fetal monitoring

VIII. Glossary

Acceleration: a visually apparent abrupt increase (onset to peak is <30 seconds) in FHR above baseline. Peak is ≥15 bpm. Duration is ≥15 seconds (from onset to return), and <2 minutes. In gestations <32 weeks, a peak of ≥10 bpm and duration of ≥10 seconds are considered an acceleration. A prolonged acceleration lasts ≥2 minutes but <10 minutes in duration. If acceleration lasts >10 minutes or longer, it is a baseline change.

Baseline: the approximate FHR rounded to increments of 5 bpm during a 10-minute segment, excluding periodic or episodic changes, periods of marked variability, and segments of baseline that differ by >25 bpm. In any 10-minute window, the minimum baseline duration must be at least 2 minutes, otherwise the baseline for that time period is indeterminate. Should this occur, reference to the prior 10-minute window for baseline determination is recommended.

Bradycardia: baseline rate of <110 bpm for ≥10 minutes.

Contraction Stress Test (CST): antepartum surveillance method using induced or spontaneous contractions to evaluate the fetal heart rate response. A negative test implies no late decelerations are seen. A suspicious test implies at least one late deceleration is seen. A positive test implies that late decelerations are seen with 50% or more contractions occurring in a 10-minute period. Synonym: Oxytocin Challenge Test.

Early Deceleration: visually apparent usually symmetrical gradual decrease and return of the FHR associated with a uterine contraction. A gradual FHR decrease is defined as from the onset to the nadir of the FHR of 30 seconds or more. The decrease in FHR is calculated from the onset to the nadir of the deceleration. The nadir of the deceleration occurs at the same time as the peak of the contraction. Generally, the onset, nadir, and recovery of the deceleration occur at the same time as the onset, peak, and recovery of the contraction, respectively.

Electronic Fetal Monitoring (EFM): instrument used to show graphically and continuously the relationship between the FHR and uterine activity.

Episodic Decelerations: Decelerations occurring with <50% of uterine contractions in any 20-minute segment

Episodic Patterns: accelerations or decelerations of the FHR that are not associated with uterine contractions.

Fetal ECG Electrode (FECG): a bipolar terminal that detects the difference in voltage between the fetal presenting part and vaginal wall of the mother. Note: May also be referred to as a fetal scalp electrode (FSE) or a fetal spiral electrode (FSE).

Fetal Heart Rate (FHR): generally refers to the fetal heart rate in beats per minute.

Intrauterine Pressure Catheter (IUPC): a fluid-filled or transducer-tipped catheter inserted transvaginally into the uterus to quantify uterine activity. Intrauterine pressure is conducted through the catheter and transformed into an electronic signal, then printed on the tracing as uterine activity.

Late Deceleration: visually apparent usually symmetrical gradual decrease and return of the FHR associated with a uterine contraction. A gradual FHR decrease is defined as from the onset to the FHR nadir of 30 seconds or more. The deceleration is delayed in timing, with the nadir of the deceleration occurring after the peak of the contraction. In most cases, the onset, nadir, and recovery of the deceleration occur after the onset, peak, and recovery of the contraction, respectively.

Montevideo Units (MVU): the sum total in mmHg of the strength of all contractions occurring during a 10-minute period, minus uterine resting tone. An IUPC is required.

Non-Stress Test (NST): antepartum surveillance method used to evaluate the biophysical status of the fetus. A *reactive test* implies that at least two accelerations of the FHR are seen within a 20-minute period. A *nonreactive test* implies that the fetus was unable to produce the desired amount of fetal heart accelerations within the allotted time period.

Oxytocin Challenge Test (OCT): antepartum surveillance method using oxytocin to induce a minimum of three contractions to evaluate the FHR response. A *negative test* implies that no late decelerations are seen. A *suspicious test* implies that at least one late deceleration is seen in a 10-minute period. A *positive test* implies that late decelerations are seen with 50% or more of the contractions occurring in a 10-minute period. Synonym: Contraction Stress Test.

Periodic Patterns: FHR changes, either accelerations or decelerations from the baseline, lasting less than 10 minutes; distinguished on the basis of the waveform's onset, either "abrupt" or "gradual." Are associated with uterine contractions.

Prolonged Acceleration: an acceleration (see definition above) that lasts longer than 2 minutes but less than 10 minutes in duration.

Prolonged Deceleration: visually apparent decrease (gradual or abrupt) in FHR below baseline. Decrease is ≥15 bpm. Duration is ≥2 minutes but <10 minutes from onset to return to baseline.

Recurrent Decelerations: decelerations (early, late, or variable) that occur with ≥50% of uterine contractions in any 20-minute window

Sinusoidal pattern: visually apparent, smooth, sine-wave-like undulating pattern in FHR baseline with a cycle frequency of 3–5 per minute, typically 5–15 bpm above or below the FHR baseline, which persists for ≥20 minutes.

Tachycardia: baseline rate of >160 bpm for ≥10 minutes.

Tachysystole: more than 5 contractions (either spontaneous or induced) in 10 minutes, averaged over a 30-minute window and should be qualified as to the presence or absence of associated FHR decelerations. This term replaces hyperstimulation and hypercontractility, which are no longer defined and should be abandoned.

Tocodynamometer (toco): external appliance used to measure uterine activity via abdominal wall enlargement.

Transducer: external devices that convert mechanical energy into electrical energy.

Uterine Contraction: a rhythmic tightening of the uterine fundus that contracts the size of the uterus to push the presenting part onto the maternal cervix. Creates intrauterine pressure. When externally palpated, may be classified as mild, moderate, or strong based on density of muscle. When internally monitored, may be quantified by frequency, duration, intensity, and resting tone or calculation of Montevideo Units (MVU).

Uterine Resting Tone: baseline intrauterine pressure measured between the contractions or when the uterus is at rest, externally evaluated by palpation as soft or firm. Internal assessment may be accomplished by IUPC. May be quantified with IUPC. Normal resting tone ranges from 5–25 mmHg and may vary depending on the type of IUPC used.

Variability: fluctuations in the baseline FHR that are irregular in amplitude and frequency. Fluctuations are visually quantified as the amplitude of peak-to-trough in beats per minute (bpm) as follows:

- Amplitude range undetectable
  - absent FHR variability
- Amplitude range >undetectable ≤5 bpm
  - minimal FHR variability
- Amplitude range 6–25 bpm
  - moderate FHR variability
- Amplitude range >25 bpm
  - marked FHR variability

Variable Deceleration: visually apparent abrupt decrease (onset to nadir is <30 seconds) in FHR below baseline. The decrease in FHR is ≥15 bpm; lasting ≥15 seconds, and <2 minutes in duration. When variable decelerations are associated with uterine contractions, their onset, depth, and duration commonly vary with successive uterine contractions.

REFERENCE

Macones, G. A, Hankins, G. D. V., Spong, C. Y., Hauth, J., & Moore, T. (2008). The 2008 National Institutes of Child Health and Human Development workshop report on electronic fetal monitoring: Update on definitions, interpretation, and research guidelines. *Obstetrics & Gynecology, 112*(3): 661–666.

Guidelines for Use of Fetal Acoustic Stimulation

Fetal acoustic stimulation (FAS) may be used as an adjunct to electronic fetal monitoring (EFM) or intermittent auscultation for the assessment of fetal well-being. This method is used to elicit a fetal heart rate (FHR) acceleration, which is defined as an abrupt increase in the FHR above the baseline that is ≥15 beats per minute (bpm) above the baseline and lasts ≥15 seconds for the term fetus; ≥10 bpm and ≥10 seconds for a fetus ≤32 weeks gestation. This fetal response to acoustic stimulation is considered a reliable indicator of fetal well-being, as an acceleration most commonly occurs if the fetus does not have a metabolic acidemia.

I. **Fetal Acoustic Stimulation (FAS)**

FAS may be used to evaluate fetal well-being for antepartum and/or intrapartum surveillance.

A. Antepartum Fetal Surveillance

FAS is used to improve the reliability of results obtained from antepartum surveillance conducted via EFM or auscultation. For example, FAS may help differentiate a nonreactive Non-Stress Test (NST) related to potential fetal compromise from a nonreactive NST associated with fetal sleep states or narcosis.

1. FAS may be performed after the FHR baseline has been assessed via EFM and a nonreactive NST obtained.

2. The acoustic stimulator is positioned on the maternal abdomen near the fetal head and the stimulus applied for a time period of 1–2 seconds. If the FHR remains nonreactive, FAS may be repeated at 1-minute intervals for a maximum of three times, progressively increasing the stimulation time to 3 seconds.

3. A subsequent reactive test is considered a valid indicator of fetal well-being. (The NST is considered reactive if two FHR accelerations [15 bpm for 15 seconds] occur in a 20-minute period.) If the estimated gestational age (EGA) is <32 weeks, the NST may be considered reactive if two FHR accelerations (10 bpm for at least 10 seconds duration) occur in a 20-minute period.

4. If the NST remains nonreactive after the 20-minute duration of testing, and the FAS does not elicit an acceleration, the NST may be extended for 20 minutes (40 minutes in total).

5. Additional fetal surveillance is considered if the NST remains nonreactive.

B. Intrapartum Fetal Surveillance

FAS may be used in labor to assess fetal well-being in the presence of Category II and Category III FHR tracings. (See *Guidelines for Fetal Heart Rate Monitoring*.) However, FAS should not be used during decelerations, nor as an adjunct to other intrauterine fetal supportive measures such as IV fluid bolus, decreasing or discontinuing oxytocin, or oxygen administration when there is deterioration in the FHR status evidenced via EFM.

1. Identify Category II or Category III FHR tracing.

2. Establish the FHR baseline.

3. Position the acoustic stimulator on the abdomen near the fetal head for a time period of 1–2 seconds. If FHR remains nonreactive, acoustic stimulation may be repeated at 1-minute intervals up to a maximum of three times, progressively increasing the stimulation time to a maximum of 3 seconds.

4. A reactive FHR is considered a reliable indicator of fetal well-being.

5. A nonreactive FHR (or other Category II tracings) is not predictive of fetal metabolic acidemia or other abnormal acid-base status. There is not yet adequate evidence to classify as a Category I or II tracing. A collaborative discussion among clinicians may help determine if additional methods for assessing fetal well-being or delivery of the fetus are warranted.

APPENDIX D

Guidelines for the Care of Patients in Labor*

I. **Initial Assessment** – See *Guidelines for the Initial Assessment and Triage of Obstetric Patients*

II. **Maternal Physical Status**

These guidelines address general clinical care of patients in spontaneous labor. Additional information may be found in other guidelines in this section of the text.

A. Vital Signs (VS)
    1. Patients without identified risk factors:
        a. Maternal blood pressure, pulse, and respirations are assessed and documented according to individual institutional guidelines (e.g., at least every 4 hours during latent phase labor; every 1 hour during active labor [expert opinion]).
        b. More frequent assessments may be warranted depending upon maternal and/or fetal condition and presence and type of analgesia or regional anesthesia.
    2. Patients with Identified Risk Factors:
        a. Blood pressure, pulse, and respirations are assessed and recorded in timed intervals individualized for patient condition (e.g., for patient with cardiac failure, vital signs may be assessed every 30 minutes in latent phase and every 15 to 30 minutes in second stage).
    3. Maternal temperature is assessed every 4 hours if membranes are intact, every 2 hours if membranes are ruptured.

B. Nutrition
    1. The ingestion of liquid and solid foods during labor is typically dependent upon the current practice of anesthesia providers at any given institution.
        a. Patients in early labor may have clear liquids (should institutional and anesthesia guidelines permit); patients in active labor are limited to ice chips (unless otherwise ordered).
    2. Intravenous (IV) access may be obtained utilizing an 18–20 gauge catheter-over-needle through which IV crystalloid fluids (e.g., D_5LR, LR, $D_5$0.9% NS 0.9% NS, etc.) may be infused either continuously per pump or intermittently via an access device (e.g., heparin or saline lock). IV solutions containing dextrose/glucose should not be used for a fluid bolus.
    3. Administration of IV fluid bolus
        a. A 500–1000cc bolus of crystalloid fluid is generally administered to the parturient without complications prior to the administration of epidural analgesia/anesthesia (if applicable).
        b. IV fluid bolus administration during labor may be indicated in selected clinical situations in response to changes in the maternal/fetal condition.
        c. IV fluids used for bolus fluid administration should not contain glucose (e.g., D_5LR, D_5 0.9% NS, etc.). Rather, bolus fluids should be isotonic without glucose added (e.g. LR, 0.9% NS)
    4. Intake and output should be assessed and documented.

C. Elimination
    1. Assess urinary output at regular intervals and encourage the patient to void.
    2. Assess for bladder distention every 2 hours, particularly following administration of a fluid bolus.

*Disclaimer: Absent prospective studies, limited data are available to support absolute prescription for assignment of maternal–fetal "risk factors" or frequency of assessments during labor and birth. Therefore, guidelines are based on appreciation for and application of individual clinical situational judgment, guidelines, and standards from professional organizations and unit-specific policies.

3. Patients with bladder distention or who are unable to void may be catheterized intermittently or with an indwelling Foley catheter in accordance with institutional policy.

D. Hygiene
   1. Oral hygiene PRN
   2. Personal hygiene – encourage to shower, or perform modified self-care. If not, provide appropriate hygiene as necessary.
   3. Perineal care PRN
      a. For patients with indwelling urinary catheters, use soap and water to clean meatus and surrounding area. Do not use antimicrobial gels or liquids. Pad for leaking fluid. Do not use antimicrobials inside the vagina.

E. Activity
   1. Following initial assessment, intrapartum patients without identified risk factors and a Category I fetal heart rate (FHR) tracing may ambulate. If out of bed, telemetry electronic fetal monitoring (EFM) should be employed when available. If telemetry not available, instruct patient in active labor to return every 30 minutes for assessment and documentation of uterine activity and FHR characteristics. (See *Guidelines for Fetal Heart Rate Monitoring.*)
   2. Laboring patients receiving epidural analgesia/anesthesia with neuromuscular blockade, narcotic analgesics, or those who have demonstrated an altered level of consciousness (LOC) should remain on strict bed rest. For select patients, if the provider orders bathroom privileges or limited movement (e.g., sitting in bedside chair), patient is accompanied by appropriate nursing staff.
   3. Patients on bed rest should be frequently encouraged to change position as necessary for comfort (e.g., lateral, semi-Fowler's, sitting) and should be reminded to avoid supine positioning to prevent potential aortocaval compression. If patient is unable to move herself for position change, place patient in alternative position every 1–2 hours.

F. Lab Data
   1. Admission laboratory evaluation is dependent upon the specific facility, complications of the patient, the orders of the primary obstetric care provider, and governing state and federal laws. Tests may include:
      a. CBC (when ordered or indicated)
      b. Blood type and antibody screen (indirect Coombs); "hold" in blood bank for potential blood transfusion
      c. Human immunodeficiency virus (HIV) status
      d. Rapid plasma reagin
   2. Consider CBC with differential, Group B *Streptococcus* (GBS) culture, and urinalysis with culture and sensitivity on patients with preterm labor and premature rupture of membranes (ROM). (See *Guidelines for Care of the Patient with Preterm Labor.*)

III. **Labor Status**
   A. Uterine Activity
      Uterine activity is typically assessed when the FHR is assessed.
      1. In the active phase of labor, assess the frequency, duration, and intensity of contractions, and uterine resting tone every 30 minutes for patients without identified risk factors and every 15 minutes for patients with identified risk factors.
      2. In the second stage of labor, assess the frequency, duration, and intensity of contractions, and uterine resting tone every 15 minutes for patients without identified risk factors and every 5 minutes for patients with identified risk factors.
      3. Interpret the external tocotransducer recording for the relative frequency and duration of uterine activity. Palpate the maternal abdomen for contraction intensity/strength and uterine resting tone.
      4. When EFM is used to record FHR and uterine contractions on a permanent record, periodic documentation may be used to summarize uterine activity that was assessed at the above frequencies. A summary note that may include FHR status may be documented at intervals less than assessment intervals.
      5. In accordance with specific state Nurse Practice Acts, when indicated, an internal intrauterine pressure catheter (IUPC) may be inserted by an RN who is competency-verified to perform the procedure. The IUPC allows the quantification of uterine resting tone, contraction frequency and duration, and uterine contraction intensity in mmHg.
      6. When inducing or augmenting labor with oxytocin or cervical ripening agents, refer to the *Guidelines for the Care of Patients Undergoing Induction of Labor.*
      7. For interpretation of the electronic fetal monitor tracing and interventions related to uterine activity, refer to the *Guidelines for Fetal Heart Rate Monitoring.*

B. Amniotic Membranes
1. Assess the patient for rupture of membranes (ROM).
2. If ROM occurs, document estimated volume (i.e., small, moderate, large), color and appearance (clear, cloudy, bloody, meconium present), unusual qualities (sediment, odor) and fetal heart rate findings proximate to the time of membrane rupture.

C. Cervical Status
1. Cervical examination via a digital vaginal exam or by speculum exam may be performed by an RN, unless contraindications are present. Relative contraindications to digital vaginal exam include (but are not limited to):
   a. Abnormal vaginal bleeding (other than bloody show)
   b. Known placenta previa
   c. Known vasa previa
   d. Preterm labor unless specifically ordered
   e. Known bulging fetal membranes with unengaged head
   f. Prolonged rupture of the membranes (PROM) unless specifically ordered (Note: PROM may also be used to abbreviate premature rupture of membranes.)
   g. Preterm prolonged rupture of membranes (PPROM) unless specifically ordered; note:
      PPROM may also be used to abbreviate preterm premature rupture of membranes
2. Perform a cervical exam to check dilation, effacement, consistency, fetal station, and fetal presentation.
3. Attempt to limit the number of cervical evaluations when membranes are ruptured (unless delivery is imminent) to decrease the potential for infection.
4. Assess for vaginal bleeding and document time, amount, and characteristics when applicable.

IV. **Fetal Status**
A. Patients without identified risk factors: Assess fetal status every 30 minutes in the active phase of the first stage of labor and every 15 minutes in the second stage of labor. (See *Guidelines for Fetal Heart Rate Monitoring*.)
B. Patients with identified risk factors: Assess fetal status every 15 minutes during the active phase of the first stage of labor and every 5 minutes during the second stage of labor.

V. **Pain Management**
A. Pain management during labor involves frequent assessment of the patient's level of pain and adequacy of coping mechanisms; provision of labor support interventions (e.g., breathing techniques, assistance with ambulation, rocking, positioning, hot shower) and support of patient's choice for analgesia and/or anesthesia.
B. Regional Analgesia/Anesthesia: When regional analgesia/anesthesia is desired, the anesthesia care provider is responsible for obtaining informed consent from the patient. This includes but is not limited to discussing the procedure, the benefits and risks, and additional information that is necessary to meet the requirements for informed consent. Nursing care for the patient receiving epidural analgesia/anesthesia includes preparation for and assistance with the procedure, assessing for side effects, (e.g. changes in maternal VS, especially maternal hypotension, changes in the FHR tracing, and "rising" epidural levels with the potential for respiratory compromise). Epidural analgesia/anesthesia during labor may also increase maternal temperature. If an elevated maternal temperature is identified, temperature is assessed every 2 hours.
C. Supportive Measures – Care for the patient may require teaching various breathing and relaxation techniques, coaching, and other nonpharmacologic comfort measures to decrease pain. Interventions based on patient assessment may include:
1. Breathing techniques
2. Relaxation, support, and comfort measures
   a. Controlled relaxation – focused relaxation of all muscle groups except the uterus during contractions, especially the neck, face, and upper body. Focusing on breathing may facilitate this process.
   b. Physical comfort measures – frequent position changes, the use of positioning supports, massage, effleurage, and the use of mild heat or cold to the back or abdomen.
   c. Environmental control measures to promote rest and relaxation include appropriate lighting, comfortable ambient temperature, minimal external noise, and limiting the number of visitors based on the patient's request.
   d. Facilitation of comfort measures should incorporate the use of family and designated support persons.

VI. **Nursing Implications**

Collaborative care includes communication with the primary care provider regarding:

A. Spontaneous ROM, unsure status of amniotic membranes, meconium or blood-tinged amniotic fluid

B. Vaginal bleeding (not bloody show)

C. Analgesia or anesthesia needs of the patient not covered by order sets

D. Blood pressure >140/90 or <80/40, repeated

E. Temperature >100.4

F. Maternal heart rate >120°F or <60, sustained

G. Maternal respirations >26 or <14

H. Imminent delivery

I. Persistent Category II FHR tracings after continued surveillance and/or interventions (when indicated) are performed.

J. Category III FHR tracings

K. Significant physical assessment findings

VII. **Psychosocial Needs – Patient/Family Teaching**

A. Plan of care

B. Unit and hospital policies and procedures

C. Methods for fetal surveillance

D. Technology used during labor and delivery

E. Support for pain management options

F. Support for treatment options

G. Interdisciplinary involvement as indicated

H. Plan of care for newborn

Guidelines for the Care of Patients with Preterm Labor

I. **Background**
- Preterm delivery accounts for 10% to 12% of all deliveries in North America and is responsible for significant neonatal morbidity and mortality.
- Preterm labor (PTL) is defined as regular uterine contractions occurring before 37 weeks gestation that are accompanied by progressive cervical change (dilation or effacement).
- Preterm uterine activity/contractions do not necessarily result in progressive cervical change, making the diagnosis of PTL a clinical challenge.
- The goal of *tocolytic* therapy is to prolong the gestation for at least 24 to 48 hours, to allow administration of corticosteroids for fetal lung maturation, and/or maternal transport to another facility with a neonatal intensive care unit.
- Although tocolytic therapy is frequently used, data are not available that support its use for greater than 48 hours.
- *Antenatal corticosteroids* significantly reduce the incidence and severity of neonatal respiratory distress syndrome, and the incidence of intraventricular hemorrhage and necrotizing enterocolitis.
- Fetal fibronectin (fFN) is a protein found in vaginal secretions of patients who typically deliver in the next 7 days. The absence of fFN is helpful to identify women who will likely *not* deliver in the next week.

II. **Initial Assessment**
A. See *Guidelines for the Initial Assessment and Triage of Obstetric Patients*
B. Determine status of amniotic membranes
   1. If amniotic membranes have ruptured, confirm rupture by:
      a. Evidence of gross rupture (witnessed "gush," large amount of fluid on clothing, shoes)
      b. AmniSure, Amnioswab (nitrazine), Fern test, visual pooling, etc.
   2. If amniotic membranes have ruptured, assess for signs and symptoms of chorioamnionitis
      a. Abdominal pain, tenderness
      b. Uterine activity
      c. Fever
      d. Foul smelling vaginal discharge/amniotic fluid
      e. Maternal and/or fetal tachycardia
C. Obtain fetal fibronectin (fFN) test sample per order *prior* to digital vaginal/cervical examination if fetal membranes have not ruptured
   1. Candidates for an fFN test are patients with signs and symptoms of PTL, intact membranes, singleton pregnancy, no cerclage, and minimal cervical dilation (<3 cm), whose pregnancy is between 22 weeks and 0 days and 34 weeks and 6 days.
   2. Collect vaginal sample for fFN per test manufacturer's instructions. Label the specimen per hospital guidelines.
   3. The test may be collected and "held" prior to the decision to order or send the test sample to the laboratory (see specific manufacturer's instructions on the maximum time the collected sample may be held).
   4. When positive after 22 weeks of gestation, fFN suggests decidual disruption and predicts variable percentages of preterm delivery at different gestational ages. The fFN has a higher negative predictive value and is generally used to identify the patient who is not likely to have a preterm delivery over the next 7 days. In a group of symptomatic patients, when the test is negative, approximately 99% of women will not deliver within 1 week.

5. Prior to fFN collection, do *not* perform procedures that may disrupt the vaginal concentration of fFN. Digital vaginal exams, lubricants, sexual intercourse, and vaginal probe ultrasound may render the test results inaccurate.

D. Laboratory tests (may be ordered based on patient history)
   1. Group beta strep cultures
   2. CBC with differential
   3. Urinalysis with culture and sensitivity if indicated
   4. Specimen collection for other aerobic and anaerobic cultures if infection is suspected

E. Speculum or digital vaginal examination if no contraindications
   1. Relative contraindications to digital vaginal examination
      a. Vaginal bleeding of uncertain etiology; exceeding bloody show
      b. Ruptured membranes (after communication with primary provider)
      c. Known placenta previa
      d. Vulvar lesions

F. External continuous electronic fetal monitor (ultrasound and/or tocodynamometer).
   1. See *Guidelines for Fetal Heart Rate Monitoring*
   2. Assess uterine activity

III. Administration of Corticosteroids

A. Administered to women at 24 to 34 weeks of gestation
B. Betamethasone 12 mg intramuscular (IM) every 24 hours for a total of two (2) doses; or
C. Dexamethasone 6 mg IM every 12 hours for a total of four (4) doses

IV. Tocolytic Therapy

A. Tocolytic therapy has not proved to be effective in stopping PTL for extended periods of time (weeks/months); however, individual tocolytics may delay labor for 2 to 7 days.
B. The goal of tocolytic therapy is to stop uterine contractions. Most commonly, this allows time to initiate maternal corticosteroid therapy to accelerate the maturation of fetal pulmonary vasculature.
C. General contraindications to tocolysis
   1. Severe preeclampsia
   2. Placental abruption
   3. Intrauterine infection
   4. Lethal congenital or chromosomal abnormalities
   5. Advanced cervical dilation
   6. Evidence of fetal compromise
   7. Placental insufficiency

D. Tocolytic drug categories
   1. Beta-adrenergic agonist
   2. Magnesium sulfate
   3. Prostaglandin synthetase inhibitor
   4. Calcium channel blocker

E. Specific tocolytics
   1. Magnesium sulfate administration
      a. Magnesium sulfate acts by decreasing the release of acetylcholine at the neuromuscular junction. This decreases the availability of acetylcholine, causing a decrease in the amplitude of electrical signals in myometrial cells. Maternal side effects include nausea, vomiting, drowsiness, lethargy, flushing, urinary retention, shortness of breath, pulmonary edema. Resultant maternal–fetal side effects include decreased fetal heart rate (FHR) variability, neonatal hypotonia, and drowsiness
      b. Intravenous (IV) dose: 4–6 gram loading dose over 20–30 minutes, then 1–3 grams/hour maintenance dose.
      c. Piggyback IV magnesium sulfate infusion into main IV fluid via infusion pump.
      d. Assess for signs and symptoms of magnesium sulfate toxicity such as absent deep tendon reflexes (DTRs), respiratory depression ($\leq$12 breaths/min), decreasing level of consciousness (LOC), decreased urinary output (<30 mL/hr). If toxicity is suspected, discontinue IV magnesium sulfate infusion, provide respiratory support if indicated, consult with the primary provider. Obtain serum magnesium level. Monitor blood pressure, pulse, respirations, LOC, and DTRs until stable.
      e. Antidote: Reversal agent for magnesium sulfate is calcium gluconate. Dose: 10 mL of a 10% solution IV push, given over 1–2 minutes.
      f. FDA off-label use as tocolytic.
   2. Terbutaline sulfate (Brethine) administration
      a. Terbutaline sulfate is a beta-adrenergic agonist agent that acts to decrease gap junction formation in uterine muscle. Terbutaline sulfate may be administered for short-term use (i.e., 48–72 hours) by oral, subcutaneous, or IV dosing. Hold medication if maternal heart rate >120 bpm. Maternal side effects include anxiety and nervousness, jitteriness, tachycardia, hypotension, hyperglycemia, hypokalemia, and pulmonary edema.

Fetal side effects include tachycardia and hyperinsulinemia. Neonatal side effects include hypoglycemia and tachycardia.

b. Oral dose: 2.5–5 mg every 4–6 hours for 48–72 hours as indicated.

c. Subcutaneous (Sub-Q) dose: 0.25 mg every 15 minutes, up to three doses or 0.25 mg every 30–60 minutes up to 1 mg

d. IV dose: 1 mg/min initially; increase by 0.5 mg/min every 10 min to maximum of 8 mg/min or until contractions stop.

e. FDA off-label use as tocolytic

3. Indomethacin administration

a. Indomethacin is a prostaglandin synthetase inhibitor with potential benefit as a tocolytic agent through its inhibition of prostaglandin formation. Prostaglandins promote uterine contractions and cervical ripening associated with labor by increasing gap junction formation. Maternal side effects include nausea and vomiting, gastrointestinal distress, gastrointestinal bleeding, and increased vaginal bleeding during all stages of labor. Fetal side effects include oligohydramnios and potential premature closure of the ductus arteriosus, which necessitates ultrasonographic follow-up with this therapeutic approach.

b. Initial dose: 50 mg PO or per rectum (PR).

c. Maintenance oral dose: 25 mg PO or PR every 6–8 hours for 72 hours.

d. With PO dose, simultaneous administration of food may decrease gastrointestinal irritation.

e. FDA pregnancy category C

f. FDA off-label use as tocolytic

4. Nifedepine (Procardia) administration

a. Nifedepine is a calcium channel blocker that inhibits myometrial activity by blocking the influx of calcium through membranes of myometrial cells. The primary tocolytic effect of nifedepine may result from a decrease in the strength of contractions rather than the frequency. Maternal side effects may include nausea, headache, facial flushing, hypotension, tachycardia, and palpitations. Fetal side effects may include tachycardia and intrauterine growth restriction.

b. Loading dose: 20 mg PO, followed by 20 mg PO after 30 minutes, if contractions persist, followed by 20 mg PO every 3–8 hours for 48–72 hours as indicated. The maximum dose is 160 mg/day.

c. Loading dose: 20 mg PO, followed by 20 mg PO after 30 minutes, if contractions persist, followed by 20 mg PO every 3–8 hours for 48–72 hours as indicated. The maximum dose is 160 mg/day.

d. FDA pregnancy category B

e. FDA off-label use as tocolytic

5. Discontinuing (weaning) intravenous tocolytics

a. Assess vital signs, FHR baseline and periodic changes, uterine activity and maternal respiratory status.

b. Reassess maternal uterine activity and FHR baseline and periodic changes every 30 minutes for the first hour.

c. During oral tocolytic therapy, vital signs and respiratory status are assessed every 4 hours, with heart rate assessed immediately prior to administration.

V. **Patient/Family Education**

A. Plan of care

B. Unit and hospital policies and procedures

C. Electronic fetal monitoring

D. Signs and symptoms of PTL

E. Treatment options

Guidelines for the Care of Patients with Diagnosed or Suspected Placenta Previa during the Peripartum Period

I. **Initial Assessment**
   A. See *Guidelines for the Initial Assessment and Triage of Obstetric Patients.*
   B. Interview patient for additional history of onset of bleeding, amount, color, and character of blood, onset of uterine contractions in relation to bleeding (if present), and presence or absence of pain associated with bleeding.
   C. Physical assessment should include presence/absence of vaginal bleeding, review of laboratory results including hematocrit/hemoglobin, and signs or symptoms of excessive blood loss.

II. **Maternal Physical Status**
   A. Vital Signs
      1. Patients with active vaginal bleeding or who are unstable: Pulse, respiration, SaO_2, and blood pressure (BP) every 5–15 minutes
      2. Patients who are stable: Vital signs every 30–60 minutes and every 4 hours thereafter during expectant management
      3. Temperature every 4 hours if membranes are intact, every 2 hours if membranes are ruptured
   B. Vaginal Bleeding
      1. Inspect perineum every 1–2 hours when stable and more frequently as indicated.
      2. Assess and document character, color, and estimated amount of all vaginal bleeding.
   C. Laboratory Tests
      1. On admission, obtain (as ordered) hematocrit/hemoglobin, type and screen/cross.
      2. Repeat type and screen every 72 hours (as ordered) or according to hospital policy, depending on patient assessment findings.
      3. Consider obtaining the following labs when profuse bleeding occurs or delivery is scheduled: CBC, PT/PTT, fibrinogen, and type and cross for red blood cells, 4 units fresh frozen plasma, and 2 platelet apheresis packs.

III. **Fetal Surveillance**
   A. Electronic Fetal Monitoring (EFM)
      1. Continuous EFM is used during the initial and subsequent episodes of vaginal bleeding in accordance with the *Guidelines for Fetal Heart Rate Monitoring.*
      2. Evaluate EFM tracing every 15 minutes in presence of active vaginal bleeding or if the patient is otherwise unstable. When stable, without vaginal bleeding, EFM evaluation may occur every 30–60 minutes.
   B. Obstetrical ultrasound is obtained to confirm placental position, estimated fetal gestational age, and fetal position.
   C. Biophysical profile may be assessed when determination of fetal reassurance is not possible by EFM.

IV. **Patient Care Management**
   A. Informed Consent and Consultation
      1. Informed consent for Cesarean delivery is obtained by the physician if active bleeding persists, if patient is unstable and/or if Category III tracing occurs.
      2. Anesthesia consult is ordered and informed consent is obtained as indicated.
      3. Neonatology is notified of potential delivery, estimated fetal gestational age, and need for consultation as ordered.
   B. Vaginal Exam
      1. Vaginal exams are not performed on patients with a known placenta previa except by the primary care provider. Patients who have a

marginal previa and are stable may be candidates for vaginal delivery. Note: Access to an operating room with resources for Cesarean delivery should be immediately available, should significant vaginal bleeding occur.

2. Sterile speculum vaginal exams may be performed by medical personnel in order to evaluate cervical dilation and obtain cervical cultures.

C. Intake and Output
1. Obtain intravenous access with an 18-gauge (or larger) angiocatheter.
2. If profuse bleeding continues or delivery is anticipated, a second large bore angiocatheter should be considered.
3. In extreme hemorrhage a central line (usually in the right internal jugular vein) and placement of a pulmonary artery catheter to assess hemodynamic /oxygen transport status and guide blood and fluid replacement should be considered.
4. An indwelling urinary catheter should be placed in the presence of active bleeding.
5. Document estimated blood loss in cc or mL.
6. Assess and document hourly intake and output and 24-hour totals.

D. Uterine Contractions
1. In the presence of uterine contractions, tocolysis with magnesium sulfate (MgSO4) or indomethacin may be considered.
2. Beta-agonists (ritodrine, terbutaline) are contraindicated in the presence of active bleeding.

E. Activity
1. Strict bed rest in presence of active vaginal bleeding or if the patient is unstable.
2. Bed rest with bathroom privileges may be ordered, depending on patient status.

3. All patients on bed rest should maintain a lateral tilt. Patients should be reminded to avoid supine positioning to prevent aorto-caval compression.

F. Recurrence of Acute Vaginal Bleeding
1. Consult with primary care provider.
2. Assess color, character, and amount of vaginal bleeding.
3. Ensure patent, large bore intravenous access.
4. Administer oxygen via non-rebreathing face mask at 10–12 L/min.
5. Monitor oxygen saturation (SaO_2) every 15 minutes, maintain SaO_2 >95%.
6. Assess pulse, respirations, BP every 15 minutes until stable.
7. Observe for signs of hypovolemic shock: tachycardia, hypotension, tachypnea, dizziness, pallor, and decreasing level of consciousness (LOC).

V. **Nursing Implications**
Consult with physician for any of the following:
A. Onset or increase of vaginal bleeding
B. BP <90/60 or MAP <65
C. Pulse >120 or <60
D. Respirations >26 or <14
E. Temperature >100.4°F.
F. Urine output <30 cc/hour
G. SaO_2 <95%
H. Decreasing LOC
I. Onset or increase in uterine contractions
J. Adverse change in fetal status

VI. **Patient/Family Teaching**
Inform patient and family regarding:
A. Orientation to facility hospital and unit
B. Plan of care
C. Purpose/method of fetal monitoring and antepartum testing
D. Bed rest and physical activity restrictions
E. Potential for Cesarean delivery

Guidelines for the Care of Obstetric Patients with Diabetic Ketoacidosis (DKA)

I. **Overview**
   A. Goals of Therapy
      1. Rehydration
      2. Correction of acidemia
      3. Normalization of serum glucose
      4. Restoration of electrolyte homeostasis
      5. Elimination of the underlying cause
   B. Initial Assessment
      1. Maternal history (if available)—Patient's diabetic history, classification of diabetes, currently prescribed insulin regimen, type of blood glucose self-monitoring utilized, daily total caloric intake, recent trends in serum blood glucose levels, recent history of nausea, vomiting, or diarrhea, recent history of infection, other medications.
      2. Maternal physical status
         a. Obtain baseline data: maternal vital signs; confirmation of fetal heart rate
         b. Current blood glucose value
         c. Presence of signs and symptoms of DKA: polyuria, polyphagia, polydypsia, dehydration, nausea, vomiting, abdominal pain, gastric stasis, ileus, increased respiratory rate, Kussmaul respiratory pattern, acetone breath, mental status changes, coma, high levels of ketonuria, glucosuria, decreased blood pH and serum bicarbonate (metabolic acidemia).
   C. Management
      1. Baseline data
         a. Assess maternal vital signs and temperature
         b. Obtain initial STAT labs: CBC, serum electrolytes, BUN, creatinine, glucose, arterial blood gases, bicarbonate, urinalysis, serum lactate, serum ketones

         c. Other assessment parameters may include: serum or capillary hydroxybutyrate level, liver function tests, chest x-ray, sepsis work-up, cultures (blood, sputum, urine)
      2. Hemodynamics
         a. Monitor blood pressure, pulse, respirations, and oxygenation status per pulse oximetry every 30–60 minutes
         b. Consider placement of arterial line for continuous blood pressure monitoring, frequent laboratory analysis, and blood gas values
         c. Assess for hypovolemia: low blood pressure, increasing pulse rate, delayed capillary refill, altered central hemodynamic values (e.g., decreased cardiac output, preload, left ventricular contractility, oxygen delivery and consumption)
      3. Respiratory
         a. Maintain patent airway
         b. Administer oxygen via tight non-rebreathing face mask at 10 L/minute if hypoxemic or abnormal SaO_2
         c. Maintain oxygen saturations of >95% per continuous pulse oximetry
         d. Anticipate need for intubation and mechanical ventilation if obtunded or if airway is compromised.
         e. Consider need for nasogastric tube if obtunded or vomiting
      4. Intake and output
         a. Obtain large-bore peripheral intravenous (IV) access
         b. Place Foley urinary catheter; obtain specimen for uninalysis and culture/sensitivity

c. Measure and record all intake and output. Calculate and document hourly and 24-hour totals; alert if urine production <30 mL/hr

5. Rehydration (initial)
   a. Administer 1–2 L of .9% NS over the first hour; 500 mL/hr over next 2 hours; 250 mL/hr over next 4–6 hours. Goal: correct fluid deficit over 12–24 hours with typical need in range of 6–8 liters.
   b. Consider need for second IV line.
   c. Initiate glucose containing solutions (i.e., D5 1/2 NS) when serum glucose levels fall to 200 mg/dL
   d. Assess for pulmonary edema: dyspnea, tachypnea, wheezing, cough

6. Insulin therapy
   a. Insulin replacement may be administered as IV bolus and/or IV infusion pump
   b. Usual dose of regular insulin IV bolus approximates 0.1 unit/kg/hr
   c. Initiate regular insulin continuous IV infusion of 5–10 units/hr. May double infusion rate if serum glucose has not decreased by 25% in 2 hours.
   d. Anticipate decreasing infusion rate to 1–2 units/hr if serum glucose levels fall below 150 mg/dL.
   e. Monitor blood glucose level hourly during insulin infusion (may use laboratory correlation with each draw)
   f. Monitor for signs and symptoms of hypoglycemia (serum glucose level <40 mg/dL), shaking; headache, severe hunger, anxiety, diaphoresis, cool and clammy skin, pallor, or confusion.
   g. Monitor for cerebral edema: headache, vomiting, deteriorating mental status, diminished pupillary light reflex, bradycardia and/or widened pulse pressure

7. Correction of electrolyte imbalances/acidosis
   a. Obtain electrocardiographic data; note ST-segment depression, T-wave alterations, QRS changes and/or arrhythmias
   b. Assess serum pH and bicarbonate levels; administration of sodium bicarbonate is rarely needed and only used if pH is <7.0
   c. Obtain hourly laboratory assessment of electrolyte levels
   d. Anticipate potassium replacement within 2–4 hours; consider adding KCl 20–40 meq/L to maintenance IV fluids after adequate urine output is established; anticipate reduction in dose by approximately 50% with persistent oliguria

8. Prophylaxis
   a. Anticipate broad spectrum antibiotic administration pending results of sepsis work-up and cultures if indicated.

9. Fetal or uterine monitoring
   a. With viable, live fetus, continuous monitoring if possible
   b. Maternal lateral positioning
   c. Monitor for uterine activity
   d. Avoid betamimetics and corticosteroids while DKA is being corrected
   e. Consider delivery of compromised fetus only after maternal metabolic stabilization

II. **Procedure for the Administration of Intravenous Insulin Infusion**
   A. Prepare a standardized solution of 100 units of regular human insulin to 100 mL of .9% normal saline such that 1 cc = 1 unit regular insulin
   B. Administer insulin solution via infusion pump, through most proximal port of main IV line at prescribed rate.
   C. Monitor patient serum glucose levels at least every hour during IV insulin infusion. Titrate insulin drip to serum glucose levels as prescribed.
   D. Hypoglycemic episodes:
      1. Consult with primary care provider.
      2. Discontinue IV insulin infusion for serum glucose levels <60 mg/dL.
      3. Administer 300 cc 5% dextrose IV solution over 15–30 minutes for serum glucose of 20–40 mg/dL in the conscious patient.
      4. If serum blood glucose <20 mg/dL and/or unconsciousness occur, administer 10 cc 50% dextrose IV push over 5 minutes. Monitor pulse, respirations, and blood pressure every 5 minutes until stable. Repeat blood glucose testing every 15 minutes until stable.
   E. Hyperglycemic episodes:
      1. Consult with primary care provider.
      2. Administer insulin as prescribed.
      3. Repeat blood glucose in 30 minutes.
      4. Monitor for signs and symptoms of DKA.
   F. Implications for care:
      1. Consult with primary care provider for:
         a. Sustained systolic blood pressure >140 mm Hg or <90 mmHg
         b. Sustained diastolic blood pressure >90 mmHg or <50 mmHg
         c. Sustained tachycardia ≥120 bpm, respirations <14 or >26
         d. Abnormal blood glucose values
         e. Signs or symptoms of hypoglycemia

　　　f.　Urine output <30 cc/hour
　　　g.　Urine ketones
　　　h.　Change in neurologic status
　　　i.　Significant system changes
　　　j.　Abnormal fetal status
　　　k.　Imminent delivery

III.　Patient/Family Education
　　　A.　Plan of care
　　　B.　Electronic fetal monitoring
　　　C.　Signs and symptoms of hypoglycemia, hyperglycemia, DKA

Guidelines for the Care of Patients with Preeclampsia/Eclampsia

I. **Background**
   A. Preeclampsia is one of the top three causes of maternal death in the United States and Canada.
   B. Preeclampsia is a disease that begins in the first few weeks of pregnancy, when abnormal placental implantation and vascular modeling are known to occur.
   C. The risk of preeclampsia increases as placental size increases (e.g., multiple gestation).
   D. The exact etiology remains unknown, but recent research points to the interplay among multiple genetic, immune, familial, endothelial, inflammatory, and cellular factors.
   E. Magnesium sulfate is the drug of choice for preventing and/or treating eclamptic seizures. It is superior to phenytoin sodium (Dilantin), and/or diazepam (Valium) in the treatment of eclamptic seizures. Magnesium sulfate does not suppress the gag reflex, decreasing the risk of maternal aspiration.
   F. The blood pressure threshold for administering antihypertensive medications to women with preeclampsia has decreased. Patients may have an intracranial hemorrhage at systolic pressures ≥160 mmHg.
   G. Common antihypertensive agents used to treat hypertensive crisis in patients with preeclampsia are hydralazine hydrochloride (Apresoline), labetalol hydrochloride (Trandate), and nifedipine (Procardia).
   H. The only "cure" for preeclampsia/eclampsia is delivery of the placenta.

II. **Diagnosis of Preeclampsia**
   A. Mild Preeclampsia:
      1. Hypertension >140 mmHg systolic *or* >90 mmHg diastolic *after the 20th week of pregnancy*, and measured on two occasions at least 4–6 hours apart; *and* proteinuria >300 mg protein in a 24-hour urine collection; or a quantitative dipstick result ≥1+.
      2. Proteinuria identified by dipstick may be quantified by a 24-hour urine collection for total protein.
   B. Severe Preeclampsia:
   Patient has preeclampsia plus one of the following:
      1. Hypertension >160 mmHg systolic or >110 mmHg diastolic *after the 20th week of pregnancy*, and measured on two occasions at least 4–6 hours apart;
      2. Proteinuria >5 grams in a 24-hour urine collection; or a dipstick result of >3+.
      3. Signs and symptoms:
         a. Oliguria of <500 mL of urine in 24 hours
         b. Cerebral or visual disturbances (headache, blurred vision, scotomata)
         c. Pulmonary edema
         d. Epigastric or right upper quadrant pain
         e. Chest pain
         f. Cyanosis
         g. Elevated liver enzymes
         h. Thrombocytopenia
         i. Fetal growth restriction

III. **Admission Assessment for Patients with Preeclampsia**
   A. See *Guidelines for the Initial Assessment and Triage of Obstetric Patients.*
   B. Admission History Adjuncts
      1. Past history of preeclampsia, eclampsia, chronic hypertension, or gestational hypertension; history of preeclampsia/eclampsia in patient's mother or a sibling.
   C. Presence of maternal risk factors
      1. Age >35 years
      2. Chronic hypertension

3. African American race
4. Renal disease
5. Obesity
6. Diabetes mellitus/insulin resistance prior to pregnancy
7. Vascular disease
8. Connective tissue disease (e.g., lupus erythematosus, rheumatoid arthritis, scleroderma)
9. Antiphospholipid antibody syndrome
10. Thrombophilia
11. Active infection (e.g., urinary tract infection, pyelonephritis, periodontal disease)
12. Multiple gestation
13. Obesity
14. Other

D. Vital Signs
E. Height, Weight
F. System Review for End-organ Involvement
   1. Presence of neurologic involvement
      a. Headache
      b. Visual disturbances (blurred vision, floaters, flashes, loss of visual field, dark spots)
      c. Blindness in one or both eyes
      d. Papilledema (swelling of the optic nerve)
      e. Seizures prior to admission
   2. Presence of hepatic involvement
      a. Epigastric pain, "heartburn"
      b. Nausea or vomiting
      c. Shoulder pain
      d. Jaundice
      e. Prolonged bleeding
      f. Bruises, recent history of bruising easily
      g. Subcapsular hematoma
   3. Presence of cardiovascular and/or pulmonary involvement
      a. Chest pain
      b. Tachycardia
      c. Irregular heart rate
      d. Shortness of breath
      e. Painful inspiration ("hurts to breathe")
      f. Adventitious breath sounds (crackles, rales)
      g. Tachypnea
      h. Edema of hands, face, body
      i. Recent weight gain
      j. SaO$_2$ <95%
   4. Presence of renal involvement
      a. Decreased urine output/oliguria
      b. Blood in urine or dark urine
      c. Severe pitting edema, generalized
      d. Sudden recent weight gain
   5. Fetal status
      a. Last menstrual period (LMP)/estimated gestational age (EGA)
      b. Other pregnancy complications
      c. Fetal movement
      d. Recent fetal growth (if results available)
      e. Recent amniotic fluid assessment
      f. Recent fetal surveillance tests (if results available)

G. Physical examination
   1. General survey
   2. Neurologic
   3. Head and neck
   4. Cardiovascular
   5. Pulmonary
   6. Abdominal
   7. Musculoskeletal
   8. Gastrointestinal
   9. Genitourinary (emphasis on pregnancy)
   10. Skin
   11. Fetal status/uterine activity

H. Initial laboratory tests (*based on institutional guidelines*)
   1. CBC with manual differential (peripheral blood smear for hemolysis, abnormal cells)
   2. If platelets <100,000, send clotting studies (DIC panel): PT, PTT, platelet assay, FSP/FDP/D-dimer, fibrinogen
   3. Liver function tests: AST, ALT, bilirubin (indirect), LDH
   4. Urine quantitative dipstick to assess for proteinuria on admission; then begin 24-hour collection for total protein, creatinine clearance.
   5. Type and screen blood for possible transfusion

IV. **Procedure for Magnesium Sulfate Administration**

A. Magnesium sulfate is recognized as a "High Alert" drug that has been associated with adverse patient outcomes from overdose, specifically respiratory arrest and maternal death. Implement institutional guidelines for High Alert medications when infusing this drug.
B. Review the order for magnesium sulfate and the specific loading and maintenance doses.
C. Magnesium sulfate solution is piggybacked into main intravenous (IV) line and the infusion should always be controlled via infusion pump.
D. Loading Dose: Infuse 4–6 grams loading dose over 15–30 minutes. Consider a decreased dosage in the presence of decreased urine output or renal disease.
E. Maintenance Dose: Infuse at 1–3 grams per hour via infusion pump.
F. Assess for signs and symptoms of magnesium sulfate toxicity such as absent deep tendon reflexes (DTRs), decreasing level of

consciousness (LOC) or decreasing respiratory rate. If toxicity is suspected, discontinue magnesium sulfate infusion, provide respiratory support (if indicated), notify physician, and consider obtaining order for magnesium sulfate level. Consider administering calcium gluconate to reverse magnesium sulfate's respiratory depressant effects. Monitor blood pressure, pulse, respirations, LOC every 5 minutes until stable.

G. Antidote: For reversal of magnesium sulfate effect, the physician or nurse midwife may order calcium gluconate. The usual dose is 10 mL of a 10% solution to be given over 1 to 2 minutes IV push.

V. Nursing Implications

A. Notify physician for any of the following:
1. Systolic blood pressure $\geq$160 mmHg or diastolic blood pressure $\geq$110 mmHg
2. Respirations <14 or >26 per minute
3. DTRs absent
4. Urine output <30 cc/hour
5. Symptoms of pulmonary edema
6. Seizure activity
7. Suspected magnesium sulfate toxicity
8. SaO_2 <96%
9. Symptoms of placental abruption
10. Change in neurologic status or development of visual disturbances or headache
11. New complaints of nausea, vomiting, epigastric pain, or heartburn
12. Significant system changes
13. Persistent category II fetal heart rate tracing
14. Category III fetal heart rate tracing
15. Imminent delivery

VI. Intrapartum Care

A. Vital signs
1. Assess blood pressure, pulse, and respirations every 15 minutes during the administration of magnesium sulfate loading dose.
2. After the loading dose, assess blood pressure, pulse, and respirations every 15 minutes during maintenance magnesium sulfate infusion.
3. If patient meets following criteria, vital sign assessment every 30 minutes.
   a. Patient has mild preeclampsia
   b. Blood pressure stable without increases for minimum of 2 hours
   c. No prior antihypertensive medications administered in past 6 hours
   d. Patient antepartum or in latent phase of labor (not in active labor)

4. Assess blood pressure every 5–15 minutes during severe hypertensive episodes with IV antihypertensive medication use. Selection of 5–15 minutes based on half-life of specific antihypertensive agent.
5. Count respirations for 60 seconds during magnesium sulfate infusion.
6. Assess temperature every 4 hours if membranes intact. Increase frequency to every 2 hours if membranes are ruptured. If fever is present, assess temperature every two hours until resolved.
7. Assess DTRs every hour during infusion.

B. Intake and output
1. Obtain IV access with an 18-gauge (or larger) angiocatheter.
2. Place all IV fluids on infusion pumps. Unless otherwise ordered, maintain total hourly IV intake to $\leq$125 mL per hour.
3. NPO with ice chips or as permitted by primary provider and/or anesthesia provider.
4. Strict intake and output.
   a. Measure and record all intake hourly. Calculate total every hour, shift, and 24 hours and document.
   b. Measure and record urine output hourly. Insert Foley catheter with urimeter. Calculate total every hour, shift, and 24 hours and document.

VII. Ongoing Assessment and Care for Patients with Preeclampsia

A. Cardiopulmonary
1. Auscultate breath sounds every 4 to 8 hours.
2. Continuous SaO_2 monitoring during magnesium sulfate infusion.
3. Assess for signs and symptoms of pulmonary edema (e.g. complaints of chest pain, SaO_2 <95%, cough, shortness of breath, tachypnea (R $\geq$26/min), tachycardia (HR >100 beats/minute, or adventitious breath sounds).

B. Neurologic
1. Assess DTRs and presence or absence of clonus every hour during continuous IV magnesium sulfate infusion prior to delivery.
2. If DTRs absent, discontinue magnesium sulfate infusion and notify the primary provider.
3. Assess patient's level of consciousness, airway, and respiratory rate. If the patient's respiratory rate is <12/min, discontinue magnesium sulfate infusion, initiate oxygen therapy if the SaO_2 value is <96%, and notify anesthesia personnel or the primary care provider. See below for treatment of magnesium toxicity.

4. Assess level of consciousness every hour during continuous magnesium sulfate infusion.
5. Assess for headache and visual disturbances every shift (8 to 12 hours). Instruct patient to alert staff if headache or visual disturbances develop.

C. Activity
1. Bed rest with side rails up during magnesium sulfate infusion.
2. Instruct patient to rest in a position to optimize cardiac output and prevent vena caval syndrome (lateral positioning, may elevate head of bed 30–45 degrees; instruct patient not to lie on her back).

D. Labs – Orders from primary provider supersede these orders.
1. Follow-up abnormal admission labs if indicated.
2. Repeat labs every 24 hours if patient is antepartum with mild preeclampsia.
3. Repeat labs every 8 to 12 hours if patient is antepartum and has severe preeclampsia.
4. For significant changes in patient condition consider sending new set of labs (see admission labs).
5. If patient's condition worsens, consider renal labs, chemistry labs, arterial blood gas, serum lactate, and others based on patient condition.

E. Fetal Status—See *Guidelines for Fetal Heart Rate Monitoring*
1. If fetus is at viable gestational age: Continuous electronic fetal monitoring (EFM) is recommended during magnesium sulfate infusion. Assessment of EFM for patients diagnosed with preeclampsia receiving a magnesium sulfate infusion:
2. First stage of labor: every 15 minutes (if fetus at viable gestational age)
3. Second stage of labor: every 5 minutes (if fetus at viable gestational age)
4. Verify medical plan of care for Category III tracings that do not resolve with interventions.

VIII. Assessment and Care of Patients with Eclamptic Seizures
A. Protect patient and call for help
1. Protect the patient's airway. Turn patient on her side and call for help.
2. Protect patient from physical harm.
3. Insert oral airway if possible. Do not force jaw open.
4. Turn suction to "on" position to prepare for patient emesis. (Connect large cannula suction tip to tubing.)

5. Notify primary care provider and nurse manager/rapid response team/anesthesia provider (depending upon individual facility guidelines)

B. Administer magnesium sulfate IV
1. For patients who are NOT on magnesium sulfate at the time of the seizure, administer a loading dose of 4–6 grams of magnesium sulfate IV over 10 to 15 minutes.
   a. Initiate infusion when drug available. Place on IV pump when equipment available. Do not delay giving magnesium sulfate to wait on an infusion pump.
   b. After loading dose is complete, begin maintenance dose at 2–3 grams per hour via an infusion pump.
2. For patients who have received a loading dose of magnesium sulfate and are on a maintenance dose when the seizure occurs, administer 2 grams of magnesium sulfate slowly over 3 to 5 minutes.
   a. If the seizure has not stopped after 2 grams of magnesium sulfate, administer 2 more grams of magnesium sulfate over 3 to 5 minutes.
3. For patients who have received a total of 6 grams magnesium sulfate during the seizure, and the seizure has not stopped, intubate and mechanically ventilate the patient. For persistent seizure activity, acquire immediate (STAT) maternal–fetal medicine, neurology, consultation.
4. After patient receives 6 grams of magnesium sulfate during the seizure or as a loading dose, begin the maintenance dose at 2–3 grams/hour. Send serum magnesium level for stat analysis.
5. Recurrent seizure dose: If patient has ≥1+ DTRs and >16 respirations/minute prior to recurrent seizure, administer 2 grams of magnesium sulfate over 3–5 minutes. Send serum magnesium level for stat analysis. Adjust dose accordingly.

C. Once seizure activity stops:
1. Turn patient on her side and prepare for emesis and secretions.
2. Administer O_2 at 10 L per minute by face mask. Do not place the mask's strap on the patient (as many will have emesis once the seizure stops).
3. Suction nose and mouth as necessary.
4. Assess blood pressure, pulse, respirations, and fetal heart rate parameters every 10–15 minutes until stable.

5. Collect and send stat serum magnesium level to the laboratory

D. Note characteristics of seizure:
   1. Presence or absence of aura
   2. Duration of seizure
   3. Tonic–clonic phases
   4. Duration of postictal phase
   5. Length of unconsciousness
   6. Maternal and fetal responses

E. Assess for evidence of placental abruption and/or imminent delivery.

F. Assess for evidence of intracranial bleed (i.e., focal neurologic deficits, may be one sided, labile vital signs)

IX.   **Patient/Family Education**

A. Plan of care

B. EFM

C. Preeclampsia disease process; signs and symptoms of disease, treatment, etc.

D. Diversional activities

E. Magnesium sulfate infusion

F. Special testing—biophysical profile, ultrasound, laboratory work

Guidelines for the Care of Patients Requiring Induction of Labor with Oxytocin

I. Background

A. Oxytocin protocols are typically divided into two categories: High dose and low dose. The differences between them are: the starting dose, the amount of, and time intervals for dosage increase.

B. There is no consensus regarding which protocol is "best" for individual patients. The *high dose* protocol is associated with less time from the start of the induction to delivery, but with more episodes of uterine tachysystole. The *low dose* protocol, more commonly used in practice, is associated with fewer episodes of tachysystole.

C. Studies that have compared high dose and low dose oxytocin protocols have found no significant difference in neonatal outcomes despite the difference in rates of tachysystole.

D. Both high dose and low dose oxytocin protocols (see the dosing schedule below) have been associated with both increased and decreased rates of cesarean deliveries.

E. Patients who receive oxytocin for induction of labor are more likely to have episodes of tachysystole compared with women who have oxytocin for augmentation of labor.

F. The effectiveness of oxytocin on uterine activity is dependent upon the number of active oxytocin receptors in the uterus. The number of uterine receptors increases prior to the onset of spontaneous labor at term. Thus, in most pregnancies, lower doses of oxytocin are required to induce labor at or near term compared with preterm pregnancies.

G. Down-regulation of oxytocin receptors may occur when oxytocin is administered at a steady rate over a long period of time. Therefore, when active phase labor is estab-lished, decreasing the rate of the oxytocin infusion may be considered.

H. Oxytocin protocols generally allow increases up to a specified dose (e.g., 20 mU/min) at the discretion of the nurse. Infusion rates greater than the specified dose usually require primary care clinician evaluation of maternal and fetal status.

I. Oxytocin is similar in structure to the antidiuretic hormone vasopressin, and may increase water retention and electrolyte disturbances.

J. If adequate fetal and/or maternal surveillance cannot be continued during the oxytocin infusion, it should be discontinued until such time as personnel are able to provide oversight.

K. Patients who have induction or augmentation with oxytocin are at increased risk for postpartum hemorrhage from uterine atony.

II. Indications for Medical Induction of Labor*

(*not an all-inclusive list*)

A. Abruptio placentae

B. Chorioamnionitis

C. Fetal demise

D. Gestational hypertension

E. Preeclampsia/eclampsia

F. Premature rupture of membranes

G. Post-term pregnancy

H. Maternal medical conditions (e.g., diabetes mellitus, renal disease, chronic pulmonary disease, chronic hypertension, antiphospholipid syndrome, cancer, etc.)

I. Fetal compromise (e.g., severe fetal growth restriction, isoimmunization, oligohydramnios, etc.)

J. Logistic considerations (e.g., history of rapid labor, distance from hospital or psychosocial indications)

III. **Contraindications of Induction of Labor*** (**not an all-inclusive list*)

Note: *Contraindications for induction of labor are the same as those for vaginal delivery.*

A. Vasa previa or complete placenta previa

B. Transverse fetal lie

C. Umbilical cord prolapse

D. Classical uterine incision scar

E. Active genital herpes infection

F. Previous myomectomy entering the endometrial cavity

IV. **Induction Considerations**

A. The primary care provider is responsible for discussing with the patient the indications, benefits, and risks, and the selected method of cervical ripening and/or induction of labor.

B. For patients scheduled for elective induction of labor, the following parameters should be met:

1. Primary provider to verify gestational age; patients scheduled for elective induction are to be ≥39 weeks gestation on the day of induction as evidenced by: ultrasound measurement at less than 20 weeks gestation supporting this assessment; fetal heart tones documented as present for 30 weeks by Doppler ultrasonography; and/or it has been 36 weeks since a positive serum or urine HCG pregnancy test result.

2. Bishop's score determination: a Bishop's score ≥8 in primigravida women and ≥6 in multiparous women is associated with significantly higher rates of vaginal delivery compared with lower scores.

C. The indication for induction of labor is documented in the medical record.

D. Admission to Labor and Delivery: See *Guidelines for the Initial Assessment and Triage of Obstetric Patients.*

E. Initiate continuous electronic fetal monitoring (EFM). *See Guidelines for Fetal Heart Rate Monitoring.*

1. Obtain a minimum of a 20- to 30-minute EFM strip recording prior to the initiation of oxytocin.

V. **Administration of Oxytocin**

A. Obtain the oxytocin intravenous (IV) solution from pharmacy. Oxytocin solutions for induction of labor should be premixed in an isotonic solution such as 0.9% NaCl (normal saline), LR (lactated Ringer's solution), and so-forth, such that an infusion rate of 1 mL/hour is equivalent to 1 mU/min when administered via an infusion pump.

B. Oxytocin solutions for induction or augmentation of labor ideally should not be mixed or further concentrated on a patient care unit.

C. For patients with insulin resistance or with diabetes mellitus who require insulin during labor, oxytocin should not be administered in the same I.V. line as insulin.

D. After priming the IV tubing and placing on an infusion pump, connect the tubing (piggyback) to the most proximal port of the patient's main IV line (i.e., port closest to the patient's vein).

E. Begin the infusion at the prescribed starting dose (see protocols in table below). Increase the infusion per protocol.

F. Vital Signs

1. Assess baseline blood pressure (BP), pulse (P), respirations (R), and temperature (Temp) prior to starting the oxytocin infusion.

2. Assess BP, P and R every 15 minutes during the initiation of oxytocin infusion until maternal–fetal stabilization; then vital signs may be assessed every 30 to 60 minutes (*for patients with no other clinical concerns*).

3. Assess temperature every 4 hours if membranes intact; every 2 hours if membranes ruptured.

G. Uterine Activity

1. Assess uterine activity every 15 minutes during the initiation of the oxytocin infusion

Oxytocin Dosing Protocols and Assessments

Regimen	Starting Dose (mU/min)	Increase (mU/min)	Time Interval for Increases (minutes)
Low-dose	0.5– 2	1–2	30–60*
High-dose	4–6	3–6	15–40

mU/min = milliunit per minute.
*AWHONN recommended.

and during further increases and/or decreases of the medication.

2. Uterine tachysystole is defined as >5 contractions in 10 minutes averaged over 30 minutes.

3. Decrease or discontinue oxytocin infusion for uterine tachysystole unrelieved by interventions.

H. Fetal Status

1. Assess fetal heart rate (FHR) every 15 to 30 minutes (depending on the medical determination of "risk" assessment) for the active phase of the first stage of labor during oxytocin infusion until second stage; then assess FHR every 5 minutes.

2. Implement fetal supportive techniques specific to Category II EFM tracings as indicated.

3. Discontinue oxytocin infusion for Category III EFM tracing.

4. If oxytocin discontinued <20–30 min; subsequent FHR reassuring and uterine activity normal, restart at one-half the rate of previous level.

5. If oxytocin discontinued >30–40 min; restart at initial dose ordered if FHR reassuring and UA normal.

VI. **Care Implications**

A. Primary care provider communication for the following:

1. Rupture of membranes, meconium or blood stained amniotic fluid

2. Vaginal bleeding beyond normal bloody show

3. Analgesia or anesthesia needs of the patient

4. Vital signs
   a. BP >140/90 or BP <90/60
   b. Temperature >100.4
   c. Maternal pulse >120 or <60
   d. Respirations >26 or <14/min

5. Category II EFM tracing unresponsive to interventions

6. Category III EFM tracing

7. Inadequate uterine response at oxytocin dose of 20 mU/min

8. Persistent tachysystole unresponsive to interventions

VII. **Collaborative Patient/Family Education (may include but is not limited to)**

A. Plan of care for cervical ripening/induction/augmentation of labor

B. Purpose of pharmacotherapy

C. Potential side effects and complications

D. Potential need for operative delivery

E. Pain management options

Guidelines for the Care of Patients Requiring Induction of Labor Due to Intrauterine Fetal Demise (IUFD)

I. **Background**
  A. Maternal Risk Factors for IUFD
    1. Non-Hispanic black race
    2. Nulliparity
    3. Advanced maternal age (>35 years)
    4. Obesity
    5. Drug and alcohol use
    6. Congenital anomalies
    7. Chromosomal and genetic defects
    8. Diabetes mellitus
    9. Chronic hypertension and preeclampsia/eclampsia
    10. Systemic lupus erythematosus
    11. Renal disease
    12. Thyroid disorders
    13. Cholestasis of pregnancy
    14. Infections – human parvovirus B19, syphilis, streptococcal infection and *Listeria monocytogenes*
    15. Smoking >10 cigarettes/day
    16. Multiple gestation
  B. Methods of Delivery
    1. Dilation and evacuation (D&E) in 2nd trimester
    2. Labor induction in 3rd trimester
    3. Vaginal misoprostol before 28 weeks of gestation
    4. Cervical ripening followed by induction of labor

    5. Rarely, Cesarean delivery for unusual circumstances
  C. Confirm Fetal Death
    1. Prior to induction of labor due to IUFD, fetal death is confirmed by the primary care provider.

II. **Methods of Cervical Ripening and Induction of Labor Based on Gestational Age**
  A. Assessment of Cervical Status: Bishop's Score
    1. At term with a "ripe"/favorable cervix (Bishop's score >8), induction of labor with oxytocin is typically the treatment of choice. Bishop's score determination: a Bishop's score ≥ 8 in primigravida women and ≥ 6 in multiparous women is associated with significantly higher rates of vaginal delivery compared with lower scores.
  B. At term with an unfavorable cervix, cervical ripening and induction of labor with vaginal misoprostol may be used.
  C. Misoprostol can also be used for cervical ripening and induction of labor in the second trimester (13 to 26 weeks).
  D. The range of dosing of misoprostol has been reported from 50 to 400 micrograms administered by various routes every 6 to 12 hours.
  E. Dosing table for misoprostol for IUFD induction:

Weeks Gestation at Fetal Death	Misoprostol – Recommended Dose	Maximum Daily Dose Should NOT Exceed	Notes
13–17	200 mcg Repeat dose every 6–12 hours for total of 4 doses	1600 mcg	• Place tablet deep within vaginal fornix.
18–26	100 mcg Repeat dose every 6–12 hours for total of 4 doses	800 mcg	• If first treatment course was not effective, the subsequent doses may be doubled.
>26	Unfavorable cervix: 25–50 mcg Repeat every 4–6 hours for total of 4 doses.	200 mcg	• Insert into posterior vaginal fornix. • If first treatment course not effective, subsequent doses may be doubled.

F. Oxytocin administration, if necessary, may begin 4 hours following administration of the last dose of misoprostol.

G. For gestations >26 weeks, hold repeated doses of misoprostol if patient has ≥2 contractions in 10 minutes. If the uterine activity decreases, a repeat dose may be administered. If uterine activity does not decrease, oxytocin may be considered.

III. Maternal Assessment

A. See *Guidelines for the Initial Assessment and Triage of Obstetric Patients* for assessment parameters.

B. Laboratory tests that may be ordered (based on patient condition)
1. CBC with differential
2. Clotting studies if platelet count is less than 100,000
3. Karyotype (amniotic fluid)

C. Observe for side effects of prostaglandins, uterine contractions
1. Gastrointestinal upset: nausea, vomiting, diarrhea
2. Fever, shivering
3. Pain/cramping
4. Placental abruption
5. Postpartum hemorrhage

D. Pain management – options may include intravenous sedation, epidural anesthesia, or patient controlled analgesia pump, other methods based on provider experience and patient request.

IV. Consultation with Primary Care Provider

A. Spontaneous rupture of membranes, questionable status of membranes
B. Vaginal bleeding in excess of normal bloody show
C. Analgesia or anesthesia needs of patient
D. Abnormal vital signs
1. BP >140/90 or <90/60
2. Temp >100.4° F (38° C)
3. Sustained pulse >120 or <60 bpm
4. SaO_2 <96%
5. Respirations >26 or <14/minute
E. Imminent delivery

V. Patient and Family Support – Grief Process

A. Plan of care
B. Unit routine
C. Pain management options
D. Medications and associated side effects
E. Anticipated length of stay
F. Components of grief process, anticipatory guidance, local support groups
G. Disposition of fetal remains, autopsy, evaluation
H. Options for viewing and holding baby, photographs, etc.

Guidelines for the Care of the Obstetric Trauma Patient

I. **Primary Survey (In Accordance with: Advanced Trauma Life Support [ATLS] Protocols)**
    A. Airway
        1. Assess airway; look, listen, and feel for air movement
        2. If conscious: assume intact airway if talking, shouting
        3. If unconscious: use modified jaw thrust maneuver to open airway and assess for obstruction
        4. Assume potential for cervical spine injury until proven otherwise
        5. Consider oropharyngeal support if patency in doubt
    B. Breathing
        1. Assess ventilatory and respiratory function:
            a. Rate and quality of respirations
            b. Signs and symptoms of respiratory distress
                • inability to move air despite presence of open airway
                • asymmetric chest excursion
                • shallow or painful respirations
                • dyspnea
                • use of accessory muscles
                • tachypnea
        2. Assess trachea:
            a. Position or deviation from midline (indication of possible pneumothorax or massive hemothorax)
        3. Visually inspect chest for:
            a. Contusions
            b. Asymmetric excursion
            c. Paradoxical breathing (indication of possible flail chest)
            d. Open sucking wounds (indicative of possible open pneumothorax)
        4. Auscultate breath sounds bilaterally for:
            a. Hyper-resonance (indicative of possible pneumothorax)
            b. Dullness (indicative of possible hemothorax), if decreased or absent breath sounds noted, percuss thorax
        5. Palpate thorax for:
            a. Presence of pain
            b. Rib instability
            c. Subcutaneous emphysema (indicative of possible flail chest)
    C. Circulation
        1. Auscultate heart sounds for:
            a. Distant heart sounds
            b. Muffled heart sounds (indicative of possible cardiac tamponade)
        2. Assess for adequacy of cardiac output
            a. Palpate pulses to estimate blood pressure (BP)
                • carotid: systolic BP approximately 60 mmHg
                • femoral: systolic BP approximately 70 mmHg
                • radial: systolic BP approximately 80 mmHg
            b. Assess neck veins:
                • flatness may indicate hypotension secondary to hypovolemia
                • distention may indicate tension pneumothorax or cardiac tamponade
            c. Assess capillary refill
            d. Note skin color and temperature
        3. Assess for bleeding
            a. External
            b. Evidence of internal
    D. Neurologic Status
        1. Assess level of consciousness
        2. Determine Glasgow coma score (GCS); a score of 8 or less may indicate ongoing neurologic pathology
    E. Visual Head to Toe Assessment
        1. Avoid hypothermia with the use of adjuncts

2. Evaluate pregnancy for approximate gestational age/viability

II. Interventions

A. Respiratory
1. Maintain cervical alignment at all times; immobilize cervical spine with collar or other device; use "log rolling" or tilting of spine board to turn patient for airway management
2. Administer oxygen at 12 L/minute by non-rebreather mask
3. Initiate pulse oximetry
4. Anticipate endotracheal intubation as necessary with pre-oxygenation if respiratory rate is >25 or <12 per minute (avoid nasal intubation, which may predispose to bleeding)
5. Consider nasogastric tube to prevent aspiration and relieve abdominal distention
6. Obtain arterial blood gases as indicated
7. Apply petrolatum gauze or airtight dressing to any open sucking chest wound

B. Circulatory Interventions to Optimize Preload and Improve Cardiac Output
1. Initiate cardiopulmonary resuscitation as indicated, with lateral uterine displacement
2. Apply direct pressure or pressure bandages to control external bleeding
3. Obtain peripheral intravenous access using large bore (14–16 gauge) catheter(s). Two lines may be necessary
4. Administer 1–2 liters of warmed normal saline or lactated Ringer's solution if needed for volume resuscitation
5. Obtain appropriate blood specimens as indicated
6. Consider transfusion of O-negative blood followed by type-specific or cross-matched packed red blood cells and fresh frozen plasma as available with continued hemorrhage and maternal instability
7. Vasopressor medications DO NOT have a primary role in the treatment of hypovolemic shock for the pregnant trauma patient but may be a last resort

III. Secondary Survey

A. Reassess Neurologic Status:
1. Level of consciousness
   a. A—alert and oriented
   b. V—responds to verbal stimulus
   c. P—responds only to pain
   d. U—unresponsive
2. Sensorimotor function
   a. Response to painful stimuli
   b. Presence of flaccid paralysis
   c. Glasgow coma scale

B. Examine head for:
1. Contusions, lacerations, and bony deformities
2. Signs and symptoms of basilar skull fracture
   a. Check for bleeding from ear or nose
   b. Check for Battle's sign: postauricular swelling and discoloration
   c. Check for "raccoon eyes": periorbital edema and ecchymosis

C. Reassess chest and circulation
D. Anticipate order for X-ray of thorax
E. Make abdominal assessment noting the following
1. Pain and tenderness
2. Distention

F. Assess musculoskeletal status noting the following
1. Soft tissue injury
2. Skeletal injury
3. Neuromuscular function of affected extremity
   a. Sensation
   b. Movement
   c. Color
   d. Swelling
   e. Capillary refill
   f. Distal pulses

IV. Uterine Assessment

A. Assess uterine activity
1. Contraction frequency, intensity, and duration
2. Resting tone

B. Assess fundal height for approximation of gestational age (fundus at level of umbilicus equal to approximately 20 weeks gestation)
C. Inspect perineum for presence of bleeding, leakage of amniotic fluid, or signs/symptoms of direct fetal or uterine injury
D. Perform speculum exam to assess for vaginal bleeding, rupture of membranes, inspection of the cervix for dilation and effacement, identification of vaginal sidewall lacerations, or injuries associated with pelvic fractures
E. Perform cervical exam (in the absence of vaginal bleeding or prematurity)
1. Cervical dilation, effacement, position, and consistency
2. Status of amniotic membranes
3. Fetal station, lie, presentation

F. Assess for signs and symptoms of placental abruption
1. Presence of frequent uterine contractions
2. Vaginal bleeding or increasing fundal height
3. Evidence of fetal hypoxemia
4. Maternal hemodynamic instability
5. Abdominal tenderness

6. Increased resting tone
7. Abnormal fetal heart rate findings
G. Evaluation of pelvic bony structures
  1. Ultrasound or radiographic assessment according to the American College of Obstetricians and Gynecologists (ACOG) to minimize exposure
H. Genitourinary system assessment
  1. Place indwelling urinary catheter absent contraindication to doing so
I. Laboratory evaluation during secondary assessment
  1. CBC, electrolytes, glucose, clotting analyses, consider Kleihauer Betke (KB) stain, consider need for Rh immune globulin (RhIG)

V. **Focused Fetal Assessment**
A. Perform a focused assessment with sonography for trauma (FAST) scan to screen for intraperitoneal hemorrhage. Also included: an OB ultrasound to assess gestational age, fetal heart motion, placental location, amount of amniotic fluid, and fetal activity. *Note:* While the ultrasound may identify a placental abruption, it is not a reliable diagnostic tool for abruption.

B. Fetal heart rate according to the *Guidelines for Fetal Heart Rate Monitoring*
C. Interventions, if necessary to promote fetal status:
  1. Displace uterus laterally and avoid supine position
  2. Correct hypovolemia with fluid resuscitation
  3. Administer oxygen as indicated
  4. Consider tocolytics as indicated if no contraindications

VI. **Psychosocial Support**
A. Identify patient's support persons. Allow for contact as soon as acute resuscitative measures are completed
B. Inform patient and family of status of fetus/baby and mother
C. Promote expression of fear and anxiety
D. Provide support and reassurance

VII. **Documentation**
A. Maternal and fetal assessment
B. Initiation of protocols used in patient care
C. Interventions and patient's responses
D. Resuscitation measures

Guidelines for the Care of the Obstetric Patient Requiring Transport

Background

- Maternal transport may be accomplished for the benefit of the mother, the fetus, or both.
- Transport may be indicated when the maternal or fetal actual or potential need for advanced resources and skilled personnel exceeds the level of care available at the current facility.
- Transport may also be indicated when the newborn requires specialized care immediately following delivery.
- Common indications for maternal transport may include:
  - Preterm labor
  - Preterm rupture of the membranes
  - Severe hypertensive complications of the mother (preeclampsia/eclampsia)
  - Severe and/or recurrent antepartum hemorrhage
  - Medical comorbidities of the mother (diabetes mellitus, renal disease, sickle cell disease, etc.)
  - Anticipated postpartum complications (e.g., maternal hemorrhage)
  - Multiple gestation
  - Severe oligo- or polyhydramnios
  - Fetal anomalies requiring immediate surgery or medical management after birth (e.g., spina bifida, diaphragmatic hernia, etc.)
  - Severe intrauterine growth restriction
  - Rh isoimmunization
- Relative contraindications to maternal transport may include:
  - Maternal hemodynamic instability – (e.g. respiratory or cardiac failure not amenable to patient movement)
  - Deteriorating fetal condition requiring immediate operative delivery
  - Advanced cervical dilation or imminent birth
  - Lack of qualified personnel available to accompany the patient during transport
  - Weather and/or road conditions that preclude safe transportation
- Communication is a key issue in providing patient safety prior to and during the transport procedure.

I. **Nursing Care Immediately Prior to Transport**
   A. General Assessment
   1. Reason(s) for transport
   2. Neurologic assessment
      a. Level of consciousness (LOC), orientation
      b. Headache/visual disturbances
      c. Further neurologic checks as indicated by patient condition
      d. Deep tendon reflexes (DTRs) if patient on magnesium sulfate infusion, or for severe preeclampsia/eclampsia
   3. Respiratory function including the following:
      a. Patency of airway
      b. Rate and quality of respirations
      c. SaO_2
      d. Signs and symptoms of respiratory compromise
      e. Determine need for oxygen supplementation during transport
   4. Hemodynamic function including the following
      a. Blood pressure
      b. Heart rate and rhythm
      c. Pulses, color of mucous membranes, capillary refill (perfusion)
      d. LOC
      e. Signs and symptoms of hemodynamic compromise
   5. Other assessments
      a. Temperature

b. Intake and output (total intake and output prior to transport; begin new count during transport)

c. Gastrointestinal/bowel sounds

6. Change in maternal condition

B. Labor Assessment

1. Estimated gestational age

2. Labor status

a. Contraction frequency, duration, and intensity

b. Uterine resting tone

c. Cervical status

d. Fetal station and presentation

e. Presence or absence of vaginal bleeding

f. Status of amniotic membranes, if ruptured note the following:

i. Date and time of rupture

ii. Color and amount of amniotic fluid

C. Fetal Assessment – Assess fetal heart rate according to the *Guidelines for Fetal Heart Rate Monitoring*

1. Assess fetal heart rate:

a. Baseline rate

b. Baseline variability

c. Presence/absence of accelerations

d. Presence/absence of episodic or periodic patterns

e. Change in fetal status over time

D. Nursing Interventions

1. Ensure patent intravenous (IV) access with appropriate gauge catheter.

2. Anticipate need for indwelling urinary catheter.

3. Measure and record all intake and output.

4. Initiate guidelines for care related to specific maternal diagnosis.

5. Obtain additional/alternative orders from primary physician for complications that may arise during transport:

a. Treatment of seizures

b. Treatment of hypertensive crisis

c. Additional or alternative medications

6. Assign transport personnel as appropriate for patient's level of care.

7. Minimally required equipment and personnel for transportation of medical patients may be regulated by individual state or regional guidelines. For maternal transports the following necessary equipment should be available and in proper working condition:

a. Free-flow oxygen in adequate quantity for both maternal and neonatal needs for duration of transport

b. Maternal (adult) airway management kit, emergency intubation equipment, bag-valve ventilation unit, and portable suction equipment

c. IV start kits in 16, 18 and 20 g sizes. IV fluids of 1000 mL D5LR, 1000 mL D5 0.9% NaCl (normal saline), 1000 mL LR, and/or 1000 mL 0.9% NaCl.

d. Infusion pumps for each intravenous line; back-up batteries for pumps

e. Medications including IV fluids and supplies; syringes and assorted needles; tape; tourniquet; alcohol wipes

f. Electrocardiographic monitor

g. SaO$_2$ monitor

h. Blood pressure cuff, sphygmomanometer, and thermometer

i. Hand-held Doppler (with numeric readout for air transports with high levels of noise)

j. Oxygen with manual control, adjustable flow meter with gauge, and humidification attachment

k. Infant delivery kit/tray with bulb suction, clamps, scissors, plastic bags for placenta and medical waste; dry infant towels and blankets

l. Neonatal resuscitation supplies and medications (when indicated)

m. Neonatal isolette with oxygen delivery system (when indicated)

n. Barrier drapes, gowns, gloves, face masks, eye protection (in the event of delivery – buttock drapes, absorbable pads for fluid control)

o. Sterile water (clean up)

E. Psychosocial Assessment and Interventions

1. Explain to patient and support persons reasons for transport and transport process.

2. Allow for expression of anxiety concerning transport and answer all questions.

3. Frequently update patient and family on maternal and fetal status.

4. Anticipate need for directions, transportation, and contact persons for patient's family at arrival to receiving hospital.

F. Documentation

1. Obtain copy of prenatal records including name, phone number, and address of prenatal caregiver if different from referring physician.

2. Obtain copies of current medical record for obstetric information including:

a. Pertinent clinical information including admission history and physical

b. Treatments

c. Laboratory tests and results

  d. Ultrasound or other diagnostic tests and results
  e. Radiology films and reports (when indicated)
  f. Medications administered
  g. Fetal status – copy of prior fetal monitor tracing when indicated
  h. Labor status
  i. Intake and output

II. **Nursing Care During Transport**
  A. Maternal Care
  1. Assess blood pressure, pulse, respirations, and temperature every 30 minutes unless otherwise indicated.
  2. Measure and record intake and output hourly.
  3. Assess DTRs, if patient receiving magnesium sulfate, every hour. Use upper extremities for reflexes if unable to assess patellar reflexes due to safety restraints.
  4. Assess for contractions by palpation noting frequency, duration, and intensity every 15–30 minutes.
  5. Assess for vaginal bleeding or leaking of amniotic fluid. If legs restrained, instruct patient to report leaking of fluid or feeling damp.
  6. Assess fetal heart rate (FHR) using handheld Doppler (preferably with a digital display of the FHR) prior to transport. Intratransport FHR per specific guideline for maternal–fetal condition.
  B. Medication Administration
  1. Administer scheduled medications during transport (e.g., corticosteroid doses, scheduled antibiotics)
  2. PRN antiemetic for "motion sickness" during transport
  3. Pain medications and other PRN medications
  C. Nursing Interventions
  1. Position patient
    a. Allow for clinicians to have clear view and access to the patient during transport
    b. Position patient in lateral position with hip wedge, or semi-Fowler's position with hip wedge (based on patient condition and preference). Avoid supine position to prevent maternal vena caval syndrome.
    c. Utilize approved safety restraints during transport.
    d. Administer oxygen via face mask (when indicated).
    e. Continue care by utilizing patient care guidelines initiated prior to transport.
    f. Initiate care guidelines as patient's condition dictates.
  D. Psychosocial Assessment and Interventions
  1. Continue to update patient regarding status.
  2. Explain all procedures and answer questions.
  3. Allow for expression of anxiety during transport and give reassurance.
  E. Documentation
  1. Initiation of transport documentation tools
  2. Maternal and fetal assessments
  3. Initiation of guidelines used in patient care
  4. Communications to referring and/or receiving providers/hospitals
  5. Nursing and medical interventions and patient's response
  6. Medications administered
  7. Complete follow-up reports sent to referring physician and hospital

BIBLIOGRAPHY

American College of Obstetricians & Gynecologists. (2009). ACOG Practice Bulletin No. 100: Critical care in pregnancy. *Obstetrics & Gynecology, 113,* 443–450.

Maternal-Fetal Transport Committee & Perinatal Advisory Committee. (2009). *Maternal/fetal transport guidelines.* Ontario, Canada: PPPESO.

Wilson, A. K., Martel, M. J., Arsenault, M.Y., Cargill, Y. M., Delaney, M., Daniels, S. (2005). Maternal transport policy. *Journal of Obstetrics and Gynaecology Canada, 27,* 956–963.

Guidelines for the Care of the Critically Ill Pregnant Patient

I.   **Cardiovascular Assessment**
  A. General Assessment
     A complete cardiovascular assessment is performed every 8 hours or more frequently dependent upon patient status.
     1. Interpret the patient's ECG from a graphic recording every 8 hours. Calculate/document heart rate, rhythm, P-R interval, and QRS width. Label with patient name, date, and time.
  B. Hemodynamic Monitoring
     1. Insertion: Record and save the pulmonary artery catheter (PAC) insertion strip recording. Begin recording while catheter tip is in the right atrium prior to balloon inflation. Label with patient name, date, and time. Insertion graphic recording of central venous pressure (CVP), right ventricular pressure, pulmonary artery pressure (PAP), and pulmonary capillary wedge pressure (PCWP) should be obtained (if possible).
     2. All waveforms should appear continuously on the digital display and be inspected frequently for configuration changes. Situations may occur that warrant intermittent interruptions in CVP waveform reading (e.g., volume resuscitation, cardiac output measurement, or medication administration).
  C. Central Pressure Assessment
     1. Assessments may be performed from the digital display if waveform configurations are appropriate. All assessments should be performed from the graphic recording for patients receiving artificial mechanical ventilation with positive end-expiratory pressure (PEEP) >10 cmH$_2$O

  2. Routine assessment frequency may be as follows:
     a. Patients who are undelivered or 12 hours post delivery—CVP and PAP every hour and PCWP every 2 hours
     b. Patients who are >12 hours post delivery—CVP and PAP every hour and PCWP every 4 hours
  3. Assessments may be performed more frequently in the following situations:
     a. The patient is hemodynamically unstable (abnormal central or arterial blood pressures)
     b. The patient is receiving intravenous vasoactive medications
  4. PAC placement may be verified daily by chest x-ray.
  5. PACs are usually repositioned and discontinued by a physician or designated advanced practice nurses. PACs displaying a spontaneous occlusion waveform may be repositioned by the physician or registered nurse by withdrawing the catheter slowly with the balloon deflated until an appropriate PAP waveform returns.
  D. Derived Hemodynamic Assessment
     1. The following derived hemodynamic and oxygen transport parameters should be obtained for all patients with a PAC. For patients without a fiberoptic continuous SvO$_2$ PAC, a mixed venous blood gas is drawn from the distal port and analyzed with a Co-Oximeter.
        a. Cardiac index (CI)
        b. Systemic vascular resistance (SVR)
        c. Pulmonary vascular resistance (PVR)
        d. Left ventricular stroke work index (LVSWI)

e. Arterial oxygen content (CaO_2)

f. Venous oxygen content (CvO_2)

g. Oxygen delivery (DO_2)

h. Oxygen consumption (VO_2)

i. Oxygen extraction ratio (O_2ER)

j. Shunt fraction (Qs/Qt)

2. Routine assessment frequency of derived hemodynamic and oxygen transport parameters may be as follows:

   a. Cardiac index (CI)

      (1) Patients who are undelivered or ≤ 12 hours post delivery—every 2 hours

      (2) Patients who are >12 hours post delivery—every 4 hours

3. Assessments may be performed more frequently if patient is hemodynamically unstable.

E. Instrumentation

1. Pulmonary artery catheter pressure line set-up

   a. Obtain from pharmacy-prepared heparin flush solution (e.g., 2500 units heparin to 500 cc bag 0.9% normal saline).

   b. Place solution in pressure bag.

   c. Prepare pressure lines for CVP and pulmonary artery (PA) ports. Flush tubing and transducer with heparin solution using gravity to remove air.

   d. Replace all stopcock ports with non-vented caps. Ensure that system is free of air.

   e. Inflate pressure bag to 300 mmHg. Pressure is maintained at 300 mmHg to ensure an infusion rate to each pressure line of 3–5 cc/hour.

   f. Zero each pressure line at the patient's phlebostatic axis.

   g. Calibrate the transducer.

   h. Ensure that informed patient consent has been obtained by the physician.

   i. Initiate continuous electrocardiographic monitoring to detect ventricular ectopy, which may occur when the catheter enters the right ventricle. Have available at the bedside lidocaine 1.0 mg/kg for suppression as needed.

   j. Test balloon for patency.

2. Hemodynamic Monitoring

   a. Hemodynamic pressure readings may be taken with the patient in a position that allows for adequate cardiac output maintenance and patient comfort. Following patient position change and prior to pressure readings, all pressure lines should be re-zeroed at the phlebostatic axis. For patients with head elevation or deep side-lying position, the location of the right atrium is used for the zero reference point.

   b. For consistency, all PAPs should be assessed at the patient's end-expiration.

   c. PCWP is assessed as a mean pressure at the patient's end-expiration.

   d. In mechanically ventilated patients, all pressure measurements will be assessed with the ventilator remaining connected to the patient unless otherwise ordered.

   e. The PAC should be secured to the patient.

   f. Pressure bags should be maintained at 300 mmHg pressure.

   g. All ports on the pressure line will be protected with occlusive port covers.

   h. Stopcocks used for blood sampling should be flushed prior to replacing the nonvented cap.

   i. No fluids except the flush solution will be infused into the distal port of the patient.

3. Cardiac Output—Thermodilution cardiac output (CO) assessment may be routinely performed and documented as follows:

   a. Patients who are undelivered or ≤ 12 hours post delivery—every 2 hours

   b. Patients who are delivered or >12 hours post delivery—every 4 hours

   c. Assessment of CO may be performed more frequently if patient is hemodynamically unstable.

   d. All CO assessments should be performed using 10 mL iced injectate (0.9 sodium chloride) at a temperature between 6° and 12° C.

   e. The computation constant for CO measurement is PAC specific and should be determined prior to the procedure.

   f. CO injectate should be recorded as intake volume.

   g. Thermodilution technique is used for measuring CO by injecting 10 cc of iced saline into the CVP port. Positioning for the obstetric patient to allow optimization of CO includes right side-lying and left side-lying.

4. Fiberoptic (SvO_2) PAC

   a. An in-vitro calibration should be performed prior to insertion of a fiberoptic catheter per manufacturer's instructions.

   b. An in-vivo calibration should be performed by obtaining a mixed venous gas sample from the PA port:

      • as soon as possible after insertion if an in-vitro calibration is not performed

- every 24 hours for all patients with AM labs, or per manufacturer's instructions.
  c. If interruption of monitoring is necessary, the cable should be disconnected at the input jack. If disconnection occurs at the optical module or continues beyond 4 hours, an in-vivo calibration should be performed. (See manufacturer's instructions for specific model of PAC.)
  d. An adequate signal quality index (SQI) should be verified (according to manufacturer's recommendation) prior to documentation of SvO_2).

5. Arterial Blood Pressure (ABP) Monitoring
  a. ABP and MAP are assessed every hour or more frequently based on patient condition.
  b. The catheter insertion site should serve as the zero-reference point for intra-arterial BP monitoring.
  c. The extremity containing the intra-arterial catheter should be assessed every 2 hours.
  d. If unexplained direct ABP changes by >20 mmHg, an indirect assessment should be performed for comparison.
  e. An indirect ABP should be obtained and documented each shift for patients with an intra-arterial catheter.

6. Deep Vein Thrombus (DVT) Prophylaxis
  a. All critical care obstetric (CCOB) patients >24 hours should be evaluated for the use of DVT prophylaxis. The type of prophylaxis (anticoagulation, compression devices, filters, etc.) is based on individual patient condition and whether the patient is postoperative.
  b. If SCD hose/device is in use, it should be removed for 1 hour every 8 hours

II. Respiratory Assessment

A. General Assessment—A complete respiratory assessment should be performed and abnormal findings documented each shift, or more frequently if evidence of respiratory compromise exists.

B. Ongoing Assessment—Routine assessment of respiratory status should be performed as follows:
  1. Respiratory rate and arterial oxygen saturation (SaO_2) every hour
  2. Venous oxygen saturation (SvO_2) every hour for patients with a fiberoptic PAC
  3. Auscultate breath sounds every 2 hours.

C. Mechanical Ventilation
  1. After intubation, the following should be assessed and documented: Endotracheal tube (ETT) size and position at the patient's teeth, date of placement, and breath sounds.
  2. Placement of ETT should be verified by a chest x-ray as soon as possible after intubation.
  3. Routine assessment should be performed as follows:
    a. Ventilator settings (mode, rate, FiO_2, Vt, PEEP, PSV, peak inspiratory pressure)—every 2 hours and after any ventilator change
    b. Arterial blood gases—after any change in ventilator settings, or more frequently as indicated by patient respiratory status
  4. Ventilator setting changes should be made according to hospital protocol. In a STAT or emergency situation, when neither a physician nor a respiratory care practitioner is immediately available, a CCOB nurse should initiate changes necessary to meet a patient's ventilatory needs.
  5. A nasogastric tube should be inserted in patients requiring mechanical ventilation >4 hours and connected to low wall suction.
  6. Suctioning of the patient via ETT or tracheotomy tube should be as follows:
    a. Performed only when indicated by respiratory assessment (increasing peak inspiratory pressure, visible secretions, patient coughing, or decreasing SaO)
    b. Preceded and followed by hyperoxygenation with FiO_2 of 1.0 as necessary to maintain adequate SaO_2 >95%)
    c. Preceded by hyperventilation if open suction technique is used
    d. Stabilization of ETT by additional personnel may be required during open suction procedure.
    e. Limit each suction episode to maximum of two catheter passes
    f. Suction containers should be changed every 24 hours and emptied every shift.
  7. A manual resuscitation bag, capable of delivering PEEP and connected to an oxygen source providing 1.0 FiO_2 should be immediately accessible at all times at the head of the bed.
  8. When the patient is intubated and on a ventilator, restraints may, in accordance with institutional policies and guidelines, be ordered by a physician and applied to patient's extremities as necessary. Application and removal should be documented in accordance with institutional policies and guidelines. The need for and expected time

of restraint must be explained to the patient and family. A physician's order must be obtained

D. ETT and Tracheotomy Care
   1. Use disposable endotracheal tube holders to secure the ETT.
   2. Assess tube holder every 8 hours. If soiled or no longer secure, apply new tube holder with assistance of another staff person.
   3. Assess breath sounds to verify tube placement per unit guidelines.
   4. An extra ETT or tracheotomy tube, identical to patient's existing tube, should be immediately accessible at all times.
   5. Respiratory therapy should be consulted when the ETT requires repositioning or alteration of length is needed. No more than 5 cm of tube should protrude from the patient's mouth.

III. **Neurologic Assessment**
A complete neurologic assessment will be performed and abnormal findings documented every 8 hours, or more frequently when neurologic instability exists.

IV. **Gastrointestinal/Genitourinary (GI/GU) Assessment**
   A. General Assessment—A GI/GU assessment will be performed and abnormal findings documented every 8 hours, or more frequently if instability exists.
   B. Nasogastric Tube (NG)
      1. Position of NG tube should be documented.
      2. Gastric pH should be assessed and documented every 4 hours.
      3. Correct placement should be verified by auscultation prior to each irrigation or administration of medication.
      4. Tape should be positioned to avoid pressure on the nares.
      5. Tape should be changed when soiled.
   C. Feeding/Drainage Tubes
      1. Feeding bag and tubing should be changed every 24 hours.
      2. Location of enteral feeding tube should be verified every 24 hours.
      3. No more than 4 hours of feeding solution will be hung to prevent risk of bacterial contamination.
      4. Feeding tubes should be irrigated with 20 mL warm water before and after feeding or every 4 hours.
      5. Gastric residuals should be assessed every 4 hours. If residuals are greater than the hourly rate, feedings should be held and the physician notified.

D. Bowel Function
   1. Passage of stool should be documented in medical record.
   2. If a rectal tube is in place, the balloon should be deflated for 10 minutes every 2 hours.
   3. Rectal bags should be changed every 48 hours or PRN. The rectal area should be cleaned and dried following bag change.
E. Urinary Output
   1. Indwelling urinary catheters should be connected to a graduated urimeter and bedside drainage bag.
   2. Urine output should be assessed and documented every hour. Twenty-four-hour total urine output should be calculated and documented.

V. **Integument Assessment**
   A. General Assessment—A skin assessment will be performed and abnormal findings documented every 8 hours.
   B. Therapeutic Mattress/Bed—Therapeutic beds should be considered for patients with special skin care needs. Use of these beds usually requires a physician order.
   C. Skin Care
      1. All patients should be repositioned/ turned at least every 2 hours unless contraindicated. Position changes should be documented.
      2. Additional skin care protection (e.g., heel, elbow pads, and decubitus care) may be ordered by the nurse as needed.
      3. A protective blanket should be applied between the skin and hyper/hypothermia blanket when in use.
      4. If the corneal reflex is absent, a saline sponge should be placed over the patient's eyes each shift or eyes may be taped closed.
      5. Patients should be bathed each day as tolerated. Hair care (combing and shampooing) should be done PRN.
      6. Perineal care PRN
   D. Mouth Care
      1. Mouth care at least daily
      2. Intubated patients should receive mouth care every 8 hours and supplemented with swabbing with sponge and mouth wash every 4 hours and PRN as part of a ventilator bundle to reduce the incidence of VAP.. Oral airways should be removed during mouth care.

VI. **Uterine Activity and Fetal Monitoring**
Most critically ill undelivered patients should have uterine activity and fetal assessments performed and documented according to institutional

policy and guidelines. (See *Guidelines for the Care of Patients in Labor* and *Guidelines for Fetal Heart Rate Monitoring.*)

VII. **Metabolic Assessment**
A. Temperature Assessment—Temperature should be assessed and documented every 4 hours. Assessment should be performed and documented every 2 hours in the following situations:
1. Temperature is >100 degrees F
2. Temperature is <97 degrees F
3. Amniotic membranes are ruptured
B. If a cooling or warming adjunct is in place, the patient's temperature should be assessed and documented every hour.

VIII. **Vascular Line Care**
A. General Assessment
1. Peripheral and central vascular line access sites should be assessed every 2 hours for integrity and documented.
2. All vascular infusion lines should be assessed every 8 hours.
3. Infusion pumps should be used for all venous infusions unless rapid volume expansion is in progress.
B. Tubing Changes
Tubing changes should be in accordance with the most current Centers for Disease Control (CDC) recommendations.
C. Dressing Changes
(Dressing changes should be in accordance with the most current CDC recommendations.)
D. Blood Sampling
1. From intra-arterial line, withdraw and discard 3 mL blood prior to obtaining sample.
2. From PA or triple lumen central catheters:
a. Turn off all infusions via catheter ports prior to blood sampling.
b. Withdraw and discard 10 mL blood if sampling port has been in use for an active infusion.
c. Withdraw and discard 5 mL blood if sampling port has been capped off or used for a pressure line.
E. Vascular Access
1. All critically ill patients should have venous access at all times. Peripheral access should be obtained prior to discontinuation of central venous access.

2. All vasoactive medications should be administered via a central line except in STAT situations or when the medication to be administered is for a short period of time.
F. Transport—Patients with PAC or requiring mechanical ventilation should be attended by a CCOB nurse and physician during transport.

IX. **Rest and Activity**
A. Every effort should be made to optimize the patient's opportunity for rest and sleep.
B. Patients with a PAC may be out of bed to a chair with assistance when stable with physician's order.

X. **Psychosocial**
A. Philosophy—It is the philosophy of nursing that all patients and their family/support system be viewed in a holistic way: mind, body, and spirit. All care should adhere to this model.
B. Visitation—Insofar as it is reasonably possible, open visitation should be implemented for critically ill obstetric patients. Every effort should be made to facilitate access between patient/family and their newborn, when applicable. If it is not possible for the newborn to leave the nursery setting, every effort should be made to provide information to patient regarding newborn status.

XI. **Nursing Implications**
Collaborative communication for any of the following, unless other specified:
A. Systolic blood pressure >160 mmHg
B. Diastolic blood pressure >110 mmHg
C. Respirations <14 or >26 per minute
D. Deep tendon reflexes absent
E. Urine output <30 cc/hour or <240 cc in 8 hours
F. Symptoms of pulmonary edema
G. SaO_2 <95%
H. Seizure activity
I. Significant system changes
J. Imminent delivery

XII. **Patient/Family Education**
A. Plan of care
B. Unit routine
C. Electronic fetal monitoring
D. Disease process
E. Bed rest and physical activity restrictions
F. Diversional activities
G. Expected length of stay
H. Special testing/equipment
I. Arterial and PAC placement
J. Delivery method

INDEX

Note: Page numbers with italicized b's, f's and t's refer to boxes, figures and tables.

A

A-a gradient. *See* Alveolar-arterial oxygen difference
Abacavir, 334*t*
Abortion
  and fetal viability, 21–2
  septic, 213, 227
  spontaneous, 298, 361
  trimester, 22
Abruptio placentae. *See* Placenta abruption of
Accidents, 352–3
Acetylcholine, 63
Acidemia
  in blood transfusion, 259
  in burn injuries, 354
  in diabetic ketoacidosis, 164
  fetal, 43, 61, 207
  maternal, 349, 389
Activase, 93*t*
Activated partial thromboplastin time, 96, 137, 253, 278, 282
Activated protein C, 102*t*, 280, 314
Activated protein C resistance, 290
Acute asthma exacerbation, 154–5
Acute fatty liver of pregnancy, 277
Acute ischemic stroke, 93*t*
Acute kidney injury. *See* Acute renal failure
Acute lung injury, 52, 311
Acute myocardial infarction, 93*t*
Acute renal failure, 213–32
  clinical management of, 228–30
  diagnosis of, 227–8
  fetal considerations, 230
  incidence of, 213–4
  intrinsic, 220–4
  kidney biopsy, 227–8
  mortality rates, 213–4
  patient at risk for, 231
  patient history, 227
  patient screening for, 231
  patients at risk for, 216
  pharmacotherapeutics for, 228
  physical examination, 227
  postrenal, 224–6
  prerenal, 218–20, 221*t*
  prevention of, 230–2
  renal replacement therapy for, 228–30
  RIFLE criteria, 217–8
  risk factors, 216–7
  in special populations, 226
Acute respiratory distress syndrome, 52, 58, 152, 311, 320
Acute tubular necrosis, 218, 220, 223, 224*t*
Adalat, 73*t*
Adaptive immunity, 306
Adenocard, 80*t*
Adenosine, 80*t*
Adenosine diphosphate, 275
Adrenaline, 90*t*
Adrenomimetic drugs, 63

Adrenoreceptors, 63
Adult respiratory distress syndrome, 179
Advance directives, 18–19
Advanced Cardiac Life Support, 238, 239*f*
Advanced Trauma Life Support protocol, 346, 402–3
Afterload, 33, 64, 309
Agenerase, 334*t*
Airbags, 353
Airways
  in cardiopulmonary resuscitation, 238–40
  protection of, 346
  recognized/anticipated difficult, 177–8
  unexpected difficult, 178–9
AKI. *See* Acute renal failure
Albuterol, 154
Aldosterone, 65
Alpha receptors, 63
Alteplase, 93*t*, 96
Alveolar-arterial oxygen difference, 56
American Association of Critical-Care Nurses, 12–13
American Medical Association, 9
American Nurses Association, 8–9
Amicar, 264
Aminocaproic acid, 264
Amiodarone, 81*t*
Amniotic fluid embolus, 152, 316–24
  abnormal fetal heart rate in, 321
  altered mental status in, 320–1
  clinical management of, 321–4
    blood component therapy, 323
    circulation, 323
    in delivery, 324
    oxygenation, 321–3
  clinical presentation, 318–21
  coagulopathy in, 320
  description of, 318
  diagnosis of, 321
  differential diagnosis of, 323*b*
  in disseminated intravascular coagulation, 277
  disseminated intravascular coagulation in, 320
  etiology of, 277, 318
  hemodynamic dysfunction in, 320
  historical perspective, 316–7
  history, 316–7
  hypoxia in, 320
  incidence of, 316
  mortality rate, 277, 316
  national registry, 317–8
  pathophysiology of, 318
  phases of, 319*t*
Ampicillin, 138*t*
Amprenavir, 334*t*
Analgesia, 382
  epidural, 362–3
  for obese gravida, 362–3
  regional, 6, 181, 181–7
  in sepsis, 313*t*
Anaphylactoid syndrome of pregnancy. *See* Amniotic fluid embolus

Anemia
  aplastic, 269*t*
  diagnosis of, 147
  fetal, 335
  in HELLP syndrome, 119, 121*t*
  physiologic, 144, 246
Anesthesia, 175–87
  combined spinal-epidural, 182
  contraindications to, 178*t*
  difficult or failed intubation, 175–9
    in obesity, 176
    pathophysiologic consequences, 175–6
    predisposing factors, 175–6
  epidural, 137
  epidural hematoma, 186–7
  epidural mediated hypotension, 182–3
  general, 175–91
  high spinal block, 183–4
  induction of, 175
  mortality rate, 175
  for obese gravida, 362–3
  regional, 181–7
  spinal, 181
  systemic local anesthetic toxicity, 184–5
Antacids, 180
Antiarrhythmic agents, 75, 80–4*t*
Antibiotics, 137, 222*t*, 310–1
Anticardiolipin antibody, 291
Anticholinergics, 154
Anticoagulants, 75, 91–5*t*, 96, 137–8
Antidiuretic hormone, 54, 65
Anti-fibrinolytics, 264–5
Antihemolytic factor, 258*t*
Antihypertensives, 72–4*t*, 120
  indications for, 71*t*
  in pregnancy, 122*t*
Antiinflammatories, 222*t*
Antiphospholipid antibodies, 291
Antiphospholipid antibody syndrome, 289–90
Antiphospholipid syndrome, 291
Antiprogestins, 192*t*
Antithrombin deficiency, 290
Antithrombin III, 276, 286
Antivirals, 222*t*
Aortic stenosis, 131–32
Aplastic anemia, 269*t*
Apresoline, 72*t*
Aptivus, 334*t*
Arachidonic acid, 318
Aramine, 67*t*
ARDS. *See* Acute respiratory distress syndrome
Arrhythmias, 80–4*t*
  in amniotic fluid embolus, 320
  in aortic stenosis, 132
  drugs for, 75, 80–4*t*
  predictors of, 126*t*
  risk factors, 126*t*
  risk of, 126*t*
Arterial blood gases, 146*t*, 235, 311
Arterial thrombosis, 94*t*
Aspiration pneumonia, 149